Essential Clinical Medicine

Essential Clinical Medicine

Symptoms, diagnosis, management

Edited by
Terence Gibson and John Rees

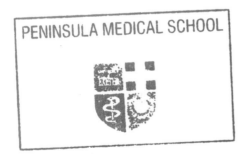
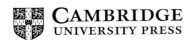
CAMBRIDGE
UNIVERSITY PRESS

CAMBRIDGE UNIVERSITY PRESS
Cambridge, New York, Melbourne, Madrid, Cape Town, Singapore,
São Paulo, Delhi, Dubai, Tokyo

Cambridge University Press
The Edinburgh Building, Cambridge CB2 8RU, UK

Published in the United States of America by
Cambridge University Press, New York

www.cambridge.org
Information on this title: www.cambridge.org/9780521835732

First published 2009

Printed in the United Kingdom at the University Press, Cambridge

A catalogue record for this publication is available from the British Library

Library of Congress Cataloging-in-Publication Data

Essential clinical medicine : symptoms, diagnosis, management / edited
by Terence Gibson and John Rees.
        p. ; cm.
    Includes bibliographical references and index.
    ISBN 978-0-521-83573-2 (hardback) – ISBN 978-0-521-54365-1
(pbk.) 1. Clinical medicine. I. Gibson, T. (Terence) II. Rees, John,
1949– III. Title.
    [DNLM: 1. Clinical Medicine–methods–Handbooks. 2. Diagnostic
Techniques and Procedures–Handbooks. 3. Patient Care–methods–
Handbooks. WB 39 E766 2009]
    RC46.E87 2009
    616–dc22
                                                            2009015598

ISBN 978-0-521-83573-2 Hardback
ISBN 978-0-521-54365-1 Paperback

To generations of medical students past, present, and future. They continue to instruct and inspire us.

J. R. and T. G.

To the memory of my late daughter Maxine Hallworth

T. G.

Contents

Contributors

Bibay Baburajan
Consultant Gastroenterologist
Maidstone and Tunbridge Wells NHS Trust
Maidstone ME16 9QQ, UK

Teresa Beynon
Consultant in Palliative Medicine
Department of Palliative Care
St Thomas' Hospital
London SE1 7EH, UK

Katia Cikurel
Consultant Neurologist
King's College Hospital
London SE5 9RS, UK

Teifion Davies
Senior Lecturer in Psychiatry
Kings College London Institute of Psychiatry
London SE1 7EH, UK

Andrew de Burgh-Thomas
Consultant in GU and HIV Medicine
Department of Sexual Health
Hope House,
Gloucestershire Royal Hospital
Gloucester GL1 3NN, UK

Charulata Deshpande
Consultant Genetecist
Guy's Hospital
London SE1 9RT, UK

Matthew Foxton
Consultant Gastroenterologist
Queen Elizabeth Hospital
Woolwich SE18 4QH, UK

Terence Gibson
Consultant Physician
Department of Rheumatology
Guy's and St. Thomas' NHS Foundation Trust
London SE1 9RT, UK

Michael Gleeson
Professor of Otolaryngology
Guy's and St. Thomas' NHS
Foundation Trust
London SE1 9RT, UK

Diana Gorog
Consultant Cardiologist
East and North Hertfordshire NHS Trust
Hertfordshire AL7 4HQ, UK

David Hausenloy
Senior Clinical Research Associate and Honorary
Consultant Cardiologist
The Hatter Cardiovascular Institute
University College London
London WC1E 6XH, UK

Shirley Hodgson
Professor of Cancer Genetics
Department of Cancer Genetics
St. George's Hospital
London SW17 0RE, UK

Simon Hogan
Higher Medical Trainee in Pharmaceutical
Medicine
Faculty of Pharmaceutical Physicians
Royal College of Physicians
London NW1 4LE, UK

Rachael Hornigold
Specialist Registrar in ENT
Guy's and St. Thomas' NHS Foundation Trust
London SE1 9RT, UK

Alison Jones
Dean of Medical School, University of Western Sydney,
Professor of Medicine and Clinical Toxicology
School of Medicine and Public Health
Faculty of Health
University of Newcastle
NSW 2310, Australia

Mark Kinirons
Consultant Physician
Department of Ageing and Health
Guy's and St. Thomas' NHS Foundation Trust
London SE1 7EH, UK

Richard Leach
Consultant Physician
Department of Respiratory Medicine
Guy's and St. Thomas' NSH Foundation Trust
London SE1 7EH, UK

Denise Mabey
Consultant Ophthalmologist
Department of Ophthalmology
Guy's and St. Thomas' NHS Foundation Trust
London SE1 7EH, UK

Michael Marber
Professor of Cardiology
Department of Cardiology
The Rayne Institute
Guy's and St. Thomas' NHS Foundation Trust
London SE1 7EH, UK

Alan Maryon-Davis
Consultant in Public Health Medicine
Division of Health & Social Care Research
King's College Medical School
London SE1 3QD, UK

David McGibbon
Consultant Dermatologist
St. John's Institute of Dermatology
Guy's and St. Thomas' NHS Foundation Trust
London SE1 9RT, UK

Lina Nashef
Consultant Neurologist
Kings College Hospital
London SE5 9RS, UK

James Pattison
Consultant Neurologist
Renal Unit Offices

Guy's and St. Thomas' NHS Foundation Trust
London SE1 9RT, UK

Jake Powrie
Consultant Endocrinologist
Diabetes & Endocrinology Unit
Guys' and St. Thomas' NHS Foundation Trust
London SE1 9RT, UK

Nicholas M. Price
Consultant Physician
Department of Microbiology
Guys' and St. Thomas' NHS Foundation Trust
London SE1 7EH, UK

John Rees
Dean of Undergraduate Medical Education
Kings College and Consultant Physician
Sherman Education Centre
Guy's and St. Thomas' NHS Foundation Trust
London SE1 9RT, UK

Leone Ridsdale
Professor of Neurology and General Practice
Division of Population Sciences and
Health Care Research
London SE11 6SP, UK

Stephen Schey
Consultant Haematologist
Department of Haematological Medicine
King's College Hospital
London SE5 9RS, UK

Jan Welch
Consultant in GU Medicine
Department of Sexual Health
The Caldecot Centre
London SE5 9RS, UK

Terry Wong
Consultant Gastroenterologist
Department of Gastroenterology
Guy's and St. Thomas' NHS Foundation Trust
London SE1 7EH, UK

Preface

This book attempts to present all the clinical topics required of a modern, clinical curriculum for medical students. Where possible, each subject has been written in a problem-oriented style starting with common presenting symptoms followed by an approach to diagnosis and management. The diagnostic possibilities are considered in relation to their probability, their context and a range of associated features. The disorders which make up the major diagnostic possibilities are then considered. For each condition a clinical description is given together with the epidemiology, pathology, investigation, management and outcome. Not all diseases and topics are presented most effectively in this way and a stylistic compromise will be evident to the reader. Each chapter is preceded by a list of the topics covered.

The order of chapters attempts a logical sequence beginning with the impact of genes on health and ending with sections devoted to the elderly and the dying patient. Some symptoms and signs are shared by multiple illnesses and an extensive cross reference system allows the reader to reach across the spectrum of diseases. We believe that the book provides easy access to information about all the important conditions relevant to a modern medical curriculum. The prominence of presenting symptoms and the clinical emphasis of the text is designed to translate ultimately into high-quality care for patients.

Terry Gibson
John Rees

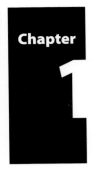

The genetic basis of disease

Charulata Deshpande and Shirley Hodgson

Contents

Introduction

Individual genetic disorders are rare but, since the advent of antibiotics, they have become the main cause of childhood morbidity and mortality in the developed world. Half of all hospital admissions are due to genetically determined conditions, including polygenic disorders. Genome-wide association studies have demonstrated genetic predispositions to breast and prostate cancer, diabetes, and coronary artery disease. These associations will continue to accumulate with the application of so called single nucleotide polymorphism (SNP) chips. With improving technology, there is also a better understanding of disease mechanisms and the possibility of new therapeutic options.

The human genome

The human genome comprises DNA that carries information for all aspects of embryogenesis, differentiation, growth, development, and reproduction. It is composed of three units: a five-carbon sugar (deoxyribose), nitrogen-containing base (purine or pyrimidine), and phosphate group. These three units polymerize into a long polynucleotide chain held together by phosphodiester bonds between adjacent sugar units. Within the cell, DNA is complexed with protein to form chromatin. During cell division, chromatin condenses and is visible as a chromosome.

A gene is a segment of DNA that codes for a functional protein. In the resting state, DNA is present as a double helix. In the process of protein production, DNA "unzips" so that messenger RNA (mRNA) can be transcribed. RNA is also composed of a five-carbon sugar (ribose), nitrogen-containing base (purine or pyrimidine), and a phosphate moiety. mRNA is produced in the nucleus and is transported into the cytoplasm where it is translated on the ribosomes to form the protein. Not all genomic DNA is transcribed into protein. The segments that are transcribed are called exons. The "silent" regions are called introns.

Members of a pair of chromosomes carry the same genes in the same order along the length of the chromosome (Fig. 1.1). The position of the gene on the chromosome is called the locus. The genes on the locus may be identical or slightly different forms of the same gene (alleles). The genetic composition of an individual is the genotype. The physical manifestation of the genotype is the phenotype.

Rearrangement involving two different chromosomes is called a translocation. A reciprocal translocation is a rearrangement of genetic material between two non-homologous chromosomes. There is usually no net gain or loss of material and no deleterious effect. There is a small risk of gene damage at the breakpoint of the chromosomes. About 1 in 1000 individuals are thought to be carriers of balanced reciprocal translocations. A Robertsonian translocation involves the short arms of acrocentric (Fig. 1.2) chromosomes. The two chromosomes are stuck together. Carriers of Robertsonian translocations are asymptomatic.

The clinical genetics appointment

Patients from all specialties are referred to the genetics clinic to establish diagnosis, arrange relevant investigations, and inform parents or relatives of the likelihood of affected children.

The genetics consultation (Table 1.1) involves a detailed history including antenatal, birth and neonatal events, developmental progress, loss of skills, at least three generation family tree with attention to inherited disorders, learning difficulties, and cancer. Clinical examination includes anthropometric measurements, risk assessment of recurrence, and management advice.

Genetic disorders
Chromosome abnormalities
Abnormalities of number

The normal chromosome complement of 46 chromosomes is called diploid. Gametes have a haploid (n) set of chromosomes. An exact multiple of the haploid

Table 1.1. When to consider an underlying genetic disorder

A child with multiple congenital anomalies
Person with learning difficulties
Family history of learning difficulties
History of recurrent miscarriages or infertility
Family history of cancer
Recognized genetic disorder in the family, e.g. polycystic kidneys

chromosome set is referred to as euploid. This could be triploidy ($3n$) or tetraploidy ($4n$) and such embryos are usually miscarried in the first trimester. Any other abnormality of chromosome number is called aneuploid.

Aneuploidy is the most significant chromosome abnormality occurring in 3%–4% of pregnancies. This may be due to an additional chromosome such as trisomy (three copies) or absence of a whole chromosome (monosomy).

Trisomy 21 (Down syndrome)

The commonest, clinically significant trisomy. The incidence is 1 in 650–1000 live births. The number of babies with Down syndrome is declining, despite increased maternal age. This reflects antenatal screening and termination of affected pregnancies. There is a correlation between the incidence of Down syndrome and maternal age.

Chromosome abnormality 95% of trisomy is due to non-disjunction at meiosis. 5% include translocation and mosaic forms.

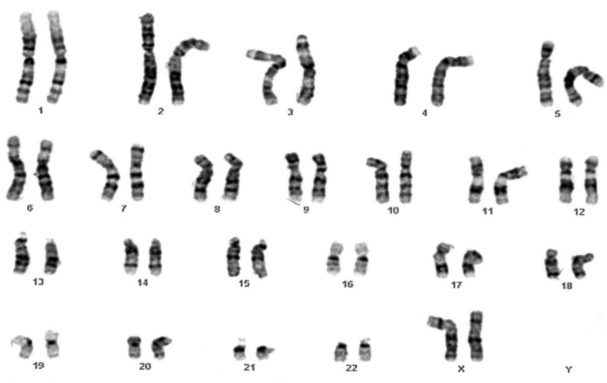

Fig. 1.1. The chromosome complement is called the karyotype. The somatic cells contain 46 (23 pairs) chromosomes. Of these, 22 pairs are common to men and women. These are called autosomes. These are conventionally numbered from 1 to 22 in decreasing order of size. The remaining chromosomes are the sex chromosomes: XX in females and XY in males. Members of the pairs of chromosomes carry matching genetic information.

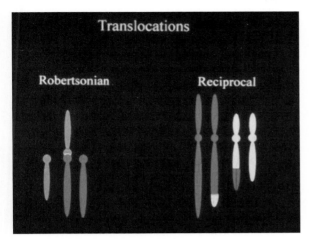

Fig. 1.2. Figurative examples of Robertsonian and reciprocal translocations.

Clinical presentation In infancy, characteristic facial features are evident. Half have congenital heart disease, the most common being atrioventricular and ventricular septal defects (50% and 40%, respectively). One third have intestinal atresia. Hypothyroidism may be a feature. Developmental delay, behavioral and visual problems, obesity, periodontal disease, deafness become apparent in childhood. There is increased risk of acute leukemia between ages 1 and 5.

Puberty proceeds normally. Folliculitis occurs in 50%. Most adults are able to carry out activities of daily living under supervision, but are unable to live independently. Few are employed. Reproduction is rare. The neuropathological changes of Alzheimer's disease usually develop in the fifth decade and 75% over 60 have dementia.

Turner syndrome
Incidence 1 in 2500 live born females. Some conceptions with Turner syndrome are lost in early pregnancy.

Chromosome abnormality Variable.

A majority have 45,X karyotype. Other X chromosome abnormalities include isochromosome Xq (duplication of the q arm of X chromosome) or ring X chromosome. The ring X is associated with a more severe phenotype. There may be more than one cell line – one 45,X and the other may be 46,XX or any of the others above. The presence of cells with different chromosome make-up in the same individual is termed mosaicism.

Infants have low birthweight, lymphedema of the dorsum of the feet, neck webbing, and puffy hands,

cardiac, and renal anomalies. Feeding problems cause failure to thrive and short stature in childhood. Ten percent have learning deficits and impaired visuospatial awareness. There is susceptibility to otitis media.

Obesity results from excessive eating. Gonadal dysgenesis occurs and most need estrogen to initiate puberty. Ten percent enter puberty spontaneously, but there is high likelihood of premature ovarian failure especially in mosaic karyotype. Hypertension and hypothyroidism occur in adults.

Klinefelter syndrome (XXY)
Incidence 1 in 1000 male births and mostly unrecognized. Diagnosis is made during prenatal testing for another reason, during the course of investigations for developmental delay or in adulthood during investigation for hypogonadism or infertility.

Increased height velocity occurs in mid childhood. Delayed speech development and reading difficulties arise in many. There is a tendency to obesity in adolescence. Most experience delayed puberty and need testosterone supplements. Half have gynecomastia.

Other sex chromosome aneuploidies
XYY and XXX.

These diagnoses are made either during prenatal testing or during investigation of developmental delay.

XYY – sudden increase of growth in mid childhood resulting in tall stature. 45% have delayed speech and behavior problems.

XXX – small at birth but height velocity increases in childhood and they are tall girls. They may have learning and behavior difficulties.

Microdeletion syndromes
In these conditions, there is deletion of part of a chromosome. The chromosome number is 46 and detailed analysis of the band pattern reveals the deletion. This can be confirmed by fluorescent *in-situ* hybridization (FISH) studies (Fig. 1.3).

Williams syndrome
The incidence is unknown. The diagnosis is based on recognition of the typical facial features and can be confirmed in 99% by FISH studies.

Chromosome anomaly 7q11 deletion.

Features in childhood are broad forehead, periorbital fullness, full cheeks, and a wide mouth with a full lower lip. Fifteen per cent have hypercalcemia. Cardiac lesions occur and supra-valvular aortic stenosis is the commonest (75%). Renal anomalies arise

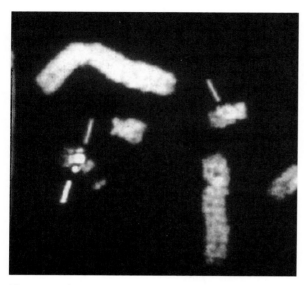

Fig. 1.3. In the FISH study, probes for specific DNA sequences on the chromosome of interest are labeled with a fluorescent dye. The probe is hybridized with the DNA sequences on a slide and analyzed under the fluorescent microscope. In a normal cell, two signals should be detected. If only one signal is present, it denotes missing information or deletion. This can be used to detect deletions at the ends of the chromosomes (telomeres) or within the chromosome (interstitial).

in 20%. There is a typical profile of better verbal and auditory compared with visuo-spatial skills. Most have ligamentous laxity (90%) which affects fine motor skills. Hyperacusis (increased sensitivity to sound) is common. Most adults have learning disability and are unable to live independently. Adult women have decreased bone density. Hypertension occurs in 50%.

Diagnosis   FISH studies to look for 7q11 deletion.

Velo-cardio-facial syndrome (also known as Di-George, Shprintzen syndrome)
Chromosome anomaly   22q11 deletion.

Congenital cardiac anomaly and cleft palate, hypocalcemia, immune defects, renal anomalies, typical facial features, and learning difficulties. Incidence 1 in 2000. Individuals present to many specialties including cardiology, immunology, and plastic surgery.

Concurrence of cleft palate and heart disease should raise suspicion. All affected children have learning difficulties and 90% speech delay. Speech has a nasal and indistinct quality (70%). Renal anomalies occur in 35%. Immunodeficiency is due to T cell dysfunction but frequent infections occur even with normal T cells. There is risk of bipolar disorder and schizophrenia in adults (20%). Recurrence risk:

children have a 50% chance of inheritance from an affected parent.

Mendelian disorders
Disorders of imprinting
Expression of some regions of the genome depend on whether they are paternally or maternally inherited. Imprinted disorders may result from chromosomal microdeletion or both alleles being inherited from the same parent (uniparental disomy).

Prader–Willi syndrome
Prader–Willi syndrome results from absent expression from the 15q11 region on the paternal allele. Prevalence is 1 in 10 000.

Genetics   Microdeletion of 15q11 on the paternal allele is the most common mechanism.

Uniparental disomy   Both alleles are maternally inherited.

Hypotonia is followed by childhood obesity due to increased appetite. Growth hormone deficiency may co-exist. Hypogonadism causes incomplete pubertal development. Short stature may respond to growth hormone treatment. All are infertile. Obesity is the major cause of morbidity and mortality. Most adults live in sheltered accommodation. There is a high frequency of psychiatric disturbance.

Diagnosis   Deletion of 15q11 region. DNA analysis is needed to check for uniparental disomy.

Angelman syndrome
Incidence is 1 in 10 000–40 000.

Genetics   Deletion of 15q11 on the maternal allele – 70%.

Uniparental disomy   Two paternal alleles only present – 2%.

Rarer mechanisms   UBE3A gene mutation, imprinting center defect.

Children have microcephaly and seizures in 80%. Some may be hypopigmented. Hyperactivity and developmental delay are common and none develops speech. Gait is ataxic and EEG characteristic. Mobility decreases due to progressive scoliosis. All adults require supervised accommodation.

Cardiovascular system
Congenital heart defect may be an isolated anomaly or part of a recognizable syndrome such as Williams or velo-cardio-facial syndromes, CHARGE association, or VACTERL association. It is the most common birth defect, affecting 0.7% of live born infants.

Atrial septal defect is mainly an isolated event. It is the characteristic heart disease of Holt–Oram syndrome, associated with an abnormal thumb or radial ray abnormalities. The left hand is affected more than the right. It is autosomal dominant and in some, mutations occur in the *TBX5* gene.

Aortic stenosis
Supravalvular aortic stenosis is seen in 75% of patients with Williams syndrome.

Coarctation of aorta
This anomaly is typically associated with Turner syndrome.

Interrupted aortic arch
About half the patients with this condition have 22q11 deletion.

Pulmonary stenosis
In Noonan syndrome, the commonest cardiac anomaly is valvular pulmonary stenosis due to dysplastic pulmonary valves. Mutations in *PTPN11* gene occur in half.

Peripheral pulmonary stenosis is seen in Alagille syndrome. Features include triangular face, down slanting palpebral fissures, posterior embryotoxon of eyes, "butterfly" vertebrae, and neonatal hepatitis. Deletions and mutations in *JAG1* have been identified. It occurs in 50% of Williams syndrome.

Hypertrophic cardiomyopathy
Is seen in Noonan syndrome and is often septal in nature. Others are familial and inheritance is often autosomal dominant.

Aortic rupture or dissection may follow dilated aorta in Marfan syndrome. Echocardiogram and abdominal ultrasound should be performed regularly.

Respiratory system
Cystic fibrosis (CF)
Autosomal recessive with a carrier frequency of 1 in 25 of Caucasians. More than 30 different mutations occur, the commonest being delta F508 (60–80%).

Failure to thrive requires pancreatic enzyme supplements to ensure weight gain. Respiratory complications start in childhood. Survival beyond the third decade is rare. Accurate prenatal testing is possible if the family mutations are known. This can be done on a CVS (chorionic villus sampling) biopsy or amniocentesis.

Alpha-1–antitrypsin
Alpha-1–antitrypsin deficiency is another autosomal recessive condition. Affected individuals may have

Table 1.2. Diagnostic criteria for autosomal dominant polycystic kidney disease (ADPKD) have been suggested based on the ultrasound features

Age at assessment	Positive family history	Negative family history
Childhood	Single cyst in both kidneys	
Adult <30 years	Two cysts in one or both kidneys	Five cysts in both kidneys
30–60 years	Four cysts in both kidneys	Five cysts in both kidneys
>60 years	Eight cysts in both kidneys	Eight cysts in both kidneys

emphysema in addition to liver disease and it is associated with the PiZZ genotype.

Gastro-intestinal tract
Structural anomalies such as gastroschisis or bowel atresia occur as sporadic events or part of a syndrome. Esophageal atresia is seen with VATER association (**v**ertebral–**a**norectal–**t**racheo–**e**sophageal–**r**enal anomalies), small bowel atresia in Down syndrome. Exomphalos or gastroschisis may occur in Beckwith–Weidemann syndrome – an overgrowth syndrome with macroglossia, hypoglycemia, and asymmetry.

Liver disease
Liver involvement may be a feature of Wilson's disease, hemochromatosis or alpha-1-antitrypsin deficiency. Zellweger syndrome presents with neonatal conjugated hyperbilirubinemia, hypotonia, and feeding difficulties. All are inherited as autosomal recessive.

Renal
Structural anomalies
Structural renal anomalies may occur as sporadic events and the recurrence risk is small.

Polycystic kidney disease
Polycystic kidney disease may be a primary disorder or part of other conditions.

Autosomal dominant polycystic kidney disease (Table 1.2)
Incidence is 1 in 1000 live births. Presentation is in adulthood. Severity is variable. There is progressive cyst formation with enlargement of the kidneys. In 25% there are additional benign adenomas. Complications include hypertension, bleeding within cysts, renal impairment, and eventual renal failure. Half develop renal failure by age 60. If an ultrasound is

normal in adulthood, the probability of carrying the faulty *ADPKD* gene is less than 5%.

Sixty percent develop hypertension even if renal function is preserved. A single cyst in a child with a positive family history is adequate for diagnosis.

Two genes are associated: *PKD1* (chromosome location 16p) and *PKD 2* (chromosome 4q). There is no relation between the mutation and clinical picture, which varies within the same family. Molecular testing is not yet possible. Risk of inheritance is 50%. Parental ultrasound should be arranged following diagnosis in children.

Autosomal recessive polycystic kidney disease
Rare with incidence 1 in 10 000.

Genetics   Autosomal recessive, mutations in *PKHD1* gene.

Cysts occur in kidney and liver. There may be oligohydramnios in pregnancy and hyperechoic kidneys identified on antenatal scans. Infants develop anuria and renal failure. Hypertension, cardiac hypertrophy, congestive cardiac failure, and renal failure happen early. Hepatic fibrosis and portal hypertension may be seen in survivors.

Mutation screening of the *PKHD1* gene is not available routinely. Linkage analysis is possible and prenatal diagnosis can be performed using this information.

Deafness
Deafness is the commonest sensory impairment worldwide. In the UK, the incidence is 1 in 1000 at birth. Thirty percent are part of a genetic syndrome. In the remaining 70%, deafness is non-syndromic.

Up to 80% of non-syndromic hearing loss is inherited as an autosomal recessive. The commonest gene implicated is *GJB2* (connexin 26). Mutations in this gene are identified in half of European patients. Profound hearing impairment is apparent from early infancy. Autosomal dominant hearing loss may present in late childhood or adults and is not severe. Mitochondrial mutations may also cause hearing loss and may be part of a more extensive neurological phenotype, e.g. MELAS and Pearson syndrome.

Testing for most of the common mutations in the *GJB2* gene is available.

Neuromuscular
Muscular dystrophies are a heterogenous group of inherited disorders characterized by progressive muscle wasting and weakness.

Duchenne muscular dystrophy
The commonest and inherited in an X linked recessive manner. Birth prevalence is 1 in 3500. It is found in affected boys during investigations for delayed walking or progressive muscle weakness in early childhood. They are wheelchair bound by age 12. Respiratory support is required by adolescence and most die in their 20s. A third develop cardiomyopathy. Female carriers require monitoring for cardiac conduction defects (41%) and dilated cardiomyopathy.

Genetics   The mutations are in the dystrophin gene – the largest human gene on Xq21. In one-third, mothers are carriers of the mutation. It is possible to detect 98% DMD mutations on molecular testing. Prenatal diagnosis is possible if the molecular defect is known.

Recurrence risk for parents with one affected child where the mother is a carrier is 1 in 4 (half the boys would be affected and half the girls would be carriers). If the mother is not a carrier, there remains a high recurrence risk (10%) probably due to gonadal mosaicism. Affected boys do not reproduce.

Becker muscular dystrophy
This is allelic to DMD and is a milder disorder. The prevalence is 1 in 18 000 males. Affected boys remain ambulant beyond age 16 and often into adult life. Progression is slow but there is risk of cardiomyopathy. Affected men may reproduce. Molecular testing and genetic counseling as for Duchenne muscular dystrophy.

Fascioscapulohumeral muscular dystrophy
Weakness of facial, scapulohumeral, anterior tibial, and pelvic girdle muscles. Many have mild weakness. Some become wheelchair bound. Inheritance is autosomal dominant and both males and females are affected. The relevant gene is linked to chromosome 4 and a large fragment is seen on RFLP analysis.

Huntington's disease
Autosomal dominant neurodegenerative condition of adult onset. Most become symptomatic in their 40s. Age of onset in an at-risk family member cannot be predicted because of anticipation. If the mutation is inherited from an affected father, symptoms may develop in adolescence (juvenile onset HD).

Genetics   Autosomal dominant affecting males and females equally. Mutation results from expansion of the CAG trinucleotide sequence in the HD gene. Affected individuals have more than 39 repeats compared with the normal of 30. It is not possible to predict the severity or age of onset based on the number of repeats.

Genetic counseling Genetic counseling is challenging and awareness of the implications of positive tests is essential. Trained genetic counselors should perform all genetic testing. It is not advisable for young people to have a predictive test before age 21.

Fragile X syndrome

Mental retardation in males and milder features in affected females. It is the most common (1 in 1000 males) cause of severe mental deficiency after Down syndrome. It derives its name from identification of the cytogenetic abnormality on the long arm of X chromosome. The diagnosis is established by demonstrating CGC expansion in the *FMR1* gene.

Genetics It is X linked. The normal allele has fewer than 45 repeats. Affected males have more than 200 repeats. Alleles between 45 and 58 repeats are referred to as intermediate alleles and are not associated with health problems. Repeats between 59 and 200 are in the premutation range and risk instability and expansion to full mutation.

Clinical features Learning and behavior problems in early childhood, high incidence of attention deficit hyperactivity disorder and autism. Premutation carriers show subtle behavior traits characterized by anxiety, obsessional thinking, and depression.

Premature ovarian failure may occur. Males with premutation have progressive intention tremor and gait ataxia (Fragile X related Tremor Ataxia Syndrome). There may be associated peripheral neuropathy. MRI reveals typical symmetrical hyperdense areas in the middle cerebellar peduncles.

Recurrence risks Females who are premutation carriers have a 1 in 4 chance of having an affected son with developmental problems and 1 in 4 probability of having a girl with milder problems.

Prenatal testing is available on a chorionic villus sampling (CVS).

Myotonic dystrophy

Multi-system disorder affecting skeletal muscle, eye, heart, and central nervous system. There is a range of severity including severe congenital or mild adult form with cataracts and mild myotonia.

Genetics Caused by CTG expansion in the *DMPK* gene. It is autosomal dominant and demonstrates anticipation. The normal allele has up to 35 repeats. Increase in the size of the gene to more than 50 repeats results in the disease. The intermediate repeat number is referred to as a premutation.

Neonatal presentation Occurs when inherited from the mother. In the pregnancy, there may be polyhydramnios. The affected child is hypotonic at birth and requires respiratory support. Affected children who survive have learning difficulties.

Mild form Usually presents as cataracts in adults. The diagnosis is often made on extended family studies.

Classic form This usually presents between 20 and 40 years of age. The main complaint is distal weakness. Males report early onset baldness. Almost all develop posterior subcapsular cataracts. Cardiac conduction defects are common. Women predispose to miscarriage and post-partum hemorrhage.

Recurrence risk is 50%. There is risk of the severe congenital myotonic dystrophy if the expansion is maternally inherited.

Prenatal testing is available.

Skeletal

Skeletal dysplasias

Diverse conditions with different patterns of inheritance including autosomal dominant, recessive, and X linked. Detailed family history including family photographs is essential. Assessment involves a full skeletal radiological survey. Prenatal testing is available where the molecular defect is identified.

Marfan syndrome

Incidence is 1–2 per 10 000. Diagnosis is based on clinical criteria (Table 1.3).

Genetics Autosomal dominant with nearly full penetrance. Causative mutations have been identified in the fibrillin 1 gene.

Clinical features Disproportionate tall stature with cardiac and eye abnormalities.

Not all features may be present at the time of diagnosis. Dilatation of the aortic root may not be apparent until adulthood but scoliosis may be manifest in adolescence. Normative data on upper segment–lower segment ratios and aortic root measurements are available for the Caucasian population at different ages. The cardiovascular manifestations of Marfan syndrome are life threatening and require follow-up.

Although mutations have been identified in *FBN1* gene, diagnosis is based on clinical examination. Prenatal testing is not offered routinely.

Recurrence 50% risk to offspring.

Table 1.3. Revised diagnostic criteria for Marfan syndrome

Index case

Major criteria in two different organ systems and involvement of a third system *or*

mutation in FBN1 gene and one major criterion and involvement of a second organ system

Relative of index case

Family history of Marfan syndrome in a first degree relative and one major criterion in one organ system and involvement of a second organ system

Diagnostic criteria (from De Paepe *et al.*)

(i) Skeletal

Major features

pectus carinatum

severe pectus excavatum (req. surgery)

wrist and thumb signs

reduced elbow extension (<170°)

scoliosis >20° or spondylolisthesis

reduced upper to lower segment ratio <0.86

arm span to height ratio >1.05

pes planus

protrusio acetabulae (from AP pelvis X-ray)

Minor features

moderate pectus excavatum

joint hypermobility

high arched palate with crowding of teeth

characteristic facies (dolichocephaly, malar hypoplasia, retrognathia)

Meets major criterion (4 or more major features)

System involved (2 major features or 1 major and 2 minor)

(ii) Cardiovascular

Major features

dilatation of ascending aorta at the sinuses of Valsalva

dissection of the ascending aorta

Minor features

mitral valve prolapse +/− regurgitation

main pulmonary artery dilatation in absence of stenosis

calcification of the mitral valve annulus

dilatation or dissection of the descending thoracic or abdominal aorta <50 years

meets major criterion (1 or more major feature)

system involved (1 minor feature)

(iii) Ocular

Major feature

ectopia lentis

Minor features

abnormally flat cornea

increased axial globe length

hypoplastic iris or hypoplastic ciliary muscle

meets major criterion (ectopia lentis)

system involved (two minor features)

(iv) Pulmonary

Minor features only

spontaneous pneumothorax

apical blebs

system involved (1 minor feature)

(v) Skin [(vi) DURA (not routine)]

Minor features

striae atrophicae with no apparent cause

recurrent incisional herniae

system involved (1 minor feature)

meets major criterion

Major criterion

lumbosacral dural ectasia on CT or MRI

Neurocutaneous syndromes

Tuberous sclerosis (TS)

This is a multi-system disorder affecting 1 in 5000 children at birth due to mutations in one of two genes involved in controlling cell growth, TSC1 and TSC2. It presents in different ways (Table 1.4). Antenatal cardiac rhabdomyoma is associated with an 80% probability of TS. The tumor regresses spontaneously within 6 months without hemodynamic compromise. In 65% infantile spasms develop and EEG shows characteristic hypsarrhythmia. Seizures in childhood, learning difficulties, and autism in 25% are characteristic. SEGA (sub-ependymal giant cell astrocytoma) manifests in late childhood. It causes hydrocephalus.

Facial angiofibromas may be obvious with sparing of the naso-labial groove. Other cutaneous manifestations are hypopigmented macules more often noted on the back over the lumbar region and shagreen patches (raised patches with a well defined margin). Periungual fibromas are fleshy outgrowths from the nail bed.

Eighty percent develop renal angiomyolipomas. These are benign hamartomas but may bleed extra- or intrarenally. Simple cysts occur in 20%. Renal cell carcinoma occurs in less than 1% and at a young age.

Table 1.4. Diagnostic criteria for tuberous sclerosis (from Roach *et al.*)

Major features

  (1) Facial angiofibroma or forehead plaque

  (2) Non-traumatic ungula or periungual fibroma

  (3) Three or more hypomelanotic macules

  (4) Shagreen patch (connective tissue nevus)

  (5) Multiple renal nodular hamartomas

  (6) Cortical tuber

  (7) Subependymal nodule

  (8) Subependymal giant cell astrocytoma

  (9) Cardiac rhabdomyoma – single or multiple

 (10) Lymphangiomyomatosis

 (11) Renal angiomyolipoma

Minor features

  (1) Multiple randomly distributed pits in the dental enamel

  (2) Hamartomatous rectal polyp

  (3) Bone cysts

  (4) Cerebral white matter radial migration lines

  (5) Gingival fibromas

  (6) Non-renal hamartoma

  (7) Retinal achromatic patch

  (8) Confetti skin lesions

  (9) Multiple renal cysts

Notes:
Definite diagnosis of TS – Either two major, or one major and two minor criteria.
Probable TS – One major and one minor.
Possible TS – Either one major or two or more minor features.

Table 1.5. NIH diagnostic criteria for neurofibromatosis Type 1 (NF1)

(Two or more of the following should be present to make a diagnosis of NF1)

  (1) Six or more café au lait macules over 5 mm in greatest diameter in prepubertal individuals and over 15 mm in greatest diameter in postpubertal individuals

  (2) Two or more neurofibromas of any type or one plexiform neurofibroma

  (3) Freckling in the axillary or inguinal regions

  (4) Optic glioma

  (5) Two or more Lisch nodules

  (6) A distinctive osseous lesion such as sphenoid dysplasia or thinning of long bone cortex with or without pseudarthrosis

  (7) A first-degree relative (parent, sib, or offspring) with NF1 as defined by the above criteria

Molecular diagnosis is possible. Parents or relatives of affected individuals can be tested.

There is 50% risk of inheritance. Parents who are clinically normal with no identifiable mutation have a 1%–2% recurrence risk due to gonadal mosaicism.

Neurofibromatosis type 1 (NF1)

A neurocutaneous syndrome characterized by café au lait spots. These are areas of increased pigmentation. Other manifestations include axillary and inguinal freckling. Multiple discrete dermal neurofibromas (tumors of the nerve sheath) may be present. If removed, abnormal scar formation may occur with risk of recurrence. Lisch nodules are hamartomas of the iris detected on slit lamp examination. Less common but more serious are plexiform neurofibromas, optic and other central nervous system gliomas, malignant peripheral nerve sheath tumors, and osseous lesions.

Genetics NF1 is autosomal dominant. NF1 gene is large and at present, diagnosis is made on clinical examination (Table 1.5). Affected individuals have a 1 in 2 chance of passing it to their children. There is variable penetrance and examination of "normal" parents or siblings for cutaneous manifestations is necessary.

Management is supportive. The plexiform neurofibromata may be disabling and impinge on normal structures necessitating surgery.

Surveillance *In childhood*: affected children should be seen annually for examination of eyes, blood pressure, and scoliosis. Blood pressure should be monitored in adults.

Cancer

Only 5% of cancers are due to a highly penetrant inherited predisposition to cancer. These may be:

(1) defects in tumor suppressor genes, such that a mutation will increase the propensity for cancer;

(2) DNA repair genes where a mutation allows accumulation of new mutations in the DNA within the cell allowing uncontrolled replication;

(3) oncogenes which increase susceptibility by cell proliferation.

These mutations can arise in cancer cells or be inherited in the germ line. It is possible to check for mutations in cancer susceptibility genes. Relatives are

Table 1.6. Guidelines for breast cancer screening. National Institute for Clinical Excellence

	Family history	Screening
Low risk	1 relative diagnosed >40 years	Not required. Clinical examination if concerns
Moderate risk	One first-degree relative diagnosed <40 years *or* One first- and one second-degree relative diagnosed >50 years *or* Two first-degree relatives diagnosed >50 years	Need to be referred for risk assessment Annual screening from 40–50 years of age and then continued screening on the National Breast Screening Program
High risk	*Breast cancer* Two first- or second-degree relatives diagnosed <50 years *or* Three first or second-degree relatives diagnosed <60 years *or* Four relatives diagnosed at any age *or* One first-degree relative with bilateral breast cancer <50 years *Ovarian cancer* One relative diagnosed at any age *and* one first- or one second-degree relative with breast cancer <50 years *or* one relative with ovarian cancer diagnosed at any age *or* two first- or second-degree relatives with breast cancer <60 years *Male breast cancer* One male breast cancer at any age *and* on the same side of family tree. One first- or second-degree relative with breast cancer before 50 years *or* Two first- or second-degree relatives with breast cancer <60 years	Formal risk assessment is necessary. High likelihood of *BRCA1/BRCA2/p53* mutation in family Surveillance tailored according to individual's genotype and family history

often anxious to understand their own risks and seek investigation and surveillance.

Breast cancer

There are about 36 000 new cases annually, 30% of all cancers in women and a rate of 114 per 100 000 women.

One in nine women in the UK will develop breast cancer at some point in their lives. Our understanding of the genetic predisposition is still limited. However, 5%–10% are thought to be due to mutations in the strongly penetrant, inherited predisposing genes, such as *BRCA1, BRCA2*, and p53.

In addition, lower penetrance, modifier genes such as *CHK2* might also influence the risk. This is modified by reproductive history, early menarche, late first pregnancy, low parity and late menopause, oral contraceptive use, hormone replacement therapy (HRT), obesity, and alcohol. A mutation in one copy of the *BRCA1* gene gives an 80% risk. *BRCA1* mutation carriers have a 40% lifetime risk of ovarian cancer and *BRCA2* carriers have a 20% risk.

Genetic testing and mammography screening are prioritized according to risk based on family history (Table 1.6).

Family members can be offered genetic (predictive) testing. Management of women who carry *BRCA1* or *2* mutation includes screening, prophylactic mastectomy, and/or oophorectomy.

Breast screening is offered every 3 years to those aged 50–64, and on request when 65 or over. For *BRCA* mutation carriers, screening is tailored to family history. Ovarian screening has been proposed.

Bowel cancer

Several hereditary autosomal dominant conditions are associated with risk of colorectal cancer. The risk to an individual can be estimated from the family tree.

Some of the genes that predispose to colorectal cancer are known.

Familial adenomatous polyposis (FAP)

This was the first pre-colorectal cancer condition where the gene *APC* was identified. The population frequency of FAP is one in 13 258.

Inheritance Autosomal dominant.

Clinical features It is defined by the presence of 100 or more polyps or microadenomas in the large intestine. Extra-intestinal manifestations may be present. These include CHRPE (congenital hypertrophy of retinal pigment epithelium), sebaceous cysts, desmoid tumors, and gastric adenomas. The association of osseous and other extra-colonic anomalies with FAP is termed Gardener syndrome.

Testing and management: molecular testing can identify the mutation in 60%. Individuals at 50% risk (if no genetic test available) are offered annual colonoscopy with dye spray from age 13–20. If polyps are identified at any stage, total colectomy is offered.

Table 1.7. Diagnostic criteria for hereditary non-polyposis cancer (HNPCC) Amsterdam Criteria (Modified)

Three or more family members with colon cancer in more than one generation *or*
Two or more individuals with colon cancer and one with endometrial cancer in more than one generation *and*
One of the affected relatives must be below 50 years of age at the time of diagnosis and
One of the affected individuals must be a first-degree relative of the other two

Hereditary non-polyposis cancer (HNPCC)

Hereditary non-polyposis colon cancer (HNPCC) is an autosomal dominant cancer syndrome characterized by increased risk of colon and related cancers that including the endometrium, ovary, stomach, small intestine, hepatobiliary tract, upper urinary tract, brain, and skin (Table 1.7). It is caused by a mutation in the mismatch repair genes.

Colon cancer   Two-thirds of the cancers develop in the proximal colon. Average age at diagnosis is 45.

Endometrial cancer may precede that of colon. Average age at diagnosis is 45. Women who have a mismatch repair gene mutation have a 20%–60% lifetime risk of endometrial cancer.

HNPCC is caused by mutations in the DNA mismatch repair genes. These include *MLH1, MSH2, MSH6*, and *PMS2*. Where identified, mutations are in *MSH2* and *MLH1*. Approximately 2.5% of all colorectal cancers fulfill the criteria for HNPCC. Analysis of the HNPCC tumors usually reveals microsatellite instability (MSI). Microsatellites are short tandem repeat sequences that are prone to mismatch in the tumors. About 15% of all colorectal cancers are MSI positive and HNPCC cancers usually demonstrate MSI. This assists in targeting screening for germline mutations in mismatch repair genes. Immunohistochemistry on tumor tissue is helpful in targeted genetic testing.

Surveillance includes colonoscopy every 2 years from age 25 and annual endometrial screening from age 35. Some choose prophylactic surgery (hysterectomy or subtotal colectomy) at the time of tumor resection. Where there is a family history of associated gastric cancer, endoscopy is recommended.

Genetic investigations

Genetic testing includes chromosome analysis as well as DNA tests.

Genetic testing

Diagnostic tests

If a test is arranged for an affected person, it is termed a diagnostic test, e.g. identifying the mutation in cystic fibrosis. If the specific mutation is identified, it is possible to offer an accurate test to family members to check carrier status.

Predictive tests

Desire to know susceptibility in advance of disease may create this need. The information has implications for physical and mental health, financial, and lifestyle decisions and risks to other family members. There are guidelines for predictive testing of Huntington's disease. Predictive testing of children for adult onset diseases or carrier testing for recessive conditions is not performed.

Prenatal testing

This refers to tests carried out on the fetus in pregnancy.

Chromosome analysis (Cytogenetics)

Chromosome analysis is carried out on blood lymphocytes. The analysis includes counting the chromosomes. International classification allows precise description of a chromosome abnormality.

Detailed studies can be carried out by fluorescent in-situ hybridizaton (FISH) studies (Fig. 1.3). Subtle rearrangements at the tips of the chromosomes (telomeres) can result in distinct dysmorphic syndromes or non-specific problems like learning disabilities. This may be done by FISH or DNA-based testing called multiple ligand probe amplification (MLPA). It is possible to analyze the genome to 1 Mb resolution by a technique called comparative genome hybridization (CGH).

Mutation detection (DNA-based tests)

A mutation is a heritable sequence change within the gene and refers to the specific underlying sequence change that leads to the clinical features (phenotype).

The mutation may be:

(a) *Deletion* – absence of a single nucleotide or a larger series of nucleotides.

(b) *Duplication* – within the gene, e.g. 17p duplication in hereditary motor and sensory neuropathy, or a region of the chromosome involving many genes.

(c) *Insertion* – of additional nucleotides alters the reading frame of the gene and results in a truncated protein that is functionally ineffective.

(d) *Missense mutation* – a change of sequence such that an alteration in a single nucleotide changes the amino acid encoded.

(e) *Nonsense mutation* – this results in termination of the transcription of the genetic sequence into mRNA.

Techniques of mutation detection

Polymerase chain reaction (PCR) – amplification of DNA. It is used for diagnosis of conditions in which there is only one common mutation (e.g. Apert syndrome) or for a limited number of mutations.

Sequencing – for small genes. It may also assist interpretation of other results.

Southern blot – a time-consuming technique. DNA is broken down into smaller fragments using restriction enzymes. The fragments are separated by electrophoresis and the distance traveled by the fragments is an indication of size.

Occasionally, microsatellite markers are used. These are runs of repeat base sequences in the DNA. The number of repeats is inherited as a family trait. Markers in the area of interest close to the gene being studied are used to trace the high-risk gene, e.g. polycystic kidney disease. The closer the marker to the gene being studied, the more reliable the information obtained. This technique is called linkage analysis.

Genetic counseling

This assists understanding of the genetic disorder, the natural course of the disease, and the management. It includes an opportunity to discuss options in a future pregnancy. The counselor must communicate these issues clearly so that the counseled can reach decisions themselves (non-directive counseling).

Genetic counseling requires:

(a) definitive diagnosis
(b) understanding the mode of inheritance
(c) risk assessment for siblings and offspring
(d) genetic testing
(e) prenatal testing.

Establishing a diagnosis and understanding the mode of inheritance

This requires detailed history and examination, an important aspect of which is constructing a family tree. Consanguinity and relationships of any other relatives similarly affected are useful as well as documenting early neonatal deaths and miscarriages. This allows an educated assessment of the mechanism of inheritance.

Risk assessment

Chromosomal anomalies The common chromosomal anomaly encountered is trisomy 21 or Down syndrome. Parents or siblings of children with chromosomal aneuploidies usually have a normal chromosome complement themselves. Recurrence risk in future pregnancies is small.

Chromosomal micro-deletions These are chance events. Parental chromosomes are often normal. Recurrence risks to parents or siblings are small. A parent may rarely have a chromosome rearrangement such as translocation. That predisposes to a deletion in the offspring. Recurrence risk in this situation is higher.

Mendelian inheritance and risk This is possible when a Mendelian pattern is recognized. This may be autosomal dominant, recessive, or X-linked.

Autosomal dominant conditions

The risk of an affected child is 1 in 2 (50%). If the genetic mutation occurred first in the affected individual and parents are normal, the risk to unaffected sibs of having an affected child is approximately 1%. This takes into account the rare possibility of gonadal mosaicism.

Gonadal mosaicism A nest of gametes within the testes or the ovary that could cause recurrence even if parents' analysis is normal. A couple may have more than one affected child with an autosomal dominant condition when neither parent is clinically affected. It is more common in some conditions, e.g. tuberous sclerosis and neurofibromatosis type I (NF1).

Variable penetrance In some conditions, e.g. tuberous sclerosis, different family members may have varying severity. Some may have normal intelligence and only skin manifestations, others learning difficulties, seizures, and skin involvement.

Autosomal recessive conditions

Both parents are carriers (one allele normal, one with the mutation) and the affected individual has a mutation in both alleles of the gene, e.g. cystic fibrosis, sickle cell anemia, many inborn errors of metabolism. The recurrence risk is 1 in 4 (25%) in both male and female offspring.

X-linked conditions

Females are usually unaffected carriers but have affected sons, e.g. Duchenne muscular dystrophy, hemophilia.

Mitochondrial inheritance Exclusively maternally inherited, e.g. MELAS, MERRF, Leber's hereditary optic neuropathy. The mutation is in the mitochondrial genome. The mitochondria are inherited exclusively from the ovum. There is more than one mitochondrial genome copy within each cell and the disease presentation and severity may vary.

Empiric risks

These are used in multifactorial conditions or where a diagnosis is unavailable. In multifactorial conditions, a genetic predisposition is suggested by clustering in families but a genetic mechanism not identified, e.g. neural tube defects and cleft lip. Risk is calculated on the basis of sex of the proband, severity of the condition and closeness of relationship to the proband.

Triplet repeat disorders

A dynamic expansion of the gene due to increased triplet repeat sequences. This renders the gene unstable and the size of the triplet repeat expands in each successive generation. With increasing size of the gene, there is a younger age of onset of symptoms in successive generations. This phenomenon is called anticipation. The triplet repeat expansion may be dominant, recessive, or X-linked:

(a) dominant triplet repeat disorders – Huntington's disease, myotonic dystrophy

(b) autosomal recessive triplet repeat – Friedreich's ataxia

(c) X-linked triplet repeat – Fragile X syndrome.

A full list of genetics services is available from www.bshg.org.uk.

Glossary

Aneuploidy: The occurrence of an additional or missing chromosome to give an unbalanced chromosome complement.

Anticipation: Occurrence of a genetic disorder at a greater severity and/or earlier onset in successive generations. This is due to a progressive expansion in the number of trinucleotide repeats in each generation.

Autosomal: Determined by a gene on one of the chromosomes other than the sex chromosomes.

Dominant: A characteristic or disorder expressed in the heterozygote (i.e. requiring only one altered copy to show itself.

Duplication: Presence of an additional copy of part of a chromosome or of a gene.

Empiric risks: Risk estimates based on those actually observed, rather than on general principles.

Genotype: The genetic constitution of an individual (either overall or referring to a specific gene locus).

Gonadal mosaicism: The occurrence of more than one genetic constitution in the precursor cells of eggs or sperm.

Homozygote: An individual with identical alleles at the same locus.

Imprinting: The differential expression of a genetic characteristic or disease depending on parent of origin.

Karyotype: The chromosome constitution as displayed by a microscopic examination.

Microdeletion: A small or invisible loss of genetic material on a chromosome preparation of dividing chromosomes.

Monosomy: The occurrence of only a single member of a chromosome pair.

Penetrance: The proportion of individuals with a particular genetic constitution that show its effect.

Phenotype: The visible expression of the action of a particular gene; the clinical picture resulting from a genetic disorder.

Recessive: A characteristic or disorder only expressed when both alleles at a genetic locus are altered.

Robertsonian translocation: The formation of a single abnormal chromosome by the joining of two chromosomes by their short arms.

Teratogen: An agent which can damage the developing embryo.

Further reading

Bitner-Glindzicz M. Hereditary deafness and phenotyping in humans. *Br Med Bull* 2002; **63**, 73–94.

De Paepe A, Devereux RB, Dietz HC, Hennekam RC, Pyeritz RE. Revised diagnostic criteria for the Marfan syndrome. *Am J Med Genet* 1996; **62**, 417–426.

Eccles DM, Evans DG, Mackay J. Guidelines for a genetic risk based approach to advising women with a family history of breast cancer. UK Cancer Family Study Group (UKCFSG). *J Med Genet* 2000; **37**(3), 203–209.

Emery A. The muscular dystrophies. *BMJ* 1998; **317**, 991–995.

McCandless SE, Brunger JW, Cassidy SB. The burden of genetic disease on inpatient care in a children's hospital. *Am J Hum Genet* 2004; **74**, 121–127.

NIH Consensus Development Conference Neurofibromatosis. Conference statement. *Arch Neurol* 1998; **45**, 575–578.

Office of National Statistics. Department of Health. www.statistics.gov.uk

Roach ES, Gomez MR, Northrup H. Tuberous sclerosis complex consensus conference: revised diagnostic criteria. *J Child Neurol* 1998; **13**(12), 624–628.

Watson JD, Crick FHC. Molecular structure of nucleic acids – a structure for deoxyribose nucleic acid. *Nature* 1953; **171**, 737–738.

Management of Genetic Syndromes. Ed. Cassidy SB, Allanson JE. Wiley-Liss. 2001.

Practical Genetic Counselling. 6th edn. Harper P. Arnold.

Useful websites

http://www.bshg.org.uk
http://www.ncbi.nih.gov
http://www.nice.org.uk
http://www.caf.org.uk
http://www.geneclinics.org

Chapter 2

Health promotion

Alan Maryon-Davis

Contents

Health promotion and public health

If the main focus of clinical medicine is about dealing with the health problems of the individual patient, then the focus of public health is about populations, the health and illness of whole groups of people.

Public health is the science and art of promoting health and preventing disease, protecting against health threats, and improving health services through population-based approaches.

Health promotion (a form of primary prevention). This is one of the four key elements of public health alongside health protection service planning and health intelligence (Fig. 2.1). Unhealthy behaviors and lifestyles are the root cause of so many diseases that a key part of the clinician's role must be to encourage and support their patients in maintaining healthy lifestyles. In this chapter we focus on five examples – stopping smoking, healthy eating, keeping active, sensible drinking, and safe sex.

Health protection (another form of primary prevention) is about protecting people against specific communicable and non-communicable disease threats, and it comprises four broad approaches: communicable disease control; environmental health; safety (home, road and workplace); and emergency planning.

Communicable disease control occurs through such means as:

- Education about basic hygiene (e.g. handwashing; food hygiene).
- Immunization and vaccination (e.g. against diphtheria, tetanus, pertussis, polio, Hib, MenC, MMR, BCG, influenza, pneumococcal pneumonia, and immunizations for travel).
- Notification of communicable diseases.
  For example:

• Acute encephalitis	• Paratyphoid fever
• Acute poliomyelitis	• Plague
• Anthrax	• Rabies
• Cholera	• Relapsing fever
• Diphtheria	• Rubella
• Dysentery	• Scarlet fever
• Food poisoning	• Smallpox
• Leptospirosis	• Tetanus
• Leprosy	• Tuberculosis
• Malaria	• Typhoid fever
• Measles	• Typhus fever
• Meningitis (all types)	• Viral hemorrhagic fever
• Meningococcal septicemia	• Viral hepatitis
• Mumps	• Whooping cough
• Ophthalmia neonatorum	• Yellow fever

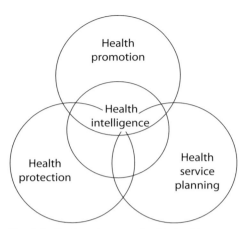

Fig. 2.1. The four elements of public health.

- Control of outbreaks (e.g. taking of samples, identification of contacts, prophylactic treatment, etc.).

Environmental health

Broader public health measures to protect populations include a wide range of interventions. To the Victorians who pushed through the great nineteenth-century "sanitary reform movement," public health was all about ensuring clean air, pure water, good sanitation, decent housing, healthy workplaces, safe neighborhoods, and safe transport. All of these remain important, most urgently in the developing world. Even in countries like the UK there are areas of relative deprivation where environmental health issues are crucial, and industries where occupational health issues continue. We also face new threats such as terrorism, SARS, pandemic flu, and natural disasters linked to global warming.

In the UK, most public health protection is backed up by laws and regulations, beginning with the famous Public Health Act of 1848, which provided for a Central Board of Health with powers to supervise street cleaning, refuse collection, water supply and sewage disposal. Today, there is a long list of legislation impacting on public health, differing slightly according to which country in the UK they apply to. Examples include:

Clean Air Act	Healthy & Safety at Work Act
Water Act	Radioactive Substances Act
Control of Pollution Act	Solvent Emissions Regulations
Environmental Protection Act	Road Traffic Act
Control of Major Accident Hazard Regulations	Motor Vehicles (Wearing of Seat Belts) Regulations
Control of Pesticides Regulations	Fire Precautions Act
Biocidal Products Regulations	Housing Act
Food Safety Act	. . . and many others

Health service planning is a public health function that is closely shared with clinicians. Health and social care services are constantly undergoing development and improvement in order to meet the needs of the population taking into account new diagnostic methods, treatments, and delivering care. The public health input into this planning process usually involves assessments of health need based on epidemiology, evidence of effectiveness, and reviews of good practice.

Health intelligence is the collation and analysis of the data and information on which all the above public health elements are based. The most commonly used routinely published types of public health information are:

- *Mortality statistics* (e.g. by age, sex, geographical area, cause of death)
- *Morbidity statistics* (e.g. prevalence of disease in general practice, prescribing data, community and social care contacts, hospital outpatient attendances, A&E attendances, hospital admissions, cancer registry notifications, infectious disease notifications, etc.)
- *Health behavior and lifestyle surveys* (e.g. eating habits, exercise participation, smoking prevalence, drinking habits, illegal drug use, sexual behavior, etc.)
- *Environmental health, hygiene and safety inspections and surveys* (e.g. compliance with the many statutory standards and regulations mentioned under Health Protection above)
- *Sociodemographic data* (e.g. resident population by age, sex, ethnicity, socioeconomic group, geographic area, conception and birth data, deprivation indices, benefits statistics, type of housing, educational achievement, employment statistics, etc.).

What is health promotion?

Health promotion is essentially about helping people to help themselves, their families and their communities to better health. It is about influencing people's health-related behaviors, also known as "health choices" – day-to-day lifestyle habits and actions that have an impact on their state of health, now or in the future. These include:

- basic physiological behaviors, e.g. nutrition, physical activity, and sex
- substance use, e.g. smoking, alcohol, and drugs
- exposure to hazards, e.g. road use, contact sports, sunbathing, poor hygiene
- use or non-use of preventive services, e.g. antenatal care, immunization, or contraception
- more general life-skill attributes such as self-esteem, self-confidence, health knowledge, and the ability to make healthy choices.

In its Ottawa Charter of 1986, the World Health Organization defined health promotion thus:

Health promotion is the process of enabling people to increase control over, and to improve, their health (WHO, 1986).

Health promotion is much more than simply giving people information and advice about healthy living. It is about helping individuals and communities to make the changes to their lives that are likely to lead to health improvement. These changes range from the "micro" individual level (e.g. one-to-one advice to stop smoking) to the "macro" socio-environmental level (e.g. increasing the tax on cigarettes or banning smoking in public places).

The range of health determinants is depicted in Fig. 2.2.

The whole population versus the targeted approach

Some approaches are aimed at the *whole population*, also known as "community-wide interventions." Others are targeted at groups of people or individuals at higher risk.

Table 2.1 lists some advantages and disadvantages of the two approaches.

Smoking and tobacco control
Problem: the patient who is a smoker

Vijay is a 55-year-old factory worker with the early stages of chronic obstructive pulmonary disease (COPD). He has smoked about 20 cigarettes a day since he was a teenager. Vijay knows how important it is for him to give up smoking and he is seeking help in doing so.

This is a typical clinical problem in which smoking plays a crucial part. It is a major risk factor for coronary heart disease (CHD), especially in combination with diabetes, and is also the prime risk factor for COPD. Giving up smoking ("smoking cessation") could greatly reduce Vijay's risk of deteriorating lung function as well as many other health benefits.

Morbidity from smoking

Smoking is associated with over 50 diseases and disorders – many of which are potentially fatal. About half of those people who take up smoking in their

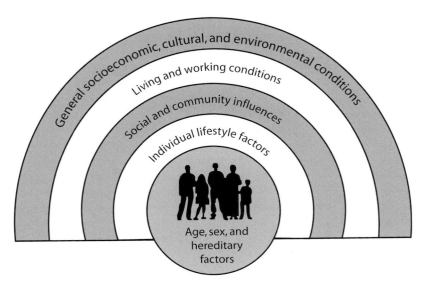

Fig. 2.2. The range of health determinants. (From Dahlgren & Whitehead, 1991. Reproduced with permission.)

General socioeconomic, cultural, and environmental conditions
Living and working conditions
Social and community influences
Individual lifestyle factors
Age, sex, and hereditary factors

Table 2.1. Advantages and disadvantages of the whole population approach and the targeted approach

Whole population approach	Targeted approach
• Aimed at larger number of people, relatively low average risk	• Aimed at fewer people, relatively high average risk
• Mass marketing techniques	• More intensive, group-based or one-to-one
• General messages aimed at a mass audience	• More individually tailored
• Economies of scale	• More costly in staff
• Relies more on self-motivation	• Relies more on concordance
• People tend to distrust the mass media	• People tend to trust health professionals
• More useful for raising general awareness	• More useful for changing behavior
• Smaller health gains, but on a larger scale	• Greater health gains, but on a smaller scale
• Only appropriate for the promotion of general good health or the primary prevention of relatively common diseases	• Useful for primary or secondary prevention of particular diseases
Example: "Five a Day" TV campaign to eat more fruit and vegetables	*Example:* HIV prevention aimed at gay males

youth and continue the habit will eventually be killed by it (i.e. die "prematurely" – under the age of 75), losing an average 16 years of life. In the UK smoking kills over 110 000 people a year and accounts for more than half the difference in life expectancy between rich and poor.

The three main causes of death linked to smoking are CHD, COPD (80% smoking related) and lung cancer. It is also a major risk factor for pharyngeal, esophageal, and bladder cancer. A third of all cancer deaths in the developed world are caused by smoking.

Social gradient
In most developed nations smoking prevalence is higher among people on lower incomes or in manual groups. Smokers in these groups also tend to smoke more cigarettes and more of each cigarette, making them generally more nicotine dependent and less easily able to give up.

Benefits of stopping smoking
See Table 2.2.

Smoking cessation methods
There are several ways to support patients who want to give up smoking (smoking cessation). These include:

PREVENTION
Many of the illnesses described in this book are preventable.
- Some can be prevented from happening in the first place (*primary prevention*).
- Some can be prevented from worsening or recurring (*secondary prevention*).

   For example, the primary prevention of coronary heart disease (CHD) involves reducing people's exposure to various *risk factors* which predispose to the development of atheromatous plaques or thrombosis in the coronary arteries.
- Some of these risk factors are inherent and fixed (*unmodifiable* risk factors), e.g. age, gender, ethnicity, family history.
- Others are linked to behavior or other influences that can be changed (*modifiable* risk factors), e.g. cigarette smoking, lack of exercise, blood pressure, serum cholesterol level. Modifiable risk factors linked to behavior are sometimes called "lifestyle" factors.

Types of prevention
There are two broad types of prevention:
- **Primary**: Any intervention that reduces the risk of a particular disease developing or becoming apparent in someone who does not yet have the disease.
- **Secondary**: Any intervention that reduces the risk of a particular disease becoming worse or recurring in someone who already has the disease (see Fig. 2.3).

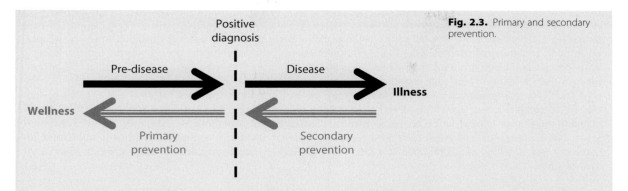

Fig. 2.3. Primary and secondary prevention.

Using the example of CHD, **primary prevention** is aimed at encouraging healthy lifestyles in children and adults who do not yet have overt signs or symptoms of the disease. Initiatives range from community-wide health campaigns to one-to-one clinical advice aimed at patients with risk factors such as hypertension, hypercholesterolemia or a strong family history of early CHD. It could also include medication to reduce specific risk factors, e.g. nicotine replacement, antihypertensives, cholesterol-lowering drugs.

Secondary prevention is aimed at patients who have been diagnosed with CHD and who receive lifestyle advice or treatment to reduce the likelihood of deterioration or further episodes. It is the essence of management of angina or post-myocardial infarct (MI) patients (Fig. 2.3).

Table 2.2. Health improvements from stopping smoking

Time since quitting	Beneficial health changes
8 hours	Nicotine and carbon monoxide levels in blood reduce by half, oxygen levels return to normal
24 hours	Carbon monoxide is eliminated from the body. Lungs start to clear out mucus and other smoking debris
48 hours	There is no nicotine left in the body. Ability to taste and smell is improved
72 hours	Breathing becomes easier. Bronchial tubes begin to relax and energy levels increase
2–12 weeks	Circulation improves
3–9 months	Coughs, wheezing and breathing problems improve as lung function is increased
1 year	Risk of a heart attack falls to about half that of a smoker
10 years	Risk of lung cancer falls to about half that of a smoker
15 years	Risk of a heart attack falls to the same as someone who has never smoked

Source: The Health Benefits of Smoking Cessation: A report of the Surgeon General, 1990.

- Brief one-to-one cessation advice and encouragement by a clinician (e.g. nurse, midwife or doctor) using motivational counseling (see below)
- Nicotine replacement therapy (NRT) using gum or patches in slowly decreasing doses
- Behavior therapy
- Hypnotherapy
- Acupuncture
- Stop smoking groups
- Telephone counseling
- Self-help leaflets

In the UK, smoking cessation services are provided locally on the NHS, including nicotine replacement therapy in appropriate cases. Patients with CHD and diabetes are likely to benefit from NRT if used under medical supervision.

Smoking prevention

Nicotine is a highly addictive drug and many smokers find giving up difficult, even with the support outlined above. Clearly, smoking prevention (i.e. stopping people starting in the first place) is preferable. Most smokers take up the habit in their early teens and preventive programs must begin at an early age. There are two broad approaches:

- Education – teaching children and young people about the disadvantages and risks of smoking
- Tobacco and smoking control – restricting access to cigarettes and opportunities to smoke

Individual behavior change and motivational counseling

In making a lifestyle behavior change, particularly one that requires an effort of will (e.g. giving up smoking), people go through a number of psychological stages. The best known theoretical model describing this process, known as the Stages of Change model, is that of Prochaska and DiClemente (1986) (see Fig. 2.4). In this model, the person may go from a stage of not even thinking about making the change (pre-contemplation) to weighing up the pros and cons (contemplation). From there they may go on to deciding they are definitely going to make the change (determination or preparation) and then making it (action, e.g. giving up smoking). Finally, they either maintain the change (maintenance) or slip back to one of the previous stages (relapse). This may all sound common sense, but it is a useful theoretical basis for a technique called motivational counseling in which the therapist or counselor (e.g. smoking cessation adviser) supports the person in moving to the next stage towards action and maintenance.

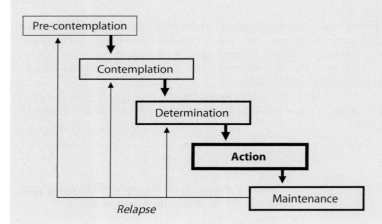

Fig. 2.4. The stages of change.

Action at national level

- Increasing tax on cigarettes and other tobacco products
- Health warnings on packs
- Restricting or ending tobacco products brand advertising, promotion, and sponsorship
- Raising the legal age for purchasing tobacco products
- Mass media campaigns
- More stringent laws on smoke-free workplaces and public places
- Increased funding for smoking education, prevention, and cessation programmes
- Reduced subsidies for tobacco farmers

Action at local level

- More smoke-free workplaces and public places
- Better controls on illegal sales to under-age purchasers
- More smoking education in schools

Promoting healthy eating and physical activity
Problem: the patient who is obese

Tony is a 42-year-old insurance salesman who has been referred to his GP by his occupational health service. He is a clearly obese and found to have a body mass index (BMI) of $34 \, \text{kg/m}^2$. He is a life-long non-smoker. His serum total cholesterol is slightly raised, and tests indicate mild type 2 diabetes. He is prescribed a weight-reducing diet and referred to the "exercise-on-prescription" service at his local leisure centre.

Overweight and obesity are terms used to describe increasing proportions of excess body fat, a contributory risk factor for a wide range of co-morbidities including:

- Hypertension
- Dyslipidemia
- Type 2 diabetes
- Coronary heart disease
- Stroke

Table 2.3. World Health Organization Classification of overweight/obesity

BMI (kg/m^2)	Classification	Risk of co-morbidities
Less than 18.5	Underweight	Low (but risk of other clinical problems increased)
18.5–24.99	Desirable, optimal or "normal"	Average
25–29.99	Overweight	Increased
30 or more	Obese	
30–34.99	Class I Obese	Moderate
35–39.99	Class II Obese	Severe
40 or more	Class III Obese (severely or morbidly obese)	Very severe

Source: WHO, 1998.

- Gall bladder disease
- Back pain
- Osteoarthritis
- Obstructive sleep dyspnea
- Gastric reflux
- Depression
- Pre-menopausal breast cancer
- Bowel cancer

Overweight and obesity are commonly assessed by using body mass index (BMI), defined as the person's weight in kilograms divided by the square of their height in meters (kg/m^2).

World Health Organization Classification of overweight/obesity. See Table 2.3.

Prevalence
In most developed countries over the past decade the prevalence of overweight and obesity has increased markedly in both children and adults. For example, surveys in the UK show that about two-thirds of men and over half of women are either overweight or obese. Among children, about 30% of boys and 25% of girls are overweight, with the proportion being highest after puberty.

What causes overweight and obesity?
Genes play some role in the metabolism and distribution of body fat – possibly contributing 25%–40%. However, the increase in the prevalence of obesity throughout the developed world has occurred too rapidly for genes to be the explanation. It is much more likely that the problem has been brought about primarily by societal and environmental changes, which have led to a more energy-dense diet and a less physically active lifestyle.

Who is most susceptible?
Overweight and obesity tend to be more prevalent in low income families and particular ethnic groups, e.g. black Caribbean women, and south Asians. Central obesity (large waist circumference) and the metabolic syndrome is especially prevalent in south Asians.

Tackling overweight and obesity
Prevention
Health promotion efforts must be aimed at encouraging healthy eating and physical activity among the whole population, but particularly the more susceptible groups, starting in early childhood. For examples of interventions, see the sections on *Promoting Healthy Eating* and *Promoting Physical Activity* below.

Weight management
This involves measuring the patient's BMI and assessing co-morbidity risk factors such as blood pressure (BP), serum lipids, smoking status, blood glucose, thyroid status, etc. The patient is given appropriate lifestyle advice and support concerning a weight-reducing diet and physical activity, plus management of other risk factors. If obese, their suitability for a course of anti-obesity drug therapy should be considered. If morbidly obese with associated risk factors, bariatric surgery (e.g. gastric banding) should be considered.

Promoting healthy eating
Even in developed countries like the UK, a poorly balanced diet is an important contributor to early death and disability and is a massive public health challenge (see Table 2.4).

Differences in everyday diet can lead to major health inequalities. Maintaining a healthy balanced diet is difficult for many, particularly those living on a low income or with poor access to healthy food choices such as fresh fruit and vegetables.

Why is it important?
A diet that is too high in fatty, sugary, or salty foods, or too low in fruit, vegetables, starchy staples, or

Table 2.4. How a poor diet can contribute to ill-health

Disease/disorder	Nutritional risk factors	Dietary contributors
Low birth weight, still birth, spinal cord defects	Low folate; lack of essential fatty acids	Low intake of vegetables, fruit, and appropriate oils and fish
Anemia in children and adults	Low iron, folate, vitamin C and vitamin B-12	Low intake of vegetables and fruit; low intake of meat
Dental caries	Low fluoride; presence of sugars in the mouth	Low level of natural fluoride in drinking water; frequent sugary snacks and drinks between meals
Obesity in childhood and adults, type 2 diabetes	High calorie intake and low physical activity levels	Too much fatty and sugary food
Hypertension	Excess sodium; low potassium, magnesium, and calcium; excess alcohol. Overweight and obesity	Too much salt in pre-prepared meals, cereals, bread, salty snacks and salt added in cooking and at table; low intake of vegetables and fruit; excess drinking
CHD, stroke and peripheral vascular disease	Excess saturated fat intake; low omega-3 fatty acids; low antioxidants. Overweight and obesity. Hypertension	Too much fatty, sugary and salty food; low intake of vegetables, fruit and fish
Breast cancer, endometrial cancer	Overweight and obesity	Too much fatty and sugary food
Colorectal cancer, pancreatic cancer	Low fiber	Low intake of vegetables, fruit and high-fiber cereals; high intake of red/processed meat
Stomach cancer	Low antioxidants	Low intake of vegetables and fruit
Osteoporosis. Bone disease in elderly people. Increased fractures	Vitamin D and calcium deficiency	Undernutrition increases the risk of falling

dietary fiber, can lead to a range of disorders including:

- Overweight or obesity, and associated problems such as type 2 diabetes, gallstones or exacerbation of back pain.
- Hypertension – linked to too much salt, alcohol or being overweight.
- Coronary heart disease and stroke – linked to a raised serum cholesterol level, high blood pressure or a lack of fruit and vegetables.
- Bowel disease including cancer – linked to a lack of fruit, vegetables and dietary fiber.
- Osteoporosis – linked to a lack of calcium and vitamin D.
- Dental caries – linked to frequent consumption of sugary food and drink.

An unhealthy diet is the main contributor to about 30% of lost life–years due to early death and disability:

- 10.9% due to high blood pressure.
- 7.6% due to high blood cholesterol.
- 7.4% due to overweight and obesity.
- 3.9% due to a lack of fruit and vegetables.

An unhealthy diet has also been estimated to contribute to:

- 33% of all cancer deaths (mainly bowel and breast).
- 30% of coronary heart disease (CHD) deaths.

Overweight and obesity (together with lack of physical activity) lead to:

- 58% of cases of type 2 diabetes.
- 21% of cases of CHD.

A poor diet also contributes to:

- Loss of independence and increased falls and fractures in older people.
- Low birth weight leading to increased mortality and morbidity throughout childhood and increased risk of cardiovascular disease (CVD) in adult life.
- Increased incidence of still births and neural tube (spinal cord) defects.

What is a healthy diet?

The basic healthy eating messages are:

- *Plenty* of fruit and vegetables.
- *Plenty* of starchy staples such as cereals, bread, potatoes, rice, pasta, cassava, preferably wholefood or wholegrain.
- *Moderate* amounts of milk and dairy products.
- *Moderate* amounts of meat, fish, eggs, or alternatives.
- *Limited* amounts of foods containing high levels of fat, sugar, or salt.

The eatwell plate

Use the eatwell plate to help you get the balance right. It shows how
much of what you eat should come from each food group.

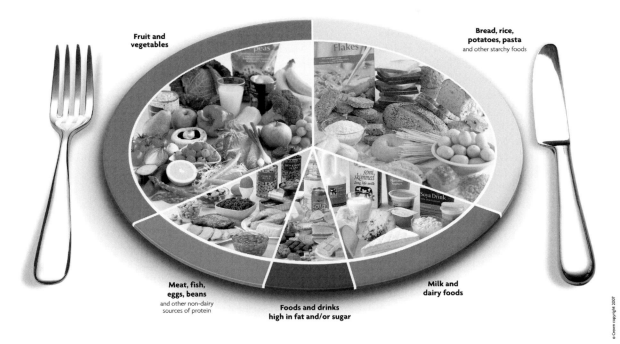

Fig. 2.5. The balance of good health – proportions of the different food groups conducive to a healthy balanced diet over a period of time. From: Food Standards Agency. © Crown copyright material is reproduced with the permission of the Controller of HMSO and Queen's Printer for Scotland.

- It is important to consume a wide variety of foods to provide adequate intakes of all the vitamins, minerals and dietary fiber which are needed to keep healthy (see Fig. 2.5).

Fruit and vegetables

Eating more fruit and vegetables can reduce the risk of many chronic diseases. For example, eating at least five portions of fruit and vegetables a day could cut the risk of dying from heart disease, stroke, or cancer by up to 20%. For most people, increasing fruit and vegetable consumption is the second most important way to prevent cancer, after avoiding smoking. Evidence also suggests an increase in fruit and vegetable intake can help lower blood pressure.

Research suggests that there are other health benefits too, including delaying the development of cataracts, reducing the symptoms of asthma, improving bowel function, and helping to manage diabetes.

The message at the heart of the 5 a day program – to eat at least five portions (400 g) of a variety of fruit

and vegetables each day – is consistent with dietary recommendations around the world, including those from the World Health Organization.

Fruit and vegetables are beneficial because, as well as vitamins and minerals, they contain flavonoids, phyto-estrogens and other substances which are anti-oxidants, destroying free radicals in the body. These free radicals are known to have a role in causing cancer as well as other harmful effects. Dietary supplements containing isolated vitamins or minerals do not appear to have the same beneficial effects as fruit and vegetables themselves.

Salt

Too much sodium can lead to hypertension, an important risk factor for stroke, coronary heart disease, and chronic kidney disease. By far the most common source of sodium in the diet is salt.

In the UK, the Food Standards Agency currently advises that adults should consume a maximum of 6 g of salt a day (about 1 teaspoon), although epidemiological studies suggest that greater benefits could be obtained by consuming even less salt, down to 3 g a day. The current average intake is about 9.5 g a day in the UK. Children should have less salt than adults on a sliding scale depending on their age. In the UK, about nine out of ten men, and seven out of ten women, currently consume more than 6 g of salt a day.

In the developed world, 75% of the salt in our food comes from processed foods, e.g. bread, breakfast cereals, savoury snacks, pizzas, sauces, canned soups, and "ready" meals. Most of the rest is added in cooking or at table. Health promotion is aimed at encouraging people to choose lower salt alternatives (e.g. an apple as a snack instead of crisps; unsalted muesli instead of a salty cereal for breakfast), to use less salt in cooking and sprinkle less on meals at table. The sense of taste can adapt to less salt, and by gradually reducing habitual salt intake, the target levels can be reached without food tasting bland and boring.

Fats

Most in the developed world eat more fat than is good for them. First, it is very high in calories – about 9 kcal per gram compared to about 4 kcal per gram for carbohydrates and proteins – and a high-fat diet, typically too many fried takeaways, is a common cause of obesity. Second, most of the fat consumed is saturated fat (high in saturated fatty acids), known to be linked to a raised serum LDL cholesterol level and hence the formation of atheromatous plaques. Saturated fats are found mostly in dairy products, meat and meat products, and also palm and coconut oil (oils are simply fats that are liquid at room temperature).

Trans fats have a similar effect on serum low density lipoproteins (LDL) cholesterol as saturated fats, perhaps to a greater degree. Trans fats are formed when liquid vegetable oils are turned into solid fats through the process of hydrogenation. Trans fats are mostly found in biscuits, pastries, and fast food.

Unsaturated fats (high in mono- or poly-unsaturated fatty acids), although just as energy dense as saturated fats, are less associated with high LDL cholesterol. Unsaturated fats are found mostly in plant oils such as sunflower, corn (maize), rapeseed, and olive oil, and fish oils. Unsaturated fats contain all the essential fatty acids the body needs and their substitution for foods high in saturated fats reduces the risk of raised LDL cholesterol and hence atheroma. Some unsaturated fatty acids raise the level of HDL cholesterol, with consequential cardiovascular benefits.

UK government guidance states that fats should provide no more than 30% of the total energy content of the average adult's diet (35% excluding alcohol), and saturated fats no more than 10% (11% excluding alcohol). There is a marked social gradient in fat consumption, with higher proportions being consumed by manual groups and people on lower incomes. Much of the fat in our diet comes from fast foods, particularly from fried takeaways.

Health promotion is aimed at encouraging people to choose low-fat dairy and meat products, switch from butter to unsaturated margarines and from saturated cooking fats to unsaturated oils, cut visible fat off meat, and grill or braise rather than fry. Children should be encouraged to eat low-fat or no-fat snacks (e.g. fruit).

Sugar

Most people in developed nations, particularly children and young people, eat and drink too many sugary things. Sugar is energy-dense (high in calories) – about 4 kcal per gram – and provides a high proportion of our total energy intake, contributing to the rise in obesity. Sugar residues in the mouth are quickly converted by oral bacteria to an acidic deposit which corrodes tooth enamel and dentine, causing dental caries (tooth decay), and irritates gum pockets, causing periodontal disease. Rapidly absorbed into the bloodstream, it makes demands on insulin production which may not be met in those with susceptibility to diabetes mellitus.

Sweets and soft drinks, biscuits, cakes, pastries, and puddings are obvious sources of sugar – but less obvious foods often contain high levels of hidden sugars: baked beans, canned peas, tomato ketchup and brown sauce, and ready meals.

Barriers to a healthier diet

- Low disposable income
- Lack of knowledge about what is a healthy diet
- Lack of awareness or concern about longer-term health consequences
- Poor access to affordable, healthy foods
- Unclear nutritional labeling on food products
- Lack of ability or interest in cooking and preparing healthy meals
- Lack of accessible information on food and health
- Poor mobility
- Poor literacy and numeracy skills

Breastfeeding

This is the best form of nutrition for infants. Breast-milk provides all the nutrients a baby needs and exclusive breastfeeding is recommended for the first 6 months of life. Babies who are breastfed are five times less likely to be admitted to hospital in the first year with infections and are less likely to become obese in later childhood. It is also beneficial to mothers.

In Scandinavia, where breastfeeding rates are consistently high, multi-faceted health education interventions have been included:

- One-to-one and group discussion in the antenatal period.
- Midwife advice before and after delivery.
- Promoting close mother–infant contact on the maternity ward.
- Mother-to-mother support groups.
- Problem-based information written mostly for and by mothers.

Health promotion is aimed at encouraging people (especially children) to choose low-sugar alternatives and avoid sipping sugary drinks or snacking sugary sweets and nibbles between meals.

Ethnicity, diet and health

- Black Caribbeans and Africans consuming a Western diet are at high risk of high blood pressure leading to increased risk of stroke. This may be linked to a greater inbuilt sensitivity to salt.
- South Asians are more susceptible to diabetes, coronary heart disease, and stroke.

Promoting healthy eating at school

The evidence supports a so-called "whole school" approach involving a combination of curricular and non-curricular interventions, for example:

- Improved teaching about nutrition and health.
- Improved teaching of cooking skills.
- Healthier school meals – national nutritional standards.
- Healthier contents of vending machines.
- Involving pupils, parents, governors, and the community.

Promoting healthy eating in adults

Healthy eating programmes aimed at motivated individuals or groups, with personally tailored advice and support, plus follow-up, can achieve sustained dietary change.

Food, drink and oral health

When people consume sugar, particularly sucrose, acid is formed as the sugar is broken down, which in turn demineralizes teeth and leads to dental caries. In the UK, the overall cost of treating dental and gum disease exceeds that of cancers and genitourinary diseases. Several studies have shown a relationship between oral health and socioeconomic determinants. The risk factors for oral health include diet, hygiene practices, smoking, and dental care.

Examples of action at national level

- Clearer nutritional labeling of foods
- Working with food industry to lower fat, sugar, and salt content in prepared foods
- Free fruit in school schemes
- Controls on advertising "junk" snacks to children
- Changes to agricultural subsidies to support fruit and vegetable production

Examples of action at local level

- Educating children and young parents in healthy eating
- Fruit and veg co-ops
- Improved school meals
- Teaching shopping and cooking skills
- School breakfast clubs for deprived children
- Healthy eating advice in primary care
- Focus on at-risk communities, e.g. low income

Promoting physical activity
The benefits of physical activity

The physical, mental, and social health benefits of an active lifestyle are well documented. Regular physical activity helps to:

- Reduce risk of cardiovascular disease, particularly coronary heart disease.
- Prevent or reduce hypertension.
- Prevent and contain type 2 diabetes.
- Regulate weight and avoid obesity.
- Reduce risk of osteoporosis.
- Reduce risk of colon cancer.
- Improve coordination, strength and balance, particularly in older people, and reduce falls and fractures.
- Reduce anxiety and lift depression.
- Avoid social isolation.

Physical activity and disease

Cardiovascular diseases

Physical inactivity is a major risk factor for coronary heart disease in both men and women, at a level similar to that of smoking, almost doubling the risk of dying from coronary heart disease. Physical activity helps to prevent stroke and peripheral vascular disease and modifies risk factors such as hypertension and high lipid profiles.

Overweight and obesity

Maintaining activity throughout life helps avoid weight gain. Physical activity by itself can result in weight loss of about 1 kg per month – but the most effective is a combination of physical activity and diet (see Obesity above).

Type 2 diabetes

Physical inactivity is a major risk factor for the development of type 2 diabetes, with active people having a 32%–50% lower risk. Not only can regular, moderate intensity physical activity help to prevent or delay the onset of type 2 diabetes, it can produce metabolic benefits that contribute to its effective management. The risk of premature death is lower in active diabetes patients.

Musculoskeletal problems

Physical activity can delay osteoporosis by slowing down the loss of bone mineral density from the late 20s onwards. It may prevent low back pain. Activities that produce high physical stresses on the bones (e.g. jogging, jumping, gymnastics, or tennis) provide optimal protection against osteoporosis, unlike low-impact exercises such as swimming.

Depression and anxiety

Physical activity helps people *feel* better by improving mood, reducing stress and anxiety and helping sleep. People who lead an active lifestyle are less likely to suffer clinical depression. Evidence is strongest for activity which lasts between 20 and 60 minutes – but shorter bouts (10–15 minutes) of brisk walking can induce significant positive changes in mood. Rhythmic aerobic forms of exercise – such as brisk walking, jogging, cycling, swimming, or dancing – appear to be most consistently effective. Group recreational sports and activities are also likely to bring social benefits.

Recommended levels of physical activity

UK recommended levels broadly agree with those of other developed countries:

- Adults: at least 30 minutes of moderate activity on at least 5 days a week
- Children: at least 1 hour of moderate activity each day

Activities can be varied and intermittent throughout the day but preferably in bouts of not less than 10 minutes. It is likely that, for many people, 45–60 minutes of moderate intensity physical activity a day are necessary to prevent obesity. For bone health, activities producing high physical stresses on the skeleton are necessary. Any movement is beneficial – and the use of pedometers/stepometers as a motivator should encourage an aim of 10 000 steps a day.

Recommendations for adults are appropriate for older adults. Older people should take care to retain mobility through daily activity. Specific activities promoting strength, coordination, and balance are particularly beneficial for older people.

For most, the easiest and most acceptable forms of physical activity are those that can be fitted into everyday life, e.g. using the stairs instead of the elevator, walking or cycling instead of driving, and taking up leisure pursuits such as gardening, DIY and sports. Individual patterns of active living should both improve physical health and promote long-term adherence to activity.

The risks associated with the recommended levels of activity are low for all ages. More intense or frequent exercise can bring further benefits but increase should be gradual to avoid sport/exercise-related injuries.

Current trends

Throughout the developed world, everyday physical activity has been steadily replaced by machinery, automation, and convenience. Jobs have become more sedentary and less physical. Elevators and escalators now whisk us effortlessly up and down buildings. Computers and TV keep us firmly in our seats. Wider car ownership has meant less active traveling – and more children being driven to and from school. Street games and football in the park are giving way to videogames and TV.

In the UK over the past 25 years, both walking (the most common form of physical activity) and cycling have declined by 25%. Children are more active than adults, but as many as one-third of boys and half of girls are failing to achieve levels of activity recommended for health – thus contributing to the so-called "obesity time-bomb." However, among adults, increased participation in leisure time activities

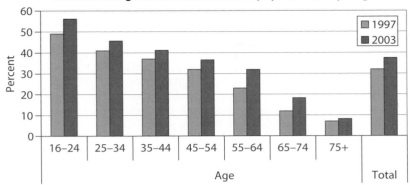

Fig. 2.6. Men achieving recommended level of physical activity, England. (Health Survey for England, 2003, published in *Primary Care* in 2004)

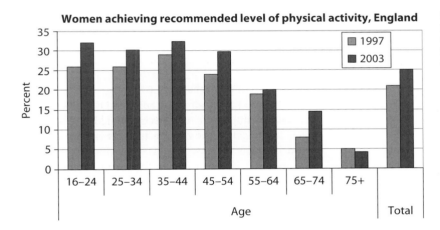

Fig. 2.7. Women achieving recommended level of physical activity, England. (Health Survey for England, 2003, published in *Primary Care* in 2004)

has led to more people achieving the recommended overall level of physical activity (see Figs. 2.6 and 2.7).

Promoting physical activity

There are many ways of encouraging and empowering people to become more physically active:

Early childhood

- Encouragement of active play through playgroups and safe play areas.

School age

- More curriculum time for physical education and sports.
- More resources for after-school clubs and games.
- More walking or cycling to school through improved street lighting and traffic calming.

Adults of working age

- More activity in the workplace, e.g. using stairs rather than elevators.
- More walking or cycling to work through improved street lighting and traffic calming.
- Fitness classes tailored to particular groups, e.g. pregnant women, disabled people.
- "Exercise-on-prescription" services for people with disorders such as obesity, hypertension or back trouble.

Older people

- Healthy walks schemes.
- Strength and stretch classes.
- Dancing, t'ai chi, balance exercises.
- Chair exercises.

Whole population

- Greater appreciation of the benefits of exercise in health and disease.
- Cheaper access to leisure facilities and sports venues.
- Safer parks and open spaces.
- More encouragement through the mass media, health days, fun-runs, etc.

Sensible drinking
Problem: the patient who has a drink problem

Julie is 34 and presented in A&E with multiple cuts and bruises due to a fall down a flight of stairs after a drinking spree. She has a long history of alcohol-related problems. She is the mother of three young children, all in care, and has been unemployed for 3 years having lost her job as a shop assistant. She is found to be mildly anemic and underweight, with moderately raised liver enzymes. After overnight observation, she is discharged and referred to her GP with advice to seek help for her alcohol dependence.

Alcohol misuse is a massive and increasing problem, particularly in the UK. Potentially harmful effects to individuals and society include:

- Alcohol-related ill health: hypertension, liver disease, peripheral neuropathy, Wernicke's encephalopathy, cognitive impairment, liver disease, cardiomyopathy.
- Injuries and accidents.
- Absenteeism and underperformance at work.
- Child neglect and family breakdown.
- Anti-social and nuisance behavior.
- Public disorder.
- Stranger violence.
- Domestic violence.
- Homelessness.
- Debt.
- Truancy and underperformance at school.

Excessive drinking accounts for nearly 10% of disability-adjusted life years (DALYs) worldwide, with only smoking and high blood pressure as higher risk factors. In Europe, mental and behavioral problems due to alcohol are the fifth highest cause of DALYs, exceeded only by depression, coronary heart disease, dementias, and stroke.

Between 15 000 and 22 000 deaths in England and Wales each year are associated with alcohol misuse.

Liver disease accounts for over 4500 of these – a 90% increase over 10 years.

Binge-drinking

Those who drink to get drunk. They are more likely to be under 25 and men, although women's drinking has been rising fast. Binge drinkers are at increased risk of accidents and alcohol poisoning. Men, in particular, are more likely both to be victims and perpetrators of violence. There is also risk of sexual assault. The impact on society is visible in the high levels of emergency hospital attendance due to alcohol.

Chronic drinking

These are more likely to be aged over 30 and two-thirds are men. They are at increased risk of a variety of health harms such as cirrhosis, cancer (particularly of the tongue, pharynx, esophagus, stomach, and liver), hemorrhagic stroke, premature death, and suicide. They are also more likely to indulge in domestic violence and drink–driving.

What is a unit of alcohol?

It is assumed that half a pint of beer or a glass of wine is equivalent to one unit of alcohol. However, this may no longer be the case because the alcohol content of drinks has increased. A glass of wine is equivalent to one unit if it is a 125 ml measure and 8% ABV (alcohol by volume) – but many bars serve wine in 175 ml measures at 13% ABV. Likewise, half a pint of beer is now more likely to be over 4% ABV than the 3% ABV on which the one unit equivalence was based. Bar measures of spirits remain broadly valid, with 25 ml of vodka, whisky, gin, bourbon, or rum, and 50 ml of port, sherry, or martini all still equivalent to one unit. Bottled "ready to drink" drinks, commonly termed "alco-pops" are equivalent to 1.5 units.

UK sensible drinking guidelines

Per week: up to 14 units for women and 21 for men. *Per day*: a maximum of 2–3 units for women and 3–4 units for men with two alcohol-free days after heavy drinking. Binge drinking is 6 or more units for women and 8 or more for men in any one day.

How the population drinks (Fig. 2.8)

Reducing the harm caused by alcohol
Prevention

- Making the "sensible drinking" message easier to understand and apply.
- Targeting messages at those most at risk, including binge- and chronic drinkers.

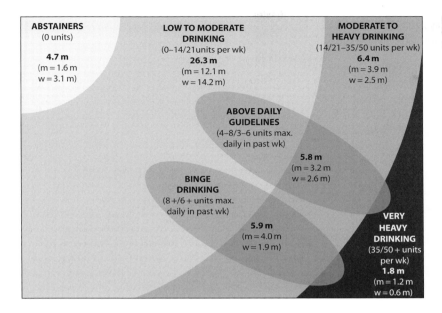

Fig. 2.8. How the adult population drinks. (The Strategy Unit, 2004, reproduced with permission)

- Providing better information for consumers, both on products and at the point of sale.
- Providing alcohol education in schools that can change attitudes and behavior.
- Providing more support and advice for employers.
- Reviewing the code of practice for TV advertising to ensure that it does not target young drinkers or glamorize irresponsible behavior.

Treatment
- Improved training of staff to increase awareness of likely signs of alcohol misuse.
- Piloting schemes to find out whether earlier identification and treatment of those with alcohol problems can improve health and lead to longer-term savings.
- Carrying out a national audit of the demand for, and provision of, alcohol treatment services, to identify any gaps between demand and provision.
- Better help for the most vulnerable – such as homeless people, drug addicts, the mentally ill, and young people. They often have multiple problems and need clear pathways for treatment from a variety of sources.

The effectiveness of treatment will depend on the degree of motivation and type of problem. Different individuals will respond to different types of treatment. Treatments need to be tailored to each individual and include:

- **Community structured counseling** motivational therapy, coping/social skills training, behavioral self-control training, marital/family therapy.
- **Community detoxification** usually takes place in the home, with the support of a GP, nurse or alcohol treatment worker.
- **Specialized residential services** for clients who are either unable or not suitable to receive community-based treatment.
- **Self-help groups** such as Alcoholics Anonymous.

Road accidents and alcohol

- In 2004, over 17 000 people in the UK were killed or injured in drink–drive accidents.
- About 7% of all road casualties and 17% of road deaths are estimated to have occurred when someone was driving whilst over the legal limit for alcohol.
- The legal limit for driving in the United Kingdom is 80 mg of alcohol per 100 ml of blood (blood alcohol concentration – BAC).
- The relative risk of a drink–drive accident increases significantly after 50 mg/100 ml BAC. There is pressure on the Government to lower the limit from 80 mg to 50 mg/100 ml BAC. Many other countries have a legal limit of 50 mg/100 ml or less.

Safer sex
Problem: the patient who has a sexually transmitted disease

Dawn is a 19-year-old student with intermittent one-sided pelvic pains. She has read about pelvic inflammatory disease and has attended the GUM clinic for a chlamydia test, which proves positive. She is prescribed a course of antibiotics and advised to use condoms in addition to the Pill. She hopes that, when the time comes, she will not have problems conceiving.

Poor sexual health can have serious consequences for the individual and the population as a whole. Effects include:

- Sexually transmitted infections (STIs) such as chlamydia, gonorrhea, and syphilis.
- Pelvic inflammatory disease which can cause ectopic pregnancies and infertility.
- HIV/AIDS.
- Cervical and other genital cancers.
- Hepatitis, chronic liver disease and liver cancer.
- Recurrent genital herpes.
- Bacterial vaginosis and premature delivery.
- Unintended pregnancies and abortions.
- Psychological consequence of sexual coercion and abuse.
- Poor educational, social and economic opportunities for teenage mothers leading to social exclusion.

Surveillance data in the UK show an increasing trend. In England, the number of visits to departments of genitourinary medicine (GUM) has doubled – while, between 2002 and 2003, new episodes seen in GUM clinics increased by 37%. Overall, between 2002 and 2003 in England:

- Genital chlamydia infection increased by 9%.
- Gonorrhea increased by 3%.
- Genital warts increased by 2%.
- Syphilis increased by 28%.

Unsafe sexual contact is undoubtedly a major contributor to these worrying trends.

Promoting safer sex

The main ways of reducing the impact of sexual health problems is by:

- Improving sex education in schools, starting at an earlier age.

The rise of HIV

The UK used to be an HIV prevention success story with one of the lowest HIV rates of any large industrialized country. Until 1999, approximately 1 in every 1000 adults had HIV, but this has now increased to one in 500, although the UK continues to maintain a prevalence rate lower than France (1 in 250) and USA (1 in 165).

The main contributors to the increase in prevalence in the UK are:

- Increased immigration from areas of the world with high prevalence.
- An increase in HIV amongst gay men.
- Increased survival of people living with HIV due to better treatment with antiretroviral drugs.

African countries with political and economic difficulties ensure a steady stream of refugees and asylum seekers to the UK from an area of the world with the highest HIV prevalence. More than two-thirds of HIV infections diagnosed in the UK in recent years were due to heterosexual sex – 90% of those infections were caught abroad, 80% in Africa.

The single public health initiative that did most to contain HIV in the 1990s was nothing to do with sex at all. It was the decision to introduce no-questions-asked needle exchange among intravenous drug users. As a result, just 7% of people currently living with HIV in the UK acquired it through needle sharing, compared with 25% in the USA.

- Providing more culturally appropriate information on the risks of unsafe sex and practical ways of reducing them.
- Promoting condom use and offering free condoms to deprived populations.
- Operating more easily accessible, young-person-friendly sexual health and contraception advisory services and clinics.
- Training primary care staff in managing sexual health problems.
- Expanding the chlamydia screening program and early diagnosis of other STIs.
- Improving contact tracing and advice.

Three approaches to health promotion

There are three broad approaches to health promotion – sometimes described as theoretical models – the so-called "medical" model, the educational model and the social model.

Medical model

Interventions aimed at reducing specific **risk factors** for a particular disease, disorder, or injury. Usually aimed at the individual, this is an essential element of prevention and is the typical approach taken by health professionals in the clinical situation. It is very much about advice, encouragement, and support, often linked to preventive treatment, e.g. dietary advice combined with cholesterol-lowering drugs; encouraging patients with diabetes to avoid smoking and supporting them with nicotine-replacement therapy.

Educational model

Interventions aimed at developing knowledge and skills to **empower** people to adopt healthy behaviors through increased self-esteem, self-confidence, life-skills, and citizenship. This approach is aimed at children and young people at school. Examples are helping young people to resist peer pressure to smoke and to know about contraceptives, what their advantages and disadvantages are and how to obtain and use them. Another example is teaching English to non-English speakers.

Socio-environmental model

Community-wide interventions aimed at making the social, cultural, environmental, or economic circumstances more **conducive** to health or healthy living. Typically, these initiatives are taken at national or local level by non-health agencies. The aim is to help make the healthier choices the easier choices. An example is a law banning smoking in enclosed public places and workplaces or a new standard to improve the nutritional quality of school meals.

These three approaches are not mutually exclusive, but work best if combined together.

Helping people change

In practical terms, a useful way of envisaging the three approaches in a combined strategy to support sustainable healthy living is by thinking of them as the "Three Es" – encouragement, empowerment and environment (see Fig. 2.9).

Encouragement

Encouragement or exhortation to make the lifestyle change (e.g. give up smoking, cut down drinking, take more exercise), usually supported by information and advice. This is the typical approach adopted by health professionals in the clinical situation (as in the "medical" model described above). However, it also includes leaflets, posters, videos, and mass media campaigns. Encouragement is a useful trigger for people to make healthy choices, but unlikely to be effective or sustainable without …

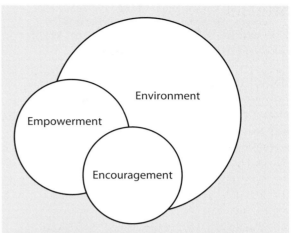

Fig. 2.9. The three Es for healthy living. (Maryon Davis 2005)

Empowerment

Education and personal or community development – the development of knowledge, life-skills and confidence to enable people to make healthy choices. This is in essence the educational model described above. Its effectiveness can be greatly boosted by …

Environment

The socio-environmental model – making changes to the social, cultural, economic, and physical surroundings within which people live, work, and play – to help make the healthy choices the easy choices.

Further reading

Dahlgren G. Whitehead M. *Policies and Strategies to Promote Social Equity in Health.* Stockholm: Institute of Futures Studies, 1991.

Department of Health. *Health Survey for England 2003.* London: TSO, 2004.

Maryon Davis A. Weight management in primary care: how can it be made more effective? *Proc Nutrit Soc* 2005; **96**, 97–103.

Prochaska JO, DiClemente CC. Toward a comprehensive model of change. In *Treating Addictive Behaviors: Processes of Change.* New York: Plenum Press. 1986.

Office of the Surgeon General. *The Health Benefits of Smoking Cessation: a Report of the Surgeon General.* US DHHS Public Health Service, 1990.

The Strategy Unit. *Alcohol Harm Reduction Strategy for England.* London: Cabinet Office, 2004.

World Health Organization. *The Ottawa Charter for Health Promotion.* Ottawa: WHO, 1986.

World Health Organization. *Obesity: Preventing and managing the global epidemic. Report of a WHO consultation.* WHO Technical Report Series 894(3), i-253. Geneva: WHO, 2000.

Useful websites

Action on Smoking & Health (ASH): www.ash.org.uk

Alcohol Concern: www.alcoholconcern.org.uk

BHF National Centre for Physical Activity & Health: www.bhfactive.org.uk

Department of Health: www.dh.gov.uk

Food Standards Agency: www.food.gov.uk

FPA (sexual and reproductive health): www.fpa.org.uk

National Institute for Health & Clinical Excellence (NICE): www.publichealth.nice.org.uk

National Obesity Forum: www.nationalobesityforum.org.uk

NHS Direct: www.nhsdirect.nhs.uk

Bijay Baburajan, Matthew Foxton and Terry Wong

Contents

Abdominal pain

Pain is the commonest presenting gastrointestinal symptom. It can be challenging to analyze due to multifactorial etiology and interpersonal variation of pain perception.

Pain is often accompanied by anxiety and, when acute, by a stress response, characterized by hypertension, tachycardia, hyperventilation, pupillary dilatation, and elevated cortisol levels.

Acute abdominal pain needs a rapid diagnosis due to the risk of a life-threatening cause requiring urgent surgical management.

Chronic abdominal pain is more gradual, developing often over weeks or months. A more methodical outpatient approach to investigations can be adopted.

Acute abdominal pain

In the assessment of a patient with acute abdominal pain the first step is to decide on the severity of the illness. A patient with a perforation of a viscus, rupture of an aneurysm, or acute pancreatitis may need immediate fluid resuscitation and urgent diagnosis and intervention.

In the differential diagnosis the character of the pain and the age and history of the patient are important factors. Characteristics of pain are shown in Table 3.1. Age is important since diagnoses such as vascular emergencies, perforated large bowel, and diverticular disease become common in older patients. In younger patients appendicitis is common, while gynecological problems and complications of pregnancy should always be considered in females.

Occasionally, problems above the diaphragm present as upper abdominal pain. This may occur in myocardial infarction or lower lobe pneumonia. Always look outside the abdominal area for obstruction associated with inguinal and femoral hernias.

The onset of the pain may be helpful. Perforation of a viscus with spillage of intestinal contents into the peritoneum often has an acute onset and leaves the patient reluctant to move.

A careful history will be helpful; gallstones, alcohol, and various drugs predispose to pancreatitis, while previous surgery will increase the risk of obstruction from intestinal adhesions.

The location of pain may aid diagnosis (Fig. 3.1).

Table 3.1. Types and mechanisms of abdominal pain

	Parietal pain	Visceral pain	Vascular pain
Cause	Inflammation of the parietal peritoneum	Obstruction of hollow viscera	Ischemia, peritonitis
Etiology	Perforated peptic ulcer Fecal peritonitis	Colonic or small bowel obstruction	Mesenteric ischemia Leaking abdominal aneurysm
Clinical features	Steady and aching pain • Movement exacerbates the pain and patients usually tend to lie still in bed • Pressure changes over the peritoneum exacerbate the pain–rebound tenderness • Reflex spasm of the abdominal wall over the affected area – rigidity and guarding • The clinical picture is highly variable and serious abdominal events such as a perforated viscus may be associated with mild pain	Colicky or "waxing and waning" • Small intestinal pain is often supra- or peri-umbilical • Colonic pain is usually infra-umbilical and may radiate to the lumbar area • Pain of distension of the biliary tree is not colicky but continuous • The intermittent nature of the pain can be masked in the progressively dilating viscus	• Pain may be severe and diffuse in conditions such as leaking aneurysm • May be mild and continuous prior to deterioration from vascular collapse or peritoneal inflammation • Mesenteric angina is typically postprandial and accompanied by weight loss

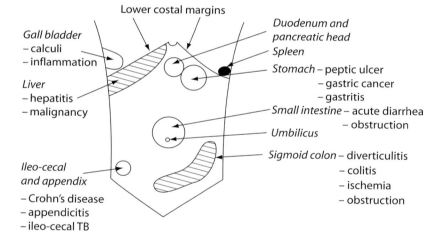

Fig. 3.1. Anterior abdominal surface projections of visceral pain.

Acute gastroenteritis

Infectious diseases are common in the gastro-intestinal tract. They have a higher incidence in developing countries and are a major cause of mortality. However, they are usually mild and self-limiting, requiring no antibiotic treatment.

Clinical manifestations vary according the predominant area of bowel involved.

Small bowel infection

Usually causes large volume, watery diarrhea. Malabsorption may be a feature, causing steatorrhea. Blood and leukocytes are not usually seen in the stool and abdominal pain tends to be diffuse. *Salmonella, V. cholerae, E. coli, Yersinia,* and Norwalk viruses are common causes.

Large bowel infections

Commonly present as lower abdominal pain, with small volume mucoid and bloody stools. Stool examination often reveals leukocytes and RBCs. *Campylobacter, Salmonella, Shigella, Yersinia, E. coli,* and *C. difficile* are frequent pathogens.

Table 3.2. Bacterial infections

Bacteria	Incubation period (in days)	Duration of infection	Blood/mucus in stools	Source of infection
Salmonella				Poultry and livestock
Gastroenteritis	1–2	3–5	0	
Colitis	1–2	14–21	++	
Typhoid, Enteric fever	7–14	28	+	
Shigella	1–2	3–5	+++	Feco-oral transmission, eggs, dairy produce
Campylobacter	1–4	5–10	++	Poultry, milk
Escherichia coli	2–7	3–8	+++	Hamburger, salami
Vibrio parahemolyticus	1–2	2–7	0	Shellfish
Vibrio cholerae	1–3	4–7	0	Water, shellfish
Yersinia	4–7	7–21	0	Pork, milk

Viral infections

In developed countries, most gastroenteritis is viral. A short-lived episode of nausea and vomiting, usually without fever, abdominal pain or bloody diarrhea, is characteristic. Symptomatic therapy is recommended with hydration and antiemetics.

Rotavirus

INTRODUCTION

Rotavirus is the commonest cause of diarrhea in children worldwide.

CLINICAL FEATURES AND EPIDEMIOLOGY

Symptoms last for 4–5 days and include mild pyrexia, vomiting, and diarrhea. Immunocompromise, malnutrition, and old age may lead to prolonged and severe illness and death due to dehydration. Rotavirus infections are commoner in winter with onset of symptoms within 72 hours of exposure to the virus. Infections are propagated by feco-oral transmission. Infection does not usually result in effective immunity.

INVESTIGATIONS

Diagnosis is usually made clinically.

MANAGEMENT

Treatment is based on oral rehydration, which stimulates mucosal recovery and attenuates the severity and duration of symptoms.

OUTCOME

It is a self-limiting illness and recovery is usually complete.

Caliciviruses

INTRODUCTION

Caliciviruses are also known as small, round, structured viruses (SRSV). They are the commonest cause of viral gastroenteritis in adults.

CLINICAL FEATURES

A short incubation period of 36–48 hours is followed by fever, headache, malaise, diarrhea, nausea, and vomiting with abdominal pain.

MANAGEMENT

Treatment is symptomatic, maintaining hydration.

OUTCOME

The course is self-limiting over 3–4 days and recovery is complete.

Bacterial infections (Table 3.2)

Most cases of bacterial gastroenteritis, particularly in the absence of fever, pain, bloody stools, and leukocytosis, are adequately managed by symptomatic treatment and hydration. In the presence of the above alarm features, in the immunocompromised and the elderly, particularly when symptoms are prolonged, stool culture should be performed.

Salmonella

INTRODUCTION

Over 2000 serotypes of salmonella have been described. A high rate of colonization of livestock and poultry causes food-borne outbreaks, particularly in the summer. Person to person transmission is important in the spread of the infection. Domestic

Table 3.3. *E. coli* infections

Type	Affected group	Pathophysiology	Clinical features
Enteropathogenic (EPEC)	Infants in developing countries, travelers	Attachment alters the brush border	Watery diarrhea
Enterotoxigenic (ETEC)	Children in developing countries, travellers	Enterotoxin-mediated secretion	Watery diarrhea
Enteroinvasive (EIEC)	Rare	Direct invasion	Usually watery diarrhea, some have dysentery
Enterohemorrhagic (EHEC)	Undercooked meat, sporadic or outbreaks	Shiga-like toxin	Watery then bloody diarrhea hemolytic uremic syndrome (HUS)/ thrombotic thrombocytopenic purpura (TTP)
Enteroaggregative (EAEC)	Infants in developing countries, HIV patients	Adherence, toxins	Prolonged watery diarrhea

pets have also been described as transmitting the disease to humans, but do not serve as reservoirs of infection.

S. typhi and *S. paratyphi* cause typhoid fever, which may be complicated by disseminated infection.

CLINICAL FEATURES

Salmonella infections present with fever, malaise, arthralgia, and headaches after a 7–10-day incubation period. Constipation rather than diarrhea is a feature. Signs include relative bradycardia, hepatosplenomegaly, lymphadenopathy, and a macular rash (rose spots).

Gastroenteritis   Nausea and vomiting are followed by abdominal pain and diarrhea. Fever is common and the stools are often bloody. This usually lasts less than a week but may be prolonged for up to 3 weeks if colitis occurs. Rarely, hematogenous spread of bacteria can lead to seeding in distant organs such as the central nervous system, kidneys, and the heart.

Typhoid fever   In typhoid there is a bacteremia.

The organism can be successfully cultured from blood, bone marrow aspirate, bile, stool, and urine.

The agglutination test (Widal test) requires a four-fold increase in serum antibody titers to be diagnostic and is therefore not helpful in diagnosis in the early stages of the illness.

MANAGEMENT

Uncomplicated gastroenteritis is treated with hydration and symptomatic therapy. Antibiotic treatment may prolong the carrier state and is not indicated in otherwise healthy individuals. However, antibiotics are indicated for colitis, patients with or at risk for bacteremia, and with severe disease.

Therapy should be guided by sensitivities to avoid antibiotic resistance. For non-typhoidal bacter-emia, ampicillin, chloramphenicol, or quinolones are effective.

For typhoid fever, quinolones, or third-generation cephalosporins are typically used while sensitivities are pending.

OUTCOME

Chronic carriers need prolonged therapy. Cholecys-tectomy may be required in some circumstances.

COMPLICATIONS

* Bowel perforation
* Hemorrhage
* Persistent bacteremia and disseminated infections
* Chronic carriage can occur in up to 3% of patients leading to fecal shedding for up to 1 year, although more commonly for 4–5 weeks
* There is a predilection for extremes of age and patients with gallstones (*S. typhi* harbored in the gall bladder)

Escherichia coli (Table 3.3)
ENTEROHEMORRHAGIC E. COLI

Introduction   The commonest cause of bacterial diarrhea in the developing world, it has become increasingly frequent in the west. Diagnosis and subsequent attribution of symptoms to *E. coli* infection are difficult as the organism is a normal commensal of the intestine.

Clinical features   After a 3–5-day incubation period, the *Shiga* toxin produced causes a colitis. The initially watery diarrhea progresses to bloody stools with systemic symptoms. Abdominal pain is usually severe but fever is unusual.

Epidemiology   Serotype O157:H7 accounts for many of the cases in the west. Ingestion of undercooked contaminated meat is usually the cause. Several outbreaks have been reported, but it is usually sporadic.

Investigations **Culture:** Identification of the organism in a culture of the stool is not indicative of an infection. However, serotyping is available in some laboratories and can identify subtypes that are pathogenic.

Successful culture from blood is indicative of hematogenous spread, which is not usually seen in acute diarrheal illness.

O157:H7 infection is easily identified as it grows in sorbitol–McConkey agar, unlike other *E. coli*.

Management Treatment is supportive with adequate hydration and nutrition. Isolation is advisable. Food handlers and healthcare workers should delay return to work until several stool cultures are negative.

Antibiotics and anti-motility agents can increase or prolong toxin release and should be avoided.

Outcome
Complications

The hemolytic–uremic syndrome (HUS) with renal failure and hemolysis can be a fatal complication, particularly in the young and the elderly. The association of neurologic symptoms in the above setting suggests thrombotic thrombocytopenic purpura (TTP).

ENTEROTOXIGENIC E. COLI

This a common cause of travelers' diarrhea in developing countries. The organism is adherent to the bowel wall and secretes enterotoxins. Diarrhea of a variable severity is the presenting symptom. Treatment is supportive. Antibiotics are not required but are often used empirically.

ENTEROPATHOGENIC E. COLI

This is a diarrheal disease of infants most often seen in developing countries. The organism attaches to the small bowel mucosa and causes villous changes. Antibiotic therapy with trimethoprim–sulfamethoxazole is effective.

Campylobacter
INTRODUCTION

The commonest cause of infectious bacterial diarrhea in developed countries; most infections are due to *C. jejuni*.

CLINICAL FEATURES
A prodrome with fever, myalgia, abdominal pain and headache follows a 1–4-day incubation period.

Bloody or watery diarrhea ensues and can last for up to 2 weeks.

EPIDEMIOLOGY
It is usually transmitted through contaminated poultry or milk.

PATHOLOGY
Campylobacter is an invasive bacterium and causes a systemic illness.

INVESTIGATIONS
The bacteria are easily identified in stool cultures.

MANAGEMENT
Antibiotics (quinolones or erythromycin) are given for worsening symptoms, persistent symptoms for a week or more, and in high-risk groups such as the elderly, pregnant women, and the immunocompromised.

OUTCOME
Complications Prolonged carriage can occur and recurrent infections can be a problem in a third of patients. Hemolytic–uremic syndrome may occur and *Campylobacter* is the commonest precipitant of Guillain–Barré syndrome. Enteropathogenic arthritis has been reported.

Parasites

Giardia lamblia
INTRODUCTION
Giardia are found all over the world, particularly in the summer months.

CLINICAL FEATURES
They cause an acute diarrheal illness and chronic small intestinal mucosal damage can cause malabsorption. An asymptomatic carrier state is recognized.

PATHOLOGY
Cysts, resistant to many forms of disinfection, are shed in the feces of affected patients. These can survive for prolonged periods. When ingested, they release the parasites which attach to the small bowel mucosa.

INVESTIGATIONS
Identification by microscopy of the trophozoites or cysts in stools during an acute diarrheal illness. In the chronic form diagnosis is more difficult and may require microscopy of a duodenal biopsy and aspirates. An enzyme-linked immuno-assay of feces is available.

MANAGEMENT
Treatment with metronidazole is effective.

OUTCOME
In immunocompetent patients treatment is usually effective, although metronidazole resistance is an

increasing problem. In immune-deficient states treatment is difficult and intestinal carriage is often chronic.

Entamoeba histolytica

INTRODUCTION

Amebiasis is the commonest parasitic infection in the world.

CLINICAL FEATURES

It causes acute diarrheal illness of varying severity with abdominal pain, fever, and bloody stools.

EPIDEMIOLOGY

In developed countries it is usually found in immigrants, travelers, and homosexual men. Transmission of infection is by fecal contamination of food and water. The incubation period is up to 3 weeks.

PATHOLOGY

Parasites invade the colon causing typical flask shaped mucosal ulcers.

INVESTIGATIONS

Parasites are difficult to identify in the stool and multiple samples may need to be studied. The identification of a live trophozoite with phagocytosed erythrocytes indicates invasive infection. Stool antigen or PCR of stool specimens may be more sensitive tests and serum antigen tests are also available.

MANAGEMENT

Metronidazole is the drug of choice and may be required intravenously in severe disease. Eradication of the cysts will need further treatment with diloxanide furoate.

OUTCOME

The prognosis is usually good but when complications such as liver abscesses occur the mortality may be as high as 40%. Complications are perforation, intestinal hemorrhage and portal dissemination resulting in liver abscesses.

Travelers' diarrhea

Infectious diarrhea is a significant problem among travelers to developing countries. Attention to food and water hygiene is preventive. Symptoms are usually self-limiting. Bacteria, chiefly *E. coli*, are the commonest cause. Prolonged symptoms or systemic features need further investigation by stool microscopy and culture for specific organisms. Giardiasis, amebiasis, or an undiagnosed immunocompromised state are occasionally found to be the cause. Mild cases need no more than supportive and symptomatic therapy. Prolonged diarrhea and systemic symptoms can be effectively treated by quinolones.

Gallstones

Introduction

Bile is secreted by the liver and partially stored in the gall bladder. It is composed of water, bile acids, phospholipids, and cholesterol. A relative imbalance among the concentrations of these substances leads to the cholesterol coming out of solution and precipitating as cholesterol gallstones. Pigment gallstones can be caused by an increase in bile pigment in bile. They are also associated with bacterial biliary infections. The anatomy of the gall bladder is shown in Fig. 3.2.

Clinical features

Many patients with gallstones are asymptomatic. Some complain of biliary colic (episodic bouts of constant right upper quadrant or epigastric pain). Often other symptoms such as dyspepsia, fat intolerance, or flatulence are prominent features and can make diagnosis difficult. Calculi in the bile ducts can produce obstructive jaundice. Some patients have chronic inflammation of the gall bladder (chronic cholecystitis) and 2%–3% of these can become symptomatic with *acute cholecystitis*.

Typically associated with biliary colic, pain lasts for more than 4 hours, initially of a peritoneal nature, evolving over hours to a non-specific right upper quadrant pain. Nausea and vomiting are frequent. Physical examination reveals a tender abdomen over the region of the gall bladder. Pain is worsened by deep inspiration during deep palpation of the right upper quadrant (Murphy's sign).

Epidemiology

Predisposing factors for cholesterol gallstones

- Caucasian race
- Advancing age
- Female sex
- Obesity
- Diet
- Drugs
  - contraceptive pill
  - clofibrate
- Crohn's disease

Gallstones are common with a prevalence of up to 20% in a Western population. The large majority are cholesterol stones.

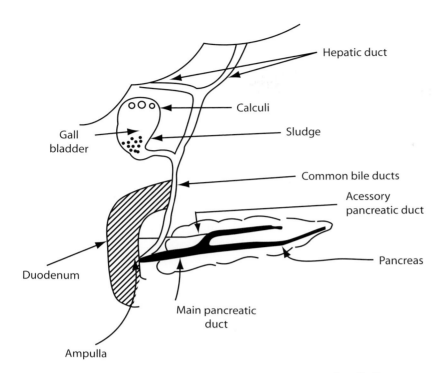

Fig. 3.2. Gall bladder and bile ducts.

(Labels: Hepatic duct, Calculi, Sludge, Common bile ducts, Acessory pancreatic duct, Pancreas, Gall bladder, Duodenum, Main pancreatic duct, Ampulla)

Investigations

Biochemical and hematological investigations are non-specific with leukocytosis, neutrophilia, transaminitis, elevated alkaline phosphatase and amylase.

Transabdominal ultrasound examination has a high sensitivity for gall bladder stones and should be the first investigation. The presence of a thickened gall bladder with surrounding fluid or edema suggests cholecystitis. Abdominal CT scanning is an effective tool for diagnosis of the complications of cholecystitis. Endoscopic ultrasound or magnetic resonance cholangio pancreatography (MRCP) is preferred for the diagnosis of common bile duct stones (Fig. 3.3).

Management

Treatment includes adequate hydration, pain relief, antibiotics, and removal or drainage of the obstructed gall bladder. A cholecystectomy can be performed after the initial acute presentation has been effectively managed with appropriate antibiotics.

Endoscopic retrograde cholangiopancreatography (ERCP) may be required if there is cholangitis (obstruction of the common bile duct by a gallstone leading to ascending sepsis of the biliary tree).

Outcome

The outcome of uncomplicated cholelithiasis is good and cholecystectomy is not indicated for asymptomatic gall bladder stones.

Complications

- **Empyema of the gall bladder**. Gallstone obstruction of the gall bladder neck leads to severe illness with symptomatic deterioration beyond 24–48 hours.
- **Gall bladder perforation** with local abscess formation may result. In the elderly, presentation may be more indolent with subacute pain and low grade pyrexia.
- **Cholecystoenteric fistulae** may decompress the abscess into neighboring bowel presenting as bile-stained diarrhea or
- **Ascending cholangitis** or ascending sepsis of the biliary tree.
- **"Gallstone ileus"**: passage of a calculus through the fistula can obstruct the bowel.
- **Mirizzi's syndrome** describes stone impaction in the distal cystic duct causing common hepatic duct compression. Complications usually will need more immediate intervention.

Acute appendicitis
Introduction

A declining incidence has been reported, but a high index of suspicion for the diagnosis should always be maintained in any presentation of an acute abdomen.

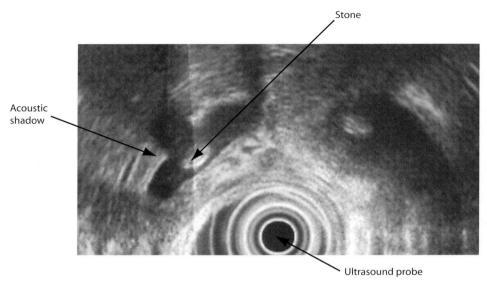

Stone

Acoustic shadow

Ultrasound probe

Fig. 3.3. Endoscopic ultrasound showing a stone in the common bile duct (bright white) casting an acoustic shadow (black).

Clinical features

Nausea and loss of appetite are common, vomiting less so. A low grade pyrexia is usual. Pain is initially diffuse epigastric or peri-umbilical, eventually shifting to the right lower quadrant of the abdomen. Either constipation or diarrhea may be a presenting feature. Guarding, rigidity, or tenderness may be absent at the outset but becomes more obvious after 24 hours. A retrocecal appendix presents atypically without pain, vomiting, or abdominal rigidity.

Investigations

The diagnosis is usually made clinically. Abdominal ultrasound and localized CT scan will often help confirm the diagnosis and the decision to operate. Leukocytosis is not usually an early feature.

Management

Urgent surgery is normally required. If an appendix mass has formed, management is adequate hydration, pain relief, and antibiotics with appendicectomy when the mass has resolved.

Outcome

The outcome of uncomplicated appendicitis is good after appendicectomy.

If left untreated, it may result in perforation and peritonitis.

Diverticular disease

Introduction

Colonic diverticulae are outward herniations of the colonic mucosa at areas of muscle wall weakness, chiefly at the site of entry of penetrating blood vessels.

Epidemiology

Diverticular disease affects 10% of the population older than 45 years in a Western population, becoming more common as the population ages. A diet low in unrefined fiber is thought to contribute to the etiology.

Clinical features

Uninflamed diverticulae are asymptomatic and pain in this setting is usually due to coincident irritable bowel syndrome. Twenty percent of those affected will have a complication such as diverticulitis (fever with left sided abdominal pain) or hemorrhage. Chronic constipation can result from a relatively fixed deformity of the colon, particularly in the sigmoid region.

Investigations

An important differential diagnosis, particularly at first presentation, is carcinoma of the colon, and colonic investigations (barium enema or colonoscopy) should be performed when symptoms have settled. Abdominal CT scanning can be helpful for suspected diverticular abscess.

Management

- **Diverticultis:** Conservative treatment with oral antibiotics is usually sufficient but surgical excision of the affected segment (usually sigmoid colon) may be needed.

- **Hemorrhage**: Usually settles spontaneously. Supportive fluid resuscitation and blood transfusions are often required. Elective surgery is sometimes needed when hemorrhage is recurrent. Emergency surgery for control of bleeding is rarely required.
- **Chronic constipation**: Often an intractable problem, see p. 59.

Outcome and complications

Outcomes are usually good, but surgical resection is sometimes needed.

Acute gastritis

This is a condition associated with gastric mucosal inflammation. It often causes abdominal pain of variable location, intensity, and nature. Recognised forms are:

Acute hemorrhagic gastritis
- NSAIDS
- Alcohol
- Trauma, burns and sepsis

Acute neutrophilic gastritis
- *Helicobacter pylori* infection

Pathology

A predisposing acute event compromises the vascular perfusion of the gastric mucosa, leading to a breach of mucosal integrity and back diffusion of H^+ ions.

An alternative, proposed mechanism is an imbalance in the prostaglandin system reducing bicarbonate release, mucus formation and blood flow, leading to a perpetuating cycle of injury.

Management

Is based on acid suppressive medication and eradication of *H. pylori*.

Acute pancreatitis

Acute pancreatitis is an important cause of severe abdominal pain and is associated with significant morbidity and mortality. Early diagnosis and aggressive, usually conservative, management has resulted in an improved outcome in recent years.

Clinical features

Severe epigastric pain radiating to the back. This is almost always associated with nausea and vomiting. Increasing severity is characterized by fever, tachycardia, tachypnea, and hypotension. Physical signs such as abdominal ecchymoses (Grey Turner's sign and Cullen's sign) are occasional features.

Table 3.4. Ranson's criteria of severity of acute pancreatitis

At admission – five criteria	After 48 hours – six criteria
Age > 55 years	Fall in PCV >10%
WBC count > 16 000 cells/l	Urea >16 mmol/l
Glucose > 10 mmol/l	Calcium <2 mmol/l
LDH > 600 U/l	PaO_2 <8 kPa
AST > 120 U/l	Base deficit >4 mmol/l
	Fluid sequestration >6 l

Diagnostic features

- Serum amylase greater than three times the upper limit of normal (limited by a low sensitivity and specificity)
- Elevated ratio of urinary lipase : amylase
- Definitive findings on CT or ultrasound of the pancreas
- Surgical biopsy (rarely required)

Classification systems based on severity of the illness are useful in risk stratification and targeted treatment for high-risk groups. The most easily used, Ranson's criteria of severity, are calculated 48 hours after admission (Table 3.4).

Number of positive criteria:
- 0–2 <5% mortality
- 3–4 20% mortality
- 5–6 40% mortality
- 7–8 100% mortality

Pathology

Acute inflammation of the pancreas is of two main types:
- Interstitial or edematous: 80% of cases, edema and inflammation without acinar cell death.
- Hemorrhagic or necrotizing: 20% of cases, extensive parenchymal destruction and pancreatic fat necrosis causes almost all of the mortality from acute pancreatitis.

Causes of acute pancreatitis in order of decreasing frequency are:
- Alcohol
- Gallstones
- Idiopathic
- After endoscopic retrograde pancreatography (ERCP)
- Pancreatic cancer causing pancreatic ductal obstruction

41

- Hyperlipidemia
- Hypercalcemia
- Drugs (alpha-methyldopa, azathioprine, cimetidine, estrogens, frusemide)
- Pancreas divisum
- Abdominal trauma
- Rare genetic syndromes

Epidemiology

The incidence in a Western population is around 400 cases per million per year and alcohol is the most common cause followed closely by gallstones.

Investigations

- Full blood count, renal function test, liver function test, amylase

    Abdominal X-ray: Although no diagnostic features may be seen, it is helpful in excluding perforation of a viscus. A "sentinel loop" (focally dilated small bowel loop) or paralytic ileus may be seen.

    Ultrasound: May be helpful in identifying stones in the gall bladder or bile duct dilatation. It is rarely a diagnostic investigation.
- *Abdominal CT:* contrast-enhanced CT scan of the abdomen is the best imaging modality and findings correlate well with prognosis and mortality.

Management

- Aggressive fluid balance and supportive treatment in an intensive care unit or high dependency unit with particular emphasis on early diagnosis and treatment of acute respiratory distress syndrome (ARDS).
- Prevention of infection with systemic antibiotics providing good penetration into pancreatic tissue (Imipenem and Cilastatin) started early in severe acute pancreatitis and continued for 2–4 weeks.
- Targeted treatment of infection with the help of CT-guided aspiration of the pancreatic lesion for culture reduces the mortality.
- ERCP with biliary sphincterotomy is reserved for patients with co-existent obstructive jaundice and cholangitis caused by an obstructing common bile duct stricture.
- Enteral feeding to provide some of the high caloric requirements should be instituted early. Naso-jejunal tube feeding is often required.

Surgery

- The mortality of sterile acute pancreatitis is relatively low at 10%. However, in infected necrotic pancreatitis and severe multi-system illness, surgical debridement or pancreatic necrosectomy can reduce mortality if performed early.
- Cholecystectomy after complete recovery to prevent further recurrences in cases of gallstone pancreatitis.

Outcome

Mortality can be as high as 30%, due to multiorgan failure in the early period. Systemic infections contribute to the late mortality.

Long-term outcome

- Although mild glucose elevations are common, overt diabetes is uncommon.
- Malabsorption can present with steatorrhea and may need treatment with pancreatic enzymes.
- Obstructive pancreatic ductal abnormalities can occur, causing intermittent abdominal pain and even recurrent episodes of pancreatitis.

    The continued consumption of alcohol in the group with an alcoholic etiology predicts a poorer long-term exocrine and endocrine function of the pancreas.

Chronic pancreatitis

(see section on chronic abdominal pain)

Acute intestinal obstruction

This dramatic condition is caused by a variety of pathologies in the small or large intestine. The speed of onset of symptoms and associated clinical features help locate the site of the affected bowel (Fig. 3.4).

Symptoms and signs: obstruction of the small bowel
Clinical features

- Epigastric abdominal cramping pain
- Vomiting (early with small-bowel and late with large-bowel obstruction)
- Absolute constipation to both gas and feces with complete obstruction
- Diarrhea is often a presenting feature of partial obstruction
- Abdominal tenderness with prominent high-pitched bowel sounds coinciding with cramps.

    Abdominal distention with tenderness, silent abdomen on auscultation, oliguria and shock are important signs of severe disease.

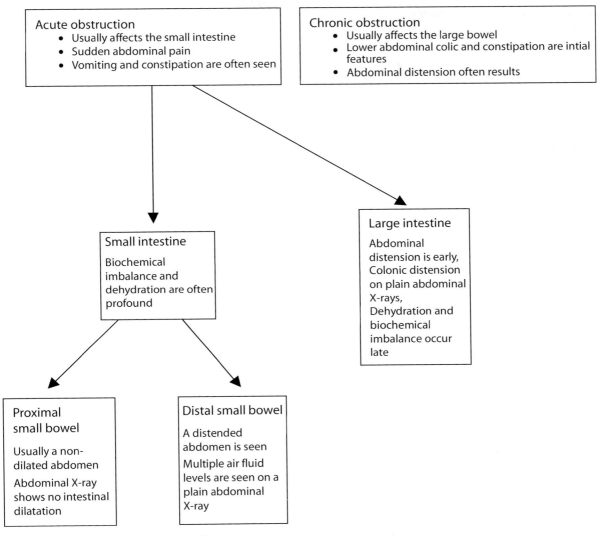

Fig. 3.4. Clinical features of intestinal obstruction.

Investigations Supine and erect plain abdominal X-rays should be obtained. Distended bowel loops with fluid levels are often very suggestive of the diagnosis.

Obstruction of the large bowel

Clinical features Presentation is usually subacute with increasing constipation and abdominal distension. Vomiting may occur several hours after onset of symptoms. Systemic symptoms with large-bowel obstruction are less common as are fluid and electrolyte imbalance.

On examination, there may be a distended abdomen with loud borborygmi and a mass palpable at the site of the obstruction. Perforation of a tumor or diverticulum may occur at the obstruction site.

Investigations

- *Abdominal X-ray*: A dilated cecum of 13 cm or more indicates a high risk of rupture and immediate operation is indicated. Preliminary endoscopy or continent enema may be performed for precise location of the obstruction (Fig. 3.5).
- Contrast-enhanced CT of the abdomen can localize the site and suggest the cause of the obstruction.
- Volvulus often has an abrupt onset and has a high risk of strangulation of blood supply. A continent enema shows the site of obstruction by a typical bird-beak deformity at the site of the twist.

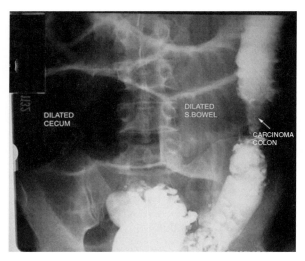

Fig. 3.5. Barium enema showing large bowel obstruction due to carcinoma of the descending colon.

Causes of intestinal obstruction

- **Duodenal obstruction**
  - Cancer of head of the pancreas
  - Duodenal ulcer
- **Small-bowel obstruction**
  - Incarceration in hernias
  - Adhesions
  - Crohn's disease
  - Intussusception
  - Meckel's diverticulum
  - Tumors
- **Large-bowel obstruction**
  - Tumors: obstructing cancer occurs most often at the splenic and sigmoid flexures
  - Fecal impaction
  - Diverticulitis: diverticulitis usually obstructs in the sigmoid

Pathology The causes of intestinal obstruction are illustrated in Fig. 3.6. Above the obstruction, food, fluids, and intestinal secretions accumulate, resulting in bowel distension and edema. This may lead to intestinal ischemia and subsequent perforation.

Strangulating obstruction can occur with hernia, volvulus, or intussusception leading to infarction of the bowel. This begins with venous obstruction followed by arterial occlusion leading to gangrene and perforation.

Management

Treatment of acute intestinal obstruction must proceed simultaneously with diagnosis, and surgery is

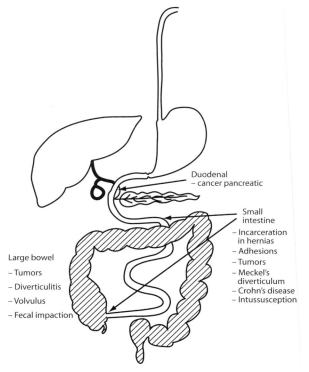

Fig. 3.6. Causes of intestinal obstruction.

often necessary to definitively diagnose strangulating obstruction.

- Small-bowel obstruction
  - A **nasogastric tube** is inserted and placed on suction.
  - **Electrolyte balance**: serum Na^+ and K^+ are likely to be depleted and must be replaced with intravenous normal saline and KCl.
  - Meticulous **fluid balance** must be maintained continuously.
  - Surgery to remove the obstructive lesion or to bypass the obstruction is definitive treatment.
- Fecal impaction usually occurs in the rectum and can be removed digitally.
- In sigmoidal volvulus, a typical distended loop of the sigmoid can be seen on the abdominal X-ray. The endoscope or a long rectal tube can usually decompress the loop, so that resection and anastomosis may be deferred for a few days. Without a resection, recurrence is almost inevitable.

Mesenteric ischemia

The arterial supply to the esophagus and the stomach is rich with collaterals and ischemia of these regions is rare. However, the bowel distal to the stomach is vulnerable, particularly at the celiac axis and the origin of the superior mesenteric artery. Even so, at least two of three mesenteric vessels need to be involved to cause ischemic symptoms.

Clinical features

In acute superior mesenteric infarction symptoms of pain are often greater than the severity of tenderness on physical examination. Systemic findings such as fever, tachycardia and hypotension indicate severity of the condition. Intestinal bleeding is due to mucosal necrosis. The condition is usually fatal without urgent surgery.

Ischemic colitis occurs at the splenic flexure, which is a watershed area between the superior mesenteric and the inferior mesenteric arteries. Left iliac fossa abdominal pain and bloody diarrhea are typical.

Chronic mesenteric ischemia presents with post-prandial abdominal pain and weight loss.

Pathology

Vascular compromise may be due to local athero-sclerosis or an embolus from a remote source, as in atrial fibrillation. Predisposing factors include those for atherosclerosis, hyperviscosity syndromes, vasculitides, cardiac arrhythmias, valvular heart disease, and infective endocarditis. Embolic phenomena are usually sudden and catastrophic.

Secondary ischemia can be caused by adhesions, strangulation, volvulus, the median arcuate ligament syndrome, etc.

Investigations

- ECG (for atrial fibrillation)
- Plain abdominal X-ray
  - Intestinal mucosal edema (thumb printing)
  - Free abdominal air (perforation)
- Transabdominal mesenteric Doppler ultrasound
- CT angiography
- Abdominal CT scan

Management

In acute superior mesenteric infarction, urgent surgery is required after the patient has been adequately resuscitated. Ischemic colitis can usually be managed expectantly. Surgery may be required in severe cases.

Chronic mesenteric ischemia can be managed effectively by angioplasty or surgery in expert hands.

Outcome

Delay in appropriate diagnosis and management is associated with a very poor outcome. Predisposing arteriosclerosis and cardiac arrhythmias are significant co-morbidities and can independently worsen the outcome.

Chronic abdominal pain

In chronic abdominal pain the pattern of pain may be more relevant than the location and severity. Emphasis is placed on aggravating and relieving factors and associated symptoms and signs. The majority of cases are caused by relatively common conditions such as gastroesophageal reflux, irritable bowel disease, and gall bladder disease, but uncommon causes need to be considered. A careful history is very important in establishing the cause. A variety of descriptions are used by patients, who often refer to cramping pain, burning or wind pain. Reflux esophagitis pain is epigastric and retrosternal, peptic ulcer pain in the epigastrium, chronic pancreatitis central and radiating to the back, and irritable bowel disease in the lower half of the abdomen, especially in the left iliac fossa.

The history should explore any relation to eating and to bowel movements. Reflux and peptic ulcer pains may have a time relationship to eating. The pain in peptic ulcer disease often occurs 2–3 hours after food. Irritable bowel disease usually has an association with bowel movements, most often relieved by defecation.

The abdominal wall can be a source of pain. Careful examination should include a search for abdominal wall hernias and local trigger points in the abdominal muscles. In children, chronic functional abdominal pain is commonly the final diagnosis once other causes have been ruled out.

Common causes are:

Gastroesophageal reflux disease (GORD)

Irritable bowel syndrome

Peptic ulcer disease

Chronic gastritis

Biliary colic

Chronic pancreatitis

Gastric cancer

Less frequent causes are:

Chronic diverticulitis

Chronic intestinal obstruction

Tuberculous peritonitis

Gastro-intestinal manifestations of systemic disease (diabetes, porphyria, connective tissue diseases, lead poisoning, etc.)

Pancreatic malignancy

AIDS

Gastroesophageal reflux disease

The term describes the abnormal reflux of gastric contents into the esophagus, leading to symptoms or visible damage to the esophageal mucosa.

Clinical features
Symptoms

- **Heartburn:** Burning retrosternal pain radiating upwards towards the neck
- **Regurgitation:** Reflux of sour or acidic contents into the mouth
- **Odynophagia:** Pain while swallowing
- **Dysphagia:** A sensation of discomfort or obstruction while swallowing
- **Chest pain:** May be difficult to distinguish from angina
- **Water brash:** Hypersalivation in the mouth associated with regurgitation

These symptoms may be associated with respiratory tract abnormalities due to acid exposure. These include cough, wheezing or hoarseness. In severe cases aspiration pneumonitis and pulmonary fibrosis may result.

The typical description of heartburn and regurgitation is specific for gastroesophageal reflux as long as alarm symptoms are absent.

Alarm symptoms

New symptoms in a patient older than 55 years

Chronic gastro-intestinal bleeding

Progressive unintentional weight loss

Progressive difficulty swallowing

Persistent vomiting

Iron deficiency anemia

Epigastric mass

An abnormal barium meal

Endoscopy of those with a typical history of GORD and without alarm symptoms is not mandatory.

Pathology

Causes of reflux

- A weak lower esophageal sphincter
- Transient lower esophageal sphincter relaxations (TLESR)
- Hiatus hernia

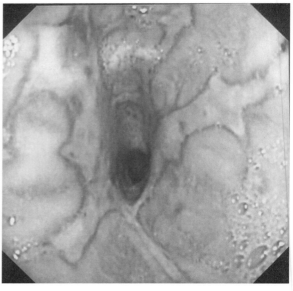

Fig. 3.7. Reflux esophagitis.

- Decreased gastric content clearance
- Increased intra-abdominal pressure

The condition is common, affecting up to 40% of a Western adult population.

Management

- Proton pump inhibitor (PPI) therapy (omeprazole, lansoprazole)
- H2 receptor antagonists (ranitidine, famotidine)
- Smooth muscle prokinetic drug (metoclopramide, domperidone)
- Responsive patients can be maintained on intermittent self-medication

Persistently unresponsive patients will require referral for further investigation.

- Esophago-gastro-duodenoscopy (OGD)
- Barium swallow
- 24-hour esophageal pH study
- Trial of PPI therapy

Upper gastro-intestinal endoscopy is the first investigation of choice. It should be performed after a 2-week period without acid suppression treatment. It identifies esophageal erosions (erosive esophagitis), hiatus hernia (predisposes to GORD), achalasia of the cardia, esophageal malignancy and complications of GORD, such as Barrett's esophagus or strictures. In 50% or more, no abnormalities will be found (Fig. 3.7).

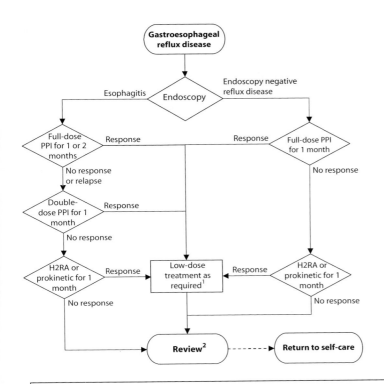

Fig. 3.8. Management of gastroesophageal reflux based on NICE guidelines for adult dyspepsia in primary care (2005) PPI = Proton Pump Inhibitor H2RA = H2 Receptor Antagonist.

[1]Offer low-dose treatment, possibly on an as-required basis, with a limited number of repeat prescriptions.

[2]Review long-term patient care at least annually to discuss medication and symptoms.
In some patients with an inadequate response to therapy or new emergent symptoms it may become appropriate to refer to a specialist for a second opinion.
Review long-term patient care at least annually to discuss medication and symptoms.
A minority of patients have persistent symptoms despite PPI therapy and this group remain a challenge to treat. Therapeutic options include doubling the dose of PPI therapy, adding an H2RA at bedtime and extending the length of treatment.

Contrast radiography is useful for identifying stricture or large hiatus hernias, but is insensitive for erosions or mucosal abnormalities.

An ambulatory 24-hr pH study is indicated when the diagnosis is in doubt or when a surgical anti-reflux procedure is being considered.

If peptic strictures requiring dilatation are present, life-long maintenance PPI treatment is recommended.

Barrett's esophagus has a risk of progression to esophageal cancer, and current guidelines advise PPI therapy and bi-annual surveillance endoscopy with histological examination of biopsies from the abnormal area to detect dysplasia.

Management
The management of gastroesophageal reflux is illustrated in Fig. 3.8.

Anti-reflux surgery
Unequivocal reflux documented by pH studies, unresponsive to PPI or H2RA therapy may be suited to surgical or endoscopic anti-reflux procedures.

Irritable bowel syndrome (IBS)
This common condition affects 10% of the population. However, not all of those affected seek treatment. Women appear to be more commonly affected than men 2 : 1, and no age predilection has been identified. Ethnic differences are widely reported.

Clinical features
The diagnosis is based on the identification of symptoms. There are no diagnostic investigations, but negative investigations may support the diagnosis.

The **Rome III criteria** are commonly used for diagnosis in a research setting but can be clinically useful.

47

At least 3 months, (not necessarily consecutive) in the preceding 6 months of abdominal discomfort or pain that has two of three features:

- Relieved by defecation
- Onset associated with a change in frequency of stool
- Onset associated with a change in form (appearance) of stool

Symptoms that support the diagnosis of IBS (but are not diagnostic in the absence of the above features):

- Abnormal stool frequency (>three bowel movements per day or <three movements per week)
- Abnormal stool form
- Abnormal stool passage (straining, urgency, or a sensation of incomplete evacuation)
- Passage of mucus
- Bloating or abdominal distension.

It is assumed that a structural or biochemical explanation for the symptoms is not present.

Clinical features

A detailed dietary history is needed, focusing on the consumption of fiber, unabsorbed sugars such as sorbitol (sugar-free chewing gum), drugs such as angiotensin converting enzyme (ACE) inhibitors, beta-blockers, proton pump inhibitors, antibiotics (ampicillin), laxatives (may be surreptitious).

Alarm features (the presence of any of these should arouse suspicion of an alternative diagnosis).

- Fever
- Weight loss
- Rectal bleeding
- Anemia
- Family history
  - Inflammatory bowel disease
  - Celiac disease
  - Bowel cancer

Pathology

Not all patients with IBS seek medical attention. In those who do, there is a higher level of psychologic dysfunction, ranging widely from anxiety to depression and hostility. Interpersonal difficulties at home or at work are also reported with a greater frequency. Stress has been shown to accelerate gut transit times and depression to decrease it. It also alters thresholds of perception of visceral pain. No psychologic

symptom predicts the likelihood of IBS as opposed to organic disease.

Patients with IBS perceive gut stimuli as unpleasant at lower intensity levels when compared with normal individuals.

An episode of acute gastroenteritis can be followed by symptoms of IBS in 25% of patients. Although the bowel mucosa appears normal, microscopic abnormalities are sometimes seen. A more severe illness or prior psychologic morbidity predicts a greater duration of IBS. A number of patients can have a persisting infection needing definitive antibiotic therapy, and stool cultures and microscopy are always advisable.

Most patients report an association of their symptoms with different constituents of their diet, and dietary exclusion testing can identify foods that precipitate symptoms. However, pre-testing beliefs about implicated foods are only confirmed in a minority of patients, implicating psychologic mechanisms. Lactose intolerance due to lactase deficiency and true food allergy manifesting as angiedema, asthma, rhinorrhea or eczema are important differential diagnoses.

Investigations

A full blood count should be performed.

Further investigations may be required in selected cases:

- Erythrocyte sedimentation rate (ESR)
- Thyroid function
- Stool microscopy and culture
- Celiac antibodies
- Lactose H2 breath testing (lactase deficiency)
- Lactulose H2 breath testing (bacterial overgrowth)
- SeHCAT (selenium labeled bile acid) scan (bile salt malabsorption)

Patients over the age of 45 at symptom onset need colonic imaging, either barium enema and sigmoidoscopy or colonoscopy, to exclude bowel cancer.

Patients under the age of 45 may require the above to exclude inflammatory bowel disease if the history or screening investigations are suggestive.

All patients with alarm symptoms (see list above), regardless of age, require colonoscopy or barium enema and flexible sigmoidoscopy.

Management

Management is based on the predominant symptoms.

Investigations are recommended if alarm symptoms of organic pathology are present. Otherwise, it is acceptable to treat empirically (Fig. 3.9).

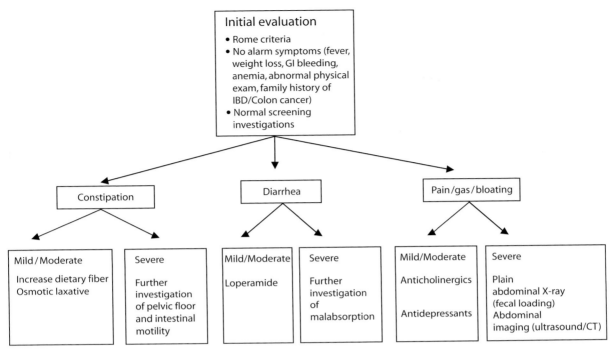

Fig. 3.9. Assessment and management of Irritable Bowel Syndrome (IBS).

Outcome

The disease is benign but the large majority of patients report chronic symptoms and effects on quality of life.

Peptic ulcer disease

This common condition is characterized by defects of the gastro-intestinal mucosa that may extend deeper. They always occur in a setting of disruption of the gastric acid secretion–inhibition mechanism. Protective features such as mucus, mucosal blood flow and tight intercellular junctions retard ulcer development. Other factors such as NSAID therapy and *H. pylori* infection, compromise mucosal defence allowing subsequent epithelial injury. The contributory ratio of *Helicobacter pylori* : NSAID varies from 95 : 5 in duodenal ulcers to 80 : 20 in gastric ulcers.

Clinical features

Dyspepsia is the commonest presentation; burning abdominal pain relieved by antacids and acid suppressive medication. Pain occurs 2–3 hours after a meal and can recur despite initial pain relief after the patient goes to bed.

Silent ulceration may present as a sudden gastro-intestinal hemorrhage or acute perforation.

Physical examination is usually normal. Occasionally, there is epigastric tenderness. Complications are gastro-intestinal hemorrhage, intestinal perforation, or gastric outlet obstruction.

Causes of peptic ulceration

- *Helicobacter pylori* infection
- NSAIDS
- Gastric cancer
- Drugs such as calcium antagaonists, nitrates, theophyllines, bisphosphonates and steroids.
- Gastrinoma (Zollinger–Ellison syndrome) and multiple endocrine neoplasia (MEN) syndromes
- Crohn's disease

Pathology

Helicobacter pylori is a fastidious, Gram-negative, flagellated, spiral bacterium, only found in gastric epithelium. The hostile acidic environment of the stomach is made inhabitable by the secretion of urease which provides resistance to acid proteolysis. The bacteria are acquired in childhood and are compatible with good health. Person-to-person transmission is probably feco-oral. In developing countries 80% of the population is infected by adulthood. In developed countries the prevalence rises throughout life to reach 60% in old age.

Table 3.5. Chronic gastritis

Type of gastritis	Causes	Associated features	Treatment	Complications
Non-atrophic (Type B)	*Helicobacter pylori* infection	Antral gastric inflammation at endoscopy Positive CLO test *H. pylori* identified on histopathology	*H. pylori* eradication	Risk of gastric malignancy
Atrophic (Type A)	Auto-immune gastritis	Achlorhydria Hypergastrinemia Anti intrinsic factor and anti-parietal cell antibodies Anemia (iron deficiency or Vitamin B12 deficiency)		Increased risk of gastric neoplasm
Special forms of gastritis: 　Chemical 　Lymphocytic gastritis	Chemical irritation (NSAIDS, alcohol) Gastric manifestation of celiac disease	Topical effects of implicated chemicals Dense T lymphocytic infiltrate Protracted course	 Gluten-free diet Omeprazole therapy	

The presence of the bacteria in the stomach leads to a chronic gastritis resulting in a loss of somatostatin-induced suppression of the antral G cells. This causes gastric acid hypersecretion and subsequent ulcer formation. They also directly cause gastric mucus barrier disruption.

Non-steroidal anti-inflammatory drugs cause prostaglandin inhibition which leads to impaired mucosal blood flow, decreased mucus secretion and inhibits bicarbonate secretion. There is also a direct topical effect on gastric epithelium causing injury. Long-term NSAID use results in duodenal ulceration in 5%–10% of patients. Prophylactic use of anti-acid secretory medication reduces risk of ulcerogenesis.

Factors increasing risk of ulcers
- Age >70 years
- Previous history of peptic ulceration
- Concurrent anti-coagulant therapy
- Concurrent *H. pylori* infection and cardiovascular disease

Investigations
- Full blood count: for anemia.
- Calcium: hypercalcemia can be associated with peptic ulceration.
- Fasting serum gastrin levels: hypergastrinemia should be considered in unusual or recurrent peptic ulceration particularly when NSAID use and *H. pylori* infection have been excluded.
- For *Helicobacter pylori*:
  - Serum *Helicobacter pylori* antibodies: these are sensitive and specific and are helpful in initial diagnosis but not in assessment of the efficacy of treatment
- *H. pylori* stool assay is a simple non-invasive test and is highly accurate. It also appears to be helpful in the monitoring of therapy.
- The urea breath test is performed with C^{13} labeled urea administered orally. In the presence of urease (not normally present in the stomach in the absence of *H. pylori*), the labeled CO_2 is split off, absorbed into the bloodstream and easily measured in the breath. False-negative tests occur in the setting of small bacterial loads or recent antibiotic or acid-suppressive medication.
- Gastric mucosal biopsies can be tested with the CLO test for urease. This provides a quick result but can be falsely negative after recent proton pump inhibitors (PPIs) or antibiotics.
- Esophago-gastro-duodenoscopy (OGD).
- Histologic analysis of mucosal biopsies is the gold standard of diagnosis of peptic ulcers.
- Barium meal examination is useful in patients unsuitable for endoscopy.

Chronic gastritis (see Table 3.5)

Chronic pancreatitis

This is a chronic painful condition sometimes associated with pancreatic endocrine deficiency (diabetes) or exocrine deficiency (malabsorption).

Clinical features

Pain is the usual presenting feature with exacerbations seen during inflammatory episodes of the pancreas. Diabetes and exocrine deficiency (manifesting as steatorrhea – pale, floating stools) are late features usually indicating significant loss of pancreatic reserve (>90%).

Causes

Alcohol

Cystic fibrosis common particularly in a Western population

Idiopathic

Tropical – rare except in parts of Asia and Africa

Rare genetic mutations

Investigations

Abdominal CT scanning has a good sensitivity for diagnosing abnormalities in moderate to severe chronic pancreatitis. CT is useful in detecting the complications of pancreatitis such as pseudocysts and in identifying mass lesions in the pancreas larger than 1 cm. Endoscopic ultrasound (EUS) may be helpful.

Pancreatic function can be tested invasively by analysis of duodenal aspirate after stimulation with secretin.

Non-invasive function testing is used more often. It has a sensitivity and specificity around 80% and consists of oral glucose tolerance testing, fecal elastase estimation and a pancreolauryl test.

Management

Management of abdominal pain is challenging. Patients requiring opiate analgesia need further investigation with imaging techniques. A high incidence of narcotic addiction and a poor understanding of the pathogenesis of the pain makes rational treatment difficult. A stepwise approach in the setting of specialist pain management clinics is preferable.

Diabetic complications are managed according to well-defined guidelines. Exocrine pancreatic deficiency needs replacement with orally administered pancreatic enzymes with every meal. Persistent pain may require surgical intervention or endoscopic retrograde cholangiopancreatography (ERCP).

Outcome

The condition is chronic but benign. Mortality is due to carcinoma of the pancreas, the complications of diabetes, or the diseases associated with alcohol abuse and cigarette smoking.

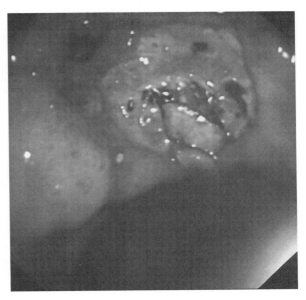

Fig. 3.10. Endoscopic appearance of gastric cancer.

Gastric cancer

The second commonest cancer in the world has seen a decreasing disease related mortality over the past seven decades. Incidence is higher in Japan and South East Asia.

Clinical features

Symptoms occur late and are associated with advanced disease. Abdominal pain, postprandial fullness, early satiety, weight loss, nausea, anorexia, and vomiting are typical symptoms. Occult blood loss may result in iron deficiency anemia. Overt bleeding may occur in advanced disease.

Etiology Diet: a diet rich in nitrates and nitrites has been shown to increase risk of gastric cancer in animal models.

> *Genetic*: Familial clustering has been noted.
> *Helicobacter pylori* infection: chronic infection is carcinogenic.
> *Pernicious anemia*: The co-existent autoimmune gastritis predisposes to gastric cancer.

Pathology

The location of the disease has now changed from a previously predominantly distal or antral distribution to a proximal gastric or esophageal location.

Adenocarcinoma is the commonest lesion (Fig. 3.10). Lymphoma (non-Hodgkin's) is an important differential diagnosis and requires separate management. Dissemination to lymph nodes (celiac), liver and lungs is common.

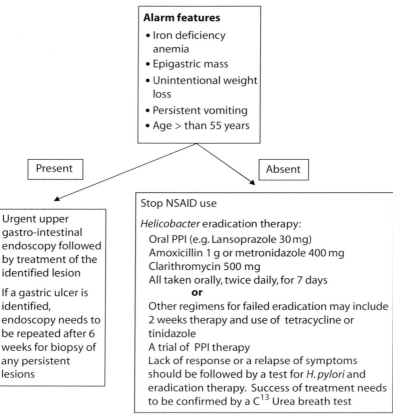

Fig. 3.11. Indications for urgent endoscopy in dyspepsia.

Alarm features
- Iron deficiency anemia
- Epigastric mass
- Unintentional weight loss
- Persistent vomiting
- Age > than 55 years

Present

Absent

Urgent upper gastro-intestinal endoscopy followed by treatment of the identified lesion

If a gastric ulcer is identified, endoscopy needs to be repeated after 6 weeks for biopsy of any persistent lesions

Stop NSAID use

Helicobacter eradication therapy:
Oral PPI (e.g. Lansoprazole 30 mg)
Amoxicillin 1 g or metronidazole 400 mg
Clarithromycin 500 mg
All taken orally, twice daily, for 7 days
      or
Other regimens for failed eradication may include 2 weeks therapy and use of tetracycline or tinidazole
A trial of PPI therapy
Lack of response or a relapse of symptoms should be followed by a test for *H. pylori* and eradication therapy. Success of treatment needs to be confirmed by a C^{13} Urea breath test

Investigations

Esophago-gastro-duodenoscopy and biopsy should be carried out for suspicious symptoms or occult blood loss (Fig. 3.11). On diagnosis, CT scanning of the chest, abdomen and pelvis for staging.

Management

Surgical resection and lymph node clearance of suitable lesions are the procedures of choice. Chemotherapy is of limited benefit and radiotherapy is only useful for symptom palliation.

Outcome

Five-year survival is dependent on the stage of disease and is 50% for stages 1–2 (loco-regional), 15% for stage 3, and 5% for stage 4 (disseminated).

Diarrhea (Fig. 3.12)
Acute diarrhea

see accounts of

Acute gastroenteritis (p 34)

Acute diverticulitis (p 40)

Ischemic colitis (p 45)

Chronic diarrhea
Clinical features

This term is subjective and is used to indicate increased frequency of stool, looseness of stool, and increased volume of stool. The type of stool is influenced by a number of factors such as diet and gender. The normal frequency is highly variable from person to person (from three per week to three per day).

A change in bowel habit, fecal incontinence, and nocturnal diarrhea are important predictors of a pathologic condition and should be actively sought.

Colonic disease is the usual cause of chronic diarrhea. In a small number of cases, malabsorption may be the cause of steatorrhea which manifests as a combination of fat, carbohydrate and protein malabsorption. Symptoms are of pale, offensive, bulky stools which are difficult to flush away and leave a greasy residue.

Investigation

- Celiac antibody testing
- Small bowel histologic analysis (biopsy at duodenoscopy or enteroscopy; this also allows for visualization of the intestinal mucosa for macroscopic abnormalities)

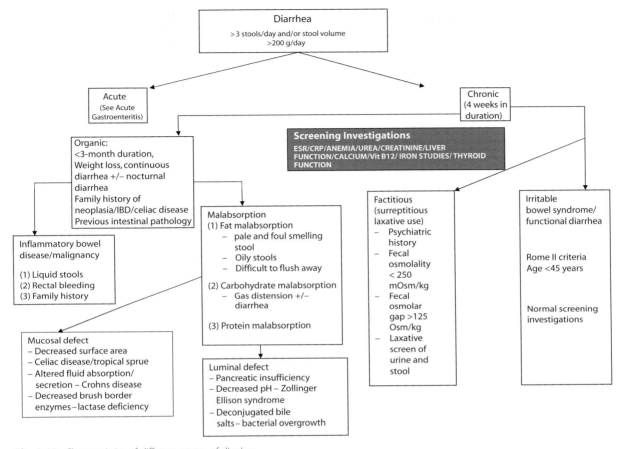

Fig. 3.12. Characteristics of different causes of diarrhea.

- Measurement of the absorptive defect
  - Test of fat loss: fat loss usually co-exists with carbohydrate and protein loss, and is easier to assess. An estimate of the absorptive defect was traditionally achieved with a 3-day fecal fat estimation but this test is unpopular with patients and laboratories
  - Breath tests for fat malabsorption are more acceptable (^{14}C-triolein or ^{13}C-labeled triglyceride), but are limited by a low sensitivity
  - Pancreatic function
- Small bowel barium follow-through examination should be considered when the endoscopy and histology are normal
- Colonoscopy

Celiac disease

This is a genetically inherited condition of disordered auto-immunity leading to small intestinal inflammation and subsequent villous atrophy. It has a prevalence of 1 : 300 in the UK.

The clinical features are non-specific.

- Gastro-intestinal symptoms are related to malabsorption
  - Diarrhea
  - Abdominal cramping and bloating
  - Weight loss
- Non-intestinal symptoms
  - Fatigue
  - Malaise
  - Growth deficiencies

- Menstrual abnormalities
- Neurological abnormalities
- A significant number of adult patients will have more insidious disease presenting as asymptomatic iron, folate, vitamin D, or vitamin K deficiency.

Investigations

Serologic screening can be performed for antibodies to tissue transglutaminase, gliadin and endomysium. IgG and IgA anti-tTG have a high sensitivity (90%). However, there is a 10% incidence of IgA deficiency in this population, which may lead to false-negatives on screening if IgA alone is being tested.

The gold standard for diagnosis is histology. Biopsies are acquired at duodenoscopy. The characteristic changes of villous atrophy, crypt hyperplasia, and lamina propria inflammation are occasionally mild leading to diagnostic confusion.

The blood film may show features of hyposplenism (target cells, spherocytes, and Howell–Jolly bodies).

Other nutritional deficiencies such as iron, folic acid, vitamin B-12, calcium, and albumin can co-exist.

Management

Absolute gluten exclusion, a gluten-free diet, is the cornerstone of therapy. This is the exclusion of food containing wheat, rye, and barley. Although oats may be consumed, there is significant contamination of commercially procured oats with wheat and they may be best avoided. This diet is restrictive and treatment needs to be lifelong.

Nutritional deficiencies may require correction with oral supplementation. Osteopenia and ostoporosis may be seen and will need treatment with calcium supplementation and bisphosphonates. Serial bone densitometry is recommended.

Outcome

Refractory celiac disease: a lack of response to compliance with an appropriate diet without any clear cause. The disease may be particularly severe in such patients with ulcerative jejunitis. Oral corticosteroid therapy and subsequent maintenance on immunosuppressive medication such as azathioprine is sometimes required.

Dermatitis herpetiformis: This distinctive skin lesion occurs in 2% of patients with celiac disease. Treatment is effective with a combination of oral dapsone and a strict gluten-free diet.

Small bowel lymphoma: There is a definite association although the effectiveness of strict adherence to a gluten-free diet is uncertain. A return of symptoms in a previously treated and compliant patient should suggest this complication. Diagnosis is difficult and prognosis is poor.

Small bowel bacterial overgrowth

Introduction

Remarkably, the small intestine in health has a very low level of bacterial colonization. This is effected by gastric acid and a competent ileo-cecal valve.

Clinical features

Patients present with diarrhea, abdominal bloating and sometimes steatorrhea.

Pathology

In states of impaired intestinal motility (diabeic autonomic neuropathy, scleroderma) previous intestinal surgery and achlorhydria, small intestinal bacterial overgrowth can occur. The resultant changes in small intestinal pH, bile salt deconjugation, and destruction of mucosal disaccharidases by bacterial proteases lead to carbohydrate, fat and protein malabsorption.

Investigations

- The culture of small bowel contents is the gold standard of diagnosis but needs invasive procedures.
- Radioisotope breath testing (^{14}C or ^{13}C-labeled xylose) or the lactulose–hydrogen breath test are easily performed but have low sensitivity and specificity.
- Small bowel imaging.

Management

Treatment with antibiotics (metronidazole, tetracycline, or quinolones) is effective, but will need to be repeated when symptoms recur. Pro-motility agents may be useful if intestinal motility is defective.

Outcome

The problem tends to be chronic and re-infection is common.

Lactose malabsorption

Introduction

An important differential diagnosis for chronic diarrhea, it should be considered in all patients with prominent diarrhea and a previous diagnosis of IBS.

Clinical features

Large volume watery diarrhea occurs and a temporal relationship with dairy consumption is usually reported.

Pathology

Dietary lactose is hydrolyzed by intestinal lactase. The activity of this enzyme declines rapidly in most non-Caucasian populations after the age of 2 years leading to relative lactase deficiency. It may also occur in celiac disease or after an episode of gastroenteritis. As many as 30% of patients with a previous diagnosis of IBS are lactase deficient.

Undigested lactose in the gut is osmotically active, leading to diarrhea.

Investigations

- The lactose–hydrogen breath test is most commonly employed when the diagnosis is suspected but has a false-negative rate of 25%.
- Trial of a lactose-free diet.

Management

Dietary lactose exclusion leads to complete recovery.

Bile salt malabsorption

Pathology

Bile salts are normally reabsorbed in the terminal ileum. However, in ileal disease (Crohn's disease, ileal resection), bile salts may be malabsorbed leading to diarrhea. A similar condition may occur following cholecystectomy and in post-infectious diarrhea.

Clinical features

Diarrhea and steatorrhea.

Investigations

- Retention of an orally administered radio-labeled analog of taurocholic acid (Se-HCAT test) is suggestive of the diagnosis.

Management

Treatment with orally administered bile salt binders such as cholestyramine is effective but poorly tolerated.

Chronic pancreatitis (see p 50)

Inflammatory bowel disease

This term is used to describe an idiopathic chronic inflammatory condition of the intestine comprising Crohn's disease and ulcerative colitis.

Crohn's disease is defined as a transmural intestinal inflammation affecting any part of the bowel, but

Table 3.6. Assessment of disease severity in ulcerative colitis

Feature	Mild	Moderate	Severe
Stool frequency	<4	4–6	>6
Pyrexia	None	Intermediate	>37.8 °C
Tachycardia	None	Intermediate	>100
Hemoglobin	>11 g/dl	Intermediate	<10.5 g/dl
ESR	<20 mm/h	Intermediate	>30 mm/h

typically the ileum and the colon. It is further typified by a patchy distribution and relative rectal sparing.

In ulcerative colitis inflammation is restricted to the intestinal mucosa and affects contiguous segments of the large bowel from the anal verge. The disease extent can vary from proctitis (isolated rectal involvement) to pancolitis (total colonic involvement).

Clinical features

Ulcerative colitis Characterized by bloody diarrhea and abdominal pain, but a minority, with rectal disease can present with constipation and rectal bleeding. The onset is usually subacute but can vary; abdominal pain, cramping, and fever are frequent symptoms. The rectum alone is involved in 50% of cases. Increased stool frequency and nocturnal urgency to stool, systemic symptoms such as anorexia and weight loss suggest severe or extensive disease (Table 3.6). Severe attacks can be fatal and require hospitalization for intensive therapy and possible surgical management.

Extra-intestinal manifestations

  Skin: pyoderma gangrenosum
  Joints: sacro-ilitis
  Biliary: primary sclerosing cholangitis
  Vascular: venous thrombosis

Crohn's disease While the condition can affect any part of the intestine from the mouth to the anus, it typically affects the ileum and the colon, either in isolation or combination. Further sub types are non-stenosing, non-penetrating, stenosing, or penetrating. Diarrhea, abdominal pain and weight loss are the commonest symptoms (Table 3.7).

Extra-intestinal manifestations

Skin: erythema nodosum
        clubbing
Eyes: conjunctivitis
        episcleritis
        iritis

Table 3.7. Features of Crohn's disease

Disease location	Type	Symptom	
Small intestine (30%)	Stenosing Penetrating (entero-enteric fistula or abscesses)	Abdominal pain, subacute intermittent intestinal obstruction, weight loss Abdominal pain, fever, anorexia, weight loss	
Colon (30%)	Crohn's colitis	Severe diarrhea, rectal sparing	
Perianal	Penetrating	Fistulae (entero-cutaneous, recto-vaginal, colo-vesical, etc.) and perianal abscesses with perianal pain and fever	Ileo-colonic disease is common and can result in a combination of these

Joints: arthralgia

       arthritis (non-deforming, seronegative)

       sacro-ilitis

Gallstones

Renal calculi

Pathology

There appears to be no predilection for the two diseases based on gender or social class. The incidence of Crohn's is higher in the age group of 15–40 years and among Jews. Smoking is a risk factor for Crohn's disease. Paradoxically, ulcerative colitis predominantly affects non-smokers. No infectious agents have been definitively correlated. There is a clear genetic basis to Crohn's disease with mutations in the *NOD2/ CARD 15* gene on chromosome 16 accounting for 40% of ileal Crohn's disease in a Caucasian population. The *HLA* genes are associated with both ulcerative colitis and Crohn's disease.

Population studies show that there is a familial aggregation of cases and that there is a concordance for Crohn's disease among monozygotic twins.

Investigations
Laboratory

    Iron deficiency anemia

    Anemia of chronic disease

    Vitamin B-12 deficiency (ileal Crohn's disease)

    Leukocytosis

    Hypoalbuminemia

    Hypokalemia

    Metabolic acidosis

    Raised ESR and CRP

Radiology (Table 3.8, Fig. 3.13)

Endoscopy This procedure is usually diagnostic in ulcerative colitis and mucosal biopsies offer further confirmation. Care should be exercised during severe exacerbations of diarrhea as the procedure can cause colonic perforation or toxic megacolon.

Table 3.8. Findings on imaging in inflammatory bowel disease

Modality	Crohn's disease	Ulcerative colitis
Plain abdominal X-ray	Displacement of intestinal loops due to mass effect of an abscess or fluid collection Subacute obstruction	Absent fecal shadows Ahaustral colon Mucosal islands/ thumb printing Toxic dilatation (≥ 6 cm) (Fig. 3.13)
Barium enema	Rose thorn ulcers Cobblestone mucosa Pseudo-polyps Skip lesions Strictures Fistula	Punctate ulcers Pseudo-polyps Back wash ileitis
CT abdomen	Abdominal collection/abscess Colonic thickening	Colonic mucosal edema
Radio-labeled leukocyte scan	Increased uptake in areas of active inflammation	
MRI scan	Perianal fistulae and abscesses	

In Crohn's disease, the procedure is less definitive but can provide valuable information and histological samples. Typical findings are shown in Table 3.9.

Histology (Table 3.10)
Differential diagnosis
Acute self-limiting colitis

    Bacterial

        E. coli

        Salmonella

        Campylobacter

        Yersinia

        Mycobacterium

        Clostridium difficile

Parasites
    Amebiasis
Viral
    Cytomegalovirus
Collagenous/lymphocytic colitis
Diverticular colitis
Drug-induced colitis (NSAIDs)
Ischemic colitis
Radiation colitis
Appendicitis
Solitary rectal ulcer
Colonic malignancy

Management

The inflammatory bowel diseases are characterized by exacerbations and remissions. Treatment algorithms are based on induction of remission of active disease by pharmacologic means and subsequent maintenance of the remission. However, surgery may be needed to treat situations not amenable to medical management (Table 3.11).

Outcome

As a chronic disease, it is characterized by a remitting and relapsing course.

Complications

Long-standing ulcerative colitis, and probably Crohn's disease, lead to an increased risk of colorectal malignancy. The cumulative risk is 15% after 20 years of disease. A greater extent of disease confers greater risk as does concurrent primary sclerosing cholangitis. A program of regular surveillance colonoscopy and biopsy in patients with pancolitis of 8 years or more in duration is recommended for early diagnosis of colonic dysplasia. If any flat dysplasia is detected, colectomy is recommended. Polypoidal dysplasia can be managed by polypectomy.

Colorectal cancer

The second most common cancer in terms of incidence and mortality in the UK, it appears to affect both sexes equally. The elderly have a greater risk of colorectal cancer. There is a very low incidence in patients below 45 years of age.

Clinical features

Typically colorectal cancer is suspected when diarrhea, constipation or rectal bleeding occur, but at this

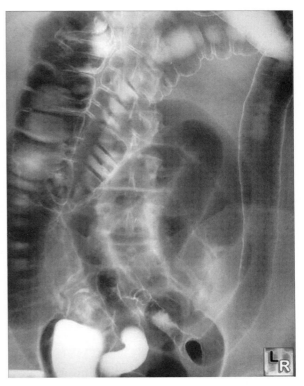

Fig. 3.13. Plain abdominal X-ray showing dilated bowel in toxic megacolon.

Table 3.9. Endoscopic findings in inflammatory bowel disease

Ulcerative colitis	Crohn's disease
Attenuated mucosal vascular pattern	Deep linear ulcers (bear claw)
Granular mucosa	Skip lesions
Focal ulceration	Ileal ulceration
Muco-pus exudate	Colonic and ileal strictures

Table 3.10. Histologic features of Crohn's disease and Ulcerative colitis

Crohn's disease	Ulcerative colitis
Mucosal architecture is well preserved	Mucosal inflammation
Transmural inflammation	Acute and chronic inflammatory cell infiltration
Granulomas (65%)	Cryptitis
Penetrating fissures	Crypt abscesses
	Distorted crypt architecture
	Crypt atrophy

Table 3.11. Treatment of IBD

Medical therapy	5-Amino salicylates	Sulfasalazine Mesalamine	For induction and maintenance of a remission in mild and moderately active disease
	Cortico-steroids	Predisolone Hydrocortisone	For induction of remission in moderately and severely active disease. Due to side effects , not to be used for maintenance of the remission
	Immuno-supression	Azathioprine 6-Mercaptopurine Methotrexate	Induction of remission in patients with moderately active disease but need frequent monitoring of blood tests for evidence of toxicity
		Cyclosporin Infliximab	Effective for severe ulcerative colitis Very effective monoclonal antibody
Surgery		Colectomy	Severely active steroid resistant, steroid dependency, colonic cancer, colonic dysplasia (pre-cancerous state)
		Intestinal resection Stricturoplasty	For stricturing Crohn's disease
		Incision and drainage of abscess Fistulotomy Setons	Fistulizing perianal disease

stage the disease is often advanced. Alarm signs for colorectal malignancy are:

- recent change in bowel habit
- rectal bleeding
- iron deficiency anemia in any adult male or a non-menstruating adult female.

Pathology

Adenocarcinoma of the colon is thought to arise from colonic polyps as part of a predictable sequence. Adenomatous polyps have the greatest risk (increasing size, number and villous histology are particularly hazardous).

There is a greater prevalence of the condition within families and first-degree relatives have a higher risk than the general population. Familial adenomatous polyposis (FAP) and hereditary non-polyposis colorectal cancer (HNPCC) are well characterized as clusters of colonic polyposis and subsequent cancer within families.

Diets high in dietary fats and red meat (particularly with heavy browning) have been identified as risk factors, as have heavy alcohol consumption and cigarette smoking. Inflammatory bowel disease, primary sclerosing cholangitis, and acromegaly confer an added risk.

Histology

Nearly all colorectal cancers are adenocarcinomas with lymphoma, carcinoid and metastases making up just 2% of tumors.

Table 3.12. Duke's staging

Duke's stage	Definition	5-year survival
A	Cancer localized within the bowel wall	83%
B	Cancer penetrating the bowel wall	64%
C	Lymph node metastasis	38%

Investigations

For diagnosis

- Colonoscopy
- Barium enema

For staging

- CT scan

Staging

Duke's staging (Table 3.12) is usually used to stratify patients into groups of advancing disease severity with worsening prognosis.

Management

Colonic resection is the preferred mode of treatment with adjuvant chemotherapy or radiotherapy, depending on the site and the staging.

In patients with advanced and incurable disease, all these modalities and certain others such as colonic stenting for obstructing cancers may be employed for palliation.

Colorectal cancer screening (Fig. 3.14)

Dependence on the clinical features for diagnosis will result in many presenting in an advanced state of

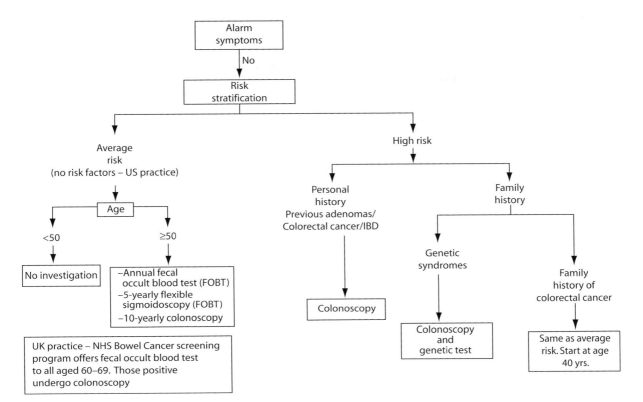

Fig. 3.14. Colorectal cancer screening.

disease. In order to prevent this, suspicion is needed in well patients who have a high risk of the disease. In countries such as the United States, screening is performed on both average and high-risk categories of patients. In the United Kingdom, the current practice is to screen only patients who have a high risk.

Patients at high risk of colorectal cancer
- Previously detected colonic adenomatous polyps
- Strong family history of colorectal cancer
- Long-standing inflammatory bowel disease
- Primary sclerosing cholangitis
- Acromegaly

Screening investigations
- Fecal occult blood testing
- Colonoscopy or flexible sigmoidoscopy
- Barium enema
- CT colography

Outcomes
Are usually good. Poor prognostic features are those associated with advanced stages of disease. Even

hepatic secondaries are considered for resection with curative intent.

Constipation
Clinical features
Complaints of constipation are common. However, like diarrhea, the symptoms are often subjective. Importantly, any recent onset of symptoms should be treated with suspicion of malignancy in patients older than 45 years of age.

Investigations
A detailed history is helpful. Recognized causes are shown in Table 3.13.

Abnormal findings on investigations such as full blood count, erythrocyte sedimentation rate (ESR)/ C-reactive protein (CRP), stool for occult blood suggest a pathologic cause.

Recent onset of symptoms in patients older than 45 requires a colonoscopy/sigmoidoscopy or a barium enema.

Table 3.13. Causes of constipation

Dietary

- Low levels of fiber

Neuromuscular

- Impairment of colonic innervation
- Impairment of colonic muscle function

Metabolic disorders

- Myxedema
- Hypercalcemia

Drugs

- Opiates
- Anticholinergics

Obstruction

- Colonic neoplasm
- Crohn's disease
- Diverticular disease

Management

A diet rich in unabsorbed fiber, increased physical activity, and adequate fluid intake is the initial management. If this is unsuccessful, an osmotic laxative such as lactulose or polyethylene glycol may be used. Neuromuscular dysfunction will often need management in specialist centers.

Chronic straining at stool can lead to anal fissures, hemorrhoidal bleeding, and rectal prolapse.

Acute gastro-intestinal hemorrhage
Acute upper gastro-intestinal hemorrhage

Bleeding in the upper gastro-intestinal tract is associated with significant morbidity and mortality.

Clinical features

Upper gastro-intestinal bleeding may be slow and result in anemia. However, acute loss of larger volumes of blood results in hematemesis, melena and risk of hemodynamic collapse with hypotension and tachycardia.

Pathology

The loss of blood proximal to the ligament of Trietz into the upper gastro-intestinal tract manifests as hematemesis or coffee ground vomitus. As the blood is passed through the gastro-intestinal tract, it is digested and results in black tarry stool or melena. The loss of large volumes of blood, usually more than 1000 ml, results in the passage of frank blood per rectum.

Causes of upper gastro-intestinal bleeding

Peptic ulcers – (commonest)	40%
Gastric erosions	15%–25%
Variceal hemorrhage	5%–30%
Mallory–Weiss tears	5%–15%
Gastric cancer	
Vascular anomalies	

Management

Upper gastro-intestinal hemorrhage has a mortality of 15%, which drops to 5% when managed in a dedicated unit. Accurate assessment of severity and goal directed resuscitation are essential. 20% of patients rebleed in hospital and these have a significantly higher mortality. This group needs to be identified early. The Rockall scoring system and early in-hospital endoscopy are used in many units to achieve these aims.

Predictors of poor outcome on treatment

Pulmonary diseases: acute respiratory failure, pneumonia, COPD

Malignancy

Liver disease (cirrhosis, alcoholic hepatitis)

Sepsis

Post-operative GI bleeding

Renal failure

Bleeding diathesis (e.g. anticoagulation, thrombocytopenia)

After adequate resuscitation, early endoscopy allows diagnosis and hemostatic therapy such as injection of epinephrine, clipping, thermal coagulation. Intravenous proton pump inhibitors reduce the risk of rebleeding e.g. omeprazole 80 mg as a bolus and a subsequent infusion for 72 hours.

Helicobacter pylori eradication should be used if infection is present and malignant lesions will need surgery for definitive management.

Variceal hemorrhage

Esophageal varices occur exclusively in patients with portal hypertension. Cirrhosis of any cause is the commonest hepatic lesion. Mortality is high in advanced cirrhosis (50% in Child–Pugh C cirrhosis) and management is complex. In addition to the hemostatic effects, these patients are at risk of infection, encephalopathy, hepatic decompensation, and renal failure. Hence management needs to address all these issues.

- *Fluid resuscitation*: Saline or colloids are commonly used but risk exacerbating ascites. 5% dextrose could worsen hyponatremia. Hence a balanced approach with a combination of these fluids and packed cell transfusion.
- *Correction of coagulopathy*: Vitamin K given parenterally corrects any reversible deficiencies of dependent factors. Fresh frozen plasma and platelet transfusions may be needed for uncontrolled hemorrhage.
- *Sepsis prophylaxis*: Bacterial translocation into the ascitic fluid causes bacterial peritonitis worsening portal hypertension. Oral ciprofloxacin 500 mg bd or a combination of a cephalosporin and metronidazole are commonly used as prophylaxis.
- There is a high risk of aspiration-associated chest infections which increase morbidity.
- *Control of bleeding*: Bleeding can be torrential, unresponsive to conservative management. 30% of patients known to have varices have a non-variceal source of hemorrhage, hence early endoscopy after adequate resuscitation is advocated. Respiratory complications are frequent and endoscopy is safest after airway protection with intubation. Endoscopic variceal band ligation for esophageal varices often controls bleeding. Intravenous terlipressin reduces the portal pressure and proton pump inhibitors can stabilize the blood clots. Early repeat endoscopy consolidates the benefits of variceal ligation.
- *Uncontrolled hemorrhage*: If endoscopy is unavailable or the procedure cannot control the hemorrhage, a Sengstaken–Blakemore tube is used for balloon tamponade of the varices. Esophageal ulceration and rupture are complications of prolonged use, so deflation of the balloon is usual after 24 hours. If bleeding recurs, a shunting procedure to decompress the portal circulation is effective. Esophageal transection can be useful as a last resort.
- *Secondary prophylaxis*: The majority will rebleed and 5-year mortality is 60%. Secondary prophylaxis with oral β-blockers and serial endoscopic band ligation reduces the risk of rebleeding. Regular antibiotics may reduce the risk of spontaneous bacterial peritonitis. Liver transplantation is the definitive treatment.
- Treatment of esophageal varices (Table 3.14).

Table 3.14. Treatment of esophageal varices

	First-line treatment	Second-line treatment
Primary prophylaxis	β-blockers	Endoscopic variceal band ligation (EVL)
Bleeding control	EVL + terlipressin	Trans-jugular intra-hepatic porto-systemic shunt (TIPSS)
Secondary prophylaxis	EVL + β-blockers	TIPSS

Lower gastrointestinal hemorrhage

Causes

Large upper GI hemorrhage
Diverticular hemorrhage (40%)
Inflammatory bowel disease (20%)
Colonic malignancy and polyps (15%)
Hemorrhoids (10%)
Arteriovenous malformations
Small bowel hemorrhage

Clinical features

The history can suggest the cause of bleeding but is not reliable. Bright red bleeding separate from the stool is thought to suggest anorectal bleeding (hemorrhoids), and dark red blood mixed with the stool to suggest colonic (malignancy or inflammatory bowel disease).

Investigation

Abdominal examination and proctosigmoidoscopy can be diagnostic in the acute setting.

Nuclear scintigraphy can localize the bleeding site in small volume bleeding. If the bleeding rate is more than 1 ml/min, selective mesenteric angiography is preferred as it offers a therapeutic option of selective embolization when a bleeding source is identified.

Colonoscopy is often performed but views are usually limited by blood. However, it can be useful in locating the site of bleeding. Capsule endoscopy is another possible investigation when the cause cannot be found.

Management

Adequate fluid resuscitation.

Expectant management is usually adequate especially in diverticular or anorectal hemorrhage. However surgical intervention is sometimes required.

Dysphagia

This term describes a sensation of food or liquid sticking in the esophagus as it is swallowed. The

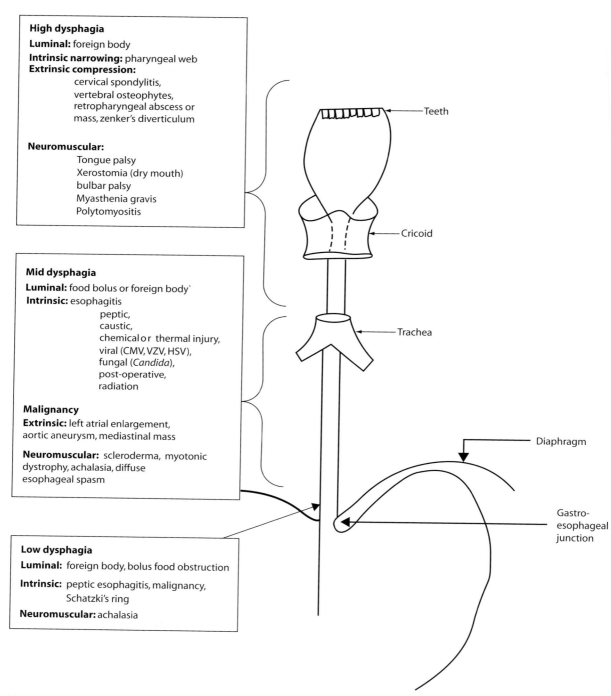

High dysphagia

Luminal: foreign body
Intrinsic narrowing: pharyngeal web
Extrinsic compression:
     cervical spondylitis,
     vertebral osteophytes,
     retropharyngeal abscess or
     mass, zenker's diverticulum

Neuromuscular:
     Tongue palsy
     Xerostomia (dry mouth)
     bulbar palsy
     Myasthenia gravis
     Polytomyositis

Mid dysphagia

Luminal: food bolus or foreign body`
Intrinsic: esophagitis
     peptic,
     caustic,
     chemical or thermal injury,
     viral (CMV, VZV, HSV),
     fungal (Candida),
     post-operative,
     radiation

Malignancy

Extrinsic: left atrial enlargement,
aortic aneurysm, mediastinal mass

Neuromuscular: scleroderma, myotonic
dystrophy, achalasia, diffuse
esophageal spasm

Low dysphagia

Luminal: foreign body, bolus food obstruction

Intrinsic: peptic esophagitis, malignancy,
     Schatzki's ring
Neuromuscular: achalasia

Teeth

Cricoid

Trachea

Diaphragm

Gastro-
esophageal
junction

Fig. 3.15. Causes of dysphagia.

obstruction may be mechanical due to an anatomic narrowing of the esophageal lumen, or motor due to an abnormality of the neuromuscular function of the swallowing mechanism (Fig. 3.15).

Achalasia
This is an idiopathic condition resulting in disordered esophageal motility.

Pathology

The depletion of the myenteric plexus of the esophagus leads to failed peristalsis and a failure of relaxation of the lower esophageal sphincter.

Secondary causes of a similar picture are recognized and include Chagas' disease, paraneoplastic syndromes and malignancy of the gastroesophageal junction.

Clinical features

There is slowly progressive dysphagia to solids and liquids with spontaneous reflux of non-digested food (non-acidic/not bile stained). Chest pain is common and there is often weight loss and halitosis.

Investigations

Esophageal manometry shows the classical features of failed peristalsis of the esophageal body and a non relaxing lower esophageal sphincter.

Barium studies are often suggestive showing a "bird-beak appearance" at the lower esophagus. Endoscopy is not diagnostic, but is required to rule out other causes of the symptoms.

Management

Balloon dilatation
Surgical myotomy
Botox injection

Esophageal cancer

Introduction

The incidence of esophageal and gastro-esophageal cancer is rising in Western Europe and in the United States. This condition is now the sixth commonest cause of cancer mortality. As symptoms appear late, most patients present in advanced stages of the disease with significant loco-regional and distant spread of the disease.

Clinical features

The major symptoms are dysphagia to solids earlier than to liquids and odynophagia (painful swallowing). However, this implies a significant burden of malignant disease and a poor prognosis.

Pathology

Adenocarcinoma is the commonest type. Barrett's esophagus is thought to predispose but probably contributes to only a minority of cases. Squamous cell carcinoma is now less frequently seen. Other histologic types are rare.

Staging

The use of the TNM classification system allows for the pre-operative identification of patients with a probability of nodal metastasis and therefore a poor prognosis.

TNM Classification

Primary tumor
TX: Primary cannot be assessed
T0: No primary found
Tis: Carcinoma *in situ*
T1: Tumor invades submucosa
T2: Tumor invades muscularis propria
T3: Tumor invades adventitia
T4: Invades adjacent structures
Lymph nodes
NX: Regional nodes cannot be assessed
N0: No regional nodes
N1: Regional nodal metastasis
Distant metastasis
MX: Distant metastasis cannot be assessed
M0: No metastasis
M1: Distant metastasis present
Staging
Stage 0: TisN0M0
Stage I: T1N0M0
Stage IIa: T2/T3 N0M0
Stage IIb: T1/T2 N1M0
Stage III: T3 or T4 N1M0
Stage IV: Any T, any N, M1

Investigations

- Upper gastro-intestinal endoscopy and targeted biopsy for diagnosis
- Histopathology
- Endoscopic ultrasound for local staging
- Contrast-enhanced CT scanning for distal staging
- PET scanning for distant metastases

Management

Pre-operative chemotherapy (neo-adjuvant) and post-operative (adjuvant) chemotherapy may be helpful but is controversial.

Patients with Stage III or higher are unsuitable for surgery.

Palliative therapy with expandable esophageal stents, radiotherapy and photodynamic therapy are used increasingly.

Outcome

In the early stages of the disease (T1–T2) primary surgery is preferred with an intent to cure. 5-year

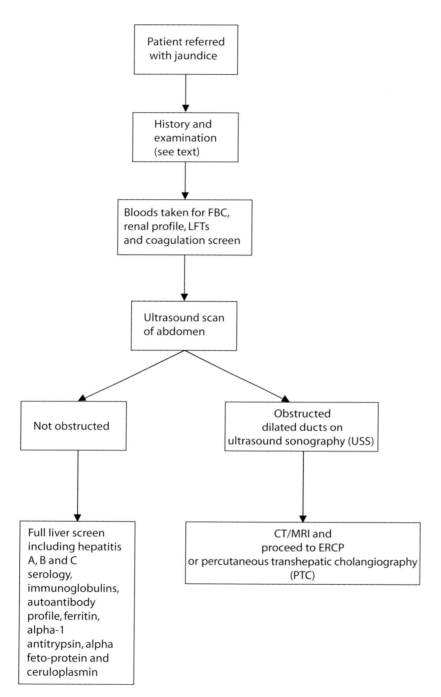

Fig. 3.16. Plan for investigation of the jaundiced patient.

survival exceeds is 60% for T2N0. This falls rapidly as the stages advance to around 10% 5-year survival.

Jaundice (Fig. 3.16)

Jaundice is the sign of yellow discoloration of the skin occurring as a result of bilirubin deposition in the subcutaneous tissues. It is usually seen initially in the sclerae. The normal serum bilirubin concentration is less than 17 μmol/litre and jaundice is usually detectable clinically once the level is greater than 50 μmol/litre. It is classically associated with liver and biliary tract disease, but there are important extra-hepatic causes.

Bilirubin is produced by the breakdown of heme products from red blood cells (70%–80%) and extra-hematopoietic tissues (20%–30%). The unconjugated bilirubin is hydrophobic and is thus transported bound to albumin in the plasma. The bilirubin is then taken up actively by the hepatocytes. Bilirubin undergoes conjugation which renders it water soluble and thus it can be readily excreted into the bile canaliculus to form bile with its other constituents. The bile is then propelled into the duodenum, where it aids in the digestion of food and is excreted into the stool.

Jaundice results from an increase in bilirubin production, abnormalities in bilirubin metabolism, liver disease or a decrease in the elimination of bilirubin from the hepatobiliary tract. The causes of this are summarized in Table 3.15.

The etiology of jaundice is multifactorial, but many clues as to the underlying diagnosis can be obtained from the history and examination.

History

The absence of any symptoms except jaundice is consistent with hemolysis or an isolated disorder of bilirubin metabolism, but does not exclude liver disease or biliary tract obstruction.

Questions should be asked regarding:

- Medication
- Alcohol use
- Risk factors for viral hepatitis, e.g. intravenous drug use, blood transfusions
- Use of illicit/herbal/complementary drugs
- Travel history including place of birth
- Previous operations including gall bladder surgery
- Exposure to toxic substances
- Family history of liver disease/hemolytic disorders

Symptoms such as anorexia, malaise, myalgias, gastro-intestinal disturbance may be suggestive of viral hepatitis. Rash and arthralgias may be a clue to a diagnosis of auto-immune hepatitis. Pruritus is suggestive of cholestatic liver disease.

Biliary tract obstruction may present with fevers, rigors and abdominal pain (especially in the right upper quadrant) indicating cholangitis. A history of weight loss in an older patient may suggest malignancy.

Examination

The signs of chronic liver disease are manifold and include signs in the hands (clubbing, palmar erythema, Dupuytren's contracture, leukonychia), upper body (spider nevi, gynecomastia, parotid

Table 3.15. Causes of jaundice

Increase in bilirubin production

Hemolysis

Ineffective erythropoiesis

Massive blood transfusion

Resorption of hematomas

Abnormalities in bilirubin metabolism

Decreased uptake of bilirubin by hepatocytes, e.g. rifampicin

Decreased bilirubin conjugation, e.g. Gilbert's syndrome, Crigler–Najjar syndrome, physiologic jaundice of the newborn

Impaired canalicular excretion of bilirubin, e.g. Dubin–Johnson syndrome, Rotor's syndrome

Liver disease

Hepatocellular injury

Acute or subacute, e.g. viral hepatitis, hepatotoxins, ethanol, acetaminophen, ischemia, Wilson's disease, acute fatty liver of pregnancy, HELLP syndrome, auto-immune hepatitis

Chronic hepatocellular injury

Viral hepatitis, ethanol, Wilson's disease, alpha-1 antitrypsin deficiency, hemochromatosis, auto-immune hepatitis

Intrahepatic cholestasis

Granulomatous disease, amyloidosis, malignancy

Inflammation of intrahepatic bile ducts and/or portal tracts, e.g. primary biliary cirrhosis, drugs

Miscellaneous conditions

Drugs, e.g. estrogens, anabolic steroids, intrahepatic cholestasis of pregnancy, total parenteral nutrition, sepsis, post-operative cholestasis

Obstruction of the bile ducts

Choledocholithiasis, e.g. gallstones

Diseases of the bile ducts

Inflammation/infection, e.g. primary sclerosing cholangitis, AIDS cholangiopathy, post-surgical strictures

Neoplasms, e.g. cholangiocarcinoma

Extrinsic compression of the biliary tree

Pancreatic carcinoma, hepatocellular carcinoma, metastatic lymphadenopathy

Pancreatitis

enlargement, loss of axillary hair) and abdomen (hepatomegaly, splenomegaly, ascites, prominent abdominal veins). Particular signs such as hyperpigmentation (hemochromatosis), Kayser–Fleischer rings (Wilson's disease) and xanthoma (primary biliary cirrhosis) may identify a particular etiology for the liver disease.

Signs that may be present on examination in cases of biliary tract obstruction are fever, abdominal tenderness, palpable abdominal mass, or a previous surgical scar, indicating previous biliary surgery.

Investigations

In order to evaluate the patient with jaundice, laboratory studies in conjunction with imaging following careful history taking and examination are crucial to formulate a working diagnosis.

Laboratory studies The initial laboratory studies are serum bilirubin, transaminases (ALT/AST), alkaline phosphatase (ALP) and prothrombin time (see section on Abnormal liver function tests).

In hemolytic disorders and isolated abnormalities in bilirubin metabolism, the bilirubin is elevated with normal alkaline phosphatase and transaminases.

Biliary tract obstruction usually produces a rise in ALP levels greater than those of the transaminases, although this is also seen in intrahepatic cholestasis.

Hepatocellular injury results in a rise of the transaminases to a level greater than that of the ALP.

Imaging studies The initial imaging study in cases of jaundice should be abdominal ultrasonography (USS). This is non-invasive, portable, and inexpensive with good sensitivity and specificity for detecting biliary obstruction. It is, however, operator dependent and images may be poor in obese individuals.

Computed tomography of the abdomen can also be used and has a higher sensitivity and specificity for the diagnosis of biliary obstruction. It can detect smaller lesions than ultrasonography and is not operator dependent. However, it does require the use of contrast, involves exposure to radiation and is unable to detect non-calcified gallstones.

Magnetic resonance cholangiopancreatography (MRCP) is a technique that uses magnetic resonance to delineate the biliary tree without the use of intravenous contrast. It has now replaced endoscopic retrograde cholangiopancreatography (ERCP) as the means of diagnosing the cause of biliary obstruction since, although it has lower sensitivity and specificity, there are not the morbidity and mortality risks.

Endoscopic ultrasound (EUS) is less widely available and more invasive than MRCP but has similar indications and better sensitivity and specificity for the detection of choledocholithiasis.

ERCP is the gold standard for the diagnosis of biliary obstruction but has disadvantages due to its invasive nature with an associated morbidity and mortality of 3% and 0.5%, respectively, due to

respiratory depression, aspiration, bleeding, perforation, cholangitis, and pancreatitis. It is still commonly used as a therapeutic procedure to relieve jaundice. It also offers the benefits of obtaining brush cytology although this has a low yield. The therapies to relieve jaundice via ERCP include sphincterotomy (cutting the sphincter of Oddi), stone extraction, dilatation, and stent insertion.

Percutaneous transhepatic cholangiography (PTC) involves the passage of a needle through the skin via liver tissue and into a bile duct. Once cannulation has occurred, radio-opaque contrast can be injected and the cause of biliary tract obstruction elucidated. The advent of non-invasive diagnostic techniques has diminished its use and its therapeutic role is similar to ERCP, although PTC is now usually reserved for cases where ERCP has failed.

Abnormal liver function tests (Fig. 3.17)

Abnormalities in the liver function tests are a common incidental finding and a common reason for referral to outpatient clinics. A good understanding of the origins of the abnormalities is essential to enable a rational approach to investigation.

The term liver function tests is usually taken to mean alanine aminotransferase (ALT), aspartate aminotransferase (AST), alkaline phosphatase (ALP), gamma-glutamyltransferase (GGT), bilirubin, albumin, and prothrombin time. The former four tests are markers of hepatic damage, whilst the latter three tests are markers of liver function.

AST and ALT are abundant hepatic enzymes that catalyze the transfer of amino groups to form the hepatic metabolites pyruvate and oxaloacetate, respectively. ALT is found in the cytosol of the liver, whereas two AST isoenzymes are located in the cytosol and mitochondria, respectively. Both ALT and AST are released from damaged hepatocytes into the blood after hepatocellular injury or death. AST also is abundantly expressed in several non-hepatic tissues including heart, skeletal muscle, and blood. ALT is found in low concentrations in tissues other than liver, so it is frequently considered specific for hepatocellular injury.

The alkaline phosphatase family of enzymes are zinc metalloenzymes that are present in nearly all tissues. In liver, the enzyme has been localized to the bile canaliculus. When evaluating serum liver chemistries, the important issue is whether the alkaline

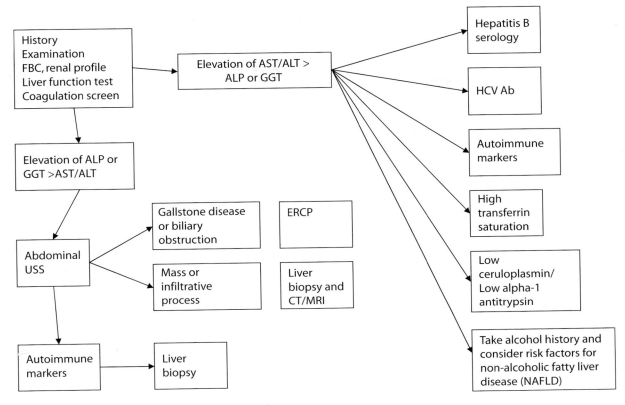

Fig. 3.17. Algorithm for management of abnormal liver function tests.

phosphatase abnormality is of hepatobiliary or non-hepatic origin. The level of gamma-glutamyltransferase (GGT) helps do this.

GGT is a glycoprotein located on membranes of cells with high secretory or absorptive activities. It is abundant in liver, kidney, pancreas, intestine, and prostate, but not in bone. Thus, serum levels may be clinically useful for determining whether an alkaline phosphatase elevation is of liver or bone origin. Serum levels also may be elevated after alcohol consumption (presumably because of enzyme induction) and in almost all types of liver disease. Elevations of this enzyme are therefore less useful for determining the cause of liver disease.

Bilirubin is a normal heme degradation product that is excreted from the body predominately via secretion into bile. Bilirubin is insoluble in water and requires conjugation (glucuronidation) into the water-soluble bilirubin mono- and di-glucuronide forms before biliary secretion. Both unconjugated and conjugated bilirubins are measurable within the serum of patients. Unconjugated bilirubin may sometimes be described as the indirect bilirubin, whereas conjugated bilirubin may be described as direct bilirubin. This is as a result of the way in which bilirubin was originally measured and describes the reaction of conjugated bilirubin, reacting directly with the Ehrlich's diazo reagent, whereas unconjugated bilirubin required the addition of alcohol for color development.

Albumin is quantitatively the most important plasma protein and its concentration reflects the rate of synthesis, the degradation, and the volume of distribution. Albumin synthesis is regulated by a variety of influences including nutritional status, serum oncotic pressure, cytokines, and hormones. The level of albumin can also be affected by loss of albumin through the glomerulus or intestine and by malnutrition and systemic inflammation. Low levels of albumin usually occur in advanced liver disease and, as a result, it is usually normal in asymptomatic patients with abnormal liver function tests.

The prothrombin time is also an important marker of the synthetic function of the liver since most of the factors are synthesized by the liver. However, as with albumin, it is not specific to the liver and can be affected by acquired and genetic conditions as well as by malabsorption and, most commonly, warfarin. Thus, its use in analysis of liver function is predominantly in patients with acute severe liver injury and advanced chronic liver disease.

The range of normal laboratory values for serum biochemical tests is defined as the mean of the distribution ±2 standard deviations of a presumably representative healthy population. As a result, 2.5% of "normal" individuals have results outside the normal range, with no underlying hepatic disease. Conversely, liver function tests within the normal range do not exclude hepatic pathology and levels may fluctuate in and out of the normal range. Hence a low threshold for repeating liver function tests is warranted.

Hepatitis A

Hepatitis A virus (HAV) was initially described in 1947 and the virus was identified in 1973.

Clinical features

HAV infection usually results in an acute, self-limited illness and only rarely leads to fulminant hepatic failure. The manifestations vary with age. Infection is usually silent or subclinical in children but in adults varies from a mild flu-like illness to fulminant hepatitis.

The incubation period is usually 4–6 weeks. Symptomatic patients develop prodromal symptoms including, fatigue, malaise, nausea, vomiting, anorexia, fever, and right upper quadrant pain. Within a few days to 1 week, these patients note dark urine, pale-colored stools, jaundice, and pruritus. The prodromal symptoms usually diminish when jaundice appears; jaundice typically peaks within 2 weeks. Patients with HAV can occasionally develop a relapsing or cholestatic clinical illness.

The two most common physical examination findings are jaundice and hepatomegaly, which occur in 70% and 80% of symptomatic patients, respectively. Less common findings include splenomegaly, cervical lymphadenopathy, evanescent rash, arthritis, and, rarely, a leukocytoclastic vasculitis.

Epidemiology

The incidence of hepatitis A is decreasing with ∼1000 cases reported each year in England and Wales. This decrease in incidence has occurred due to the widespread use of vaccination in at-risk groups. It still remains a major problem in the developing world especially Central/South America, Asia and Africa with intermediate rates of prevalence in Eastern Europe. Spread is via the feco-oral route with highest prevalence in areas with lower socioeconomic development and poor sanitary conditions. It is most commonly contracted from contaminated water or food (especially shellfish) or transmitted from person to person. The virus is excreted in the feces and the patient is most contagious prior to jaundice appearing.

Pathogenesis

Injury to the liver is secondary to the host's immune response. Replication of HAV occurs exclusively within the cytoplasm of the hepatocyte, where the virus causes a non-cytopathic infection. Hepatocellular damage and destruction of infected hepatocytes is mediated by HLA-restricted, HAV-specific CD8+ T lymphocytes and natural killer cells. An excessive host response (observable clinically by a marked degree of reduction of HAV RNA during acute infection) is associated with severe hepatitis.

Investigations

Laboratory findings in symptomatic patients are notable for marked elevations of serum aminotransferases (usually >1000 U/l), serum total and direct bilirubin, and alkaline phosphatase. The elevations in ALT/AST precede the bilirubin elevation, with the peak bilirubin concentration occurring after the peak aminotransferase elevations. Serum bilirubin levels above 170 μmol/l are common (Fig. 3.18).

The diagnosis of acute HAV infection is made by identifying HAV-IgM in the serum, although this can persist for up to 6 months. Immunity to infection with hepatitis A is demonstrated with the presence of HAV IgG in the serum.

Management

The disease is usually self-limiting, although up to 20% of patients may require hospital admission. Patients who develop signs of severe liver dysfunction (rising prothrombin time), particularly if older, should be referred to a liver transplant center.

Prevention can be aided by improved sanitary conditions, handwashing, heating foods appropriately, and avoidance of water and foods from endemic areas. Close contacts of patients (household and sexual contacts) should be offered prophylaxis with human normal immunoglobulin (HNIG) or HAV vaccine. HNIG can be given within 14 days and offers 50–90% protective efficacy for up to 4 months. HAV vaccine must be given within 1 week and offers ∼80% protective efficacy 10 days after administration.

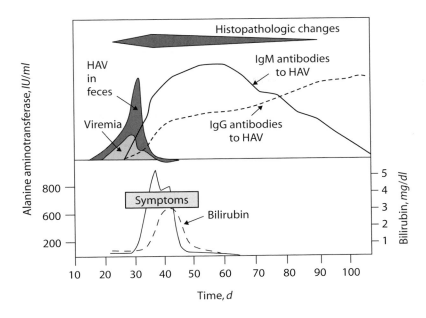

Fig. 3.18. Hepatitis A virus (HAV) serologic evolution.

Table 3.16. Vaccination against hepatitis A

Travelers to countries with high or intermediate hepatitis A endemicity

Homosexual and bisexual men and adolescents

Users of illicit injection drugs

Patients with chronic liver disease

Patients with clotting disorders

Individuals working with hepatitis A virus in research laboratories or working with infected non-human primates

Sewage workers at high risk of regular contact with raw sewage

Vaccination against hepatitis A is extremely effective with a seroconversion rate approaching 100%. The vaccine is inactive and administered at 0 and at 6–12 months. The indications for vaccination are shown in Table 3.16.

Outcome

Almost all patients make a complete recovery with liver function tests back to normal within 6 months. However, fatal cases of hepatitis A occur in 0.4% of patients between 15 and 39 years of age and 1.1% of patients older than 40 years old. The severity of hepatitis A is also increased in patients with chronic liver disease.

Hepatitis E

Clinical features

The incubation period for HEV is 4–6 weeks and the risk of person-to-person transmission is low. In keeping with other acute viral hepatitis, the symptoms are those of jaundice accompanied by malaise, anorexia, nausea, vomiting, abdominal pain, fever, and hepatomegaly. Other less common features include diarrhea, arthralgia, pruritus, and urticarial rash.

Epidemiology

HEV is a waterborne virus, transmitted via the feco-oral route and is a common cause of acute hepatitis in developing countries. Most cases within the UK result from travel to endemic areas, although there are reports of zoonotic transmission in the UK.

Investigations

The laboratory features are those of elevated bilirubin, ALT/AST and the diagnostic test is the detection of anti-HEV IgM in the serum.

Management

Treatment of HEV infection is supportive. Travelers to endemic areas should avoid impure drinking water, uncooked shellfish, fruit, and vegetables.

Outcome

Fulminant hepatitis can occur, resulting in an overall case fatality rate of 0.5% to 3%. Acute liver failure occurs more frequently during pregnancy, resulting in a mortality rate of 15 to 25%, primarily affecting women in the third trimester. The risk of hepatic

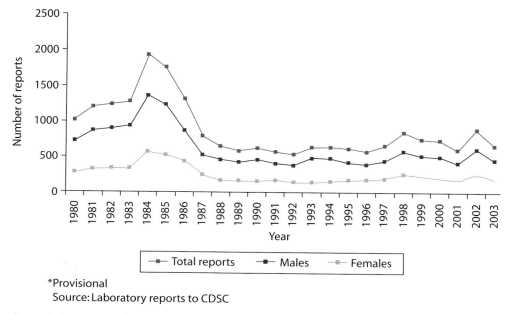

*Provisional
Source: Laboratory reports to CDSC

Fig. 3.19. Acute hepatitis B laboratory reports for England and Wales by sex, 1980–2003.

decompensation is also increased in HEV infection if there is pre-existing liver disease.

Hepatitis B

Hepatitis B is the commonest viral hepatitis with 400 million people worldwide having chronic infection.

Acute hepatitis B

Clinical features

The clinical features of acute HBV infection depend upon the age at infection with infection in neonates and children generally being subclinical. The incubation period is 1 to 4 months. The mode of infection usually depends on the geographic region with most perinatal and childhood infection occurring in high prevalence areas such as sub-Saharan Africa and South East Asia, while most cases in developed countries occur in adults as a result of sexual contact and percutaneous transmission (e.g. intravenous drug use). Acutely infected adults develop jaundice in ~30%–50% of cases. In common with other acute viral hepatitis, patients often have constitutional symptoms of anorexia, fatigue, malaise and right upper quadrant discomfort. The jaundice usually disappears within 3 months.

Persistence of HBsAg, HBeAg and high titer HBV DNA for more than 6 months implies progression to chronic HBV infection. Age at the time of infection is the best determinant of chronicity. Up to 90% of infants of highly infectious HBsAg and HBeAg positive mothers become chronic HBV carriers, compared with approx. 30% of children infected in the next 5 years. However, only 1%–5% of adults become chronically infected.

Epidemiology

The majority of cases of acute hepatitis B in the United Kingdom have no identifiable risk factor identified, with the remainder occurring in intravenous drug users, homosexual males, and heterosexual contacts (Fig. 3.19).

Pathogenesis

Hepatitis B virus does not usually cause direct cell injury except in unusual circumstances. The immune response determines the course of infection and the degree of liver injury. Recognition of hepatitis B virus determinants by cytotoxic T lymphocytes (CD8+ cells) leads to destruction specific to infected hepatocytes, with augmentation by CD4+ cellular responses. In conditions such as immunosuppression, control of infection may be lost, hepatitis B virus replication exaggerated, and a direct cytopathic effect produced, leading to fibrosing cholestatic hepatitis. On the other hand, severe hepatitis is sometimes observed on withdrawal of immunosuppression, presumably the result of an enhanced immune response.

Investigations

Elevations in ALT and AST of 1000–2000 IU/l are typically seen during the acute phase. Serum bilirubin may be normal. The prothrombin time is the best indicator of prognosis and should be monitored at short intervals. In patients who recover, serum aminotransferases usually return to normal within 1 to 4 months. Elevation of ALT for more than 6 months indicates progression to chronic hepatitis. The diagnosis of acute HBV infection is made by the presence of HBsAg and hepatitis B core IgM in the serum.

Management

The management of acute hepatitis B infection is primarily supportive with close monitoring of the prothrombin time (PT). Patients with a rising PT should be transferred to a specialist center because of the risk of acute liver failure.

Outcome

Patients who recover from acute hepatitis B acquire protective levels of anti-HBs with lifelong immunity. However, a proportion of patients will be chronically infected and acute liver failure occurs in approximately 0.1% to 0.5% of patients. Fulminant hepatitis B is believed to be due to massive immune-mediated lysis of infected hepatocytes and resulting in inhibition of viral replication. This may explain the absence of HBV serological markers in these patients. Co-infection with hepatitis delta virus (HDV) or hepatitis C virus (HCV) has been reported to increase the risk of acute liver failure in the setting of acute HBV infection.

Hepatitis B serology (Fig. 3.20)

The understanding of the serologic tests available for hepatitis B is essential in understanding the management.

Hepatitis B surface antigen (HBsAg) is a viral protein found in the blood of patients with acute or chronic hepatitis B. It can appear in the serum of patients within 1 week of exposure to HBV and becomes undetectable in patients after 4–6 months. Its persistence for greater than 6 months defines cases of chronic hepatitis B.

Hepatitis B surface antibody (HBsAb or anti-HBs) are antibodies to HBsAg and appear in the serum as HBsAg disappears and confer long-term immunity.

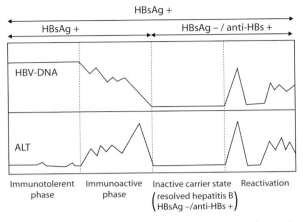

Fig. 3.20. Natural history of serologic and liver function changes in hepatitis B infection. Reprinted from Fattovich, G., J Hepatol 2003; 39: Suppl 1 S50–58. With permission from Elsevier.

They are also present in individuals vaccinated against HBV.

Hepatitis B core antigen (HBcAg) is an intracellular antigen that is only present in infected hepatocytes and cannot be measured in the serum.

Hepatitis B core antibody (HBcAb or anti-HBc) is present at every stage of HBV infection and comprises both IgM and IgG. The presence of HBcIgM is the hallmark of acute HBV infection with the subsequent development of HBcIgG and loss of HBcIgM. HBcAb is only present in the serum if a patient has been exposed to HBV rather than HBV vaccine.

Hepatitis B e antigen (HBeAg) is a secretory protein that is processed by the precore protein and its function is unknown. Its presence usually indicates active viral replication.

Hepatitis B e antibody (HBeAb or anti-HBe) appearing in the serum is usually associated with a reduction in HBV DNA. In about 20%–30% of patients with chronic HBV infection, however, it can be associated with hepatitis and elevated levels of HBV DNA. This occurs due to a mutation creating a stop codon in the precore region of the HBV genome, which means that the virus cannot produce HBeAg.

HBV DNA is detectable early in the acute episode and gradually disappears from the serum upon recovery. However, with more sensitive assays, some patients who have cleared the virus serologically may still have detectable DNA. With the increase in sensitivity of HBV DNA assays has come improved understanding of the natural history of HBV infection.

71

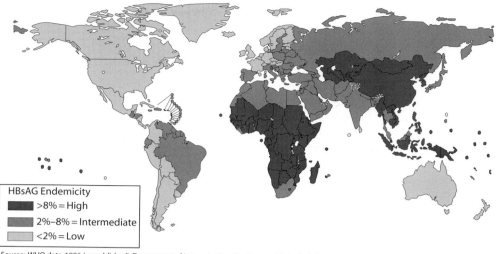

HBsAG Endemicity
■ >8% = High
■ 2%–8% = Intermediate
□ <2% = Low

Source: WHO data, 1996 (unpublished), Department of Immunization, Vaccines and Biologicals (IVB)

Fig. 3.21. Geographic distribution of hepatitis B infection, with permission from WHO.

Chronic hepatitis B

Epidemiology

Around 180 000 people in the UK have chronic hepatitis B, with 7700 new cases each year. Of these, around 300 people were infected within the UK; most of the remainder come from areas of high prevalence where transmission from mother to child is frequent (Fig. 3.21).

Pathogenesis

There are four phases in the pathology of chronic HBV infection, although not all patients go through each phase (Fig. 3.22).

(1) *Immune tolerant* – This is usually present in patients who acquire HBV perinatally and is characterized by the presence of HBeAg, high levels of HBV DNA in the serum, normal serum transaminases, and minimal inflammation on liver biopsy. This stage usually lasts one to four decades. In patients who acquire HBV after the perinatal period, this phase is absent or short-lived.

(2) *Immune clearance* – This is characterized by the presence of HBeAg, high or fluctuating serum HBV DNA levels, persistent or intermittent elevated transaminases and active inflammation on liver biopsy. The duration of this phase and the severity and frequency of elevated transaminases correlate with the risk of progression to cirrhosis and the development of

hepatocellular carcinoma. It is during this phase that seroconversion occurs from HBeAg to HBeAb positivity

(3) *Inactive carrier state* – This is characterized by the absence of HBeAg, the presence of HBeAb, normal transaminases and low HBV DNA levels. If patients arrive at this stage early in their disease and it persists, then they have a favorable long-term outcome. However, approximately 25%–30% of patients will reactivate.

(4) *Reactivation of HBV replication/ HBeAg-negative chronic hepatitis B* – this is characterized by negative HBeAg, positive HBeAb, detectable HBV DNA, elevated transaminases and continued inflammation on liver biopsy.

Investigations

The investigations required are those necessary to determine the stage of disease. Liver biopsy should be performed every 3–5 years in patients at risk of progression to cirrhosis (see below). Patients should also have abdominal ultrasound and alpha fetoprotein levels to screen for the development of hepatocellular carcinoma.

Management

The goals of treatment in chronic hepatitis B virus infection are sustained viral suppression, normalization of serum alanine aminotransferase (ALT), and improvement in liver histology, leading to long-term

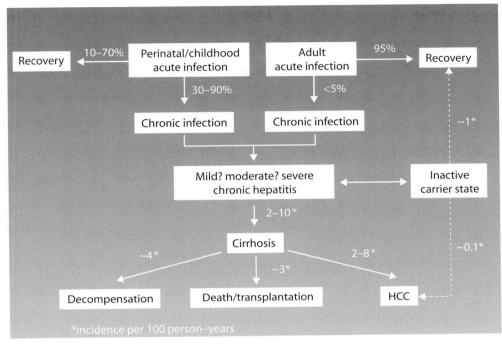

Fig. 3.22. Summary of the natural history of HBV infection. European Association for the Study of the Liver (EASL) Consensus Statement, 2003.

reduction in the risk of cirrhosis and hepatocellular carcinoma (HCC).

The advantages of therapy with pegylated interferon, the finite duration of treatment and durable response with the low but real chance of HBeAg clearance, must be balanced against the risk of side effects and costs of administration. Although lamivudine is well tolerated and easily administered, the high risk of development of resistance limits its long-term use. Adefovir and entecavir are also well tolerated and exhibit lower rates of resistance at 1 year, but they are expensive especially since they may require long-term use.

The advantages and disadvantages of the treatments for chronic hepatitis B infection are shown in Table 3.17.

Outcome
Patients with chronic HBV infection can seroconvert from HBsAg to HBsAb at a rate of 0.5%–1% per year. This is usually associated with a good prognosis.

The risk factors associated with progression to cirrhosis are older age, male gender, immunosuppression, high levels of HBV replication, alcohol consumption, concurrent infection with HBV, HDV, HCV or HIV, diabetes mellitus and obesity. The incidence of cirrhosis

is estimated at 2%–6% for HBeAg positive patients and 8%–10% for HBeAg negative patients.

Hepatitis B virus is a recognized carcinogen and the incidence of hepatocellular carcinoma (HCC) in patients with chronic HBV infection is <1% for non-cirrhotics and 2%–3% for patients with cirrhosis. Increasing levels of HBV DNA are associated with an increase in the risk of developing HCC.

The recognition that suppression of HBV DNA levels can prevent the development of cirrhosis and HCC, along with the development of the antiviral agents, has led to the realization that the natural history of chronic hepatitis B infection can be changed. However, the risk of drug resistance and cost associated with the antiviral agents means that careful consideration must be given before initiating these drugs.

Hepatitis C
Clinical features
People are often asymptomatic after exposure to the virus, but about 20% will develop acute hepatitis. Up to 85% of those exposed do not clear the virus and go on to develop chronic hepatitis C. Progression of the disease occurs over 20–50 years. About 5%–30% of

Table 3.17. Advantages and disadvantages of chronic hepatitis B treatments

	Pegylated IFN	Lamivudine	Adefovir	Entecavir
Dose	Weekly	Daily	Daily	Daily
Route	Subcutaneous	Oral	Oral	Oral
Duration of treatment	48 weeks	>1 year	>1 year	>1 year
Safety	Supervision autoimmunity	Excellent	Excellent	Excellent
Tolerability	Inferior	Superior	Superior	Superior
Cost	Expensive	Inexpensive	Expensive	Expensive
HBeAg seroconversion	Superior	Inferior	Inferior	Inferior
HBsAg seroconversion	Superior	Inferior	Inferior	Inferior
Prolonged suppression	Inferior	Superior unless resistance	Superior unless resistance	Superior unless resistance
Resistance	None	20% at 1 year 70% at 4 years	0% at 1 year 15% at 4 years	0% in previously untreated except with lamivudine

people initially infected will develop cirrhosis within 20 years and a small percentage of these are at high risk of developing hepatocellular carcinoma. One-third may never progress to cirrhosis or will not progress for at least 50 years. Some people with end-stage liver disease or hepatocellular carcinoma may require liver transplantation.

In patients with chronic hepatitis C, it is difficult to predict who will have a relatively benign course and who will go on to develop cirrhosis or cancer. Factors associated with progression to cirrhosis are concurrent alcohol abuse, male gender, increasing age, and obesity. Certain findings on liver biopsy can also be helpful in predicting a relatively benign or progressive course. Viral genotype may also play a role.

Many individuals with HCV infection do not display symptoms. However, non-specific symptoms, such as fatigue, irritability, nausea, muscle ache, anorexia, abdominal discomfort, and pain in the upper right quadrant, have been reported even in the absence of secondary pathology. If cirrhosis develops, there may be severe symptoms and complications.

Hepatitis C has also been associated with extra-hepatic manifestations. These include essential mixed cryoglobulinemia, non-Hodgkin's lymphoma, membranoproliferative glomerulonephritis, and porphyria cutanea tarda. Other associated conditions, with a wide range of reported frequencies, include lichen planus, autoimmune thyroiditis, diabetes mellitus, and Sjögren's syndrome.

Epidemiology

Hepatitis C infection is common with an estimated 400 000 people affected within the UK. It is transmitted via blood with the majority of people infected due to intravenous drug use or use of blood products prior to the introduction of screening in 1991. HCV infection is more common in sexually promiscuous individuals. Perinatal transmission from mother to fetus or infant is also relatively low but possible (less than 10%). Many individuals infected with HCV have no obvious risk factors. Most of these have probably been exposed to contaminated blood or blood products inadvertently. There is a small risk of infection associated with tattooing, electrolysis, body piercing and acupuncture. Concomitant HIV infection is thought to increase the risk of transmission.

Investigations

The initial screening test for hepatitis C infection is the HCV antibody test. Patients who should be screened for hepatitis C are those with symptoms of chronic liver disease, those at risk for hepatitis C infection, e.g. past or current intravenous drug use or blood transfusions prior to 1990, and those with abnormal liver function tests. If the HCV antibody test is positive, then qualitative polymerase chain reaction (PCR) for HCV RNA should be performed. A positive HCV RNA test indicates active infection and is present in 85% of those with a positive HCV antibody test. In those with positive HCV

RNA, a liver biopsy should be performed to assess the inflammation and stage of fibrosis within the liver. Other investigations include quantitative PCR to assess the HCV viral load and viral genotyping. These tests are useful in patients being considered for treatment.

Management

Those with positive antibody test and negative PCR should have this repeated. If still negative they have cleared the virus.

Patients with positive PCR should undergo liver biopsy and genotype testing. Liver biopsy is not required in people with hemophilia, complications from a previous liver biopsy, and those with extra-hepatic manifestations of HCV infection. Moderate/severe scarring and/or significant necrotic inflammation in the liver biopsy should prompt consideration for treatment with pegylated interferon and ribavirin. The HCV RNA should be measured 6 months after the completion of treatment to assess whether there has been a sustained viral response. Patients with a negative test have cleared the virus.

Outcome

Factors that favor a good outcome with treatment are genotypes 2 and 3, low viral load, young age, absence of obesity, less fibrosis in liver biopsy, and non-black racial origin.

Approximately 20% of patients with chronic hepatitis C will develop cirrhosis 20 years after infection. After development of cirrhosis, 4% will decompensate with the development of ascites, variceal bleeding, encephalopathy, or jaundice. The mortality of decompensated HCV cirrhosis is 50% at 5 years. Decompensated cirrhosis is an indication for liver transplantation. HCV is now the commonest indication worldwide.

The risk of developing hepatocellular carcinoma in patients with HCV cirrhosis is 1%–3% per year.

Autoimmune hepatitis (AIH)

Autoimmune hepatitis is a chronic inflammation of the liver of unknown etiology. It is characterized by hepatitis with hypergammaglobulinemia and autoantibodies. Since its first description, it has been known by a variety of terms, including chronic active hepatitis, lupoid hepatitis, plasma cell hepatitis, and, most commonly, autoimmune chronic active hepatitis. It is now known as autoimmune hepatitis (AIH).

Clinical features

It is a heterogeneous condition with a fluctuating course.

Manifestations range from asymptomatic patients identified only with an elevated ALT/AST to acute liver failure. Physical examination may be normal or show hepatomegaly, splenomegaly, stigmata of chronic liver disease, and/or deep jaundice.

Patients who present acutely may have profound jaundice, an elevated prothrombin time, and aminotransferase values in the thousands. Many patients with an acute presentation have established cirrhosis when biopsied suggesting subclinical disease for some time.

Some patients present with non-specific symptoms, such as fatigue, lethargy, malaise, anorexia, nausea, abdominal pain, itching, and arthralgia involving the small joints.

There are often associated autoimmune conditions such as hemolytic anemia, idiopathic thrombocytopenic purpura, type 1 diabetes mellitus, thyroiditis, and celiac disease.

Epidemiology

The mean annual incidence of AIH among white Northern Europeans is 1.9 per 100 000, and its prevalence is 16.9 per 100 000. It accounts for 2.6% of the transplantations in Europe and 5.9% in the United States. Women are affected more than men (gender ratio, 3.6:1), and all ages and ethnic groups are susceptible.

Pathogenesis

The pathogenesis of autoimmune hepatitis is thought to be due to an environmental agent that triggers a cascade of T-cell–mediated events directed at liver antigens in a host genetically predisposed to this disease, leading to a progressive necroinflammatory and fibrotic process in the liver.

The environmental agents commonly implicated are measles, hepatitis viruses, Epstein–Barr virus, or cytomegalovirus. Drugs such as methyldopa, nitrofurantoin, diclofenac, interferon, minocycline, and atorvastatin have also been implicated. HLA-DR3 and DR4 are the commonest serotypes associated with AIH.

Investigations

Elevated ALT/AST levels up to 5–10 times the upper limit of normal are the commonest abnormalities. Other investigations necessary to make the diagnosis are immunoglobulin levels and auto-antibody profile.

Immunoglobulin G (IgG) is commonly raised 1.2–3 times the upper limit of normal. The characteristic auto-antibodies seen in AIH are anti-nuclear (ANA), anti-smooth muscle (SMA), anti-liver–kidney microsomal (LKM), and soluble liver antigen (SLA).

Liver biopsy in patients with AIH may reveal plasma cell infiltrate, hepatocyte rosetting and interface hepatitis. Advanced cases may demonstrate fibrosis and cirrhosis.

Management

Treatment should be instituted in patients with serum ALT levels greater than tenfold the upper limit of normal or in patients with serum ALT levels that are fivefold the upper limit of normal in conjunction with a serum IgG level at least twice the upper limit of normal. Treatment is also warranted in patients with features of necrosis on their liver biopsy. Treatment may not be indicated in patients with inactive cirrhosis, pre-existent co-morbid conditions, or drug intolerances.

The initial drug for treatment is high dose prednisolone, or prednisolone with azathioprine. Response to treatment is defined as resolution of symptoms, reduction in serum ALT levels to less than twice the upper limit of normal, normalization of serum bilirubin and gamma globulin levels or improvement in liver histology to normal or only mild hepatitis.

The aim of treatment is sustained remission without drug therapy but this is only achievable in 10%–40% of patients. Most need control with monotherapy, usually azathioprine.

In patients who have AIH that does not respond to this approach, cyclosporin, methotrexate, tacrolimus, and mycophenolate mofetil have been used.

Outcome

Untreated severe AIH results in 40% mortality at 6 months with a further 40% developing cirrhosis. Forty-nine percent of patients with less severe disease develop cirrhosis within 15 years and death from liver failure occurs in 10%. The 20-year life expectancy for all treated patients exceeds 80%, and survival is similar to that of age- and sex-matched normal subjects from the same geographic region.

Primary biliary cirrhosis

PBC is a presumed autoimmune disease of the liver, which predominantly affects middle-aged women. PBC is caused by granulomatous destruction of the interlobular bile ducts, which leads to progressive ductopenia. The consequent cholestasis is slowly progressive, and fibrosis, cirrhosis, and eventual liver failure occur. Currently, the diagnosis of PBC is most often made when the patient is still asymptomatic, with abnormal liver biochemistry and/or anti-mitochondrial antibodies (AMA) noted incidentally.

Clinical features

Most patients are asymptomatic at diagnosis with fatigue (50%) and pruritus (30%) the most common presenting symptoms. Itching is worse at night especially under constricting, coarse garments, in association with dry skin, and in hot, humid weather. Hyperpigmentation of the skin may be present in 25%–50%. Patients may also have musculoskeletal complaints. There are also associations with Sjögren's syndrome and limited scleroderma. Rarely, patients present with advanced disease manifest by hemorrhage from esophageal varices, ascites, or hepatic encephalopathy. Patients with PBC are at risk of osteoporosis and osteomalacia.

Examination may reveal hyperpigmentation, excoriations from scratching, jaundice, xanthomas and xanthelasmas from hyperlipidemia. Hepatomegaly, splenomegaly, spider nevi, temporal and proximal limb muscle wasting, ascites, and edema are all late manifestations of disease.

Epidemiology

Ninety-five percent are women. The onset is usually between ages 30 and 65.

The incidence in the UK is 32 cases per million and appears to be increasing. The cause of the increase is unclear, but it may be due to better detection and increased awareness rather than a true change in disease incidence.

Pathogenesis

Current data suggest that PBC is an autoimmune disease and there appear to be at least two distinct requirements for PBC to develop: genetic susceptibility and a triggering event that initiates the autoimmune attack on bile duct cells. There is a strong familial link.

Investigations

The serum alkaline phosphatase concentration is elevated, often to striking levels. The serum ALT is usually normal or slightly elevated. The serum bilirubin is usually normal but rises as the disease progresses and is a poor prognostic sign.

Antimitochondrial antibodies are the serologic hallmark of PBC and are present in 95% of patients.

Serum lipids are usually elevated without increased risk of cardiovascular disease.

Patients with PBC often have an elevated IgM level.

The characteristic findings on biopsy are portal hepatitis with granulomatous inflammation. More advanced cases have bile duct proliferation, fibrosis, and cirrhosis.

Management

The mainstay of treatment for PBC is ursodeoxycholic acid (UDCA). It improves bile acid transport and has been shown to improve survival. It also improves liver biochemistry but has little effect on fatigue or pruritus. The symptomatic treatment of pruritus is difficult but cholestyramine, rifampicin, and naloxone have all been used. In view of the high risk of osteoporosis, bone densitometry should be performed regularly, with supplementation of vitamin D and calcium. Hormone replacement therapy, where appropriate, or bisphosphonates should be used if osteoporosis is present.

Outcome

Patients with early-stage disease who are treated do not have increased mortality compared with the general population. Cirrhosis is associated with a worse prognosis and identifies a group of patients at risk of variceal bleeding and development of hepatocellular carcinoma (HCC). HCC develops in 6% of patients with advanced disease over 20 years.

Hemochromatosis (HH)

Clinical features

The clinical features occur as a result of excess iron deposition within tissues. The organs predominantly affected are the liver, pancreas, heart, joints, skin, and pituitary. The commonest presenting features are liver function abnormalities, weakness and lethargy, skin hyperpigmentation, diabetes mellitus, arthralgia, impotence in males, and ECG abnormalities.

Progressive iron deposition is associated with hepatomegaly, elevated liver enzymes, and the eventual development of cirrhosis. Development of cirrhosis is associated with variceal hemorrhage and a 20-fold increased risk of HCC. Iron is also deposited in the beta cells of the pancreas resulting in decreased insulin secretion and the development of diabetes mellitus. HH is associated with pseudogout, chondrocalcinosis, and chronic arthropathy. Iron is deposited

in the myocardium resulting in conduction abnormalities such as sick sinus syndrome and a dilated cardiomyopathy.

Males may present with decreased libido and impotence. This occurs as a result of excess iron deposition in pituitary cells, leading to reduced serum levels of a number of trophic hormones and resultant secondary hypogonadism. Skin hyperpigmentation occurs as a result of iron deposition and increased melanin.

Epidemiology

Hereditary hemochromatosis (HH) is the most common, identified, genetic disorder in the Caucasian population. It is concentrated predominantly in individuals of northern European origin, particularly of Nordic or Celtic ancestry, in whom it occurs with prevalence close to 1 per 200 of the population.

Pathology

The gene defect, described in 1996, is a G to A missense mutation (C282Y) leading to the substitution of tyrosine for cysteine at the 282 amino acid position of the protein product of the newly discovered *HFE* gene located on the short arm of chromosome 6 (6p). In most studies to date, C282Y/C282Y homozygosity has been found in more than 90% of patients. A compound heterozygosity (C282Y/H63D) accounts for 3%–5%.

The absorption of iron via the gut is controlled by the body's iron stores. This control is lost with hemochromatosis. Accumulation of iron occurs over many years with deposition in many tissues leading to the clinical features. The body has no mechanism to excrete excess iron except via blood loss. This leads to the protective effect of menstruation and the late development of the condition in women.

Investigations

The routine tests for iron overload are serum iron levels, transferrin concentration (total iron binding capacity), and serum ferritin. These are all elevated in HH, but can be raised in other conditions. A transferrin saturation (serum iron divided by the total iron binding capacity) >50% for women and 60% for men gives a positive predictive value of 86% for the diagnosis of HH.

Liver biopsy is useful to document the presence of cirrhosis, to rule out significant iron overload and to investigate other possible causes of liver disease but the diagnosis is best confirmed by genetic profiling rather than invasive procedures.

The presence of C282Y and H63D can now be detected by polymerase chain reaction and if HH is suspected it is important to document the patient's genotype to enable family screening.

Management

The mainstay of treatment remains phlebotomy. One unit of blood should be removed once or twice per week as tolerated. This regimen may take up to 3 years to reduce iron stores to just short of iron deficiency. The iron stores should be monitored with hematocrit and serum ferritin. Once the ferritin is at the lower end of the normal range, maintenance phlebotomy should be performed. The frequency of maintenance phlebotomies varies.

Outcome

Certain clinical features may be ameliorated by phlebotomy (malaise, fatigue, skin pigmentation, insulin requirements in diabetes, abdominal pain), whereas others are either less responsive to iron removal or do not respond at all (arthropathy, hypogonadism, cirrhosis). Once cirrhosis develops, patients must be screened for HCC since this accounts for 30% of deaths in patients with HH. Other causes of death in patients with HH are cirrhosis, cardiomyopathy and diabetes mellitus.

Primary sclerosing cholangitis

Primary sclerosing cholangitis (PSC) is a chronic cholestatic disease of the liver and bile ducts that is frequently progressive and can lead to end-stage liver disease.

Clinical features

Patients are commonly asymptomatic at diagnosis and PSC is often diagnosed during investigation of patients with inflammatory bowel disease and a raised alkaline phosphatase. Other features include fatigue, lethargy, fevers, chills, night sweats, and right upper quadrant pain. Other manifestations of the disease include pruritus, steatorrhea and fat-soluble vitamin malabsorption, osteoporosis, and gallstone disease. As the disease progresses, intra- and extra-hepatic strictures develop that lead to jaundice and episodes of cholangitis. Patients have a 10%–15% of lifetime risk of developing cholangiocarcinoma.

Epidemiology

PSC is rare, with a prevalence of 20.9 cases per 100 000 men, and 6.3 cases per 100 000 women. The mean age at diagnosis is 40 years. There is an association with inflammatory bowel disease (mostly ulcerative colitis) in 70%. Approximately 4% of patients with ulcerative colitis have PSC and 3% of those with Crohn's disease.

Pathogenesis

The exact mechanism causing PSC is not well understood but theories include an autoimmune component, chronic bacterial translocation through the bowel wall into the portal circulation, or ischemic damage to the bile ducts.

Investigations

Elevations of ALP levels are the commonest finding in PSC with a raised bilirubin occurring in advanced disease or in the presence of dominant strictures. Other findings include elevated IgM and a positive p-ANCA in 30%–80%.

Cholangiography, either with ERCP or MRCP, demonstrating characteristic multifocal stricturing and dilation of intra-hepatic and/or extra-hepatic bile ducts is required to establish the diagnosis of PSC.

Liver biopsy may show fibrous obliteration of small bile ducts, with concentric replacement by connective tissue in an "onion skin" pattern. This investigation is useful to stage the disease, particularly if cirrhosis is present.

Management

Management focuses on slowing progression, treatment of symptoms, and managing progressive disease and complications.

Ursodeoxycholic acid (UDCA) improves liver biochemistry and stabilizes hepatic inflammation but has no effect on survival.

Treatment for pruritus includes cholestyramine, rifampicin, and naloxone. Fat-soluble vitamin deficiency should be treated with supplementation as necessary. In patients with bone disease, supplementation with calcium and vitamin D is necessary and treatment of osteoporosis with bisphosphonates.

Dominant strictures should be dilated by balloon and stented endoscopically with antibiotic cover. These strictures should also be investigated with radiologic imaging and cytology/histology to exclude cholangiocarcinoma. Surgical treatment of strictures is not recommended.

Liver transplantation is the treatment of choice in advanced disease. Indications include intractable ascites, recurrent cholangitis and encephalopathy.

Outcome

Median survival without liver transplantation is 12 years from diagnosis. Factors known to worsen prognosis are increasing age, bilirubin, AST, decreasing albumin, and the presence of variceal bleeding.

Ascites

Ascites is defined as the presence of fluid within the peritoneal cavity.

Clinical features

The etiology of ascites may be readily apparent from the history. Particular attention needs to be paid to alcohol consumption, risk factors for viral hepatitis, family history of liver disease, risk factors for non-alcoholic steatohepatitis (obesity, diabetes, and hyperlipidemia). If there are no obvious causes of liver disease, attention to the non-cirrhotic causes for ascites is necessary.

On examination, most patients with ascites due to cirrhosis will have the stigmata of chronic liver disease (spider nevi, palmar erythema, clubbing, leukonychia, icterus, loss of axillary hair, gynecomastia, splenomegaly, and hepatomegaly). The presence of ascites is determined by percussion to demonstrate shifting dullness. Those with gross ascites may exhibit a fluid thrill across the abdomen.

Epidemiology

Cirrhosis accounts for 80% of cases but there are multiple other causes as shown in Table 3.18.

Ascites is the commonest complication of cirrhosis and is of major importance, since it is associated with 50% mortality over 2 years. The cause of ascites is ascertained by analysis of the fluid. The total protein concentration of the fluid was previously used to classify the fluid into a transudate (low protein content: <25 g/l) and an exudate (high protein content: >25 g/l). However, this has only moderate sensitivity and more detailed analysis is required to define the etiology.

Pathogenesis

In cirrhosis, the pathogenesis of ascites formation is due to a combination of sodium and water retention and portal hypertension.

The cause of sodium and water retention is multifactorial involving systemic vasodilatation and an increase in cardiac output, renal vasoconstriction with an increase in renal sympathetic activity and activation of the renin–angiotensin system to maintain

Table 3.18. Causes of ascites

Cause	Frequency
Cirrhosis	80%
Malignancy	10%
Heart failure	3%
Tuberculosis	2%
Pancreatitis	1%
Dialysis	1%
Nephrotic syndrome	<1%
Budd–Chiari syndrome	<1%
Constrictive pericarditis	<1%
Bile ascites	<1%
Chylous ascites	<1%
Myxedema	<1%
Meig's syndrome	<1%

blood pressure during systemic vasodilatation. This renal vasoconstriction, in turn, leads to a decrease in glomerular filtration rate and a resultant decrease in sodium excretion. This is further exacerbated by enhanced reabsorption of sodium at both the proximal and distal tubule in cirrhosis. Increased reabsorption of sodium in the distal tubule is due to increased circulating concentrations of aldosterone.

Portal hypertension increases the hydrostatic pressure within the hepatic sinusoids and favors transudation of fluid into the peritoneal cavity. This occurs as a consequence of structural changes within the liver in cirrhosis and increased splanchnic blood flow. Progressive collagen deposition and formation of nodules alter the normal vascular architecture of the liver and increase resistance to portal flow.

The pathogenesis of the other causes of ascites is defined by the same principles as edema formation at other sites, i.e. net capillary permeability and the hydraulic and oncotic pressure gradients. Inflammatory processes involving the peritoneum also cause ascites.

Investigations

Although the cause of ascites may be obvious from the history and examination, other causes must be excluded. Blood tests should be taken for measurement of urea and electrolytes, liver function tests, prothrombin time, and full blood count. Abdominal ultrasound is required to evaluate the appearance of the liver, pancreas, and lymph nodes and the

Table 3.19. The causes of ascites based on SAAG

SAAG ≥11 g/l	SAAG <11 g/l
Cirrhosis	Peritoneal malignancy
Cardiac failure	Tuberculous peritonitis
Myxedema	Pancreatitis
Budd–Chiari syndrome	Nephrotic syndrome Bile ascites

presence of splenomegaly, which may signify portal hypertension.

The essential investigations on admission include a diagnostic paracentesis with measurement of ascitic fluid albumin and protein, ascitic fluid neutrophil count and culture, and ascitic fluid amylase. Ascitic fluid cytology should be requested when there is a clinical suspicion of underlying malignancy.

Diagnostic paracentesis is performed under aseptic conditions, usually in the lower left quadrant.

Ascitic white blood cell count and culture An absolute neutrophil count of >250 cells/mm³ is a good indication of spontaneous bacterial peritonitis (SBP). This diagnosis is imperative to make since, untreated, it has significant mortality and warrants initiation of empirical antibiotics. An elevated ascitic lymphocyte count is suggestive of peritoneal carcinomatosis or tuberculous peritonitis.

Blood culture bottles should be inoculated at the bedside. This improves the diagnostic yield when compared to specimens without culture medium.

Ascitic protein and albumin concentration Patients with a protein concentration of <10 g/l are at risk of SBP and prophylactic antibiotics may be used, although this can lead to bacterial resistance.

The albumin concentration enables calculation of the serum–ascites albumin gradient (SAAG).

$$SAAG = albumin_{serum} - albumin_{ascites}$$

Patients with values ≥ 11 g/l have portal hypertension, whereas those with gradients <11 g/l do not. The causes of ascites based upon the SAAG are shown in Table 3.19.

Amylase activity This is markedly elevated in pancreatic ascites and gut perforation into ascites.

Gram stain
This is usually negative in early SBP but if multiple types of bacteria are seen, this is suggestive of gut perforation.

Cytology
This is useful in diagnosing malignant ascites. However, a large volume is required with concentration techniques to increase the diagnostic yield. It is not of use in the diagnosis of hepatocellular carcinoma.

Management
Bed rest There is a theoretical benefit to bed rest in patients with ascites since the upright position leads to activation of the renin–angiotensin–aldosterone and sympathetic nervous system, a reduction in glomerular filtration rate and sodium excretion, as well as a decreased response to diuretics. However, there are no clinical studies that demonstrate improved diuresis or decreased hospitalization with bed rest and hence it is not recommended.

Dietary salt restriction Sodium restriction has been associated with lower diuretic requirement, faster resolution of ascites, and shorter hospitalization. Stringent sodium restriction (<50 mmol/day) is difficult due to the unpalatable nature of the diet and a diet with <90 mmol/day is recommended. This means no salt added to food and avoidance of salty foods (crisps, cheese, soups, gravy, etc.). The use of normal saline as fluid replacement and volume expanders should be avoided in patients with uncomplicated ascites.

Diuretics Spironolactone is an aldosterone antagonist, acting mainly on the distal tubules to increase natriuresis and conserve potassium. The dose may have to be increased up to 400 mg to achieve adequate natriuresis. The side effects of spironolactone are due to its antiandrogenic activity, such as decreased libido, impotence, and gynecomastia in men and menstrual irregularity in women. Hyperkalemia is another complication that limits its use.

Furosemide is a loop diuretic, which causes marked natriuresis and diuresis in normal subjects. However, it has low efficacy when used alone in cirrhosis and is usually used in combination with spironolactone. High doses of furosemide are associated with severe electrolyte disturbance and metabolic alkalosis, and should be used cautiously.

Fluid restriction The role of water restriction in the management of ascites is controversial and there are no studies to support or refute the use of this strategy. However, fluid restriction may exacerbate the underlying hypovolemia and worsen renal function.

Therapeutic paracentesis This procedure involves the removal of a large volume of ascites with a catheter inserted through the abdominal wall. It is indicated for patients with severe ascites who are in discomfort, have respiratory compromise, or who are resistant to diuretics.

The drain should be left *in situ* for up to 4 hours, aiming to drain as much fluid as possible. Removal of ascitic fluid can cause circulatory dysfunction, particularly in volumes >5 liters, leading to renal impairment and hyponatremia. To avoid this, 20% human albumin solution should be given at a dose of 8 g/l after paracentesis of 5 liters or more.

Transjugular intrahepatic portosystemic shunt (TIPS) This is a radiologically placed shunt between the hepatic vein and the portal vein that results in lowering of portal pressure. It has been shown to be better at controlling ascites than repeated therapeutic paracentesis. The risks of the procedure include hepatic encephalopathy in 25% and cardiac dysfunction.

Outcome

The development of ascites is associated with a mortality of 50% within 2 years of diagnosis. Once ascites becomes refractory to medical therapy, 50% die within 6 months. In patients who have an episode of spontaneous bacterial peritonitis, survival is 30%–50% at 1 year and 25%–30% at 2 years. In the light of these poor outcomes, patients with cirrhosis and ascites should be considered for liver transplantation.

Further reading

Collins P, *Gastroenterology* 3rd edition, Elsevier Health Sciences, Mosby, 2008.

de Franchis R, Hadenque A, Lau G, *et al.* EASL Consensus Conference on Hepatitis B, 13–14 Sept. 2002, Geneva. Consensus Statement. *J. Hepatol.* 2003; **39** Suppl. 1: 53–55.

Langmead L, Irving P. *Inflammatory Bowel Disease.* Oxford University Press, 2008.

Moore K P, Wong T, Gines P, *et al.* The management of ascites in cirrhosis: report on the consensus conference of the International Ascites Club. *Hepatology* 2003; **38**(1): 258–266.

Thomsen T W, Shaffer R W, White B, Setnik G S. Videos in clinical medicine. Paracentesis. *N Engl J Med* 2006; **355**(19), e21.

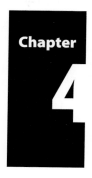

Kidney

James Pattison

Contents

Peripheral edema

Edema is caused by accumulation of excess fluid in the extravascular interstitial compartment. It is gravitational in nature, so that it is often evident in the morning as puffy eyes, and in the evening as swollen ankles. It may be very mild or very severe extending up the legs, abdomen, and thorax. Edema needs to be distinguished from lymphedema, which is due to abnormal lymphatic drainage. True edema is "pitting," whereas lymphedema is "non-pitting." This is assessed by firmly pressing the area of swelling. If pitting is present, an indentation will be present for several seconds after the release of pressure.

Edema may be caused by cardiac failure, cirrhosis, renal disease, and severe malnutrition. Associated features helpful in the differential diagnosis of edema are given in Table 4.1. Cardiac edema is related to right heart failure which may be combined with left heart failure or secondary to pulmonary or pericardial disease. Too often, physicians assume edema in elderly patients is cardiac in origin. Urinalysis detecting proteinuria, and a blood test showing a raised serum creatinine, will often reveal the presence of renal disease. Renal disease may cause edema either because of nephrotic syndrome or renal failure. Edema that is symmetric is likely to be of systemic origin, e.g. cardiac failure or hypoproteinemia. Edema that is asymmetric may have a systemic contribution, but is likely to be due mainly to peripheral pathology, i.e. impaired local venous or lymph drainage. Edema may be caused by a combination of pathologies, for example, patients with cardiac failure commonly have impaired renal function. Certain drugs may cause edema, notably the calcium antagonists class of antihypertensive drugs and minoxidil. Edema commonly occurs in the setting of sepsis due to a combination of hypoalbuminemia, "leaky microvasculature," and fluid loading by clinicians.

Common causes of edema are listed below:

Cardiac failure

Chronic liver disease

Nephrotic syndrome

Severe renal failure

The investigations required to establish the diagnosis depend on the clinical picture, and can be limited to the relevant tests (Table 4.2).

Nephrotic syndrome

Nephrotic syndrome is defined as the presence of edema together with the excretion of greater than

Table 4.1. Associated features helpful in the differential diagnosis of edema

Associated feature	Likely diagnosis	Other common features
Shortness of breath	Cardiac failure	History of heart disease Elderly Chest pain Raised JVP
Confusion	Cirrhosis	Hepatitis B/C infection Heavy alcohol use Signs of chronic liver disease
Muscle wasting	Kwashiorkor	Protein malnutrition
Rapid onset	Nephrotic syndrome	Children most often Previous episodes
Diabetes mellitus	Nephrotic syndrome	Diabetic retinopathy Peripheral neuropathy Diabetes >10 years
Nausea/vomiting	Chronic renal failure	Known previous renal disease Itching; cramps Anemia Skin pigmentation
Ankle sparing	Idiopathic edema	Depression Diuretic abuse
Asymmetric	Local venous/ lymph obstruction	Previous surgery Lymphadenopathy

Table 4.2. Important investigations used in the diagnosis of patients with edema

Suspected diagnosis	Investigation
Heart failure	Electrocardiogram Chest X-ray Echocardiogram
Cirrhosis	Liver function tests Coagulation screen Abdominal ultrasound
Nephrotic syndrome	Urinalysis 24-hour protein collection Serum albumin Serum cholesterol

Table 4.3. Examples of renal diseases that are relatively frequent in different age groups

Child	Young adult	Elderly
Minimal change	SLE	Membranous
FSGS	HIV	Amyloid/myeloma
Mesangiocapillary	Type 1 diabetes	Type 2 diabetes

3 g protein per day in the urine, a serum albumin <30 g/l and a raised serum cholesterol.

The major causes of nephrotic syndrome are listed below:

No systemic disease	Minimal change disease Primary focal segmental glomerulosclerosis (FSGS) Membranous nephropathy IgA nephropathy Mesangiocapillary glomerulonephritis
Systemic disease	Diabetes mellitus Systemic lupus erythematosus (SLE) HIV nephropathy Myeloma Amyloid

Certain conditions are much more prevalent in different age groups (Table 4.3).

Minimal change disease is much the commonest disease in children age 2–12 years. As a result, standard practice in this age group is not to perform a renal biopsy but to give the child a course of steroids and to perform a renal biopsy only if the child fails to respond to treatment or if there are atypical features on presentation. In adult patients a renal biopsy is usually necessary to discriminate between the various primary forms of glomerulonephritis. Secondary causes can sometimes be diagnosed by blood tests, for example, SLE (Lupus) by the presence of antinuclear antibodies, and myeloma by the presence of a monoclonal para-protein, although a renal biopsy is usually necessary to define the severity of renal involvement. SLE is much commoner in Black and Far Eastern patients than in Caucasians. HIV-associated nephropathy occurs almost exclusively in Afro-Caribbean patients.

It is difficult to discriminate the cause of nephrotic syndrome based on the mode of onset. However, minimal change disease and FSGS are primary glo-merular diseases which may present with rapid onset of proteinuria. Likewise, Lupus nephritis and HIV-associated nephropathy often present acutely. Patients with diabetic nephropathy have a long history of diabetes and microalbuminuria and proteinuria before developing frank nephrotic syndrome. Diabetic retinopathy is almost invariably found in patients with diabetic nephropathy as both diseases are due to abnormalities of the microvasculature.

Indeed, if diabetic retinopathy is not present in a diabetic with nephrotic syndrome, an alternative cause for the proteinuria should be considered.

The presence of microscopic hematuria in a patient with nephrotic syndrome suggests that the patient does not have minimal change disease, and that alternatives such as focal and segmental glomerulosclerosis should be considered.

Minimal change disease (MCD)

MCD usually presents as nephrotic syndrome with marked edema. It typically remits rapidly with corticosteroid therapy.

Clinical features

Patients with MCD usually have edema as their presenting complaint. They may notice puffy eyes in the morning and ankle swelling in the evenings. The swelling may be massive with edema up to the trunk. Some patients may have lesser degrees of proteinuria and no edema, and may present because of proteinuria being detected on urinalysis. Rarely, patients present in acute renal failure. They usually have massive edema, and one theory is that the kidneys themselves are so swollen that the renal intracapsular pressure has risen to the point where glomerular filtration stops.

Epidemiology

MCD is commonest in children but can occur in any age group. It occurs in all ethnic groups.

Pathology

The underlying cause is not clearly defined. The disease is associated with allergies and rarely with lymphoma. It has been reported to remit with measles infection, and is responsive to steroids and cyclosporine. This all suggests that there is an immune basis to the condition, and that T cells may play an important role. The kidney appears normal at the light microscope level, but on electron microscopy there is effacement of the epithelial cell foot processes, which is the anatomic explanation for the proteinuria. Proteinuria leads in turn to hypoalbuminemia. The low albumin leads to changes in the osmotic forces controlling extravascular fluid distribution, and edema develops. Hypoalbuminemia also triggers hypercholesterolemia by stimulating VLDL production by the liver.

Investigations

Serum creatinine, electrolytes, albumin, and lipids are measured. Urinary protein can be measured on a spot sample measuring the protein/creatinine ratio or by a 24-hour urinary protein collection. A renal biopsy is performed in adults to exclude alternative diagnoses but is not necessary in children with a typical presentation.

Management

Specific treatment involves the initial use of corticosteroids. Most patients will respond extremely rapidly with resolution of the peripheral edema as the serum albumin returns to normal. The corticosteroid dose is then tapered. Some patients will relapse as the steroids are reduced or discontinued whereas others will remain in remission. The calcineurin inhibitors ciclosporin and tacrolimus, and also mycophenolate mofetil, have all been used as second-line agents in patients who frequently relapse. Cyclophosphamide can be used in an 8–12-week course in the most difficult cases, but its use is tempered by concerns about gonadal function and increased risk of late malignancies especially hematological and bladder cancers.

Patients usually require symptomatic control of their edema with diuretics. Care must be taken not to over-diurese these patients as they are at risk of hypovolemia induced acute renal failure. If the patient is very hypoalbuminemic, consideration should be given to anticoagulation to reduce the risk of thromboembolic events. Deep vein thrombosis, renal vein thrombosis (Fig. 4.1), and pulmonary emboli are common in patients with nephrotic syndrome, and children with nephrotic syndrome may also develop arterial thromboses.

Outcome

The outcome is extremely variable with some patients having a single episode of nephrotic syndrome, and others having a lifelong tendency to relapse. Patients with this condition usually do not develop end-stage renal failure, although calcineurin inhibitors may

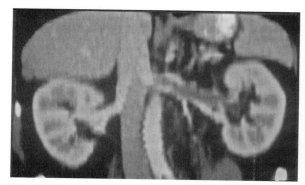

Fig. 4.1. CT scan with contrast showing a left renal vein thrombus in a patient with nephrotic syndrome.

cause renal fibrosis if used for many years. Serial renal biopsies may be necessary to monitor for signs of these drugs causing structural renal damage. The long-term use of steroids may cause considerable morbidity, especially in children by reducing growth and causing weight gain.

Primary focal and segmental glomerulosclerosis (FSGS)

Primary FSGS usually presents with nephrotic syndrome in the same way as minimal change disease. However, it is less responsive to treatment, and frequently progresses to end-stage renal failure.

Clinical features

Patients may present with abnormalities on urinalysis, or with nephrotic syndrome or renal impairment. Microscopic hematuria is usually present. Hypertension is common.

Epidemiology

Primary FSGS can occur in any age group. It is commonest in Blacks. Secondary causes of FSGS include obesity, sickle cell disease, reduced nephron number, e.g. after partial nephrectomy of a single kidney, and viral infections such as HIV or parvovirus.

Pathology

At the light microscope level, there is segmental sclerosis affecting some of the glomeruli. Foot process effacement is seen on electron microscopy. There is thought to be a circulating factor produced by the immune system which triggers the renal injury. Evidence for this factor's existence includes the fact that FSGS often recurs rapidly following renal transplantation, and that plasma exchange, possibly by removing the factor, can reverse the development of proteinuria. Injecting a patient's serum into rats can induce the lesion in the rats' kidneys.

Investigations

Serum creatinine, albumin, electrolytes, and lipids are measured together with urinary protein quantitation. Renal biopsy confirms the diagnosis, and the extent of renal damage.

Management

Nephrotic syndrome is managed symptomatically using diuretics, anticoagulants, and statins. Angiotensin-converting enzyme (ACE) inhibitors and angiotensin receptor blockers also should be used as there is good evidence that they reduce proteinuria and slow down progression of renal disease.

Specific treatment involves the use of corticosteroids and ciclosporin. Patients need to be treated for several months with high dose steroids to obtain a response. The patients who show a response to corticosteroid therapy have a better renal prognosis than those who do not.

Outcome

Patients with massive proteinuria (>10 g/day) or impaired renal function at presentation, and those who fail to respond to corticosteroid therapy, will usually progress to end-stage renal failure. Renal transplantation is complicated by the fact that the FSGS recurs in the graft in 30%–50% of cases.

Membranous nephropathy (MN)

MN causes nephrotic syndrome in adults of all ages. It may be idiopathic or secondary to a variety of diseases, or the use of certain medications.

Clinical features

Patients may present with subnephrotic range proteinuria, nephrotic syndrome or renal impairment. The clinical course of the condition is extremely variable with some cases remitting spontaneously, while others develop increasing levels of proteinuria and progression to end-stage renal failure. Recurrence occurs (rarely) after renal transplantation. Patients with MN appear particularly susceptible to thromboembolic complications.

Epidemiology

The underlying cause of idiopathic MN is not understood. MN occurs commonly in patients with systemic lupus erythematosus (SLE). It can occur secondary to hepatitis B and C virus infection. It can be associated with solid malignancies, especially colon and lung neoplasms. The proteinuria can remit after removal of the tumor and relapse after recurrence of the tumor. Gold salts, penicillamine, and NSAIDs can all cause MN, and in these cases the lesion remits after discontinuation of the drug.

Pathology

On light microscopy the capillary walls appear thickened, and on silver stain "spikes" are seen in the capillary wall. The spikes represent normal glomerular basement membrane surrounding immune complexes. On electron microscopy subepithelial deposits are seen (Fig. 4.2). Immunoperoxidase staining is positive for C3 and IgG. Cases of MN secondary to SLE may also

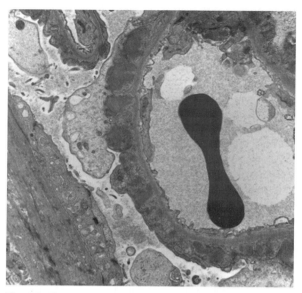

Fig. 4.2. Electron micrograph of a capillary wall from a patient with membranous nephropathy demonstrating subepithelial and intramembranous electron dense deposits (×10 000).

have a proliferative glomerulonephritis, a "full house" of complement and immunoglobulins deposited, and mesangial and subendothelial deposits.

Investigations
Renal function and proteinuria need to be quantitated. A renal biopsy is necessary to make the diagnosis. In patients aged over 60 consideration should be given to screening for an occult carcinoma with a chest X-ray and colonoscopy.

Management
The management of idiopathic MN is challenging given the variable clinical course of individual patients. Nephrotic syndrome is managed supportively with diuretics, ACE inhibitors or angiotensin receptor blockers, statins, and anticoagulants as necessary. Specific treatment with immunosuppressive drugs is usually reserved for patients with increasing levels of proteinuria or deteriorating renal function. Immunosuppressive agents that have been used in this condition include corticosteroids, azathioprine, ciclosporin, and most recently anti-B cell monoclonal antibodies (rituximab).

Outcome
The outcome is variable. The majority have a benign renal prognosis but a minority will progress to end-stage renal failure.

IgA nephropathy
(see Hematuria section).

Mesangiocapillary glomerulonephritis (MCGN)
MCGN is a relatively rare form of glomerulonephritis. It occurs most frequently in children, and type 2 MCGN is associated with partial lipodystrophy. There is a variable response to immunosuppression. It tends to recur following renal transplantation.

Diabetic nephropathy
Diabetic nephropathy is a common complication in patients who have had diabetes mellitus for many years. It is progressive and leads to end-stage renal failure.

Clinical features
The earliest phase occurs in patients who have had diabetes mellitus (either type 1 or type 2) for many years (typically 10–15 years). The initial manifestation is asymptomatic, with microalbuminuria and an increased glomerular filtration rate. Subsequently, proteinuria develops and evolves into nephrotic range proteinuria. During this time glomerular filtration rate falls, and eventually the patient reaches end-stage renal failure. The rate of progression to end-stage renal failure is variable, but typically takes about 5–10 years from the initial development of proteinuria. Patients with diabetic nephropathy almost invariably have retinopathy and neuropathy. There is a high incidence of vascular disease in these patients.

Epidemiology
Diabetic nephropathy occurs in patients with type 1 or 2 diabetes mellitus. Diabetic nephropathy occurs in young patients who have had type 1 diabetes since childhood, and older patients who have developed type 2 diabetes in middle age. Type 2 diabetes mellitus is much commoner than type 1 because of the epidemic of obesity in the Western world. Patients with type 2 diabetes are living longer because of treatments for hypertension and ischemic heart disease, and thus many patients are surviving long enough to reach end-stage renal failure. Diabetic nephropathy is the commonest cause of end-stage renal failure in the Western world. For reasons that are not well understood some diabetics never develop diabetic nephropathy. Risk factors for developing diabetic nephropathy include a positive family history of diabetic nephropathy, hypertension, poor glycemic control, and race (increased risk especially in Blacks).

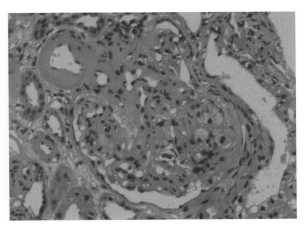

Fig. 4.3. Glomerulus from a patient with diabetic nephropathy showing hyalinosis of the afferent and efferent arterioles (top left), diffuse mesangial expansion, and a secondary sclerosing lesion (bottom right) (H and E ×200).

Pathology

Hyperglycemia stimulates mesangial cell matrix formation and the accumulation of advanced glycosylation end products which cross-link with collagen. In the earliest stage of the disease there is glomerular hypertrophy, and thickening of the glomerular basement membrane. There is hyalinosis of the afferent and efferent arterioles (Fig. 4.3). Progressive mesangial expansion causes diffuse diabetic glomerulosclerosis, and Kimmelstiel–Wilson nodules. The extra-mesangial matrix stains positively with silver and periodic acid Schiff stain (PAS). Electron microscopy shows thickened glomerular basement membranes.

Investigations

The earliest abnormality is microalbuminuria detected by a sensitive radioimmunoassay. Albumin excretion rate in normoalbuminuria is <30 mg/24 h, microalbuminuria 30–300 mg/24 h, and proteinuria >300 mg/24 h. Because of daily variations in albumin excretion, the diagnosis of microalbuminuria depends on finding increased rates of excretion in three collections over a 6-month period.

Management

The rate of progression of diabetic nephropathy can be slowed with optimal glycemic control, good blood pressure control, and the use of angiotensin-converting enzyme inhibitors and angiotensin receptor blockers.

Outcome

The rate of decline of renal function is variable but typically patients take 5–10 years from the onset of

proteinuria to the development of end-stage renal failure. Renal transplantation, simultaneous kidney–pancreas transplantation, and pancreas after kidney transplantation are potential management options.

Lupus nephritis

Systemic Lupus Erythematosus (SLE) is a multisystem disease, which usually affects the skin and joints, and in more severe cases causes inflammation in the kidneys, brain, and lungs.

Clinical features

Lupus nephritis varies in severity. At the mild end of the spectrum patients may have microscopic hematuria, and minimal proteinuria. Severe renal involvement is manifested by nephrotic syndrome and/or acute renal failure. In severe cases accelerated phase hypertension occurs and these patients may have evidence of a microangiopathic hemolytic anemia. A proportion of patients with lupus nephritis will have anticardiolipin antibodies, and these patients may have a history of thrombotic events or miscarriages.

Epidemiology

SLE is much commoner in Afro-Caribbean and Far Eastern ethnic groups than Caucasians. It is also much more prevalent in women than men (9:1). A small proportion of cases are familial, and may be associated with complement deficiency.

Pathology

The histologic appearances of lupus nephritis are variable depending on the severity of renal involvement. Mild cases have mesangial hypercellularity or a membranous appearance. Severe cases have a diffuse proliferative glomerulonephritis, with crescent formation (Fig. 4.4). A full house of staining for IgG, IgM, IgA, C3, C1q, and C4 is characteristic. Electron microscopy will show subendothelial deposits, which underlie the wire-loop lesion seen on light microscopy. There will often also be subepithelial and intramembranous deposits.

Investigations

Most cases will have a positive antinuclear factor, anti-DNA antibodies, and reduced complement levels. Antiphospholipid antibodies are found in about a third of patients. A renal biopsy is usually necessary to assess the relative degrees of active inflammation and chronic damage.

Management

Lupus nephritis is treated with immunosuppressive therapy. The key is to treat acute flares aggressively to

87

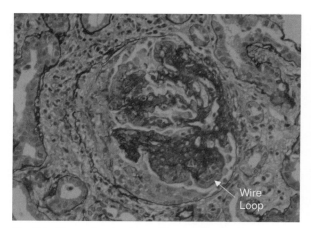

Fig. 4.4. Glomerulus showing a diffuse proliferative lupus nephritis with a wire loop in the capillary wall (arrow), and a crescent (PAMS ×200).

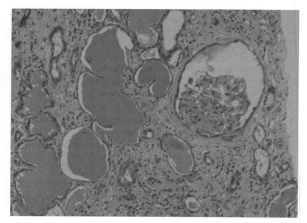

Fig. 4.5. Renal biopsy of a case of HIV-associated nephropathy (HIVAN). The glomerulus is collapsed leaving a large acellular Bowman's space. The tubules show gross microcystic dilatation and contain pink amorphous casts. There is marked tubulointerstitial fibrosis (H and E ×100).

minimize permanent tissue damage, and minimize maintenance treatment to reduce the long-term toxicity associated with the medication. Serial renal biopsies may be helpful to allow tailoring of treatment. Milder cases are managed with prednisolone and azathioprine or mycophenolate mofetil. More severe cases require high dose corticosteroids and cyclophosphamide. For resistant cases intravenous immunoglobulin, plasma exchange or monoclonal anti-B cell antibodies may be used.

Outcome

The outcome is extremely variable depending on the severity of renal involvement. The condition runs a remitting and relapsing course. Severe lupus nephritis recurs rarely following renal transplantation. Much of the morbidity and mortality in this condition is related to infection due to the immunosuppression, and ischemic heart disease.

HIV-associated nephropathy (HIVAN)

HIV infection can affect the kidneys in many ways. Electrolyte, acid–base disorders, and acute renal failure may occur due to sepsis related to opportunistic infections or chemotherapy. Many glomerular diseases and hemolytic–uremic syndrome have been described in association with HIV infection. However, HIVAN is the commonest lesion in this condition.

Clinical features

Patients usually present with nephrotic range proteinuria and rapidly deteriorating renal function. Edema is often minimal. The presence of hypertension is variable. There may be physical signs suggestive of

HIV infection, e.g. hairy leukoplakia, herpetic lesions or Kaposi's sarcoma.

Epidemiology

HIVAN is much more common in Blacks than Whites (about 10:1).

Pathology

Typically there is a focal and segmental collapsing glomerulopathy manifested by shrinkage and sclerosis of the entire glomerulus (Fig. 4.5). There may be crescent formation. There is a striking focal microcystic dilatation of the renal tubules filled with casts. On electron microscopy tubuloreticular inclusions are found in endothelial cells.

Investigations

Renal ultrasound characteristically shows enlarged echobright kidneys. Renal biopsy is diagnostic, but is not always necessary.

Management

Angiotensin converting enzyme inhibitors and angiotensin 2 receptor antagonists reduce proteinuria and reduce the rate of progression of renal failure. Antiretroviral medication can stabilize or improve renal function in patients with HIVAN, and it is important to start these drugs as early as possible once a diagnosis of HIVAN has been made.

Outcome

Without treatment there is rapid progression to end-stage renal failure over a matter of weeks or months.

Antiretroviral treatment can lead to dramatic improvement of renal function.

Myeloma

Renal disease occurs commonly in multiple myeloma, primary amyloidosis and light chain deposit disease. These diseases are caused by clonal proliferation of plasma cells and their precursors, activated cells, which secrete unique immunoglobulin proteins or light or heavy chains.

Clinical features

Myeloma classically presents with skeletal pain, pathologic fractures, or infection. Renal disease in myeloma can present as mild proteinuria with or without hematuria, nephrotic syndrome, slowly progressive renal insufficiemcy or acute renal failure. Patients are usually anemic, and bruise easily.

Epidemiology

Myeloma is usually found in the elderly, reaching a peak incidence in the eighth decade.

Pathology

Myeloma can affect kidney function by different mechanisms. Myeloma kidney is the commonest type of renal injury in which large intratubular casts are formed. The tubular injury is caused by Bence–Jones proteins. The tubular injury leads to interstitial inflammation and fibrosis. Light chains may form nodular deposits in the glomeruli (light chain deposit disease), or be enzymatically degraded into amyloid proteins which polymerize into amyloid fibrils. Myeloma commonly causes hypercalcemia. Acute renal failure is common in patients with myeloma following the administration of intravenous contrast.

Investigations

These should include a full blood count, serum creatinine, and calcium, serum protein electrophoresis, a 24-hour urine collection for immunofixation, a bone marrow examination, and a skeletal survey. A renal biopsy is usually necessary in patients with nephrotic syndrome or renal impairment to define the type of renal involvement and the degree of chronic damage.

Management

Volume depletion and hypercalcemia should be corrected. In patients with rapidly deteriorating renal function plasma exchange is combined with chemotherapy to rapidly lower the level of the light chains which are causing the tubular injury.

Outcome

The renal outcome is variable. Many patients will eventually require renal replacement therapy.

Amyloidosis

Amyloidosis consists of the deposition in the extracellular space of an insoluble protein which progressively destroys the involved organ. Amyloidosis can affect almost any organ or tissue.

Clinical features

Renal involvement usually presents with nephrotic syndrome, which persists despite progression to renal insufficiency. Renal vein thrombosis is a common complication. Weight loss and fatigue are common. There may be symptoms and signs of cardiac failure, gastro-intestinal involvement, peripheral neuropathy, or carpal tunnel syndrome. Periorbital purpura is common.

Epidemiology

Primary amyloidosis (AL) can occur in patients with or without overt multiple myeloma. The underlying disease process is the clonal proliferation of plasma cells in both groups. A paraprotein is found in 90% of patients without myeloma. The median age at presentation is 65 years.

Secondary amyloidosis (AA) complicates chronic inflammatory conditions such as rheumatoid arthritis, ankylosing spondylitis, bronchiectasis, osteomyelitis, paraplegia with chronic skin ulceration, malignancies such as Hodgkin's disease, and familial Mediterranean fever.

Pathology

Generally amyloid first deposits in the glomerular mesangium, and then the capillary loops, eventually forming nodules. It is also found along the tubular basement membrane. Amyloid stains red with Congo red (Fig. 4.6) and shows a characteristic green/orange birefringence when viewed with polarized light. Electron microscopy shows regular non-branched fibrils.

Investigations

A monoclonal protein is found in serum and urine by immunofixation in 90% cases of AL amyloid. Tissue biopsy is necessary to reach a precise diagnosis. Positive immunochemistry staining with anti-AA antibodies confirms AA amyloid. Negative staining implies AL amyloid. Serum C-reactive protein (CRP) or serum amyloid A (SAA) concentrations can be used to follow the activity of the underlying inflammatory

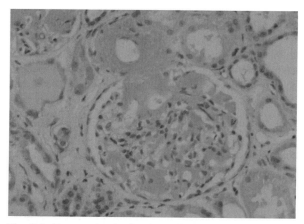

Fig. 4.6. Congo red stain of a glomerulus in a case of amyloidosis demonstrating amyloid deposition in the arteriole and mesangium (Congo red ×200).

process. Radioiodinated SAP specifically localizes to amyloid deposits and can be used to measure the total amyloid burden (amount and organ distribution) and serial scans can be used to follow progression or regression with treatment.

Management

The goal of treatment in AL patients is to decrease the synthesis of amyloidogenic protein with chemotherapy. In AA amyloid, therapy is aimed at controlling the underlying inflammatory disease. Colchicine is used to treat familial Mediterranean fever.

Outcome

The median survival for AL patients is about 2 years. Cardiac failure is a common cause of death. Most patients with renal involvement progress rapidly to end-stage renal failure.

Chronic renal failure

Patients with significant renal impairment may develop peripheral edema. Generally the glomerular filtration rate is below about 20 ml/min before edema develops unless there is co-existing cardiac or liver disease. Fluid overload can also present as pulmonary edema. Patients with chronic renal failure have symptoms related to reduced excretion of waste products of metabolism. Symptoms include fatigue, loss of appetite, nausea, vomiting, a metallic taste in the mouth, itching, cramps, and restless legs. On examination, patients are anemic and the skin has a diffuse lemon–brown pigmentation. Typically there are "half-and-half" nails with pale proximal nail bed, and distal pigmentation.

The major causes of chronic renal failure are listed below:

Diabetes mellitus
Glomerulonephritis
Reflux nephropathy
Polycystic kidney disease
Renovascular disease
Essential hypertension
Alport's syndrome
HIV-associated nephropathy
Systemic lupus erythematosus
Myeloma/amyloidosis

These causes can be crudely divided according to age at presentation with renal impairment (Table 4.4).

Chronic renal failure is much more prevalent in Afro-Caribbean and Indo-Asian ethnic groups. Essential hypertension is a rare cause of renal failure in Caucasians, but is a relatively common cause in these other ethnic groups. SLE is much more prevalent in Afro-Caribbeans and Far Eastern Asians. HIV-associated nephropathy occurs almost exclusively in Afro-Caribbeans. Some of the individual conditions described above will be discussed in other sections.

The progression of most renal diseases can be modified by medical treatment. Blood pressure should be tightly controlled to maintain a target of less than 130/85. Angiotensin converting enzyme inhibitors and angiotensin 2 receptor blockers have been shown in large studies to retard the progression of renal disease. End-stage renal failure is managed either by dialysis or renal transplantation. Renal transplantation is the optimal treatment both in terms of life expectancy and quality of life.

Diabetic nephropathy, glomerulonephritis, hypertension, HIVAN, lupus nephritis and myeloma are discussed in the nephrotic syndrome section.

Table 4.4. Causes of CRF by age

Children	Young adults	Older adults
Congenital anomalies	Hypertension	Type 2 diabetes
FSGS	Polycystic kidneys	Renovascular
Hemolytic–uremic syndrome	SLE	Myeloma
Reflux nephropathy	Glomerulonephritis HIV nephropathy Type 1 diabetes Alport's syndrome	Amyloid

Reflux nephropathy

Primary vesicoureteric reflux is a common congenital condition which leads to small, irregularly scarred kidneys which can present with urinary tract infections, hypertension, proteinuria, or renal impairment.

Clinical features

Reflux nephropathy may present with recurrent urinary tract infections, nocturnal enuresis, hypertension, proteinuria, renal impairment, or with asymmetric kidneys on renal imaging. Those patients who develop renal impairment usually need renal replacement therapy in the second or third decade of life.

Epidemiology

Vesicoureteric reflux is inherited as an autosomal dominant trait with a variable penetrance. The prevalence is uncertain with studies quoting 0.4%–9.0% of the normal infant population. Reflux nephropathy is probably responsible for about 10% of patients reaching end-stage renal failure.

Pathology

Primary vesicoureteric reflux is the back flow of urine due to an abnormally short submucosal bladder segment of ureter. As the child grows, the intravesical ureter lengthens and reflux decreases with age. Renal damage is associated with intrarenal reflux and is accelerated by bacterial infection. Macroscopically there is coarse segmental scarring overlying the dilated calyx, most prominent at the poles. In the scarred areas there is tubulointerstitial fibrosis and often a lymphocytic infiltrate. There may be focal and segmental glomerulosclerosis secondary to hyperfiltration in the remnant glomeruli.

Investigations

Renal ultrasound and intravenous urography (IVU) will detect the reduced renal size and scarring in this condition. DMSA scans are very sensitive for detecting scars and measuring individual kidney function.

Management

Children with vesicoureteric reflux should have long-term antibiotic prophylaxis as this retards progression to renal failure. Surgery to prevent reflux is only of proven benefit in the most severe cases. Family members should be screened for the condition.

Outcome

Some kidneys subjected to vesicoureteric reflux will become progressively damaged, whereas others will

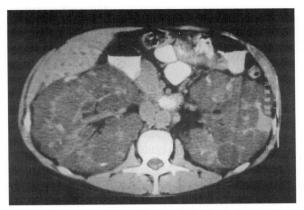

Fig. 4.7. CT scan showing massively enlarged polycystic kidneys (autosomal dominant).

be unaffected. The severity of reflux is the major risk factor for parenchymal damage.

Polycystic kidney disease (Fig. 4.7)

The commonest form of cystic kidney disease is autosomal dominant polycystic kidney disease (ADPKD). Apart from causing renal cysts, it can affect many other organs.

Clinical features

Manifestations of renal involvement include pain, hematuria, urinary tract infection, hypertension and renal impairment. Multiple liver cysts are common, but liver function is preserved. Intracranial berry aneurysms are associated with ADPKD, and are more likely to occur in patients with a family history of intracranial aneurysm or subarachnoid hemorrhage. Other disease associations are aortic aneurysms, valvular heart disease, pancreatic cysts, diverticular disease, and hernias.

Epidemiology

ADPKD is a common disease with an incidence of approximately 1 : 500. The *PKD1* gene is on the short arm of chromosome 16 and is responsible for 85%–90% of cases. The *PKD2* gene is found on chromosome 4.

Pathology

PKD1 codes for polycystin 1, which may function as a cell membrane receptor involved in cell–cell or cell–matrix interaction, and interacts with *PKD2*'s product polycystin 2, which has similarities to a calcium channel. Renal failure is caused by cyst growth,

91

hypertension and production of inflammatory mediators by the cysts.

Investigations

Ultrasound will detect large cysts, but MRI is more sensitive for smaller cysts.

Management

There is, as yet, no specific treatment to retard cyst growth. Hypertension needs to be optimally managed, and urinary tract infections treated. Screening for intracranial aneurysms is indicated in patients with a family history of subarachnoid hemorrhage.

Outcome

There is significant variability in the rate of progression of renal disease. Risk factors associated with progressive renal failure include *PKD1* genotype, male gender, African race, and onset of hypertension before age 35 years.

Renovascular disease

Atheromatous renovascular disease is a relatively common cause of chronic renal failure in the elderly. Fibromuscular hyperplasia presents as hypertension in young patients, but is a rare cause of renal failure and will not be discussed further in this section.

Clinical features

Patients with atheromatous renovascular disease usually present with hypertension and/or renal impairment. Patients may present after deterioration of renal function after starting an ACE inhibitor or angiotensin receptor blocker. Rarely, patients present with recurrent, sudden onset pulmonary edema. Renal artery bruits may be audible. There is commonly evidence of generalized atherosclerosis. Patients usually have evidence of coronary artery disease or peripheral vascular disease.

Epidemiology

Renovascular disease is a disease of the elderly. Diabetes mellitus, hypertension, hypercholesterolemia, and smoking are major risk factors.

Pathology

There is usually eccentric plaque formation in the renal arteries, which may be unilateral or bilateral. If the stenosis is sufficiently narrow, the kidney distal to the stenosis may atrophy. The atrophied kidney secretes increased renin which enhances angiotensin II production, which causes systemic hypertension. Cholesterol emboli may be found downstream of a significant renal artery stenosis, and may contribute to intravascular and interstitial fibrosis.

Investigations

Ultrasound is useful for raising the clinical suspicion of renovascular disease if the renal size is asymmetric. Doppler ultrasound is not a reliable screening investigation in most centers. CT or MR angiography are good non-invasive imaging methods, although MRA tends to overestimate the degree of stenosis. Renal angiography with pressure gradient measurements remains the gold standard investigation.

Management

Medical management consists of optimizing blood pressure control, stopping ACE inhibitors and angiotensin receptor blockers, and lowering serum cholesterol levels. The role of angioplasty and stenting is controversial (Fig. 4.8). In some patients it may improve blood pressure control and renal function. Patients most likely to benefit are those with very critical stenoses, rapidly deteriorating renal function, and a kidney which measures more than 9 cm in length beyond the stenosis.

Outcome

Atheromatous renovascular disease is progressive so stenoses tend to become more critical over time. As

(a)   (b)

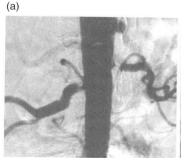 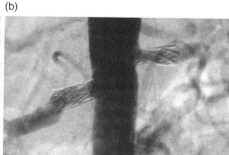

Fig. 4.8. Renal angiography in a case of bilateral renal artery stenosis before (left panel) and after (right panel) angioplasty and stenting.

this happens, renal function deteriorates. Renovascular disease is the cause of end-stage renal failure in approximately 10% of UK dialysis patients. As renovascular disease is part of a generalized atherosclerotic process, patients often die of a vascular event before reaching end-stage renal failure.

Alport's syndrome

Alport's syndrome is characterized by glomerulonephritis manifested by hematuria and progressive renal impairment, deafness, and in some cases ocular abnormalities.

Clinical features

Microscopic hematuria, together with episodes of macroscopic hematuria, is found in most affected males. Proteinuria progressing to nephrotic syndrome occurs in 30%. Most will progress to end-stage renal failure by age 16–35 years. Females have milder disease, but some will develop end-stage renal failure after age 50. High-frequency sensorineural deafness is common. Anterior lenticonus and retinal flecks occur in 15%–30% of cases.

Epidemiology

The incidence is 1 in 10 000. The most common form is X-linked, although autosomal recessive and dominant types of inheritance are also seen.

Pathology

The X-linked form is caused by mutations in the *COL4A5* gene. This causes an absence of the α3 chain of type IV collagen in the glomerular basement membrane. The diagnosic features are seen on electron microscopy. Initially, there is thinning of the basement membrane, which progresses to thickening with a characteristic "basket weave" appearance.

Investigations

Electron microscopy on the renal biopsy is necessary to make the diagnosis. Audiograms and ophthalmologic assessment should also be performed.

Management

There is no specific treatment for Alport's syndrome. Transplanted patients frequently develop anti-GBM antibodies, but only 5%–10% will develop a crescentic nephritis.

Outcome

Virtually all males will progress to end-stage renal failure. In heterozygous females, the prognosis is usually benign with most maintaining preserved good renal function.

Idiopathic edema

This is a condition in which fluid retention occurs in the absence of cardiac, hepatic, renal, hypoproteinemic, obstructive venous, or lymphatic disease. There is episodic or constant fluid retention which may accumulate in the face, hands, breasts, thighs, and abdominal wall tissues. Ankle edema is relatively uncommon. Triggers for fluid retention include emotional stress, obesity, food high in carbohydrate, and prolonged standing. It is most common in women, and often is associated with depression. Some women have features of anorexia nervosa and abuse diuretics. Patients should be advised to avoid long periods of standing, and to elevate the legs rather than use diuretics to relieve edema. However, most patients' symptoms are unacceptable without some diuretic treatment.

Lymphedema

This may be idiopathic or may occur secondary to damage to the lymphatics either by surgery or radiotherapy. It occurs commonly in the arm after an axillary lymph node dissection for breast cancer. Lymphedema does not pit easily after digital pressure. Lymphedema can also be distinguished from edema by a relative lack of response to elevation and diuretics. Treatment is problematic, but involves elevation of affected limbs, isotonic muscle exercise to stimulate lymph transport, and compression dressings.

Polyuria

The symptom polyuria means the patient is passing more urine than they consider normal. This must be distinguished from frequency, which is an increased number of episodes of bladder voiding usually due to lower urinary tract pathology. A 24-hour urine collection measuring urine volume, and a diary record, is helpful in distinguishing frequency from true polyuria. Polyuria in a fully conscious patient usually leads to polydipsia.

Causes of polyuria and polydipsia (Table 4.5):
(1) Decreased vasopressin production
   Cranial diabetes insipidus
(2) Decreased renal tubular response to vasopressin
   (i) **Hypercalemia or hypokalemia**
   (ii) **Chronic renal failure**
   (iii) **Obstructive uropathy**
   (iv) **Recovery phase of acute tubular necrosis**
   (v) **Congenital nephrogenic diabetes insipidus**
   (vi) **Lithium therapy**

93

Table 4.5. Associated features useful in the diagnosis of polyuria

Associated feature	Likely diagnosis	Other common features
Weight loss	Diabetes mellitus	Recurrent infection Family history
Fatigue	Chronic renal failure	Nausea Loss of appetite Itching Cramps Edema
Acute illness	Acute renal failure (recovery phase)	Use of diuretics Aminoglycosides
Psychiatric illness	Psychogenic polydipsia	Varying severity Absent nocturnal symptoms
Abdominal pain	Hypercalcemia	Nausea Bone pain Confusion
Muscle weakness	Hypokalemia	Drug history Laxative abuse
Headaches/ head injury	Cranial diabetes insipidus	Visual field defect Hypopituitarism
Manic depression	Lithium therapy	
Neonates	Nephrogenic diabetes insipidus	Dehydration Failure to thrive X-linked

(3) Drinking abnormalities
  Psychogenic polydipsia
(4) Osmotic diuresis

Diabetes mellitus

Diabetes mellitus, hypercalcemia, hypokalemia, and renal failure are discussed in other sections.

Cranial diabetes insipidus

There is a disturbance of vasopressin (ADH) secretion, leading to an inability to concentrate the urine. The normal role for ADH in the regulation of water homeostasis is shown in Fig. 4.9. There may be partial, moderate or total loss of neurosecretory function giving a wide range of severity.

Clinical features

The onset of polyuria and polydipsia is often sudden in contrast to patients with psychogenic polydipsia. There may be symptoms and signs of a space-occupying lesion such as a visual field defect, or a disturbance in anterior pituitary function. In severe cases urine volumes may be 10–20 liters per 24 hours.

Table 4.6. Important investigations used in the diagnosis of patients with polyuria

Suspected diagnosis	Investigation
Diabetes mellitus	Blood sugar
Renal failure	Serum creatinine
Hypercalcemia	Serum calcium
Hypokalemia	Serum potassium
Cranial diabetes insipidus	Water deprivation test

Urinary osmolality is low (50–100 mosmol/kg) but, provided the patient drinks normally, plasma sodium and osmolality remain within the normal range. Disturbances of thirst lead to hypernatremia.

Patients with psychogenic polydipsia often have psychiatric illnesses. Drinking is episodic compared with the constant intake in cranial diabetes insipidus, and nocturnal polyuria may be absent. Water intake may exceed 40 liters per day. Plasma osmolality tends to be lower (265–280 mosmol/kg) than in diabetes insipidus (290–295 mosmol/kg).

Epidemiology

Idiopathic disease is one of the commonest diagnoses made in cranial diabetes insipidus. Other common causes include head injury, pituitary surgery, meningitis and metastatic pituitary deposits (especially lung and breast). Rarer causes include craniopharyngioma, sarcoidosis, histiocytosis-X, and Sheehan's syndrome.

Pathology

There is damage to the hypothalamus or pituitary stalk.

Investigations

Water deprivation test with serial measurement of weight, plasma osmolality, urine volume and osmolality, and plasma ADH levels. The test is completed by giving desmopressin to assess the renal tubular response.

Management

A number of ADH analogs are available as replacement therapy.

Outcome

This depends on the underlying intracranial cause of the diabetes insipidus. A high fluid intake is essential to prevent dehydration.

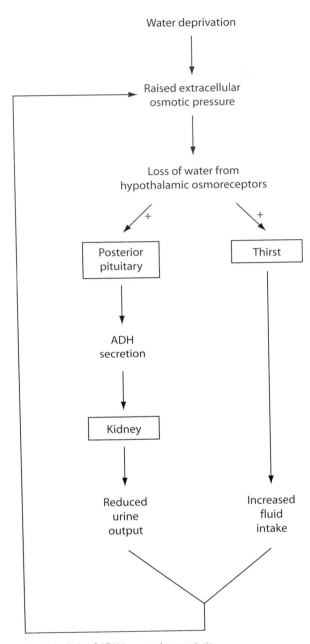

Water deprivation

Raised extracellular osmotic pressure

Loss of water from hypothalamic osmoreceptors

Posterior pituitary

Thirst

ADH secretion

Kidney

Reduced urine output

Increased fluid intake

Fig. 4.9. Role of ADH in water homeostasis.

Oliguria

Oliguria is defined as the passage of less than 500 ml urine per 24 hours. Anuria is defined as urine output of less than 100 ml/day. This section will be devoted to acute renal failure. Acute renal failure is defined as a sudden decline in excretory renal function and commonly presents with oligoanuria. However, some cases of acute renal failure may have a normal urine output or even be polyuric; this is classically seen in aminoglycoside toxicity. Some patients may not be aware that they are oliguric. They may present with shortness of breath due to pulmonary edema or metabolic acidosis. Alternatively, acute renal failure may be first detected on a set of blood tests showing a raised creatinine or hyperkalemia.

When determining the cause of a patient's oliguria, it is worth dividing the potential causes into pre-renal, renal, and post-renal accepting that in many cases acute renal failure may be due to a combination of factors. For example, a patient may be admitted to hospital with acute renal failure secondary to obstruction caused by bladder outflow obstruction, and then after initial improvement in renal function following catheterization, develop worsening renal function due to bacteremia and use of gentamicin. The major causes of acute renal failure are listed in Table 4.7 and associated features for diagnosis in Table 4.8.

Acute renal failure

In the following section some of the commoner causes of acute renal failure are discussed:

Acute tubular necrosis
Rhabdomyolysis
Systemic vasculitis
Interstitial nephritis
Hemolytic–uremic syndrome
Obstructive nephropathy

Acute tubular necrosis (ATN)

Acute tubular necrosis is the histologic appearance seen on renal biopsy caused by a period of renal hypoperfusion. The degree of renal impairment depends on the severity and duration of the period of hypoperfusion.

Clinical features

Patients with acute tubular necrosis will usually have an identifiable cause, e.g. hypovolemia related to protracted vomiting or septicemia. Acute tubular necrosis is common in patients with multiorgan failure in intensive care. Patients with cardiac failure, cirrhosis, nephrotic syndrome, or renal artery stenosis can develop acute tubular necrosis if diuresed over-aggressively or if given NSAIDS, ACE inhibitors or angiotensin 2 receptor blockers. Radiologic contrast or aminoglycoside antibiotics are common causes of acute tubular necrosis in hospital practice.

Table 4.7. Causes of acute renal failure

Pre-renal	Diarrhea/vomiting Excessive urinary losses Excessive sweating Reduced fluid intake Hypotension Septicemia Post-cardiac/aortic aneurysm surgery Renal artery thrombosis/embolus
Renal	Pre-renal causes leading to acute tubular necrosis Tubular toxins, e.g. aminoglycosides, myoglobin from rhabdomyolysis and hemoglobin from intravascular hemolysis Glomerulonephritis, e.g. vasculitis, lupus Interstitial nephritis Vascular damage, e.g. accelerated phase hypertension, hemolytic–uremic syndrome
Post-renal	Ureteric stones Papillary necrosis Retroperitoneal fibrosis Bladder carcinoma Prostate carcinoma Cervical carcinoma Pelvic radiotherapy

Table 4.8. Associated features helpful in the differential diagnosis of acute renal failure

Associated feature	Likely diagnosis	Other common features
Anuria	Bilateral obstruction Renal artery thrombosis Anti-glomerular basement membrane disease (Goodpasture's disease)	
Postural hypotension	Pre-renal	Tachycardia Low jugulovenous pressure (JVP) Reduced skin turgor History of fluid loss
Crush injury	Rhabdomyolysis	Brown urine Raised creatine kinase
Hemoptysis	Vasculitis	Skin rash Joint pains Weight loss
Certain drugs, e.g. NSAIDs	Interstitial nephritis	Skin rash Eosinophilia Eosinophiluria
Headaches	Accelerated hypertension	Blurred vision Retinopathy Cardiac failure
Bloody diarrhea	Hemolytic–uremic	Case cluster Thrombocytopenia Anemia
Loin pain	Obstruction	Hematuria Urinary symptoms Enlarged prostate
Back pain	Myeloma	Hypercalcemia Pathologic fractures

There is a rise in serum creatinine, and usually a reduced urine output. Hyponatremia occurs due to reduced water excretion, and hyperkalemia is common and can cause life-threatening cardiac arrhythmias. Metabolic acidosis, hypocalcemia, and hyperphosphatemia are the other usual biochemical abnormalities. Uremia is associated with an acquired platelet functional defect quantified as a prolonged bleeding time. This leads to bleeding commonly from the gastro-intestinal tract.

Epidemiology

The incidence of acute renal failure is about 200–300/million population per year (about 50/million will require temporary dialysis). Acute tubular necrosis is most common in the elderly population who are particularly susceptible after procedures such as coronary artery bypass grafting or aortic aneurysm repair.

Pathology

The proximal tubule and medullary thick ascending loop of Henle are the most susceptible to injury, because these parts of the nephron are relatively hypoxic in health. Necrosis and apoptosis occur, and cellular debris blocks the renal tubular lumen. The peritubular capillaries are filled with polymorphs, lymphocytes, and platelets. Renal biopsy is not routinely performed if the clinical setting is of acute tubular necrosis because a biopsy does not alter management.

Investigations

The patient's circulating volume status is assessed clinically by measuring pulse rate, postural blood pressure, and examining the jugular venous pressure (JVP). If necessary central venous pressure is measured via an indwelling line. Urinary sodium may be measured to attempt to distinguish between the pre-renal state (low urinary sodium), and acute tubular necrosis (high urinary sodium). However, the prior use of intravenous saline and/or diuretics confounds this interpretation. Renal ultrasound is necessary to assess the size of the kidneys and exclude obstruction.

Management

Acute tubular necrosis can be avoided in hospital practice by careful management of the patient. A patient who becomes oliguric due to hypovolemia should be given intravenous fluid to correct volume status as rapidly as possible to prevent the establishment of acute tubular necrosis. Intravenous contrast used for radiologic and interventional vascular and cardiologic procedures should be minimized in high-risk cases; such patients should be prehydrated with intravenous fluids. There is some evidence that *N*-acetylcysteine is renoprotective. Aminoglycosides should be used with respect and therapeutic levels monitored.

Once patients have developed acute renal failure, many nephrologists will use furosemide and dopamine for a period of time. Although there is no convincing evidence that this improves the eventual outcome, it is easier to manage fluid restriction if the patient is not oliguric. Patients in established acute tubular necrosis need to be fluid restricted to prevent fluid overload and need to have their weight measured daily together with an accurate fluid balance chart. Renal replacement therapy may be necessary in the presence of uremic symptoms and signs, rapidly rising creatinine, hyperkalemia, fluid overload, or metabolic acidosis. Hemodialysis is generally performed if the patient has acute renal failure only, whereas continuous hemofiltration is used in patients in the intensive care setting because it is more suitable in patients with circulatory instability. Gastro-intestinal bleeding is prevented by the use of proton pump inhibitors.

During the recovery phase, oliguric patients may become polyuric for a brief period, and may require intravenous fluids to prevent hypovolemia.

Outcome

In most cases, renal function will recover within a period of a few days to 4 weeks as the renal tubular cells regenerate. The time to recovery depends on the severity of the primary renal insult. Young patients will usually recover renal function completely, whereas elderly patients may be left with significant renal impairment. The main causes of death in patients with acute renal failure are the original disease and septicemia.

Rhabdomyolysis

Rhabdomyolysis is the breakdown of skeletal muscle. The myoglobin released is directly toxic to renal tubular cells and causes acute renal failure.

Clinical features

Following the damage to skeletal muscle, oliguria develops. The urine produced is a dark brown color due to presence of myoglobin. Renal function usually takes 1–3 weeks to recover. If the patient has sustained a muscle injury to a large group of muscles, the muscles may swell within the surrounding fascia and decompressive fasciotomies may be necessary to retain viability.

Epidemiology

Rhabdomyolysis is seen in acute crush injuries, for example following earthquakes. It is also seen in patients who have been unconscious at home on the floor, where they have been lying on one side for many hours, making the tissues ischemic. It can also rarely occur after viral infections, use of statins, or severe exercise. Patients with certain inborn errors of metabolism such as McArdle's syndrome are particularly susceptible.

Pathology

Myoglobin precipitates in acid urine in the distal tubule and causes oxidative damage. Patients are often severely volume depleted as the damaged muscles sequester large amounts of fluid.

Investigations

Urine will contain myoglobin, which causes a false-positive dipstick test for blood. Creatine phosphokinase levels will be grossly elevated. Levels of creatinine, phosphate, potassium, and urate will be very high as these molecules are released by dead muscle.

Management

Establishment of acute renal failure can be prevented by aggressive volume replacement. A forced alkaline diuresis minimizes the damage to the renal tubules.

Outcome

Renal replacement may be necessary for approximately 1–3 weeks, until renal function recovers.

Systemic vasculitis

Vasculitis is an autoimmune condition causing inflammation of the blood vessels. Large caliber arteries are involved in conditions such as Takayasu's arteritis and giant cell arteritis. Medium-sized vessels are affected in polyarteritis nodosa. Renal involvement occurs predominantly in small vessel vasculitis, in conditions such as microscopic polyarteritis (MPA) and Wegener's granulomatosis (WG).

Clinical features

Patients with WG and MPA can present with fever, weight loss, joint pains, skin rash, acute renal failure, hemoptysis, and respiratory failure. Patients may have a long prodromal illness or present with fulminant respiratory or renal failure. WG patients may

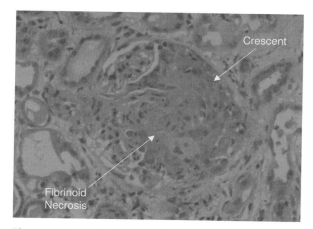

Crescent

Fibrinoid
Necrosis

Fig. 4.10. Glomerulus in a case of systemic vasculitis showing fibrinoid necrosis (long arrow) and a crescent (short arrow) (H and E ×200).

have cavitating lung lesions, tracheal stenosis, sinusitis, episcleritis, and deafness. Some WG patients may have no renal involvement and present to ENT specialists. Arthritis, rash, scleritis, or uveitis may be present. Collapse of the bridge of the nose may occur in WG.

Epidemiology

Small vessel vasculitis can occur in any age group, but occurs most commonly in the middle aged and elderly, with peak incidence in the 65–74 age group.

Pathology

The primary abnormality is an inflammation in the wall of the small arterioles. In the kidneys there is a crescentic glomerulonephritis (Fig 4.10). Immunostaining is negative for complement and immunoglobulin components. This contrasts with Goodpasture's disease where there is linear staining for IgG along the glomerular basement membrane. Granulomas are occasionally seen in renal biopsies in WG patients but are more commonly seen in nasal or bronchial biopsies.

Investigations

The urine of patients with renal involvement will contain red cell casts. Most patients will have positive anti-neutrophil cytoplasmic antibodies (ANCA) and the titer of these antibodies often correlates with disease activity. An indirect immunofluorescence assay on ethanol-fixed neutrophils distinguishes between two patterns of staining by vasculitis sera. Cytoplasmic or c-ANCA is a diffuse granular staining of the neutrophil cytoplasm and corresponds to

antibodies directed against the enzyme proteinase-3, and is usually associated with WG. Perinuclear or p-ANCA staining around the nucleus, is due to antibodies directed against the neutrophil granule enzyme myeloperoxidase (MPA). ESR and CRP can also be used to monitor disease activity. A renal biopsy is necessary to assess the relative degrees of acute inflammation and chronic damage.

Management

The initial management of a patient with acute renal failure is with steroids, cyclophosphamide and plasma exchange. Maintenance treatment is usually with steroids and azathioprine or mycophenolate mofetil. Treatment options in refractory cases include intravenous immunoglobulin, methotrexate and anti-B cell monoclonal antibodies.

Outcome

The renal outcome depends on the degree of inflammation and permanent scarring at presentation. If aggressive treatment is given before tissue necrosis occurs, renal function can be salvaged. Indeed, patients who are dialysis dependent at presentation may recover significant renal function. Much of the morbidity is due to infection related to the immunosuppressive treatment given to treat this condition. Patients who develop end-stage renal failure have a satisfactory prognosis on dialysis. Kidney transplantation can be complicated by a recurrence of vasculitis.

Acute interstitial nephritis

Acute interstitial nephritis is characterized by the presence of an inflammatory cellular infiltrate involving the renal tubules. It usually occurs as an allergic reaction to drugs, but may also be triggered by certain infections and occur as part of an autoimmune disease process.

Clinical features

Patients present with renal impairment. Oliguria occurs in about 40% of cases. Urinalysis is often negative for blood and protein. In patients with drug-induced interstitial nephritis, fever, maculopapular rash, and arthralgias may occur.

Epidemiology

Almost every drug has been associated with interstitial nephritis, but non-steroidal anti-inflammatory drugs, penicillin, sulfonamides, mesalazine, allopurinol, and frusemide are common culprits.

Pathology

There is a lymphocytic infiltrate affecting the renal tubules. Eosinophils may also be present. In some cases granulomas may be a feature.

Investigations

A peripheral blood eosinophilia or eosinophiluria is a clue that a patient with acute renal failure may have an interstitial nephritis. Renal biopsy is necessary to confirm the diagnosis.

Management

The offending drug is discontinued. A course of steroids is generally given in cases of drug-induced or autoimmune interstitial nephritis, as it probably hastens recovery of renal function.

Outcome

Renal function generally recovers if the duration of inflammation has been short. However, if the interstitial nephritis has been long-standing, there may be significant residual renal impairment. Predictors of poor outcome include the presence of interstitial fibrosis, granuloma formation, and diffuse infiltrates.

Hemolytic–uremic syndrome (HUS)

Patients with HUS typically have a microangiopathic hemolytic anemia, thrombocytopenia, and acute renal failure. Most sporadic cases are caused by the ingestion of meat containing *E.coli* 0157 : H7.

Clinical features

HUS often occurs after bloody diarrhea has started to improve. Patients are often anemic with purpura. Oliguria, fluid overload, and hypertension develop.

Epidemiology

Diarrhea-associated HUS occurs mainly in young children, but can occur in adults. The *E.coli* 0157 strain produces Shiga-like toxins which trigger endothelial cell damage. HUS may also be caused by pregnancy, oral contraceptives, SLE, ciclosporin and tacrolimus, HIV, certain mucin-secreting carcinomas, and mitomycin-C. Familial cases are often due to Factor H deficiency.

Pathology

Endothelial injury leads to a prothrombotic state, and thrombosis of intrarenal vessels in the absence of cellular inflammation. The intravascular thrombosis leads to red cell fragmentation and thrombocytopenia.

Investigations

Thrombocytopenia and hemolytic anemia are found. Fragmented red cells are seen in the peripheral blood film. Renal biopsy will confirm the diagnosis. In diarrheal cases antibodies to *E.coli* 0157 are found.

Management

Anemia is managed by blood transfusion and renal failure by dialysis if necessary. Diarrheal-associated HUS does not respond to fresh frozen plasma (FFP) or plasma exchange, whereas cases with other causes should be managed by treating any underlying disease and with plasma exchange.

Outcome

In children with diarrheal-associated HUS, complete renal recovery normally occurs within 2 or 3 weeks. Renal prognosis is worse in adults.

Obstructive nephropathy

Obstructive nephropathy describes the renal disease that results from an impaired flow of urine.

Clinical features

Acute upper tract obstruction causes pain in the loin radiating into the groin. Pain is worsened by a high fluid intake, alcohol, or diuretics. In the presence of infection there is fever and loin tenderness. Anuria only develops if there is complete bilateral obstruction or obstruction of a single functioning kidney. Polyuria may even occur in cases of intermittent obstruction. Lower urinary tract obstruction usually causes symptoms of hesitancy starting micturition, poor stream, terminal dribbling, and acute urinary retention. Patients with chronic retention may present with a large bladder and renal failure which resolves after bladder catheterization. Repeated urinary tract infections in a male should raise the possibility of obstruction.

Epidemiology

Obstructive nephropathy is most common at the extremes of life. In early childhood there may be congenital anomalies. In elderly men obstruction due to prostatic hypertrophy or carcinoma is common. Other causes of obstruction include calculi, sloughed renal papillae, blood clot, fungal balls, tumor, radiation damage, and extrinsic compression by retroperitoneal fibrosis.

Pathology

Acute obstruction causes raised ureteric pressure, and decreased renal blood flow and glomerular filtration.

The kidney becomes edematous and hemorrhagic. Chronic obstruction causes thinning of the renal parenchyma. The presence of bacterial infection and obstruction can lead to rapid and permanent loss of renal function.

Investigations

Ultrasound will usually show a dilated renal pelvis in cases of obstruction. Spiral CT is sensitive for detection of renal calculi and defining retroperitoneal and pelvic lesions.

Management

If infection is suspected, obstruction must be relieved, usually by the insertion of a percutaneous antegrade nephrostomy. Stones larger than 7 mm usually require urologic intervention. In patients with malignant disease, decisions are made on an individual basis about the appropriateness of intervention.

Outcome

This clearly depends on the site, duration, and cause of obstruction. In general, the sooner obstruction is relieved, the better the renal function recovers.

Difficulty passing urine

Micturition is the medical term for passing urine. Patients with difficulty passing urine may have localized pathology affecting the lower urinary tract, i.e. bladder, prostate, or urethra, or may have a central or peripheral neurologic lesion such as diabetic neuropathy, which affects bladder innervation.

Patients should be asked if they have urinary frequency, and this is most clearly expressed by writing down how often the patient passes urine during the day and night. Increased frequency due to lower urinary tract causes must be distinguished from polyuria where a patient passes an increased volume of urine due to a condition such as diabetes mellitus (see section on polyuria). Elderly men may mistakenly be referred for prostatectomy because they have to get up to pass urine at night. Such patients, in fact, have a good flow rate, no residual urine, and a fluid chart shows that they are passing relatively large volumes throughout the night. In fact, these patients have mild heart failure, and edema fluid which accumulates during the day is being excreted as the patient is recumbent at night.

Male patients should be asked how strong their urinary stream is, and in elderly patients compared to how strong it was in their youth. Hesitancy describes

Table 4.9. Associated features helpful in the differential diagnosis of urinary frequency

Associated feature	Likely diagnoses	Other common features
Dysuria	Acute cystitis	Hematuria Sudden onset Smelly urine
Hesitancy	Benign prostatic hypertrophy	Over age 40 Poor stream Chronic retention Acute retention Overflow incontinence Urinary infection Renal failure
Weight loss	Prostate carcinoma	Shorter history Bony pain Ureteric obstruction Hard prostate Elderly
Hematuria	Bladder carcinoma	Sterile pyuria Urine infection Pelvic pain Suprapubic mass
Urge incontinence	Overactive bladder	Diabetes mellitus Elderly Pelvic surgery
Daytime only	Anxiety	Psychiatric history
Night time only	Cardiac failure	Elderly Good flow rate No residual urine

the symptom of difficulty starting to pass urine. Patients may also describe the symptom of incomplete bladder evacuation after micturition. Patients should also be asked if there is associated incontinence or pain on passing urine. Associated hematuria is an important symptom that suggests the presence of carcinoma of the bladder or prostate until proven otherwise.

Patient diaries are helpful to record the frequency, volume, and pattern of voiding.

Physical examination includes palpation and percussion of the bladder and a rectal examination. A midstream urine should be performed to screen for hematuria and infection. Ultrasound is a noninvasive test for residual urine volume (Table 4.9, Table 4.10).

The major causes of increased urinary frequency are listed below:

Acute cystitis

Benign prostatic hypertrophy

Prostate cancer

Table 4.10. Important investigations used in the diagnosis of patients with increased urinary frequency

Suspected diagnosis	Investigation
Acute cystitis	Midstream urine culture
Benign prostatic hypertrophy	Rectal examination Ultrasound prostate/renal Urine flow rate PSA (to exclude carcinoma)
Prostate cancer	Prostate specific antigen (PSA) Prostate biopsy CT pelvis/abdomen Bone scan
Bladder carcinoma	IVU/CT pelvis Cystoscopy (+biopsy)
Overactive bladder	Cystoscopy Urodynamics

Bladder cancer
Overactive bladder
Cardiac failure
The major causes of poor urinary flow are:
Benign prostatic hypertrophy
Prostate cancer
Diabetic neuropathy
Urethral stricture
Neurologic lesions

Acute cystitis

Acute cystitis is a very common problem especially in women. It is acute inflammation of the bladder usually caused by bacterial infection. Chemical cystitis may be caused by cyclophosphamide.

Clinical features

There is a sudden onset of suprapubic pain, frequency, and burning on passing urine. The urine may smell fishy and frank hematuria may occur. Fever may not be present if infection is confined to the bladder.

Epidemiology

Bacterial cystitis is usually caused by bowel organisms such as *Escherichia coli*, *Klebsiella*, or *Streptococcus faecalis*. In patients with indwelling catheters, other infections such as *Staphylococcus aureus* are more common.

Pathology

The bladder mucosa is inflamed. This stimulates the afferent arc of micturition causing the patient to wish to pass urine, even though the bladder is not full. In some patients infection may ascend the ureters to cause pyelonephritis.

Investigations

Urine microscopy will show numerous leukocytes and bacteria. Culture will reveal the species and antibiotic sensitivity. Urine dipsticks for nitrites and leukocyte esterase are helpful tests for the presence of infection.

Management

Treatment is started before the culture and sensitivity results are available. Ciprofloxacin and trimethoprim are commonly used first-line agents. A short course (3 days) is probably as effective as a more prolonged course in uncomplicated cases. Patients should be encouraged to drink copious amounts of fluid, and to empty the bladder regularly.

Outcome

Most cases will resolve with a course of antibiotics. A male with cystitis should be investigated for an underlying urologic abnormality. Women with recurrent episodes or hematuria should be investigated to rule out a stone or bladder tumor.

Bladder carcinoma

Transitional cell carcinoma is the commonest form of bladder tumor. Less often seen are squamous cell and adenocarcinoma which occur in the context of chronic infection or inflammation.

Clinical features

Macroscopic hematuria occurs in about 80% of cases. The tumor irritates the surrounding urothelium leading to frequency and sometimes pain on voiding. The presence of white cells but absence of infection (sterile pyuria) suggests the possibility of bladder tumor or tuberculosis until proven otherwise. If the bladder tumor extends outside the bladder, there may be severe pelvic pain. Urinary tract infection may occur as the bacteria multiply in the necrotic tumor. In advanced cases there may be a palpable mass.

Epidemiology

Bladder carcinoma usually occurs in middle-aged and elderly age groups. Risk factors include smoking and occupational exposure to aniline dyes in the chemical and rubber industries. Schistosomiasis is the major cause for squamous cell carcinoma due to the prolonged irritation of the bladder wall.

Pathology

Bladder tumors may be single or multiple. They may be a superficial papillary lesion, a solid lump, or an ulcer. Direct spread occurs through the wall of the bladder into other pelvic organs. Lymphatic spread is common once the tumor has infiltrated the muscle wall. Hematogenous spread to brain, lung, or liver is less common.

Investigations

Urine is sent for cytology. Malignant cells have a large nucleus and little cytoplasm. Cystoscopy and biopsy will confirm the diagnosis. CT images of the bladder are necessary to image the bladder wall, and assess whether there has been any lymphatic spread.

Management

Management depends on the stage and grade of the tumor. Superficial tumors can be removed cystoscopically. Repeat cystoscopies are necessary to screen for recurrence. Intravesical chemotherapy or immunotherapy with BCG have beneficial effects of reducing the number of recurrences. Cases of invasive bladder cancer are managed by three main methods: total cystectomy, radiotherapy, and combination chemotherapy.

Outcome

If the tumor has invaded into the muscle wall of the bladder, the prognosis is much worse. Advanced bladder cancer is very miserable for the patient because of severe pelvic pain, bowel obstruction, and extreme urinary frequency. A palliative urinary diversion may give considerable relief from the painful urinary frequency.

Benign prostatic hypertrophy (BPH)

BPH occurs in all men over age 40, but only about 10% will experience symptoms of obstruction. It is a major cause of morbidity in middle-aged and elderly men.

Clinical features

At an early stage, patients may notice difficulty initiating urination, with some frequency, but have a good stream. During this time, there is bladder wall hypertrophy and detrusor instability. At a later stage, the detrusor muscle fails and the bladder fails to empty. The residual volume increases and chronic retention occurs. Overflow incontinence may occur. The urinary stream becomes very poor. Renal failure may occur due to obstruction. Urinary infection is common due to the residual volume. Acute retention may occur often in association with an intercurrent illness. Rectal examination is essential to detect carcinoma, but the size of the prostate is not related to the severity of outflow obstruction.

Pathology

Obstruction is caused by hyperplasia of the inner cranial zone of the prostate. The bulky adenomas on either side of the urethra become the enlarged lobes of the prostate. Obstruction causes structural changes in the bladder wall. The bladder wall becomes trabeculated and also contains more fibrous tissue. The ureters become dilated and obstructive uropathy occurs.

Investigations

Urine is sent for cytology and microbiology. Serum creatinine and prostate specific antigen (PSA) are measured. Renal and bladder ultrasound will detect upper tract dilatation and residual bladder volume. Cystoscopy is done to exclude bladder cancer.

Management

Medical management includes the use of alpha blockers and anti-androgens. Finasteride is a specific inhibitor of the enzyme 5α-reductase which metabolizes testosterone into the more potent androgen, dihydrotestosterone. This leads to reduction in prostate size, with improvement in urinary flow rate and in obstructive symptoms. The selective alpha blockers such as tamsulosin and terazosin relax smooth muscle in benign prostatic hyperplasia, producing an increased flow rate. The main side effects are drowsiness, and fainting due to postural hypotension. Surgical management involves prostatectomy. Open prostatectomy is now rarely performed, and various techniques for transurethral prostatectomy, including laser resection, are now available. Complications include bleeding, thromboembolism, infection, retrograde ejaculation, and erectile dysfunction.

Outcome

Modern management with medical therapy will delay the need for surgical treatment in many cases. Obstructive uropathy is an important cause of chronic renal failure in elderly men.

Prostate carcinoma

Prostate cancer is the commonest cancer in men, with over 27 000 new cases diagnosed each year in the UK.

Clinical features

Disease confined to the prostate gland is usually diagnosed in asymptomatic men undergoing screening with a PSA test or in men undergoing investigation of lower urinary tract symptoms or by histologic diagnosis following transurethral prostatectomy for presumed benign prostatic hypertrophy. A short history of outflow tract obstruction should increase suspicion of prostate cancer. Advanced prostate cancer may present with widespread bony pain due to skeletal metastases. Intestinal or ureteric obstruction may occur.

A hard nodule on rectal examination of a man suggests prostate cancer until proven otherwise.

Epidemiology

Small foci of prostate carcinoma are found in 14% of glands of 50 year olds, and 100% of men at age 80. It is rare in the Japanese and more common in Africans. There is an inherited predisposition.

Pathology

The histologic characteristics of prostate cancer are described using the Gleason score (potential score 2–10). Gleason scores of up to 4 represent well-differentiated tumors, 5–7 moderately differentiated, and 8–10 poorly differentiated (and the poorer the differentiation, the worse the prognosis).

Investigations

Men with an abnormal rectal examination and a PSA above 4 ng/ml should have a prostate biopsy under transrectal ultrasound guidance. When advanced prostate cancer is suspected CT or MRI pelvis and bone scans are performed.

Management

The management options for localized prostate cancer are conservative management or potentially curative radical treatment. Conservative management strategies can be divided into watchful waiting or active surveillance. Watchful waiting means giving no treatment while the patient is ay\mptomatic, but monitoring every 6–12 months for onset of symptoms of metastases, and then giving palliative hormonal treatment. It is intended for older patients, with co-morbid illnesses, limited life expectancy, and well-differentiated prostate cancer. Such patients are more likely to die with, rather than from, the prostate cancer. Active surveillance involves 3-monthly clinical review with PSA and rectal examination. If the PSA rises rapidly, the patient can be offered radical treatment while the disease is still curable. Patients with a Gleason score above 4 should be offered radical treatments. The options include radical prostatectomy, external beam radiotherapy, brachytherapy (inserting

radioactive implants into the prostate), or hormonal therapy using luteinizing hormone-releasing hormone, gonadorelin analogs or anti-androgens. There is much controversy over which treatments are best for an individual patient, and whether combination treatments should be used. It is important to involve patients actively in treatment decisions. Hormone therapy is used in patients with advanced prostate cancer but side effects include loss of libido, hot flushes, weight gain, gynecomastia, and osteoporosis.

Outcome

The clinical outcome for patients is extremely heterogeneous with some men living for decades after the diagnosis and other men succumbing rapidly to aggressive metastatic disease. Men with clinically localized prostate cancer usually have a life expectancy of greater than 10 years. Adverse prognostic features are raised PSA, high Gleason score, spread beyond the capsule, and evidence of distant spread. In one study 13% of patients with well-differentiated prostate cancer were dead at 10 years, compared to 66% with poorly differentiated cancer.

Overactive bladder

Overactive bladder is a symptom complex that includes urinary urgency with or without urge incontinence, urinary frequency, and nocturia. The symptoms are associated with involuntary contractions of the detrusor muscle (detrusor instability).

Clinical features

The symptoms of overactive bladder have many potential causes. Lower urinary tract conditions which can cause or contribute to symptoms of overactive bladder include urinary tract infection, outflow tract obstruction, bladder tumors or stones, and prostate enlargement. Stroke, dementia, or Parkinson's disease can impair higher cortical inhibition of the bladder as can spinal cord injury leading to detrusor overactivity. Constipation, impaired mobility, and anxiety can all cause symptoms of overactive bladder.

Patients with symptoms of overactive bladder often reduce their social activities and are prone to isolation and depression. Patients with nocturia have sleep disruption. There is an increased incidence of falls.

Epidemiology

In a survey of 16 776 adults aged over 40 years, 16% of men and 17% of women reported symptoms of overactive bladder. The numbers rose in the over 75 year olds to 42% of men and 31% of women.

Pathology

There is a complex interplay between the bladder myocytes, afferent and efferent neural pathways, and central nervous system. Disturbance of any of these can lead to symptoms of an overactive bladder.

Investigations

In selected patients residual urine volume should be measured by ultrasound. Cystoscopy is necessary in older age groups and in those with hematuria to exclude bladder carcinoma. Formal urodynamic tests are expensive and invasive and are recommended only where they will alter management, such as after the failure of initial therapy.

Management

Educating patients about bladder function, appropriate fluid intake, and avoiding constipation is important in all patients. Surgical procedures such as augmentation cystoplasty are used only in patients with the most severe symptoms. Pharmacologic treatment includes anticholinergic drugs such as oxybutynin and tolterodine and alpha-blockers. Anticholinergic drugs can have side effects of dry mouth, constipation, urinary retention, blurred vision, and cognitive side effects. Alpha-blockers are used in men with symptoms of overactive bladder caused by benign prostatic hypertrophy.

Outcome

The outcome depends on the cause of the detrusor instability and the severity of the symptoms.

Loin pain

Loin pain may sometimes be difficult to differentiate from pain originating from the vertebral column. Loin pain may be unilateral or bilateral. Bilateral loin pain may be caused by bilateral obstruction, acute glomerulonephritis, or acute pyelonephritis. Unilateral pain can be caused by a renal tumor, unilateral obstruction due to calculi, papillary necrosis, renal arterial or venous thrombosis. If the pain radiates from the loin into the groin and is very severe, it is called renal colic and is most commonly caused by the passage of a renal calculus down the ureter. Hematuria, either macroscopic or microscopic, can occur with all the causes of loin pain mentioned above. Acute loin pain can occur in acute glomerulonephritis and acute interstitial nephritis probably due to renal

Table 4.11. Associated features helpful in the differential diagnosis of loin pain.

Associated feature	Likely diagnosis	Other common features
Sudden onset	Renal calculus	Previous calculus history Severe pain Passage of grit/stone Sudden resolution
Fever	Pyelonephritis	Frequency, urgency Rigors Sudden onset
Recurrent symptoms	Renal calculus Papillary necrosis	Previous imaging
Weight loss	Renal cell carcinoma	Palpable mass Pain for weeks/months
Edema	Renal vein thrombosis	Nephrotic syndrome Pulmonary embolus
Atrial fibrillation	Renal artery embolism	Ischemic heart disease
Psychiatric history	Loin pain/hematuria	Opiate use Multiple hospitalization

edema stretching the renal capsule. Patients with chronic glomerular diseases usually do not have loin pain, although a minority do complain of bilateral loin pain. Patients with polycystic kidneys may report no pain from the kidneys or may have a chronic pain. Acute pain may develop if there is a bleed into a renal cyst or an infected cyst.

Loin-pain hematuria syndrome occurs in patients who often have a background of psychologic problems. They may complain of severe loin pain and crave analgesia and even ask the surgeon to remove the kidney. Some patients may cause factitious blood to appear in the urine. The treatment should involve psychologic counseling and patient pressure to have surgery should be resisted (Tables 4.11 and 4.12).

Acute pyelonephritis

Acute pyelonephritis is an infection of the renal parenchyma usually caused by bacteria which have ascended the urinary tract.

Clinical features

Typically, patients present with high fever, rigors and loin pain. Some patients, but not all, also have symptoms of acute cystitis. Bacteremia and septicemia may develop, especially in patients with obstructed kidneys or who are immunosuppressed.

Table 4.12. Causes of loin pain according to duration of symptoms

Minutes/hours
    Renal calculus
    Papillary necrosis
    Renal artery embolism
    Renal vein thrombosis

Days/weeks
    Acute pyelonephritis
    Renal cell carcinoma
    Acute glomerulonephritis, e.g. post-streptococcal
    Retroperitoneal fibrosis

Months/years
    Chronic glomerulonephritis, e.g. IgA nephropathy
    Loin-pain hematuria syndrome
    Medullary sponge kidney
    Polycystic kidney disease

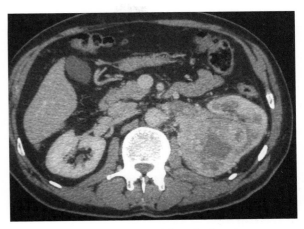

Fig. 4.11. CT scan showing large left renal cell carcinoma.

Epidemiology

Acute pyelonephritis is much more common in women than in men. The most common pathogens are Gram-negative organisms that are normally found in the bowel. Risk factors for acute pyelonephritis include sexual intercourse, instrumentation of the urinary tract, structural abnormalities of the urinary tract including obstruction and vesicoureteric reflux, pregnancy, and diabetes mellitus.

Pathology

There is a neutrophil infiltrate of the renal tubules.

Investigations

Urine microscopy shows an excess of white cells, white cell casts and bacteria on Gram staining. Renal ultrasound is important to exclude obstruction. Intravenous urography is indicated after acute pyelonephritis has been treated if the episode has been severe, slow to resolve or relapsing. It can detect obstruction, stones or papillary necrosis. In severe cases, intrarenal and perirenal abscess formation may occur which is best imaged by CT.

Management

Intravenous rather than oral antibiotics are indicated for patients with vomiting, obstruction or stones. A nephrostomy should be inserted into an obstructed infected kidney as a matter of urgency.

Outcome

Acute pyelonephritis in patients with normal kidneys usually leaves no long-term scarring or functional impairment. However, if the kidneys are already scarred repeated bouts of infection can lead to worsening renal function. Perirenal abscess is a rare complication of acute pyelonephritis usually occurring when there has been an inadequate course of treatment with antibiotics.

Renal cancer

Most renal tumors are malignant in childhood and adult life. Renal cell carcinoma is the commonest renal cancer in adults. In children, Wilm's tumors are commonest at the age of 2, but can occur from age 1–10 years.

Clinical features

Loin pain, macroscopic hematuria, and weight loss are the commonest symptoms of renal tumors. There may be a unilateral hard mass present on palpation of the loin. Other presenting symptoms and signs include fever, hypercalcemia, venous thrombosis, and polycythemia.

Epidemiology

Renal cell carcinoma has an annual incidence of 5/100 000 population. Peak incidence is between the fifth and seventh decades of life, but can occur earlier especially in the context of von Hippel–Lindau disease.

Pathology

The typical histology of a renal cell carcinoma is of tumor cells with abundant clear cytoplasm. Other histologic patterns include a papillary and an anaplastic sarcoma-like pattern. A transitional cell carcinoma may arise in the renal pelvis and infiltrate the kidney.

Investigations

Ultrasound, CT (Fig. 4.11) and MRI scanning define the primary tumor, and local spread to lymph nodes and along the renal vein and inferior vena cava.

Management

Surgical management is generally by radical nephrectomy. In cases of small tumors where it is important to preserve renal function partial nephrectomy may be possible. Radiotherapy, chemotherapy, and immunotherapy with interferon or interleukin-2 are used in selected cases.

Outcome

Outcome for renal cell carcinoma depends largely on whether the tumour has spread outside the kidney by the time of surgery. The cure rate for Wilm's tumors is in the order of 80%–90%.

Renal calculi

Stones are a common cause of severe loin pain when they migrate from the renal pelvis down the ureter.

Clinical features

Calculi may be asymptomatic and discovered by chance when renal imaging is performed. They may be the cause of hematuria. Renal colic occurs as the stone passes down the ureter. Typically, this is severe pain which radiates into the groin. Vomiting may occur. There may be tenderness in the loin. The pain resolves suddenly when the stone passes into the bladder. Stones can cause acute renal failure if they are bilateral or if they obstruct a single functioning kidney.

Epidemiology

Stones occur in over 10% of the population in the industrialized world. They are commoner in men, and the highest incidence is in the fifth and sixth decades. About 75% of stones are composed of calcium oxalate alone or calcium oxalate together with calcium phosphate. Pure calcium phosphate stones occur in about 5%. 10%–20% of stones are made of magnesium ammonium phosphate (struvite) as a result of urinary infection. Urate stones make up 5%–10% of stones and cystine 1%. Risk factors for calcium stone disease include living in hot climates with low fluid intake, high protein intake, hyperoxaluria, hypercalciuria, primary hyperparathyroidism, and medullary sponge kidney.

Pathology

Calcium-containing stones initially form when the urine is supersaturated. Calcium phosphate may form a nucleus for calcium oxalate crystallization in the collecting ducts of the renal papillae. Struvite stones are caused by urinary tract infection by bacteria such as *Proteus mirabilis*, which split urea to ammonia and carbon dioxide and cause urine to be alkaline. These stones may be very large and have the shape of the renal

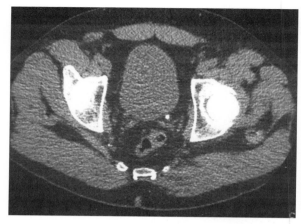

Fig. 4.12. CT showing renal calculus at left vesicoureteric junction.

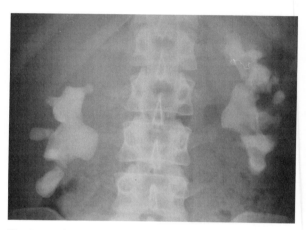

Fig. 4.13. Plain kidney ureter bladder (KUB) film showing bilateral staghorn calculi.

pelvis and calyces (staghorn calculi); chronic infection leads to chronic pyelonephritis. Urate stones occur in Western populations with a high purine intake.

Investigations

Spiral CT is now the imaging modality of choice for renal calculi (Fig. 4.12). Plain abdominal X-ray will detect most calcium-containing stones (Fig. 4.13), but not uric acid stones. Ultrasound will image non-calcium-containing stones but can miss small stones, and ureteric stones. Serum calcium measurement, urine culture and a 24-hour urine collection for calcium, urate, oxalate, and cystine should be performed to identify a metabolic reason for stone formation.

Management

Renal colic requires analgesia usually with opiates and non-steroidal anti-inflammatory drugs. Stones less than 5 mm in diameter will usually spontaneously pass down the ureter. Stones can be removed by a variety of techniques including percutaneous nephrolithotomy, extracorporeal shockwave lithotripsy, and ureteroscopy. Open surgery is now rarely needed except in certain cases of staghorn calculi or to correct a complication that has occurred during lithotripsy or ureteroscopy.

Outcome

Calculi may pass spontaneously or may require urologic intervention. For a group of first time calcium stone formers, the expected risk of stone formation during a 10-year period is 30% and, in those who had formed at least two stones at the start of follow-up, the corresponding figure was 70%.

Papillary necrosis

Dead renal papillae can detach, pass into the ureter and cause loin pain.

Clinical features

Patients present with recurrent episodes of loin pain, and may report passing fleshy tissue in the urine which is the necrotic renal papilla.

Epidemiology

Renal papillary necrosis occurs in diabetes mellitus, sickle cell disease, obstructive uropathy, and chronic analgesic abuse.

Pathology

There is usually cortical atrophy over the area of papillary necrosis.

Investigations

The radiologic changes of papillary necrosis are classically shown on IVP.

Management

If a renal papilla is causing ureteric obstruction, ureteroscopy and stenting are required.

Outcome

Recurrent episodes of infection and obstruction may lead to chronic renal failure.

Hematuria

Hematuria may be microscopic or macroscopic. Healthy subjects excrete approximately 1.2 million red cells per day, or approximately one erythrocyte per microliter of urine. Microscopic hematuria is detected with urine dipsticks, and confirmed by urine microscopy. Urine samples should be obtained from women when they are not menstruating as

Table 4.13. Some discriminatory features in the diagnosis of a patient with hematuria

Associated feature	Likely diagnosis	Other common features
Proteinuria	Glomerulonephritis	Red cell casts Hypertension Impaired renal function
Family history	Alport's syndrome	X-linked Renal failure
	Thin basement membrane	Autosomal dominant
	Polycystic kidney	Autosomal dominant Loin pain Renal failure
Rash	Systemic vasculitis	Joint pains Hemoptysis Renal failure
Sore throat	Post-streptococcal	10–14 days post-tonsilitis
	IgA disease	Contemporaneous with sore throat
Renal mass	Polycystic kidney	Family history Renal failure Bilateral
	Renal tumor	Weight loss Unilateral
Frequency	Bladder tumor	Pelvic pain

contamination with blood will otherwise cause a positive result. Jogging and heavy physical exercise can cause hematuria. Dark urine can also be caused by pigments such as bilirubin, hemoglobin, porphyrins, and consuming large amounts of beetroot.

Hematuria can originate from anywhere in the urinary tract. A tumor must be excluded if macroscopic hematuria develops in a middle aged or elderly person. However, tumors can also present with microscopic hematuria. Conversely glomerulonephritis can present with macroscopic hematuria. Some IgA nephropathy patients will pass clots of blood at the start of an upper respiratory tract infection. Even patients with thin basement membrane disease can develop loin pain and macroscopic hematuria. However, if macroscopic hematuria only occurs at the start or the end of the stream, a bladder or urethral malignancy should be suspected.

Microscopic hematuria is often detected at an insurance or job medical examination. If it has been present for many years, then the diagnosis is very likely to be glomerulonephritis. If there is a strong family history, thin basement membrane disease is the most likely diagnosis (Tables 4.13, 4.14).

Table 4.14. Major causes of hematuria

Bladder carcinoma

Prostate carcinoma

Renal carcinoma

Renal calculi

Polycystic kidney disease

Acute cystitis

IgA nephropathy

Thin basement membrane disease

Post-streptococcal glomerulonephritis

Systemic vasculitis

Systemic lupus erythematosus

Alport's syndrome

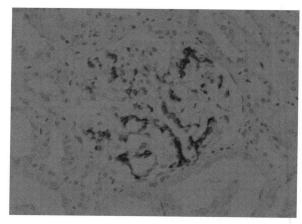

Fig. 4.15. IgA mesangial deposits (immunoperoxidase ×200).

In general patients aged over 40 years with microscopic hematuria should initially be referred to a urologist because it is mandatory to exclude a renal, bladder, or prostatic carcinoma (Fig. 4.14). The urologic assessment will include a rectal examination, urine cytology, ultrasound, IVP, and cystoscopy. Patients aged under 40 years are more likely to have some form of glomerulonephritis and should be referred to a nephrologist. These patients need to have their renal function measured and proteinuria quantified. Renal biopsy is only recommended if renal function is reduced or proteinuria is greater than 1 g/24 hours.

IgA nephropathy, thin basement membrane disease, and post-streptococcal glomerulonephritis are dealt with in the following sections.

IgA nephropathy

IgA nephropathy is a mesangial proliferative glomerulonephritis with a diffuse deposition of IgA in the mesangium. It is one of the commonest forms of glomerulonephritis, and is the leading primary glomerular cause of end-stage renal failure.

Clinical features

Most patients present with asymptomatic microscopic hematuria with or without proteinuria. Patients may also present with hypertension which may be in accelerated phase, or with renal impairment. The classic presentation is with episodes of macroscopic hematuria triggered by upper respiratory tract infections. This presentation only occurs in about 10% of patients with this condition. It may also occur as part of the manifestations of Henoch–

Schonlein purpura, which include a vasculitic rash on the extensor aspects of the legs, joint and abdominal pain, and sometimes bloody diarrhea.

Epidemiology

IgA nephropathy is the cause of about 10% of cases of end-stage renal failure. It occurs in all age groups but is most commonly diagnosed between the ages of 16 and 35. Men are more commonly affected. It is commoner in Asians and Europeans than in Africans.

Pathology

There is mesangial expansion with tubulointerstitial scarring in proportion to the degree of glomerular damage. In very severe cases there may be crescent formation. IgA deposits are found in the mesangium and capillary loops (Fig. 4.15).

Investigations

A renal biopsy is indicated if renal function is reduced or there is significant proteinuria.

Management

Hypertension needs to be well controlled and there is evidence that ACE inhibitors and angiotensin 2 receptor blockers are renoprotective. In some studies tonsillectomy, fish oil, and steroids have been shown to improve renal prognosis, but these results have not been confirmed by other investigators.

Outcome

The incidence of end-stage renal failure at 20 years after diagnosis is approximately 15%–30%. Adverse prognostic markers include baseline 24-hour urinary protein excretion rates exceeding 1 g, hypertension,

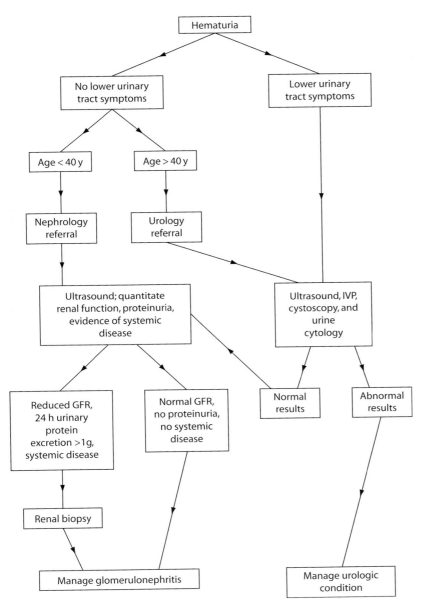

Fig. 4.14. Algorithm for the investigation of patients presenting with hematuria.

impaired renal function, and glomerular obsolescence, or interstitial fibrosis on renal biopsy. IgA nephropathy commonly recurs after renal transplantation but rarely causes early graft loss.

Thin basement membrane disease

Thin basement membrane disease presents with asymptomatic microscopic hematuria, and is due to abnormally thin glomerular basement membranes.

Epidemiology

It is a major cause of persistent asymptomatic microscopic hematuria. It is inherited as an autosomal dominant trait.

Clinical features

Most patients have isolated asymptomatic microscopic hematuria. A few patients have macroscopic hematuria, loin pain, or low grade proteinuria.

Pathology

Glomeruli appear normal on light and immuno-fluorescence microscopy. On electron microscopy, there is diffuse thinning of the lamina densa of the glomerular basement membrane.

Investigations

Electron microscopic examination of a renal biopsy is the only definitive method of making this diagnosis. However, an autosomal dominant pattern of inheritance in a family is very suggestive of the diagnosis.

Management

There is no specific management.

Outcome

The long-term outcome for renal function is the same as in the general population.

Post-streptococcal glomerulonephritis

Post-streptococcal glomerulonephritis is an acute nephritis that develops secondary to a pharyngitis or skin infection with specific strains of group A β-hemolytic streptococci.

Clinical features

Nephritis is preceded by a streptococcal infection by 1–4 weeks. The typical presentation is with hematuria, oliguria, hypertension, edema, proteinuria, and renal impairment. Children may develop vomiting, abdominal pain, headache, encephalopathy, and seizures.

Pathology

There is an endocapillary proliferative glomerulonephritis, with a granular deposition of IgG, C3, and IgM. Electron microscopy shows dome-shaped subepithelial deposits in the glomerular basement membrane.

Investigations

Anti-streptolysin O titers rise at 10–14 days after infection and peak at 4 weeks with a subsequent fall. C3 is reduced with normal C4 levels. Renal biopsy is generally performed to confirm the diagnosis.

Management

Antibiotics are given to eradicate persistent infection. Salt restriction and loop diuretics reduce fluid overload and control hypertension. Renal function improves spontaneously in most patients.

Outcome

In children the renal prognosis is excellent with most patients recovering normal renal function within 1–2 months. Adults are more commonly left with hypertension, proteinuria, and renal impairment.

Asymptomatic kidney problems

(a) Hypertension
(b) High serum creatinine
(c) Microscopic hematuria
(d) Proteinuria
(e) Hypokalemia
(f) Hyperkalemia
(g) Hyponatremia
(h) Hypernatremia

Some patients may be completely asymptomatic but discovered to have a clinical problem such as hypertension or microscopic hematuria. Others may be in hospital and during treatment may develop an abnormality such as hyperkalemia, which may be related to the underlying condition or medication.

Hypertension

Most are asymptomatic. However mild–moderate hypertension accelerates atherosclerosis and increases the risk of sudden death from coronary artery or cerebrovascular disease.

Treatment of mild hypertension reduces mortality and morbidity.

Hypertension is the commonest reason for seeing a physician in the United States. What constitutes hypertension depends on arbitrary definitions of normality. The level of blood pressure in a defined population is a continuously distributed variable. Such definitions differ according to patient groups, e.g. children, elderly, pregnant. One definition is the level of blood pressure at which benefits of intervention exceed the risks of non-intervention. An operational definition is tabulated in the 1997 report of the Sixth Joint National Committee on the Detection, Evaluation and Treatment of High Blood Pressure in Adults (Table 4.15).

There is evidence that pulse pressure (the difference between the systolic and diastolic pressures) correlates with clinical outcomes better than does the absolute level of the systolic and diastolic pressures. A further difficulty arises because blood pressure varies throughout the day. In some patients readings increase when blood pressure is taken by a doctor – so-called white coat hypertension. Twenty-four-hour

Table 4.15. Operational definitions of hypertension

Category	Systolic		Diastolic
Optimal	<120	and	<80
Normal	<130	and	<85
High normal	130–139	or	85–89
Hypertension			
Stage 1	140–159	or	90–99
Stage 2	160–179	or	100–109
Stage 3	>180	or	>110

Table 4.16. Associated features and age in the diagnosis of hypertension

Children	Young adults	Older adults
Chronic renal failure	Chronic renal failure	Chronic renal failure
Coarctation of aorta	Polycystic kidneys Conn's syndrome Cushing's syndrome Pheochromocytoma	Renovascular disease
Associated features	**Likely diagnosis**	**Other common features**
Family history	Essential hypertension	High salt intake Obesity Western population
Raised creatinine	Glomerulonephritis	Proteinuria Hematuria
Childhood urinary infections	Pyelonephritis	Loin pain
Bilateral renal masses	Polycystic kidneys	Family history
Renal bruits	Renovascular disease	Peripheral vascular disease
Radiofemoral delay	Coarctation of aorta	
Hypokalemia	Conn's syndrome	Alkalosis
Obesity	Cushing's syndrome	Striae Moon facies Glycosuria
Palpitations	Pheochromocytoma	Headache Sweating Anxiety Tremor

ambulatory blood pressure monitoring gives a truer reflection and can assist in a decision to initiate and monitor efficacy of treatment in borderline cases.

The assessment of the newly diagnosed patient with asymptomatic hypertension should consider:
(1) Is there a cause?
(2) How severe in terms of end-organ damage?
(3) Are there other risk factors for vascular disease?
Most have essential hypertension. This is a diagnosis of exclusion. Only approximately 5% of cases have a secondary cause.

The principal secondary causes of hypertension are:

Renal parenchymal disease
Renovascular disease
Pheochromocytoma
Conn's syndrome
Cushing's syndrome
Coarctation of the aorta
Drugs, e.g. ciclosporin, prednisolone, oral contraceptives

The secondary causes can be divided according to age at presentation (Table 4.16).

Essential hypertension
Clinical features
Most patients are symptomless unless they enter an accelerated phase, as discussed above. Shortness of breath is the one symptom that is more common compared with normotensive controls. If end-organ damage occurs, then symptoms begin to accrue: heart failure (dyspnea, orthopnea, nocturia), renal failure (nausea, vomiting, edema), or cerebral dysfunction (stroke, headache). Severe hypertension (accelerated phase or "malignant"), which is relatively rare, causes blurred vision, headache, confusion, seizures, and shortness of breath. It causes death from cerebral hemorrhage, heart failure, ruptured aortic aneurysm, or renal failure. The fundus is examined for retinopathy, papilledema; soft exudates and hemorrhages indicate accelerated phase hypertension. The heart is examined for cardiac enlargement. The apex beat is usually forceful and displaced laterally due to left ventricular hypertrophy.

Epidemiology
A family history is common in essential hypertension. The precise genetic basis is poorly understood but involves several genes. A high salt intake in Western populations has been linked to prevalence. Women tolerate hypertension better than men. Blacks have higher blood pressure than non-Blacks and hypertension related mortality is higher especially from cerebrovascular accidents.

Pathology

Accelerated atherosclerosis with coronary artery disease, cerebrovascular disease, and peripheral vascular disease occur. There is left ventricular hypertrophy and thickening of the renal arterioles with nephrosclerosis. If accelerated phase hypertension supervenes, fibrinoid necrosis of small arteries and arterioles develops.

Investigations

Electrocardiography and echocardiography assess the degree of left ventricular hypertrophy. Urinalysis and creatinine determine if there is any renal damage or evidence of a renal cause for hypertension. Renal ultrasound is advised. This will detect the small, irregularly scarred kidneys of chronic pyelonephritis or enlarged polycystic kidneys. Asymmetric kidneys in an elderly person suggest renovascular disease.

Management

Advice should be given about lifestyle. Weight reduction, low salt diet, and exercise will all lower blood pressure. Antihypertensive agents include beta-blockers, diuretics, calcium channel blockers, alpha-blockers, ACE inhibitors, angiotensin 2 receptor blockers, methyldopa, moxonidine, hydralazine, and minoxidil. The choice of drug or which combination to use depends on the individual patient's condition, how effective the drug is, and its side effects. Once started, in general treatment is lifelong.

Outcome

There is a clear linear correlation between arterial pressure and risk of death. The risk of morbidity or death at any level of arterial pressure is affected by other adverse factors such as hypercholesterolemia, smoking, and diabetes.

Renal parenchymal diseases

These have been discussed. Glomerulonephritis, chronic pyelonephritis, and polycystic kidney disease can all present with hypertension. One common diagnostic dilemma is whether a patient with hypertension and proteinuria has a primary renal disease or essential hypertension with proteinuria secondary to end-organ damage. If the proteinuria resolves with optimal blood pressure control, the latter is the most likely diagnosis. However, a renal biopsy may be necessary to discriminate between these possibilities. Microscopic hematuria and renal impairment usually only occur secondary to accelerated phase hypertension.

Renovascular disease

Atherosclerotic renovascular disease was covered above and is a common cause of hypertension in the elderly. Fibromuscular hyperplasia is a disease that tends to affect mainly young females and can cause severe hypertension. It is curable with renal artery angioplasty. For this reason if a young woman presents with hypertension and no strong family history of essential hypertension or obvious secondary cause, consideration should be given to imaging the renal arteries.

Pheochromocytoma

Pheochromocytomas secrete catecholamines to cause hypertension.

Clinical features

These tumors arise at any age but most commonly between ages 20 and 50. Some patients may have sustained hypertension, whereas others have paroxysmal attacks of severe hypertension caused by catecholamine release. During this time patients may describe symptoms of headache, anxiety, palpitations, sweating, and tremor. Attacks last between 15 minutes and 1 hour.

Epidemiology

Pheochromocytomas account for 0.5%–1% of all hypertension. They may be sporadic, familial, or be part of a wider syndrome such as neurofibromatosis or von Hippel–Lindau disease.

Pathology

Pheochromocytomas arise from chromaffin cells of neuroectodermal origin. They are most commonly found in the adrenal medulla, but can be anywhere in the sympathetic nervous system from the neck to the bladder. They are bilateral in 10% of cases, and malignant in 10% of cases.

Investigations

24-hour urinary excretion rates of norepinephrine, epinephrine, and their metabolites are measured as are plasma levels. Localization is with CT and ^{131}I meta-iodo-benzyl-guanidine (MIBG) scanning (Fig. 4.16).

Management

Surgical removal of the pheochromocytoma cures hypertension in 75%. Careful preparation with alpha and beta blockade is important in preparation for surgery.

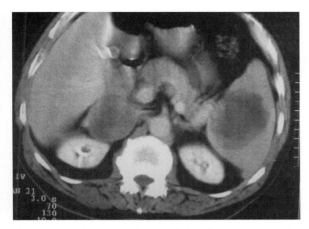

Fig. 4.16. CT showing a right adrenal pheochromocytoma and a left splenic metastasis.

Outcome

The outcome is good if surgery is successful. In patients with malignant tumors, radiotherapy and targeted treatment with ^{131}I MIBG can be given. The tumors tend to be very slow growing.

Conn's syndrome

Primary hyperaldosteronism (Conn's syndrome) causes hypertension by excessive production of aldosterone from the adrenal cortex, presumably due to excess sodium retention and volume expansion (Fig. 4.17).

Clinical features

Hypokalaemia with alkalosis is usually found, and thirst and polyuria occur secondary to the effect of hypokalemia on the urinary concentrating mechanism. Accelerated phase hypertension may occur.

Hypokalemia commonly occurs in essential hypertension due to the use of diuretics, and in accelerated phase hypertension due to secondary hyperaldosteronism.

Pathology

Excess aldosterone production may be from an adrenal adenoma, or from bilateral micronodular hyperplasia.

Investigations

Plasma sodium is at the upper limit of the normal range in contrast to the hyponatremia of secondary hyperaldosteronism. Plasma aldosterone level is raised, and plasma renin level suppressed. The normal aldosterone/renin ratio is 10, but in primary hyperaldosteronism the ratio is greater than 20. Renin levels fail to rise in response to standing up or sodium depletion, and aldosterone levels fail to suppress after saline infusion. Imaging is by CT and labeled cholesterol scintiscans.

Management

Surgical removal of an adrenal adenoma results in cure of the hypertension in 50%–60% of cases. The treatment of choice for bilateral adrenal hyperplasia is medical with spironolactone or amiloride.

Cushing's syndrome

This is covered in Chapter 12. Moderate hypertension is common in Cushing's syndrome, and it may develop into the accelerated phase in a few cases. Cardiovascular disease is a common cause of death in this condition.

Coarctation of the aorta

This is usually diagnosed during childhood, but can be missed and present later in life with severe hypertension. There may be tiredness in the legs on exertion. There is radiofemoral delay, and enlarged collateral vessels which may be visible around the scapulae. Imaging is by aortography. Treatment is surgical and is best performed before the age of 5. Hypertension is improved but not often cured by surgery.

Drugs

Cocaine can cause accelerated phase hypertension and myocardial infarction. Therapeutic drugs such as prednisolone, ciclosporin, and tacrolimus all cause hypertension in renal transplant recipients. Estrogen containing oral contraceptive pills can induce hypertension which takes 3 months to correct after discontinuing the drug.

High serum creatinine

Serum creatinine is the blood test generally used to measure renal function. Creatinine is secreted by skeletal muscles and excreted by the kidneys. Serum creatinine level is dependent on two variables: muscle mass and renal function. In a very muscular individual serum creatinine may be slightly above the normal range even with normal renal function. However, in most cases an elevated creatinine is due to impaired renal function. It is also important to appreciate that a slight reduction in glomerular filtration rate may not be reflected in a rise in serum creatinine above the normal range. For this reason, if subtle decrements in renal function need to be detected, a ^{51}Cr-EDTA GFR is performed.

A rise in serum creatinine may be due to permanent renal damage (chronic renal failure) or to a

113

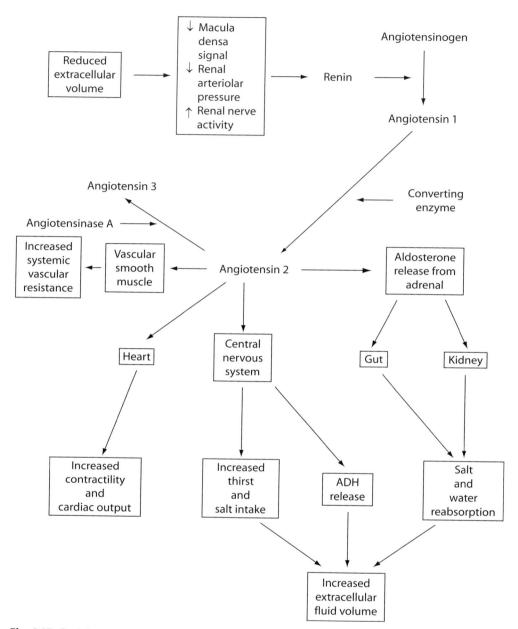

Fig. 4.17. Renin/angiotensin/aldosterone axis.

temporary reduction in renal function (acute renal failure).

Microscopic hematuria

Asymptomatic microscopic hematuria is commonly detected at routine medical check-ups. It is extremely common, with some estimates suggesting 2%–3% of the general population having dipstick positive hematuria. The approach to the

investigation and management of this presentation is discussed above.

Proteinuria

Asymptomatic proteinuria is often detected during routine examination. In women it may be discovered for the first time at an antenatal clinic. The approach to a patient with nephrotic syndrome is discussed in the peripheral edema section. All the conditions discussed in that section can also cause subnephrotic range proteinuria.

The normal 24-hour urinary excretion rate of protein is <0.15 g. If a young adult presents with a marginally increased level of proteinuria it is worth measuring lying and standing protein excretion rates. If proteinuria is greater on standing than lying, the patient has orthostatic proteinuria and no further investigation is required. The renal prognosis for orthostatic proteinuria is excellent.

Patients with severe cardiac failure or accelerated phase hypertension often have proteinuria, which resolves completely after controlling the blood pressure or treating the cardiac failure.

The threshold for performing a renal biopsy is arbitrary but most nephrologists would perform a biopsy if the protein excretion rate is greater than 1 g per day. Other indications for a renal biopsy include the presence of impaired renal function or the suspicion of a systemic disease such as vasculitis or myeloma.

Hypokalemia

Mild hypokalemia is asymptomatic. Muscle weakness progressing to paralysis and respiratory failure occurs only with severe hypokalaemia. Severe hypokalemia can also cause a paralytic ileus, atrial and ventricular arrhythmias, and enhance digitalis toxicity. Chronic hypokalemia causes renal tubular vacuolation and is a rare cause of chronic renal failure.

The causes of hypokalemia are listed below:

Vomiting	Gastroenteritis
	Pyloric stenosis
	Bulimia nervosa
Diarrhea	Gastroenteritis
	Ileostomy
	Purgative abuse
	Villous adenoma of rectum
Urinary losses	Diuretics
	Diuretic phase of acute renal failure
	Diabetes mellitus
	Primary hyperaldosteronism (Conn's)
	Secondary hyperaldosteronism
	Cushing's syndrome
	Bartter's syndrome
	Gitelman's syndrome
	Liddle's syndrome
	Renal tubular acidosis

Most of these conditions are considered elsewhere in this book. The cause of hypokalemia in an individual patient is usually obvious. Secondary hyperaldosteronism with hypokalemia can be a feature of common conditions such as accelerated phase hypertension, cardiac failure, and cirrhosis. Self-induced vomiting and purgative abuse is usually covert and part of the syndromes of anorexia/bulimia nervosa. These are eating disorders where the individual has an abnormal perception of their body weight, and is trying to reduce weight despite the fact he or she is very underweight. The condition usually affects young adult women. They may have scars on their hands, which are acid burns as a consequence of vomiting. They usually stop menstruating and lanugo hair grows on their limbs. Treatment often requires admission to an eating disorder unit with psychotherapy and a careful dietary program designed to increase body weight.

Bartter's, Gitelman's, and Liddle's syndromes are very rare but extremely interesting because the underlying pathophysiology has been elucidated in recent years. Bartter's syndrome causes a hypokalemic metabolic alkalosis. There is deficient renal reabsorption of sodium and chloride with hyperreninemia and hyperaldosteronism. Classic Bartter's syndrome is due to mutations in the chloride channel CLC-Kb in the thick ascending limb of the renal tubule. Neonatal Bartter's syndrome is caused by mutations in the NKCC2 (bumetanide-sensitive sodium–potassium–chloride cotransporter) or ROMK (potassium channel). Gitelman's syndrome causes hypokalemia, but differs from Bartter's syndrome by causing hypomagnesemia. The defect is in the *NCCT* gene coding for the thiazide-sensitive sodium chloride cotransporter in the distal convoluted tubule. Liddle's syndrome is a rare autosomal dominant condition presenting with hypertension and hypokalemia due to mutations in the amiloride-sensitive epithelial sodium channel.

The treatment of hypokalemia involves managing the underlying disease. Hypokalemia can be corrected using oral or intravenous potassium supplements. Potassium-sparing diuretics such as amiloride and spironolactone can be used.

Hyperkalemia

Hyperkalemia is usually asymptomatic. Severe hyperkalemia may present with fatigue, muscle weakness, and cardiac arrest. Pseudohyperkalemia is usually due to leakage of potassium from red cells if there is a delay between venepuncture and the sample being analyzed.

The major causes of hyperkalemia are listed below:

Acute and chronic renal failure

Drugs

Addison's disease

Isolated hypoaldosteronism

Renal tubular acidosis

These conditions are considered elsewhere in the book. Most cases of severe hyperkalemia occur in association with renal failure. Severe hyperkalemia can complicate renal failure when there is a large amount of tissue necrosis, for example in rhabdomyolysis or tumor lysis following chemotherapy.

The commonest causes of hyperkalemia are drugs, especially when a patient has pre-existing renal impairment. Angiotensin converting enzyme inhibitors, angiotensin 2 receptor blockers and spironolactone are commonly used in combination to treat patients with cardiac failure, but may induce severe hyperkalemia. These drugs need to be used with care and potassium levels need to be monitored. The immunosuppressive medications ciclosporin and tacrolimus also can cause hyperkalemia.

Adrenal insufficiency (Addison's disease) usually causes modest hyperkalemia (plasma potassium 5.0–6.5 mmol/l), hyponatremia and a slightly raised creatinine. The commonest cause of chronic hyperkalemia without severe renal failure is hyporeninemic hypoaldosteronism, which usually occurs in elderly diabetics.

ECG abnormalities in order of severity include tenting of T waves, absent P waves, widening of the QRS complex, slurring of the ST segment into the T waves, and a sine wave pattern immediately preceding cardiac arrest.

In severe cases, calcium gluconate given intravenously protects against cardiac arrhythmias. Dextrose and insulin, sodium bicarbonate, and beta 2 agonists will all temporarily lower potassium levels, but renal replacement therapy may be necessary. In milder cases oral or rectal calcium resonium can be given, but this is unpleasant to take and may cause constipation or fecal impaction.

Hyponatremia

Hyponatremia is commonly found in hospital patients. Mild cases are asymptomatic, but more severe cases may have symptoms of fatigue, loss of appetite, headache, confusion, muscle twitching, and coma.

Pseudohyponatremia is caused by severe hyperlipidemia or paraproteinemia. The true plasma sodium is normal, as is plasma osmolality.

Hyponatremia may be caused by:

(1) Massive sodium depletion

(2) Dilution due to excess water intake

(3) Syndrome of inappropriate ADH secretion

Sodium depletion

Severe sodium depletion stimulates ADH release and thirst. if water intake is increased without replacing sodium losses hyponatremia will result. Massive sodium losses can occur from the gut or kidneys. Gastro-intestinal losses occur as a result of diarrhea, vomiting, or sequestration of fluid within the bowel. Renal sodium losses may occur in chronic renal failure due to the impaired concentrating ability of the kidney, the recovery phase of acute tubular necrosis, after relief of bilateral ureteric obstruction, poorly controlled diabetes mellitus, and use of large doses of diuretics.

Sodium depletion sufficient to cause hyponatremia will usually cause signs of hypovolemia: tachycardia, postural hypotension, and reduced skin turgor. Hematocrit, creatinine, urea, and plasma proteins are raised. Urinary sodium concentration is less than 20 mmol/l if renal function is normal.

Management is with intravenous 0.9% sodium chloride with monitoring of renal function and venous pressure either clinically or via a central line.

Excessive water intake

Dilutional hyponatremia most commonly occurs in patients with impaired renal function, cardiac failure, cirrhosis, and nephrotic syndrome. In all these conditions there is an inability to excrete free water.

In hospital practice over generous fluid replacement with 5% dextrose after surgery commonly causes hyponatremia.

Some patients with acute psychoses or psychogenic polydipsia drink enough water in a short period of time to overwhelm the maximal rate of excretion of free water of a normal adult kidney, which is 10–20 ml/min.

Syndrome of inappropriate ADH secretion (SIADH)

SIADH is diagnosed if both renal and adrenal function are normal, and if there is no evidence of hypovolemia which might indicate sodium depletion. There is evidence of hypervolemia with low hematocrit, urea, creatinine and plasma protein levels. Urinary sodium excretion exceeds 20 mmol/l. Urinary osmolality is greater than that of plasma.

Major causes of SIADH are listed below:

(1) Carcinoma; most often small cell carcinoma of bronchus
(2) Central nervous system pathology
(3) Lung pathology, e.g. pneumonia, tumor
(4) Metabolic, e.g. acute porphyria
(5) Drugs, e.g. carbamazepine, vincristine, and cyclophosphamide

Management is by fluid restriction, and by treating the underlying pathology.

Hypernatremia

Hypernatremia is almost always due to massive depletion of water. This may be due to deficient water intake because the patient has no access to fluid or is unconscious. Excessive water losses can occur with protracted diarrhea and vomiting, sweating in hot climates and burns patients, and urinary losses in diabetes insipidus and a solute diuresis.

Acute hypernatremia causes cerebral dehydration, which can cause intracerebral hemorrhage. Symptoms include lethargy, muscle twitching, and coma. The aim of treatment is a gradual correction of the hypernatremia. Over-rapid correction may cause cerebral edema.

Further reading

ABC of Kidney Disease D Goldsmith *et al.* Blackwell Publishing, 2007.

Comprehensive Clinical Nephrology J Feehally *et al.* 3rd edn, Mosby Publishers, 2007.

Oxford Handbook of Nephrology and Hypertension S Steddon *et al.* Oxford University Press, 2006.

Oxford Textbook of Clinical Nephrology A Davison *et al.* 3rd edn, Oxford University Press, 2005.

The Kidney at a Glance C O'Callaghan *et al.* Blackwell Publishing, 2000.

Cardiovascular

Derek Hausenloy, Diana Gorog and Michael Marber

Contents

Chest pain

This is one of the cardinal symptoms of cardiovascular disease. However, many presenting to an emergency department with chest pain have a non-cardiovascular cause (Box 5.1).

Also see Table 5.1.

Ischemic heart disease (IHD)

This is the leading cause of mortality and morbidity in the Western world. It encompasses a spectrum of disease states including:

(1) chronic stable angina

(2) unstable angina, and

(3) acute myocardial infarction.

Clinical features

Symptoms Angina is chest discomfort due to myocardial ischemia. Chest pain can be classified into three categories according to the likelihood of IHD:

- **Typical** angina (definite):
   (1) Substernal chest discomfort with a characteristic quality and duration that is
   (2) provoked by exertion or emotional stress and is
   (3) relieved promptly (within 5 minutes) by rest or nitroglycerin
- **Atypical** angina (probable): Meets two of the above requirements
- **Non-cardiac** chest pain: Meets one or none of the above requirements

Depending on the presentation, patients can be considered to have chronic stable angina or acute coronary syndrome (ACS), which comprises the conditions of unstable angina and acute myocardial infarction. Making the distinction is essential for appropriate treatment. It is also important to identify risk IHD factors (Box 5.2).

- **Stable angina**
   The anginal chest pain only comes on with exertion or emotional stress and lasts 2–10 minutes.
- **Unstable angina**
   The anginal chest pain occurs at rest and lasts more that 20 minutes or is new in onset and occurring with increasing frequency.
- **Acute myocardial infarction**
   Prolonged severe anginal chest pain lasting more than 30 minutes, often associated with nausea, vomiting, and perspiration.

Anginal severity can be classified according to the Canadian Cardiovascular Society:

I   "Ordinary physical activity does not cause angina"
   Angina occurs with strenuous, rapid or prolonged exertion.

Box 5.1 Causes of chest pain	
Cardiovascular	
Cardiac	Ischemic heart disease
Aorta	Aortic dissection Thoracic aortic aneurysm
Pericardium	Pericarditis Cardiac tamponade
Pulmonary artery	Pulmonary embolus Pulmonary artery hypertension
Non-cardiovascular	
Pulmonary	Pleurisy Pneumothorax Pneumonia
Gastro-esophageal	Hiatus hernia Esophagitis or esophageal spasm Esophageal reflux Peptic ulcer Mallory Weiss syndrome/esophageal rupture
Chest wall	Chest injury or rib fracture Costochondritis or myositis Herpes zoster
Psychogenic	Da Costa's syndrome (stabbing discomfort localized to apex lasting 1–2 seconds and associated with anxiety)

II "Slight limitation of ordinary activity"
Angina occurs on walking more than two blocks on the level or climbing more than one flight of stairs.

III "Marked limitation of ordinary activity"
Angina occurs on walking one to two blocks on the level or climbing one flight of stairs.

IV Angina occurs either at rest or with any physical activity.

Examination Usually no helpful clinical features but, if still in pain or unstable angina or myocardial infarction, there may be anxiety and signs of distress, diaphoresis, nausea and vomiting, sinus tachycardia, and signs of ischemic mitral regurgitation.

Epidemiology
12% of the UK population live with IHD, costing the economy £7055 million a year. It is the leading cause of death in the UK with more than one in five men and one in six women dying from the disease. Since the early 1970s, death rates from IHD have fallen, and by 44% in those under age 65, because of reduction in major risk factors, especially smoking. However, by 2020 the World Health Organization predicts that IHD will be the leading cause of death worldwide.

Pathology
Atherosclerotic plaques within walls of coronary arteries are the predominant cause of coronary artery obstruction and comprise a relatively cell-free fibrin cap overlying a cholesterol-rich lipid core of macrophages, foam cells (modified macrophages), and leukocytes.

- **Stable angina.** Atherosclerotic plaques (Fig. 5.1) produce fixed coronary artery obstructions. This may allow sufficient blood flow to meet myocardial oxygen demand at rest but there is insufficient to meet increased requirements during exercise.
- **Unstable angina.** Rupture of an atherosclerotic plaque and formation of non-occlusive thrombus causes acute myocardial ischemia.
- **An acute myocardial infarction.** Rupture of an atherosclerotic plaque and thrombus formation causes complete occlusion of a major coronary artery.

Investigations
Patients presenting with chest pain should be managed according to the treatment pathways depicted in Fig. 5.2, and with investigations shown below.

(1) **Electrocardiogram**
- **Stable angina.** Normal in 50% of patients.
- **Unstable angina.** ST-segment depression and/or T wave inversion (Fig. 5.3).
- **Non ST-elevation MI (NSTEMI).** ST-segment depression and/or T wave inversion with raised cardiac biomarkers.
- **ST-elevation MI (STEMI).** ST-elevation of ≥ 2 mm in two contiguous precordial (V1–V6) leads or ST elevation of ≥ 1 mm in two contiguous limb leads.

(2) **Chest X-ray**
- Usually normal.
- Widening of the upper mediastinum may indicate aortic dissection.

(3) **Blood tests**
- **Hemoglobin** to exclude anemia.
- **Blood glucose** to exclude diabetes mellitus.

119

Table 5.1. Features of history and examination helpful in differentiating the cause of chest pain

Differential diagnosis						
	Ischemic heart disease	Aortic dissection	Pericarditis	Pulmonary embolus	Gastroesophageal	Others
Nature	Crushing/heaviness Pressure/discomfort	Sudden onset Tearing, knife-like	Sharp/stabbing Knife-like	Pleuritic Sharp/stabbing	Sharp or dull	Sharp Stabbing
Location	Retrosternal	Anterior chest	Over sternum Over cardiac apex	Anywhere in chest	Substernal Epigastric	Anywhere
Radiation	Left arm/jaw/back	Back	Neck or left shoulder	None	Back	None
Precipitating factors	Exertion Cold weather Emotion	Constant	Lying down Inspiration	Inspiration Coughing	Food In between meals Lying down	Constant Movement Palpation
Relieving factors	Rest Nitroglycerin	Constant	Sitting forward	None	Food/antacids Nitroglycerin (esophageal spasm) Belching	Position Belching
Duration	<2–10 minutes (angina) <20 minutes (unstable) >30 minutes (MI)	Constant	Constant	Minutes to 1 hour	Constant	Constant Fleeting <15 seconds
Associated features	Nausea/vomiting Perspiration Shortness of breath Risk factors for IHD	Hypertension Predisposition (Marfan's) Aortic regurgitation BP asymmetry Neurologic deficit	Pericardial friction rub Fever History of viral illness	Pleural rub Hemoptysis Shortness of breath Hypotension Raised JVP Left parasternal heave Tachycardia	Epigastric pain Dysphagia Acid reflux	Emotional stress Chest wall tender

Box 5.2 Risk factors for ischemic heart disease

Risk factors	Fold increase in IHD risk	
Non-modifiable		
Age		
Gender	2:1	Men : women
Family history (primary relatives <60 years)		
Ethnicity	1.5	South Asian
	0.5	Afro-Caribbean
Previous cerebrovascular or peripheral vascular disease	2.5–6	
Modifiable		
Smoking	3.0	Active smoking
	1.25	Passive smoking
Hypertension	2	
Diabetes mellitus	2–4	Men
	3–5	Women
Obesity (especially centripetal)	2	BMI 25–29 kg/m^2
	3.6	BMI >29 kg/m^2
Hypercholesterolemia (total chol >5 mmol/l)	10% increase in cholesterol is associated with 20–30% increase in risk	
Alcohol excess		
Physical inactivity (<30 minutes/week)	2	

Table 5.2. Localization of a myocardial infarction according to the ECG leads involved

ST elevation in leads	Classification of MI
II, III and aVF	Inferior left ventricle (Fig. 5.4)
V1–V6	Anterolateral left ventricle
V1–V3	Anteroseptal left ventricle (Fig. 5.5)
V4–V6	Apical or lateral left ventricle
V6, I, and aVL	Lateral left ventricle
V7–V9 (back of heart)	Posterior left ventricle (ST depression in V1–V3)
V1, V_3R–V_6R	Right ventricle

- **Full lipid profile** to exclude dyslipidemia
- **Cardiac biomarkers:** Raised Troponin I or T or raised CK-MB, 12 hours following the onset of chest pain, may indicate an acute myocardial infarction.

(4) *Echocardiography*
- Hypokinesia (reduced) or akinesia (absent) movement and thickening of the ventricular wall may indicate acute myocardial ischemia.

Depending on which ECG leads demonstrate the ST elevation, the area of myocardial infarction can be identified (see Table 5.2).

If diagnosis of stable angina is suspected, the standard investigations are in Figs. 5.6 and 5.7.

Investigating patients presenting with chest pain suggestive of stable angina:

(1) *Exercise ECG testing* on treadmill until either a standard percentage (usually 85%) of the age-determined maximum heart rate is reached, or an absolute indication for stopping.

Criteria for a positive exercise test

Horizontal or down-sloping ST-segment depression ≥1 mm for ≥ 60–80 ms after the end of the QRS complex.

Absolute contraindications to exercise testing
- Acute MI within 2 days
- Arrhythmias causing symptoms or hemodynamic compromise
- Severe aortic stenosis
- Acute pulmonary embolus, myocarditis, or pericarditis

Management

Management of stable angina (Box 5.3)

(1) Pharmacologic agents which control anginal symptoms.
(2) Pharmacologic agents which improve morbidity and mortality.
(3) Modification of risk factors for IHD to prevent progression of disease.

Where there is suspicion of ST-elevation myocardial infarction, unstable angina or non-ST elevation myocardial infarction, the investigation and treatment are summarized in Fig. 5.7.

An example of a coronary angiogram is shown in Fig. 5.8.

Percutaneous coronary intervention (PCI) The revascularization of coronary arteries using an angioplasty

121

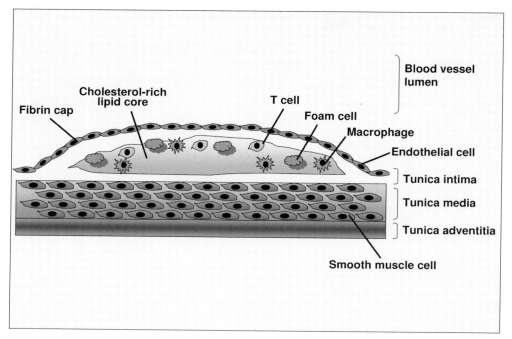

Fig. 5.1. A diagram depicting an atherosclerotic plaque.

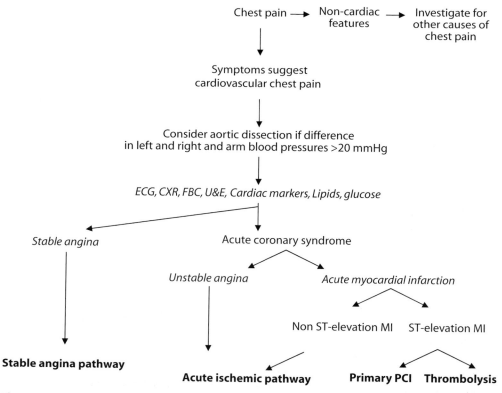

Fig. 5.2. Initial management of chest pain.

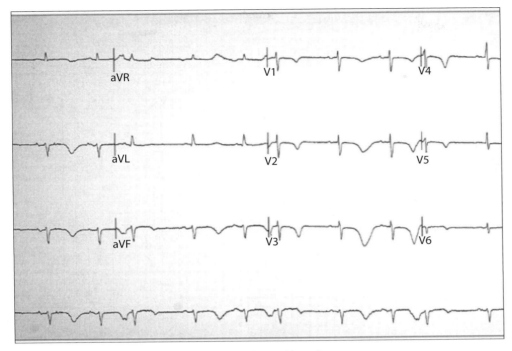

Fig. 5.3. Electrocardiogram of a patient presenting with unstable angina.

balloon and stents (Fig. 5.9), in patients presenting acutely with an ACS or elective patients with stable angina who have coronary artery stenoses amenable to PCI. Newer stents are coated with drugs (drug-eluting stents), which reduce the rate of stent restenosis to 5%–10%.

ST-elevation myocardial infarction ST elevation MI (STEMI), requires immediate reperfusion using primary PCI (Fig. 5.9) or thrombolysis to limit infarct size, which determines prognosis. Primary PCI is more effective than thrombolysis in achieving sustained reperfusion and risk of CVA is lower. Where primary PCI is unavailable, patients should be thrombolyzed or transferred to a tertiary center.

Thrombolysis Breaks down thrombus, restoring blood flow to the ischemic myocardium, and reduces mortality by 25% if given within 12 hours of pain onset. Limitations to rapid thrombolysis include:
- Time from experiencing chest pain to calling the emergency medical services – patient education should improve this.
- Time to hospital – pre-hospital thrombolysis by GPs or paramedics should improve this.

- Time to administer thrombolysis in hospital (door-to-needle time should be <20 minutes) – thrombolysis in the emergency department improves this.
- Time from receiving the call for emergency services to thrombolysis should be less than 60 minutes (call-to-needle time).

The main thrombolytic agents are streptokinase, alteplase (recombinant human tissue plasminogen activator), reteplase, and tenecteplase. Complications of thrombolysis include: hemorrhagic stroke (<1.0%), bleeding, hypotension, allergic reaction, and arrhythmias.

Contraindications
Absolute
  Previous hemorrhagic stroke at any time
  Previous CVA within 1 year
  Intracranial neoplasm
  Active internal bleeding (not including menses)
  Suspected aortic dissection

Relative
  Severe uncontrolled hypertension (BP >180/110)
  History of CVA

123

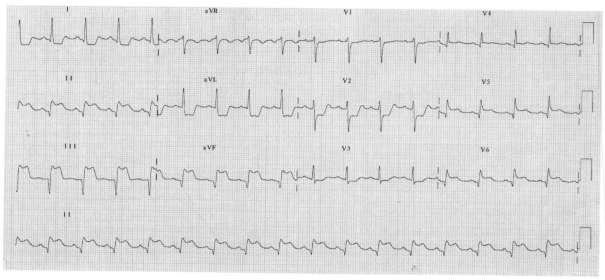

Fig. 5.4. Electrocardiogram of a patient presenting with an acute inferior myocardial infarction.

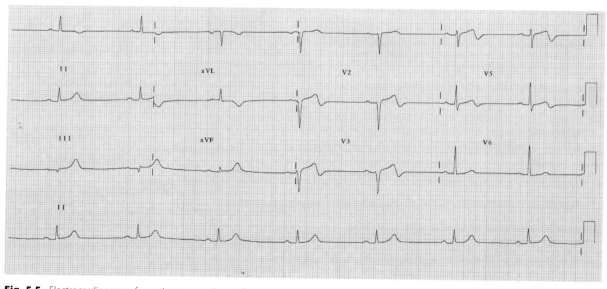

Fig. 5.5. Electrocardiogram of a patient presenting with an acute anterior myocardial infarction.

Current use of anticoagulants (INR 2–3)

Recent trauma (within 2–4 weeks) or prolonged (>10 minutes) traumatic cardio-pulmonary resuscitation

Non-compressible vascular puncture

Recent (within 2–4 weeks) internal bleeding

For streptokinase, prior exposure within 5 days to 2 years, or prior allergic reaction

Pregnancy

Active peptic ulcer

Chronic severe hypertension

Complications of myocardial infarction (MI)
(1) Arrhythmias
(2) Heart failure
(3) Pericarditis with or without pericardial effusion
(4) Acute mitral regurgitation due to rupture of papillary muscle

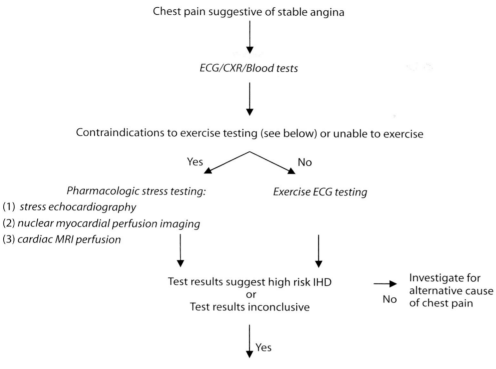

Chest pain suggestive of stable angina

ECG/CXR/Blood tests

Contraindications to exercise testing (see below) or unable to exercise

Yes   No

Pharmacologic stress testing: *Exercise ECG testing*
(1) *stress echocardiography*
(2) *nuclear myocardial perfusion imaging*
(3) *cardiac MRI perfusion*

Test results suggest high risk IHD   Investigate for
                        or   No   alternative cause
Test results inconclusive   of chest pain

Yes

(1) Medical treatment which controls symptoms and improves prognosis
(2) Modify IHD risk factors
(3) Coronary angiography/revascularization should be undertaken
     unless contraindicated

Fig. 5.6. Investigation and management of stable angina.

(5) Ventricular septal defect
(6) Free wall rupture and cardiac tamponade
(7) Dressler's syndrome – recurrent pericarditis usually 1–4 weeks following MI
(8) Venous thrombosis and pulmonary embolism
(9) Left ventricular aneurysm
(10) Left ventricular thrombus and arterial embolism

Post-MI care
- Physical activity gently increasing over 4–6 weeks.
- Most return to work within 2–3 months.
- Sexual activity is best avoided for 2 weeks and car driving 4 weeks.

Cardiac rehabilitation
Multidisciplinary approach: patient education and counseling, secondary prevention of recurrent MI, exercise to improve functional capacity and cardiovascular efficiency. The aim is to alleviate psychosocial effects and return to normal life.

Secondary prevention of recurrent MI
Lifestyle modification, lipid-lowering therapy, antiplatelet agents, beta-blockers, and ACE inhibitors.

Outcome
Half die before reaching hospital and post-hospital, discharge mortality rates are 5%–10% for ages 50–70 compared with a population mortality rate of 1% per year.

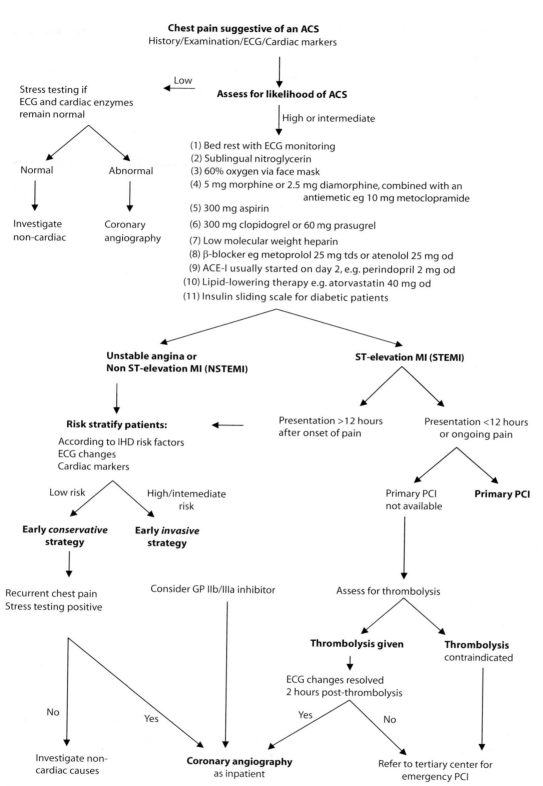

Fig. 5.7. Treatment pathway for acute coronary syndrome (ACS).

Box 5.3 Treatment of stable angina

A. Pharmacologic agents which have anti-anginal and anti-ischemic properties

(1) Beta-blockers
Decrease myocardial oxygen demand by decreasing heart rate, contractility, and arterial pressure.

(2) Calcium antagonists
Attenuate transmembrane calcium entry into the cell, decrease myocardial and smooth muscle contraction, reducing myocardial oxygen demand, heart rate, and producing vasodilatation.

(3) Long-acting nitrates
Coronary arterial vasodilatation and reduce venous return.

(4) Nicorandil
Opens the ATP-dependent potassium channel, releasing nitric oxide, causing vasodilatation.

(5) Ivabradine
Sinus node channel antagonist reduces heart rate. Best for patients intolerant of beta blockers.

B. Pharmacologic agents which reduce death/MI

(1) Aspirin
Inhibits cyclooxygenase and synthesis of platelet thromboxane A2, preventing platelet aggregation. Reduces risk of MI/death by about a third in IHD.

(2) Clopidogrel
Inhibits platelet aggregation by preventing adenosine diphosphate-mediated activation of platelets, and should be used if aspirin is contraindicated or has had to be stopped due to side effects.

(3) HMG-CoA reductase inhibitors ("statins")
Reduce MI/death by 30% in IHD.

(4) ACE Inhibitors
Reduce MI/death by 17% in IHD.

(5) Omega-3 polyunsaturated fatty acids (fatty fish oils)
Reduce MI/death by about 20% in IHD.

C. Modification of IHD risk factors

(1) Stop smoking
(2) Exercise (at least 30 minutes 3–4 times a week)
(3) Weight loss (attain BMI 20–25)
(4) Diet (5 portions of fruit or vegetables daily)
(5) Tight control of blood pressure (BP<130/80 mmHg)
(6) Tight control of diabetes mellitus (Hb1AC<7%)

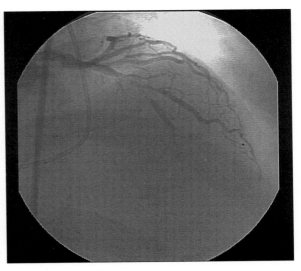

Fig. 5.8. Example of a coronary angiogram.

Aortic dissection

Etiology of aortic dissection

Medial degeneration	Cystic medial degeneration (Marfan's and Ehlers–Danlos syndromes) Advanced age Hypertension
Hypertension	Present in 80% of patients
Pregnancy	
Bicuspid aortic valve	
Unicuspid aortic valve	
Coarctation of the aorta	
Noonan syndrome	
Turner syndrome	
Aortitis	Especially giant cell arteritis
Trauma	
Cardiac surgery	

Aortic dissection is classified using either the DeBakey, Stanford or Descriptive system, according to the site of origin of the dissection (either proximal or distal to the origin of the left subclavian artery) and its propagation (Fig. 5.10).

Clinical features

History Sudden onset severe "tearing," "ripping," or "stabbing" anterior or interscapular chest pain in 70%–90% accompanied by diverse symptoms and signs.

Symptoms

- Chest pain or interscapular pain
- Syncope
- Acute myocardial infarction
- Leg weakness

Examination

Blood pressure	Difference between right and left arm blood pressures
Pulses	Loss of peripheral pulses
Added sounds	Aortic regurgitation murmur Bruits over subclavian artery
Lungs	Pleural effusion
Others	CVA or paraplegia Congestive cardiac failure

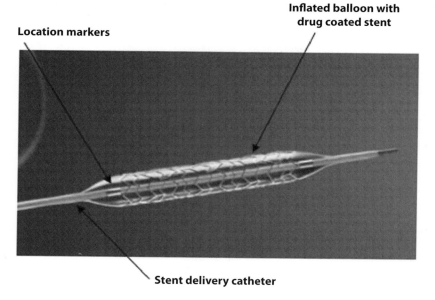

Location markers

Inflated balloon with drug coated stent

Stent delivery catheter

Fig. 5.9. Close-up view of a coronary artery stent.

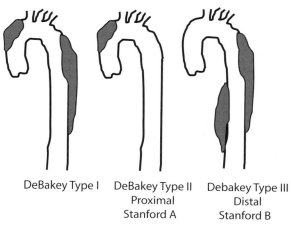

DeBakey Type I

DeBakey Type II
Proximal
Stanford A

Debakey Type III
Distal
Stanford B

Fig. 5.10. Types of aortic dissection.

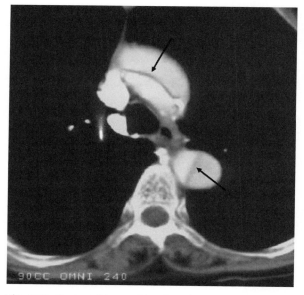

Fig. 5.11. Contrast CT scan of the chest demonstrating an aortic dissection of the ascending aorta.

Epidemiology

Marfan's syndrome accounts for 6%–9%. Peak incidence is sixth and seventh decades and three times more common in men. Bicuspid aortic valves are associated with 7%–14% of cases. In women less than 40 years half occur during pregnancy, usually in the third trimester.

Pathology

A tear in the aortic intima allows blood to penetrate the media layer forming a false lumen, or rupture of a vasa vasorum within the media causes intramural hematoma rupturing the intimal layer.

Investigations

Investigation of chest pain suggestive of an aortic dissection

(1) **Contrast CT** – investigation of choice with diagnosis based on presence of two aortic lumens separated by an intimal flap (see Fig. 5.11).

(2) **Echocardiography** – diagnosis based on the finding of an intimal flap within the aortic lumen, and colour flow demonstrating two lumens.

Aortic regurgitation due to dilatation of the aortic annulus may be present.

(3) **Chest X-ray** – Widened mediastinum due to widening of the aortic silhouette (81%–90% of cases). Pleural effusion (usually on the left side). Up to 12% of patients may have a normal chest X-ray.

(4) **ECG** – If the proximal aortic dissection has involved the coronary arteries, evidence of acute myocardial ischemia may be seen.

(5) **MRI** – MRI is the gold standard for diagnosing aortic dissection but its availability is restricted.

Management

To stop progression of dissection, vascular compromise and aortic rupture, aggressive blood pressure control maintains systolic blood pressure between 100 and 120 mmHg. For proximal aortic dissections, surgical repair is the best choice. For distal dissections, medical therapy is indicated but vital organ compromise also demands surgery.

Outcome

Untreated, mortality is 25% within first 24 hours 50% first week, 75% within 1 month and 90% within a year.

Pericarditis

Most acute cases are viral and may be preceded by upper respiratory tract infection.

Etiology of acute pericarditis

Idiopathic

Viral infections	(Coxsackie A and B, echovirus, adenovirus, mumps virus, infectious ononucleosis, varicella, hepatitis B, and AIDS)
Acute bacterial infection	(*Pneumococcus, Staphylococcus, Streptococcus, Neisseria meningitidis, Neisseria gonorrheae, Legionella, Pasteurella*)

Acute myocardial infarction
Uremia
Neoplasm
Trauma to the chest
Cardiac trauma (following cardiac surgery, pacemaker insertion, angioplasty)
Tuberculosis
Fungal infections
Radiation

Autoimmune disorders	(acute rheumatic fever, SLE, rheumatoid arthritis, scleroderma, Wegener's granulomatosis, polyarteritis nodosa)
Drugs	(hydralazine, procainamide, phenytoin, isoniazid, dantrolene, doxorubicin, methysergide, penicillin)
Dressler's syndrome	(post-myocardial infarction)

Dissecting aortic aneurysm
Myxedema

Clinical features

Features to elicit in the history and examination findings in acute pericarditis

Chest pain	Often localized to retrosternal and left precordial regions and frequently radiates to the neck. May be precipitated by lying flat, coughing, inspiration, swallowing and alleviated by sitting up and leaning forward.
Dyspnea	Due to pleuritic chest pain, a pericardial effusion or the associated fever.
Fever	

Examination
A pericardial friction rub is pathognomonic and is best heard at the lower left sternal edge, with the patient leaning forward. It sounds like a scratching, grating, high pitched sound, which is unrelated to the heart sounds.

Epidemiology

Commoner in males, and commonest in adolescents and young adults.

Pathology

Acute inflammation with infiltration of polymorphonuclear leukocytes, increased pericardial vascularity, and deposition of fibrin.

Investigations

(1) **ECG** – 90% have changes
 - Widespread "saddle-shaped" (concave-upwards) ST-elevation.
 - T wave inversion.

(2) **Chest X-ray**
 - Cardiac silhouette may be increased and globular.
 - Pleural effusions in 25%, usually on left side.
 - Evidence of pulmonary disease may be present, such as tuberculosis or neoplasm.

129

(3) Blood tests
- An acute inflammatory response with raised white cell count, ESR and C-reactive protein.
- Modest increase in cardiac markers due to myocardial inflammation injury.

(4) Echocardiography
- The most accurate method for detecting and quantifying pericardial fluid, which may develop following an episode of pericarditis.

Management
- Bed rest and overnight observation if serious disease apparent.
- Monitor for cardiac tamponade which develops in 15%.
- Non-steroidal anti-inflammatory agents.

Outcome

Most are self-limiting, resolving within 2–6 weeks. Acute pericarditis can be complicated by recurrent pericarditis, pericardial effusion, cardiac tamponade, and fibrosis, and/or calcification of pericardium resulting in constriction.

Palpitations

Awareness of forceful or rapid heart beating. The patient may describe it as a "pounding, fluttering, jumping, racing, or irregularity" of the heart. Palpitations are usually due to intermittent arrhythmias as below:

Atrial or ventricular ectopy

Junctional or ventricular paced rhythm

Tachyarrhythmias

Sinus tachycardia

Atrio-ventricular nodal reciprocal tachycardia (AVNRT)

Atrio-ventricular reciprocal tachycardia (AVRT)

Atrial fibrillation

Atrial tachycardias including atrial flutter

Ventricular tachycardia

History

Crucial information required from the history is listed below.

(1) Description
- Description in patient's own words.
- "Skipped beats" may be describing atrial or ventricular premature contractions.
- The patient is usually aware of the compensatory pause that follows an ectopic

beat, or the forceful post-extrasystolic beat which follows the pause.
- Ask the patient to tap the palpitations out on the table.
- Irregular arrhythmias include atrial fibrillation and atrial tachycardias (including atrial flutter with variable block and multi-focal atrial tachycardia).

(2) The rapidity
- Fast or slow   Slow palpitations may represent an increased awareness of normal sinus rhythm, relatively slow tachycardias or infrequent premature contractions. Rapid palpitations may suggest a tachyarrhythmia.

(3) Onset and offset
- Paroxysmal tachycardias begin and end suddenly.
- Palpitations which begin and stop gradually may be due to a sinus tachycardia.

(4) Precipitating factors
- Atrial and ventricular ectopy are most often experienced at rest.
- Some arrhythmias may be brought on by alcohol, heavy smoking, caffeine, or drugs such as cocaine and amphetamine.

(5) Relieving factors
- Benign atrial and ventricular ectopy usually decreases on exercise.
- Junctional re-entrant tachycardias such as AVNRT can often be terminated by the patient themselves with vagal maneuvers, such as swallowing, drinking cold water, coughing, or straining or rubbing one side of the neck.

(6) Co-morbid conditions
- Such as pheochromocytoma, thyrotoxicosis, anemia, hypokalemia, hyperkalemia, postural hypotension, the menopause, anxiety, hypoglycemia, pulmonary embolus, mitral valve prolapse, or febrile states.
- A previous history of myocardial infarction or heart failure may suggest that the arrhythmia is due to ventricular tachycardia.

(7) Associated features and symptoms
- Polyuria following the palpitations may occur in a paroxysmal supraventricular tachycardia, due to the release of atrial natriuretic peptide

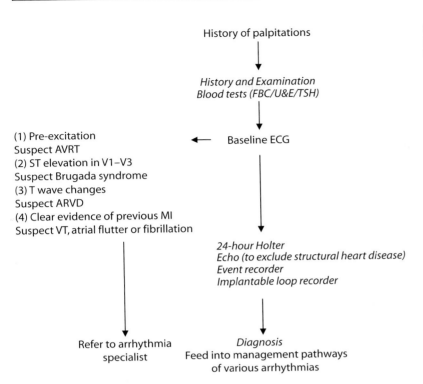

Fig. 5.12. General diagnostic pathway for patients giving a history of palpitations. For details see relevant sections in text.

History of palpitations

↓

History and Examination
Blood tests (FBC/U&E/TSH)

↓

(1) Pre-excitation
Suspect AVRT
(2) ST elevation in V1–V3
Suspect Brugada syndrome
(3) T wave changes
Suspect ARVD
(4) Clear evidence of previous MI
Suspect VT, atrial flutter or fibrillation

← Baseline ECG

↓

24-hour Holter
Echo (to exclude structural heart disease)
Event recorder
Implantable loop recorder

↓

Refer to arrhythmia specialist   *Diagnosis*
Feed into management pathways of various arrhythmias

---

from atria contracting against closed atrioventricular valves.

- *Chest pain* may occur before, during or after the onset of palpitations, an important distinction, as chest pain preceding the palpitation may suggest an ischemic etiology for the arrhythmia (such as a ventricular arrhythmia), whereas chest pain that is secondary to the palpitation may be due to tachycardia-induced myocardial ischemia.
- Pre-syncope and syncope may accompany palpitations and may suggest a ventricular arrhythmia.

General diagnostic approach to palpitations

The diagnostic pathway in Fig. 5.12 can be used for initial identification of causes in patients between episodes. The diagnostic pathway depicted in Fig. 5.13 applies to those presenting with palpitations. Once the diagnosis is established or suspected, management is outlined by the pathways specific to that type of arrhythmia.

General investigations used to identify the cause of palpitations

(1) **Blood tests**
- Electrolytes, hemoglobin, and thyroid function tests.

(2) **Baseline ECG**
- Pre-excitation (a PR interval <0.12 seconds) with a delta wave (slurred upstroke on QRS complex) in a patient with paroxysmal regular palpitations should suggest atrioventricular reciprocal tachycardia (AVRT).
- The presence of pre-excitation in a patient with paroxysmal irregular palpitations should suggest a diagnosis of Wolff-Parkinson-White syndrome. ECG changes suggesting previous myocardial infarction may increase the likelihood of ventricular arrhythmia.
- A prolonged QT interval could suggest a ventricular arrhythmia.

(3) **ECG during arrhythmia**
- Heart rate >100 bpm.
- Irregular tachycardias include atrial fibrillation, atrial tachycardia/flutter with variable atrioventricular block, and multifocal atrial tachycardia.
- Regular narrow complex (QRS duration <120 ms) tachycardias include AVNRT, AVRT, atrial tachycardia and atrial flutter.
- Regular wide complex (QRS duration >120 ms) tachycardias, include ventricular

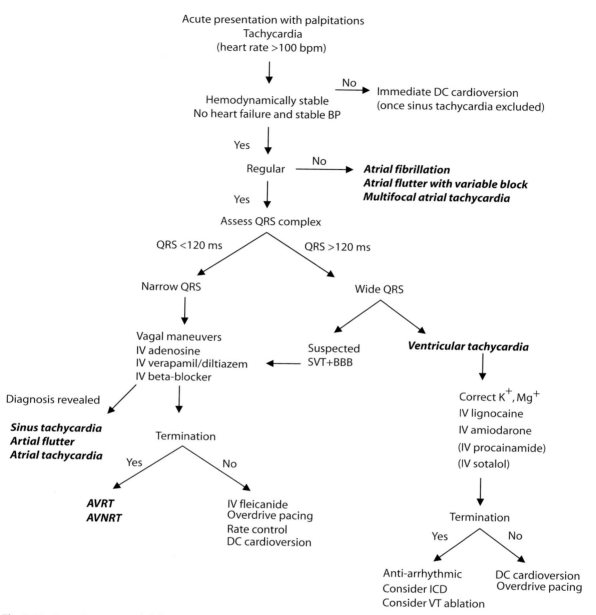

Fig. 5.13. General diagnostic/treatment pathway for acute tachyarrhythmias. For details see relevant sections in text.

tachycardia or supraventricular tachycardia (SVT) with aberrant conduction.

(4) **Response to vagal maneuvers, carotid sinus massage, or adenosine**

- Vagal maneuvers such as swallowing, coughing, straining, carotid sinus massage and administering i.v. adenosine, beta-blockers or calcium-channel blockers delay atrio-ventricular conduction, resulting in the termination of some

arrhythmias involving the atrio-ventricular node, such as AVRT and AVNRT.

- The slowing of the heart rate may also reveal atrial flutter waves, sinus tachycardia or atrial fibrillation without terminating the arrhythmia.

(5) **Exercise testing**

- Exercise testing can be useful for patients who describe palpitations on exercise,

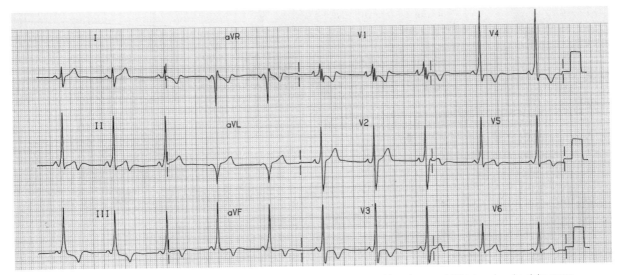

Fig. 5.14. Baseline electrocardiogram demonstrating the features of pre-excitation with a shortened PR interval and a delta wave (slurred upstroke of the QRS complex).

and may induce various types of supraventricular and ventricular arrhythmias.

(6) Echocardiography

- To exclude structural heart disease as a substrate for the arrhythmia.

(7) Cardiac MRI

- To exclude cardiomyopathy such as ARUD

(8) Ambulatory Holter recording

- 24–72 hour ambulatory Holter recording may be used to capture the arrhythmia, in patients experiencing palpitations two to three times a week.
- Should be accompanied by a patient diary describing their symptoms.

(9) Event recorders

- For those patients experiencing palpitations less frequently (about two episodes a month), these are more effective in capturing the arrhythmia.

These "loop" recorders monitor the ECG continuously; pressing the event button records the ECG for 30–60 seconds.

(10) Implantable loop recorders

- Used for infrequent palpitations (less than two episodes per month).
- Inserted beneath the skin they are capable of automatic or patient-activated event recording.

(11) Invasive electrophysiologic investigation and catheter ablation

- Involves the insertion of multi-polar catheters into the heart and positioning electrodes at various positions within the heart to record electrical activity.
- The heart is stimulated at various points and electrical activity is recorded at various intra-cardiac positions.
- Once the arrhythmia mechanism/circuit has been identified, radio-frequency ablation of this site can be performed to cure the arrhythmia (Fig. 5.14).

General mechanisms responsible for generation of cardiac tachyarrhythmias

Most cardiac arrhythmias are produced by one of three mechanisms:

(1) *Increased automaticity*

- Cells almost anywhere in the heart have the capacity to fire faster than the sinoatrial node and take over as the pacemaker of the heart when provoked by ischemia, changes in autonomic tone, hypoxemia, hypokalemia, hypomagnesemia, acid–base disorders, high sympathetic tone, anesthesia, and acute pulmonary disease. This mechanism accounts for about 10% of tachyarrhythmias and includes multifocal atrial tachycardias and junction rhythms.

(2) Re-entry
- Most common arrhythmia mechanism.
- Comprises the repetitive excitation of a region of the heart, due to the conduction of an electrical impulse between or around an electrical obstacle in the heart.
- This re-entrant circuit is initiated by a unidirectional conduction block in one arm of the circuit, due to the acceleration of heart rate or a premature impulse.
- Slow conduction is often present in part of the circuit, allowing initiation and perpetuation of the arrhythmia.
- Re-entry is the mechanism for SVTs such as AVRT, AVNRT, and atrial flutter.

(3) Triggered activity
- This has features in common with both automaticity and re-entry.

Anti-arrhythmic drugs have been traditionally categorized using the Vaughan-Williams classification, depending on their presumed mechanism of action.

Vaughan-Williams classification of anti-arrhythmic drugs

Class I	**Rapid sodium channel blockers** (this is the ion channel which opens allowing the rapid depolarization of membrane potential)
	(a) *Agents which prolong action potential duration* Quinidine Procainamide Disopyramide
	(b) *Agents that shorten duration of action potential* Mexiletine Phenytoin Lignocaine
	(c) *Agents which slow conduction* Fleicanide Propafenone
Class II	**Beta-blockers** (decrease sympathetic tone reducing conduction through SA and AV nodes).
Class III	*Agents which prolong repolarization and duration of action potential* Sotalol Amiodarone Dronedarone Bretylium

Class IV	**Calcium channel blockers** (reduce conduction through SA and AV nodes). Verapamil Diltiazem
Class V	**Digitalis agents** (increase vagal tone, reducing conduction through SA and AV nodes). Digoxin

Atrial or ventricular ectopy

Atrial or ventricular ectopy is the commonest cause of an irregular heart rhythm. The premature beat may originate from the ventricles, atria, or pulmonary veins. They can arise in both normal and structurally abnormal hearts.

Clinical features
In the patient with no structural heart disease, this is a benign condition. The patient often experiences a "skipped" or "missed" beat due to the pause that follows the extra-systolic beat. They typically occur at rest and decrease in frequency on exercise, if benign.

Investigations
ECG The atrial ectopic may have a P wave of different morphology from the sinus beat, but the QRS complex has the same morphology. The ventricular ectopic is characterized by a broad complex (QRS duration is usually >120 ms) that is of a different morphology from the sinus beat (Fig. 5.15)

Management and outcome
Premature atrial and ventricular complexes do not require therapy. If symptoms cause anxiety, a beta-blocker may be given.

Tachyarrhythmias
Sinus tachycardia
Increase in sinus rate greater than 100 bpm; it is the physiologic response to a variety of conditions.

Etiology of sinus tachycardia

Physiologic	Emotional stress
	Exercise
Pathologic	Thyrotoxicosis
	Pheochromocytoma
	Fever and sepsis
	Hypovolemia
	Anemia
	Pulmonary emboli
	Stimulants (caffeine, cocaine, alcohol, amphetamines, cannabis)

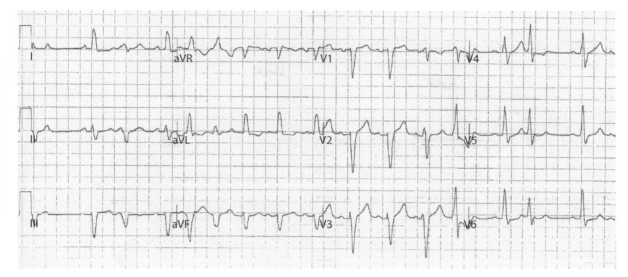

Fig. 5.15. Electrocardiogram demonstrating both atrial (supraventricular) and ventricular ectopic beats.

Medications (salbutamol, atropine, aminophyllines, catecholamines)
Anticancer treatments (doxorubicin, adriamycin, daunorubicin)
Heart failure
Cardiac tamponade
Inappropriate sinus tachycardia

Clinical features

The palpitations of sinus tachycardia are usually gradual in onset and cessation, distinguishing it from paroxysmal tachycardias, in which palpitations are sudden at start and finish.

Inappropriate sinus tachycardia may occur in health and is a persistent increase of resting sinus heart rate out of proportion to physical, emotional, pathologic, or pharmacologic stress. The two main mechanisms are increased automaticity of the sinus node and imbalance of autonomic regulation of the sinus node with reduced parasympathetic and excess sympathetic tone. A high proportion with inappropriate sinus tachycardia are healthcare professionals and 90% are female, from 30–40 years old.

Investigations, management, outcome

Investigations are undertaken to exclude the conditions listed above. Treatment of inappropriate sinus tachycardia includes beta-blockers, calcium channel blockers, or in severe cases catheter modification of the sinus node.

Atrio-ventricular nodal reciprocating tachycardia (AVNRT)

Clinical features
- Sudden onset, and terminate abruptly.
- Other symptoms may include dizziness, neck pulsations, dyspnea, chest pain, and more rarely syncope and polyuria.
- May be terminated by vagal maneuvers.

Epidemiology
Most common form of paroxysmal junctional tachycardia and occurs more often in women.

Pathology
The AVNRT is due to the re-entrant circuit involving two functionally and anatomically distinct pathways of a re-entrant circuit (Fig. 5.16):

(1) the *slow-conducting* pathway, which extends inferoposterior to the compact AV node and stretches along the septal margin of the tricuspid annulus at the level of the coronary sinus. This pathway usually acts as the anterograde limb of the circuit.

(2) the *fast-conducting* pathway, which is located near the apex of the Koch's triangle. This pathway usually acts as the retrograde limb of the circuit.

Investigations
The ECG during the arrhythmia shows a regular tachycardia (often at rates between 150 and 250 bpm).

135

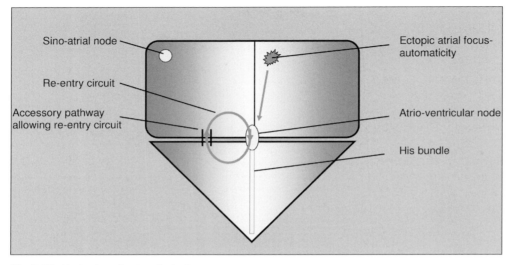

Fig. 5.16. Mechanism of tachyarrhythmias.

P waves are not usually visible as they are hidden within the QRS complex.

Management

For patients experiencing recurrent sustained episodes of tachycardia, the treatment options are:

(1) *Prophylactic pharmacologic therapy*

Oral therapy is only 30%–50% successful and requires lifelong therapy.

(a) Calcium channel blockers

(b) Beta-blockers

(c) Class I drugs such as fleicanide or propafenone

(2) *Catheter ablation*

Radio-frequency catheter ablation of the slow-conducting pathway is the treatment of choice and is 96% successful. There is a 1% risk of inducing second or third-degree heart block requiring a permanent pacemaker.

Atrioventricular reciprocating tachycardia (AVRT)

In this condition, there is an accessory pathway, usually remote from the AV node, which links the atria and ventricles.

Clinical features

The clinical features are as for AVNRT. Patients who have pre-excitation on resting ECG and also experience tachyarrhythmias are said to have *Wolff-Parkinson-White (WPW)* syndrome. Some accessory pathways are only capable of conducting in

the retrograde direction and are not apparent on a sinus rhythm ECG. This is a concealed accessory pathway.

Investigations

The resting ECG may demonstrate pre-excitation (PR interval <0.12 s) with delta waves (slurred upstroke of QRS complex). During the arrhythmia there may be a regular, narrow, complex tachycardia, often at rates between 150 and 250 bpm or *potentially* life-threatening fast atrial fibrillation. The P wave may be visible, usually after the QRS complex.

Management

Symptomatic patients For patients experiencing recurrent sustained episodes of tachycardia, the treatment options are:

(1) **Prophylactic pharmacologic therapy**

Usually a class Ic agent such as fleicanide with a beta-blocker.

(2) **Catheter ablation**

● Because of the risk of sudden death in WPW, radio-frequency catheter ablation of the accessory pathway is the treatment of choice and is curative in 96%.

● Recurrence rate is 5%.

● Major complications are complete AV block (1.0%), and cardiac tamponade (1.1%).

Outcome

The risk of death in WPW is 0.15%–0.39% over 3–10 years. Cardiac arrest may be the initial presentation in up to 50%. Asymptomatic patients should be offered assessment of the accessory pathway.

Atrial fibrillation (AF)

- A supraventricular tachycardia characterized by rapid and uncoordinated atrial activity with loss of atrial mechanical function.
- Most common arrhythmia.
- Usually associated with cardiopulmonary disease but not in 30% (so-called lone AF).
- AF is classified according to its temporal pattern as follows:

(1) Paroxysmal: terminates spontaneously.
(2) Persistent: sustained for more than 1 week.
(3) Permanent: sustained despite attempts at cardioversion.

Etiology of atrial fibrillation (AF)

Heart disease	Hypertension (especially when left ventricular hypertrophy is present)
	Valvular heart disease (usually mitral valve disease)
	Ischemic heart disease
	Congestive heart failure
	Hypertrophic cardiomyopathy
	Dilated cardiomyopathy
	Congenital heart disease (especially atrial septal defect)
	Sinus node disease
	Ventricular pre-excitation
	Restrictive cardiomyopathies (amyloidosis, hemochromatosis, endomyocardial fibrosis)
	Cardiac tumors
	Constrictive pericarditis
	Cor pulmonale
Lone AF	No evidence of cardiopulmonary abnormality in patients under 60 years of age
Secondary	Alcohol intake ("holiday heart syndrome")
	Myocardial infarction
	Cardiac surgery
	Pericarditis
	Myocarditis
	Hyperthyroidism
	Pulmonary embolism
	Pneumonia
	Acute pulmonary disease
	Diabetes mellitus
Familial	Familial AF

Clinical features

History

Symptoms of thyroid disease	
Alcohol history	
Chest pain	
Palpitations	Sudden onset, fast and irregular
Thromboembolism	CVA and arterial emboli
Polyuria	Due to the atrial release of atrial natriuretic peptide
Heart failure	
Fatigue/dyspnea	Due to reduced cardiac output associated with loss of AV synchrony, irregularity of the ventricular response, rapid ventricular rates, and loss of atrial filling.

Findings on examination

Pulse character	Irregularly irregular
Blood pressure	Hypertensive
JVP	Irregular venous pulsations
Heart sounds	Variation in the loudness of the first heart sound
Added sounds	Associated valvular lesions particularly mitral
Others	Evidence of congestive heart failure

Epidemiology

Below age 60, prevalence of AF is <1%, over 80 it is >6%. Lifetime risk is 26% for men and women over 40. Familial AF, although well characterized, is not common.

Pathology

In persistent AF, there is patchy fibrosis with normal and diseased atrial fibers juxtaposed, which may account for the heterogeneity in atrial refractoriness.

Mechanisms of AF

(1) *Enhanced automaticity in one or several rapidly depolarizing foci (focal initiation)*
(2) *Re-entry involving one or more circuits (multiple wavelets)*

Atrial electrical and mechanical remodeling

When AF becomes persistent, the likelihood of restoring and maintaining sinus rhythm is reduced due to shortening of the atrial refractory period and sometimes changes in conduction velocity. Atrial contractions contribute 20% of total cardiac output and AF

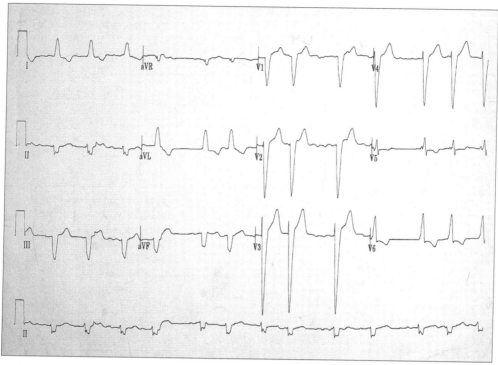

Fig. 5.17. Electrocardiogram demonstrating atrial fibrillation.

may further reduce cardiac output when LV function is impaired.

Investigations
Investigating atrial fibrillation

(1) Blood tests

Full blood count, serum electrolytes, and thyroid function tests.

(2) ECG (Fig. 5.17)

The rhythm is irregular and the P waves are replaced by rapid oscillations or fibrillatory waves, associated with a variable ventricular response.

(3) Chest X-ray

To detect cardiac enlargement and assess for pulmonary disease.

(4) Echocardiography

To assess for valvular disease, atrial size, LV dimensions and systolic/diastolic function, pulmonary artery pressure, LVH, LA thrombus, and pericardial disease.

(5) Exercise testing

This may be useful:

- If the adequacy of rate control in permanent AF needs to be determined

- To reproduce exercise-induced AF, and
- To exclude ischemia as a cause of AF or when a type IC anti-arrhythmic drug is being considered for treatment of AF.

(6) Holter monitoring/Event recorder

This is useful to assess adequacy of rate control in persistent or permanent AF and to detect AF in patients with suspected paroxysmal AF.

(7) Electrophysiologic study

This may be useful to help define the mechanism of AF, when curative radio-frequency ablation is being considered. The cause of AF may be a focus of activation in the vicinity of the pulmonary veins.

Management

The three main objectives in the long-term management of atrial fibrillation are listed below.

(1) Prevention of thromboembolism

The risk of a patient with AF developing thromboembolism is about 6 times that of patients in sinus rhythm. Risk factors for thromboembolism in patients with AF include:

(a) Previous stroke or transient ischemic attack (TIA)

(b) Diabetes mellitus

(c) Hypertension

(d) Impaired LV systolic function

(e) Advanced age (especially >75 years)

(f) Ischemic heart disease

(g) Hypertrophic cardiomyopathy

(h) Thrombus, spontaneous contrast, reduced blood flow velocity in the left atrial appendage (LAA)

Patients with AF over 65 years old or those with any of these risk factors for thromboembolism should be anticoagulated with warfarin, whereas all others should be given aspirin.

(2) *Rhythm control*

Restore and maintain sinus rhythm.

For patients over 65 years old this approach does not reduce thromboembolism and should only be considered for symptomatic AF.

Methods:

(a) ***Pharmacologic cardioversion*** using fleicanide, ibutilide, propafenone, or amiodarone.

(b) ***Synchronized electrical DC cardioversion***
Complications of electrical cardioversion include thromboembolism and arrhythmias (especially in the presence of hypokalemia or digoxin toxicity).

(c) ***Surgical ablation***

(d) ***Catheter ablation***
Anticoagulation is required for 3–4 weeks before DC cardio-version for AF of unknown duration, or for AF of more than 48 hours, and should be continued for at least 8 weeks after successful cardioversion to allow atrial contractility to return to normal.

For patients who are likely to relapse after successful cardioversion, maintenance drug therapy to maintain sinus rhythm may be indicated.

(3) *Rate control*

The aim is to accept the arrhythmia but to control the ventricular rate between 60 and 80 bpm at rest and 90–115 bpm during moderate exertion.

(a) ***Pharmacologic agents*** for controlling the ventricular rate in AF include: verapamil or diltiazem, digoxin, beta-blockers, or amiodarone.

(b) Patients with symptomatic rapid ventricular rates not controlled with conventional medical therapy may benefit from ***AV node ablation and permanent pacemaker implantation***.

An overview of the management of AF is outlined in Fig. 5.18.

Outcome

The risk of transient ischemic attacks (TIAs) and ischemic stroke in patients with non-rheumatic AF is 7% per year. One in every six strokes occurs in patients with AF. In patients with both AF and rheumatic heart disease, the risk of stroke increases 17 times. The mortality rate of patients with AF is almost double that of patients in sinus rhythm and is increased by 50% after adjustment for co-morbid illnesses.

Atrial flutter

An organized atrial rhythm of 250–300 bpm. Electrophysiologic studies have shown that there are large re-entry circuits within the right atrium.

Clinical features

Patients may present overtly with palpitations, dyspnea, chest pain, and fatigue, or more insidiously with impaired exercise tolerance, worsening heart failure or pulmonary disease.

Investigations (Fig. 5.19)

ECG The ventricular rate is determined by the extent of AV block with a 2 : 1 AV block being most common, resulting in a rate of 150 bpm. Patients may also be in atrial flutter with variable block in which case the ventricular rhythm is irregular. "Saw-tooth" flutter ('f') waves are best seen in the inferior leads.

Management

An overview of the management of atrial flutter is outlined in Fig. 5.20. Compared to atrial fibrillation, rate control and chemical cardioversion of atrial flutter is often more difficult.

Atrial tachycardia

Focal atrial tachycardias (AT) are characterized by regular atrial activation, at rates of 100–250 bpm. They may occur either in the presence or absence of underlying cardiac abnormalities and occasionally in digoxin excess, especially with hypokalemia.

Investigations

ECG P waves are often visible, but may be obscured by the T wave of the preceding QRS complex. The presence of an isoelectric line between P waves suggests focal AT rather than atrial flutter. Definitive diagnosis of AT rests with intracardiac mapping and diagnostic electrophysiological studies. The P wave morphology of the atrial tachycardia is often different from that of sinus rhythm.

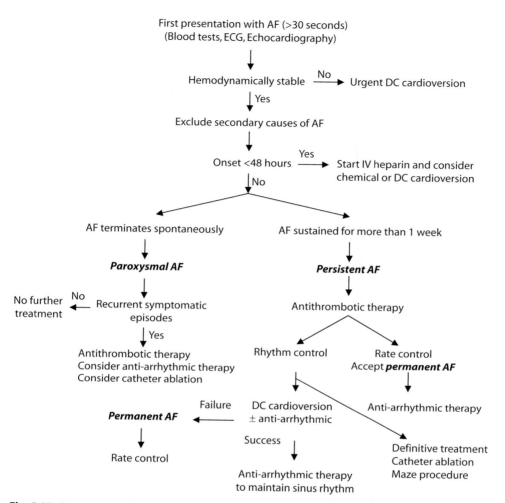

First presentation with AF (>30 seconds)
(Blood tests, ECG, Echocardiography)

Hemodynamically stable —No→ Urgent DC cardioversion

↓Yes

Exclude secondary causes of AF

Onset <48 hours —Yes→ Start IV heparin and consider chemical or DC cardioversion

↓No

AF terminates spontaneously / **AF sustained for more than 1 week**

Paroxysmal AF / *Persistent AF*

Recurrent symptomatic episodes —No→ No further treatment

↓Yes

Antithrombotic therapy
Consider anti-arrhythmic therapy
Consider catheter ablation

Persistent AF → Antithrombotic therapy → Rhythm control / Rate control Accept *permanent AF*

Rhythm control → DC cardioversion ± anti-arrhythmic

Rate control → Anti-arrhythmic therapy

DC cardioversion ± anti-arrhythmic —Failure→ *Permanent AF* → Rate control

Success ↓ Anti-arrhythmic therapy to maintain sinus rhythm

Definitive treatment
Catheter ablation
Maze procedure

Fig. 5.18. Management pathway for atrial fibrillation (AF).

Management

(1) *Pharmacologic therapy*

Rarely, acute AT will terminate with vagal maneuvers, IV adenosine, verapamil, or beta-blockers. Class IA or IC drugs may be effective in some patients by suppressing automaticity. In drug-resistant AT, DC cardioversion should be attempted. For long-term pharmacologic therapy, calcium-channel blockers, beta-blockers, fleicanide, propafenone, sotalol, or amiodarone may be used.

(2) *Catheter ablation*

Localization of the focus of activation and catheter ablation is successful in 86% of cases, but carries the risks of ablation, noted in previous sections.

Outcome

Usually benign, although the sustained intractable forms can lead to tachycardia-induced cardiomyopathy.

Ventricular tachycardia (VT)

This can be life-threatening and is defined as the presence of three or more consecutive beats arising from either ventricle.

- Episodes can be non-sustained (terminating spontaneously within 30 seconds) or sustained (>30 seconds).

- Distinguishing VT from an SVT with aberrant conduction can be difficult. A diagnosis of VT is more likely with previous myocardial infarction or heart failure. If doubt the arrhythmia should be treated as VT.

- 50% with recurrent symptomatic VT have underlying ischemic heart disease.

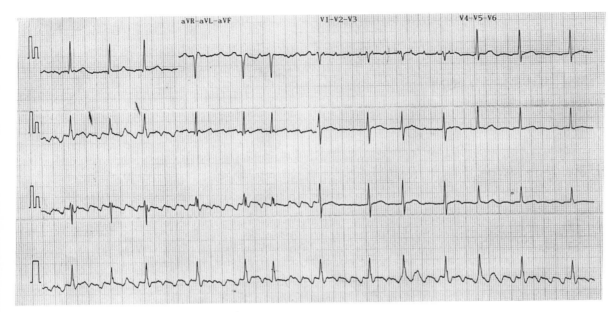

Fig. 5.19. Electrocardiogram demonstrating atrial flutter.

Fig. 5.20. Management pathway for atrial flutter.

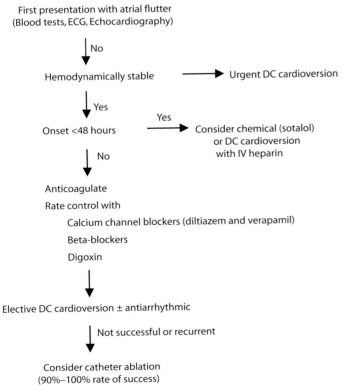

First presentation with atrial flutter
(Blood tests, ECG, Echocardiography)

↓ No

Hemodynamically stable ——→ Urgent DC cardioversion

↓ Yes

Onset <48 hours ——→ Consider chemical (sotalol)
or DC cardioversion
with IV heparin
(Yes)

↓ No

Anticoagulate

Rate control with

    Calcium channel blockers (diltiazem and verapamil)

    Beta-blockers

    Digoxin

↓

Elective DC cardioversion ± antiarrhythmic

↓ Not successful or recurrent

Consider catheter ablation
(90%–100% rate of success)

Etiology

Acquired

Ischemic heart disease

Congestive heart failure

Dilated cardiomyopathy

Congenital heart disease

Drug-induced, such as anti-arrhythmic therapy

Familial

Hypertrophic cardiomyopathy

Long QT syndrome

Arrhythmogenic right ventricular cardiomyopathy (ARVC)

Repair of Tetralogy of Fallot

Clinical features

History Patients may present overtly with palpitations, dyspnea, chest pain, dizziness, syncope, or sudden cardiac death, or more insidiously with worsening heart failure.

Epidemiology

- Sudden cardiac death (SCD), which occurs within 1 hour of onset of symptoms, is responsible for 25%–30% of deaths due to cardiovascular disease in the UK, claiming an estimated 70 000–90 000 lives each year.
- Eighty percent of SCD are due to VT and VF.

Investigations

ECG

- Three or more consecutive abnormally shaped QRS complexes (each of more than 120 ms).
- Atrial activity may be dissociated from ventricular activity.
- The R–R interval can be regular or punctuated by fusion beats (the result of fusion between a sinus beat conducted through the AV node and one emanating from the ventricle) or capture beats (a QRS complex captured by a sinus beat).
- The morphology of the different QRS complexes may be identical (monomorphic VT) or the VT may originate from multiple foci and the QRS morphology may vary (polymorphic VT) (Fig. 5.21).

Management

Acute management of VT Prompt DC cardioversion if the patient is hemodynamically unstable, has angina or is in congestive heart failure.

Long-term management of VT Amiodarone has an important role but patients at high risk of sudden

cardiac death due to severely impaired LV systolic function or a potentially serious congenital disorder such as long QT syndrome or ARVD, may benefit from an internal cardiovertor defibrillator (ICD), which can sense and terminate ventricular arrhythmias. ICD implantation can treat episodes with either anti-tachycardic pacing (89%–91%) or with shock therapy (98%).

Catheter ablation is used to cure VT arising in normal hearts such as right ventricular outflow tract tachycardia.

Outcome

In the absence of an ICD, patients with previous myocardial infarction and an episode of non-sustained VT or inducible VT have a 2-year mortality of 30% and 50%, respectively.

Shortness of breath

A cardinal symptom of both cardiovascular and respiratory disease. A thorough history and examination are essential to elucidate the many causes listed:

Cardiovascular:

- Heart failure (including cardiomyopathies)
- Valvular disease (including infective endocarditis)
- Arrhythmias
- Ischemic heart disease
- Pericardial effusion/cardiac tamponade
- Pulmonary embolism (see *Respiratory disease*)
- Pulmonary hypertension

Other pulmonary conditions and chest wall problems (see *Respiratory disease*)

Other:

- Anemia
- Obesity
- Deconditioning
- Psychogenic
- Metabolic acidosis (acute renal or hepatic failure, diabetic ketoacidosis)
- Bilateral renal artery stenosis (flash pulmonary edema)

Evaluating the cause of dyspnea

Cardiovascular causes can be divided into those that present suddenly such as acute pulmonary edema, arrhythmias, or those which present slowly, such as valvular disease, ischemic heart disease, or chronic heart failure.

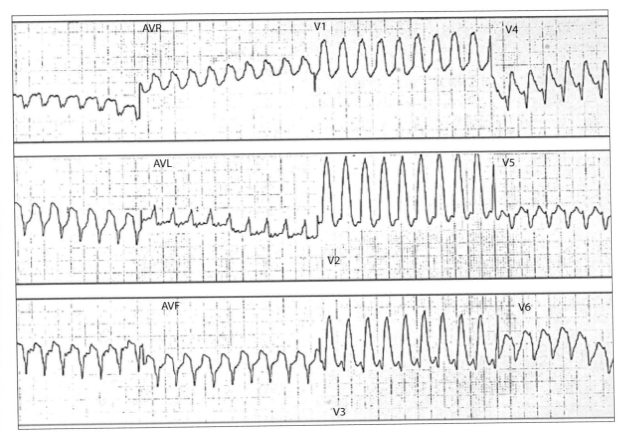

Fig. 5.21. Electrocardiogram demonstrating a ventricular tachycardia.

Features of cardiac dyspnea

- Exertional
- Shortness of breath may be exacerbated when lying flat (orthopnea)
- Patient may wake up in the middle of the night gasping for air (paroxysmal nocturnal dyspnea, PND)
- Severity of the exertional dyspnea can be gauged by walking distance on the flat before stopping
- Exertional dyspnea may be an "anginal equivalent," due to exertional angina, in the absence of chest pain. This is seen in elderly and diabetic patients. Such dyspnea is relieved by rest or sublingual nitroglycerin

Investigations for evaluating the cause of dyspnea

(1) **Blood tests**

FBC to exclude anemia and thyroid function tests to exclude thyrotoxicosis.

(2) **Oximetry**

If oximetry shows evidence of desaturation (SaO_2 < 94%), an arterial blood gas should be performed.

(3) **Chest X-ray**

This can assess cardiac size and demonstrate pulmonary edema. It can also exclude pulmonary causes of dyspnea.

(4) **ECG**

This may demonstrate an underlying arrhythmia. Features of old myocardial infarction or bundle branch block may indicate underlying CAD

(5) **Echocardiography**

This may demonstrate valvular disease, LV and RV systolic and diastolic function, and pulmonary hypertension. It can also exclude a pericardial effusion.

(6) **Pulmonary function tests**

(7) **Cardio-pulmonary exercise testing**

Determining the maximal VO_2 (oxygen consumption) and VCO_2 (carbon dioxide

143

production) during exercise testing can establish whether underlying cardiac or pulmonary disease limits exercise.

Heart failure

Heart failure is a complex syndrome that is the result of an abnormality of cardiac function such that it is unable to pump blood at a rate which meets the physiologic demands of the body or when the heart can only do so with an elevated filling pressure. Heart failure may be the result of impaired myocardial contraction (systolic dysfunction) or impaired ventricular filling (diastolic dysfunction).

Types of heart failure
Systolic heart failure
Most heart failure is due to impaired LV systolic function. The cardiomyopathies can be classified according to the predominant functional impairment, those associated with a specific disease and those forming part of a systemic disease, as outlined below.

Classification of cardiomyopathies
(A) Morphological types

Dilated cardiomyopathy	Dilatation and impaired contraction of both ventricles, which can be idiopathic or due to viral, immune, alcoholic and/or toxic factors
Hypertrophic cardiomyopathy	Left ventricular hypertrophy, often asymmetric and involving the interventricular septum
Restrictive cardiomyopathy	Restricted filling and reduced diastolic cavity dimensions with normal systolic function, can be idiopathic or due to infiltrative diseases such as amyloidosis or endomyocardial fibrosis

(B) Associated with specific diseases
Arrhythmogenic right ventricular cardiomyopathy (ARVC)

Unclassified	(including mitochondrial disease and fibroelastosis)

(C) Specific cardiomyopathies

Ischemic cardiomyopathy	(ventricular dysfunction due to CAD)
Hypertensive cardiomyopathy	(LVH with features of systolic and diastolic dysfunction)
Viral cardiomyopathy	(due to viral myocarditis)
Infiltrative cardiomyopathy	(including glycogen storage disease, sarcoidosis, amyloidosis)
Muscular dystrophies	(including Duchenne, Becker-type, and myotonic dystrophies)
Neuromuscular disorders	(including Noonan syndrome and Friedreich's ataxia)
Sensitivity and toxins	(including alcohol, catecholamines, anthracyclines, and irradiation)
Peripartum cardiomyopathy	

Diastolic heart failure
- Up to one-third with congestive heart failure have normal or only minimally impaired systolic function (ejection fraction >50%), and are believed to have diastolic heart failure.
- The underlying pathology of the condition is an abnormality of diastolic distensibility, filling or relaxation of the left ventricle, such that the left ventricle has a limited capacity to fill at normal left atrial pressures.
- There are numerous causes of diastolic dysfunction. The major causes are age and left ventricular hypertrophy.

Causes of diastolic dysfunction
Left ventricular hypertrophy
Aging
Restrictive and infiltrative cardiomyopathies
Hypothyroidism
Diffuse fibrosis
Post-infarct scarring
Fibroelastosis
Mitral or tricuspid stenosis
Pericardial constriction or tamponade
Extrinsic compression by tumor

Restrictive and infiltrative cardiomyopathies
Restrictive cardiomyopathy (RCM) is characterized by diastolic dysfunction and rigid ventricular walls, which impair filling. Systolic function is often normal. Various causes of RCM are listed. Cause remains unknown in many cases.
Causes of restrictive cardiomyopathy:

Myocardial (non-infiltrative)
Idiopathic cardiomyopathy
Familial cardiomyopathy

Hypertrophic cardiomyopathy
Scleroderma
Pseudoxanthoma elasticum
Diabetic cardiomyopathy

Myocardial (infiltrative)
Amyloidosis
Sarcoidosis
Gaucher disease
Hurler disease
Fatty infiltration

Myocardial (storage)
Hemochromatosis
Fabry disease
Glycogen storage disease

Endomyocardial
Endomyocardial fibrosis
Hypereosinophilic syndrome
Carcinoid heart disease
Metastatic cancers
Radiation
Anthracycline toxicity
Drugs such as serotonin, methysergide, ergotamine, busulphan

Clinical features of heart failure

History Breathlessness, acute or insidious is the predominant symptom of heart failure. The severity of the dyspnea can be classified according to the New York Heart Association (NYHA) Classification below.

I "Ordinary physical activity does not cause dyspnea"
II "Slight limitation of physical activity"
III "Marked limitation of physical activity"
IV "Inability to carry out any physical activity without discomfort"

Features to elicit in the history
  Exertional dyspnea
  Orthopnea
  Cough may be due to pulmonary edema.
  Paroxysmal nocturnal dyspnea (PND) is characterized by waking gasping for air due to interstitial edema.
  Reduced exercise capacity is due to pulmonary venous congestion and insufficient blood flow to skeletal muscles.

Fatigue and weakness due to poor perfusion of skeletal muscles, sodium depletion and/or hypovolemia, or from beta-blocker treatment.
Symptoms of predominant right-sided heart failure include hepatic congestion, anorexia, nausea, bloating, constipation, sense of fullness after meals, ankle edema.

Features to find on examination

General	Cachexia of chronic heart failure
	Peripheral vasoconstriction (poor capillary perfusion) and peripheral cyanosis
Pulse	Tachycardia
Blood pressure	May be low
JVP	Neck vein distension with JVP > 4 cm
Apex beat	Displaced
Heart sounds	Third heart sound and gallop rhythm
Added sounds	Pansystolic murmurs of functional tricuspid or mitral regurgitation
Lungs	Basal crepitations
	Pleural effusions, usually bilateral, but when unilateral it is usually on the right
Abdomen	Hepatomegaly
	Ascites
Others	Bilateral pitting ankle edema and sacral edema

Epidemiology

- 900 000 people in the UK have heart failure and numbers are increasing with life expectancy and improved survival after myocardial infarction.
- Average age at diagnosis is 76.
- Risk is higher in men.
- Most common cause is ischemic heart disease (two-thirds) followed by hypertension, valvular disease and atrial fibrillation.
- Idiopathic dilated cardiomyopathy (heart failure of unknown cause) accounts for 15% under age 75.

Causes of heart failure

Ischemic heart disease
Hypertension
Valvular disease
Atrial fibrillation
Idiopathic dilated cardiomyopathy
Hypertrophic cardiomyopathy
Other cardiomyopathies

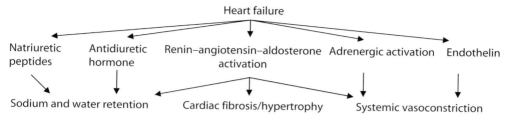

Fig. 5.22. Neurohormonal activation during heart failure.

Pathophysiology

- Left ventricular failure eventually leads to raised ventricular end-diastolic pressure, which in turn raises left atrial and pulmonary venous pressure causing pulmonary edema.
- Left ventricular failure or sustained pulmonary arterial hypertension will eventually result in right ventricular failure with systemic venous congestion, jugular venous distension, hepatomegaly, ascites, and peripheral edema.
- Low cardiac output results in hypoperfusion of vital organs and neurohormonal activation, which is initially compensatory but subsequently has deleterious effects (Fig. 5.22).

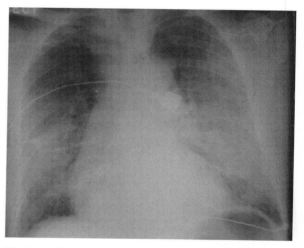

Fig. 5.23. Chest radiograph demonstrating the features of cardiac failure including upper lobe blood diversion and pulmonary edema and fluid in the horizontal fissure.

Investigations

(1) Blood tests

Dilutional hyponatremia, increased urea and creatinine due to renal hypoperfusion, and diuretic treatment. Hypokalemia due to diuretic use. Abnormal liver function tests due to hepatic congestion.

(2) Brain natriuretic peptide (BNP)

Heart failure is unlikely in a patient with a normal plasma BNP (sensitivity 90%–97%).

(3) ECG

Heart failure is unlikely in a patient with a normal ECG (sensitivity over 90%). The following features may be present in heart failure: sinus tachycardia; atrial and ventricular arrhythmias; poor R wave progression and intraventricular conduction defects especially left bundle branch block (LBBB).

(4) Chest X-ray (CXR) (see Fig. 5.23)

Cardiomegaly (cardiothoracic ratio >50%).

Upper lobe diversion due to raised pulmonary capillary pressure.

Septal or Kerley B-lines appear as sharp linear densities of interlobular interstitial edema.

Perivascular cuffing due to interstitial edema.

"Butterfly" or "bat's wing" of alveolar edema concentrated around the hila.

Pleural effusions.

(5) Echocardiography

To document ventricular dimensions and systolic and diastolic function, valvular function, and pulmonary artery pressure.

(6) Cardiac MRI

To diagnose dilated or restrictive cardiomyopathy, hypertrophic cardiomyopathy or ARVD.

(7) Cardiac catheterization

Cardiac catheterization is useful to determine the presence and severity of coronary artery disease in patients with congestive heart failure, as well as to assess LV function.

Management

Once patients have been treated for acute left ventricular failure (Fig. 5.24) management is as for chronic heart failure. The goals of treatment for

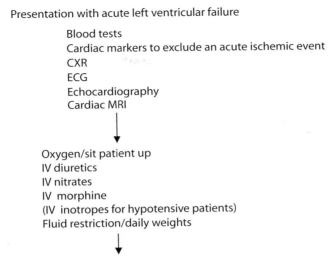

Presentation with acute left ventricular failure

Blood tests
Cardiac markers to exclude an acute ischemic event
CXR
ECG
Echocardiography
Cardiac MRI

Oxygen/sit patient up
IV diuretics
IV nitrates
IV morphine
(IV inotropes for hypotensive patients)
Fluid restriction/daily weights

Look for and treat cause of HF if possible

(e.g. non-compliance with medication, valve replacement for severe valvular regurgitation or revascularization for underlying CAD)

Management of chronic heart failure

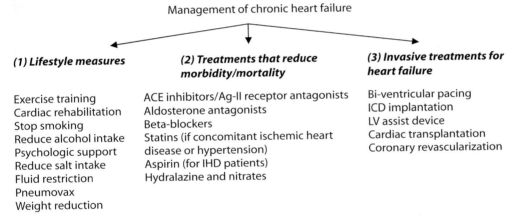

(1) Lifestyle measures

Exercise training
Cardiac rehabilitation
Stop smoking
Reduce alcohol intake
Psychologic support
Reduce salt intake
Fluid restriction
Pneumovax
Weight reduction

(2) Treatments that reduce morbidity/mortality

ACE inhibitors/Ag-II receptor antagonists
Aldosterone antagonists
Beta-blockers
Statins (if concomitant ischemic heart disease or hypertension)
Aspirin (for IHD patients)
Hydralazine and nitrates

(3) Invasive treatments for heart failure

Bi-ventricular pacing
ICD implantation
LV assist device
Cardiac transplantation
Coronary revascularization

Fig. 5.24. Management pathway for heart failure.

congestive cardiac failure are to control symptoms, prolong survival and improve quality of life.

Pharmacologic treatment of heart failure

The number of recommended drugs expanded considerably following several large clinical studies. NICE guidelines propose the algorithm depicted in Table 5.3

Invasive treatment of heart failure

(1) Coronary revascularization

Patients with heart failure and intractable angina, and those with known non-contractile viable ("hibernating") myocardium, may benefit from coronary revascularization.

(2) Cardiac-resynchronization therapy (CRT) also known as bi-ventricular pacing

CRT or bi-ventricular pacing reduces mortality, in the 30% of patients with heart failure who have incoordinate electrical activation resulting in impaired contraction of the ventricles.

(3) Implantable cardioverter-defibrillators (ICDs)

ICDs reduce mortality in heart failure patients with ejection fraction <35%.

(4) Left ventricular assist device (LVAD)

The LVAD may be used for circulatory support, as a "bridge" to cardiac transplantation.

Table 5.3. Management pathway for heart failure

Drug class	Examples	Indication and benefit
Diuretics	Furosemide Bumetanide	Fluid overload
↓		
ACE inhibitor	Enalapril Perindropil	All patients Blocks activation of the Renin–Angiotensin– aldosterone axis
Angiotensin II receptor blocker	Losartan Candesartan	If side effect with ACE-I or intolerant of beta-blocker
↓		
Beta-blockers	Carvedilol Bisoprolol	All patients Blocks adrenergic activation
↓		
Digoxin		Patients with AF or those in sinus rhythm who are still symptomatic despite above treatment
↓		
Aldosterone blocker	Spironolactone Eprenelone	Patients with NYHA III/IV heart failure Blocks effects of aldosterone
Other drugs in heart failure:		
Statins	Atorvastatin Simvastatin	Statins are beneficial irrespective of whether there is IHD.
Hydralazine/ Nitrates		Patients unable to take ACE-I or Angiotensin II receptor blockers
Anticoagulation	Warfarin	Patients with atrial fibrillation, previous thromboembolic event, intracardiac thrombus, or left ventricular aneurysm
Antiplatelet therapy	Aspirin	Patients with IHD

(5) Cardiac transplantation

Cardiac transplantation improves the quality of life and has a 70%–80% survival rate at five years.

Outcome

Heart failure has a poor prognosis, 40% dying within a year of diagnosis, and 10% per year thereafter.

Hypertrophic cardiomyopathy

- Hypertrophic cardiomyopathy (HCM) is the presence of left ventricular hypertrophy without detectable cause.

- Variable presentation, clinical course and outcome, and most cases in the adult are due to a genetic mutation.
- Most common genetic cardiovascular disease, inherited in an autosomal dominant manner.
- Commonest cardiac cause of sudden death in young adults and trained athletes.
- 25% of patients manifest a dynamic subaortic LV outflow obstruction.

Clinical features

Many are asymptomatic

- **Chest pain** – on exertion or at rest.
- **Dyspnea** – this is often exertional in nature.
- **Pre-syncope or syncope** – on exertion or at rest, and may be due to cardiac arrhythmias.
- **Sudden cardiac death** – due to a lethal ventricular arrhythmia.
  - **Pulse** – Rapid upstroke and downstroke.
  - **JVP** – Prominent "a" wave due to reduced right ventricular compliance.
  - **Apex** – Sustained LV impulse with palpable atrial beat.
  - **Added sounds** – Systolic murmur at left sternal edge radiating to the mitral and aortic areas but not the neck or axilla. The intensity of murmur increases with maneuvers which reduce preload or afterload, such as standing or the Valsalva maneuver.

  There may be a pan-systolic murmur of mitral regurgitation.

Epidemiology

1 : 500 adults have HCM. In adolescents and adults with left ventricular hypertrophy, the familial causes predominate with 50%–60% having mutations in one of ten genes that encode for different components of the cardiac sarcomeric protein.

Causes of left ventricular hypertrophy

(1) Hypertension
(2) HCM-cardiac sarcomeric protein disease (including)
  Troponins I, C and T
  Myosin light and heavy chains, and myosin binding proteins
  α actin
  α tropomyosin
(3) Athlete's heart

(4) Metabolic disease, e.g. glycogen storage diseases
Hurler's syndrome
Syndromes associated with LVH:
Noonan
LEOPARD
Friedrich's ataxia

Pathology

- The mechanism through which mutations in genes encoding cardiac sarcomeric proteins result in left ventricular hypertrophy (LVH) is unknown
- There is myocyte disarray as well as interstitial fibrosis and narrowing of intramural coronary vessels due to medial hypertrophy.

Investigations

ECG

- Left atrial enlargement (P wave duration greater than 120 ms).
- Repolarization abnormalities (such as T wave inversion).
- Pathologic Q waves (especially in the inferolateral leads).

Holter recording

- Ventricular ectopy.
- Non-sustained ventricular tachycardia.
- Supraventricular arrhythmias (such as atrial fibrillation or flutter).

Echocardiography

- Left ventricular thickness >15 mm.
- 25% have dynamic LV outflow obstruction (LV outflow tract pressure gradient ≥30 mmHg). Patients with no gradient at rest should be exercised.
- Systolic anterior movement of the mitral valve (SAM) and a posteriorly directed jet of mitral regurgitation.
- Diastolic dysfunction is present as evidenced by impaired LV filling.

Cardiac MRI

- Confirmation of HCM provides information on systolic and diastolic function and can detect associated myocardial fibrosis.

Management

Given the variable presentation, clinical course and outcome of HCM, the approach has three aims.

(1) *Symptom control*
Pharmacologic treatment of symptoms due to LV outflow obstruction (gradient of ≥30 mmHg)

- *Beta-blockers* can relieve symptoms of exertional chest pain, dyspnea, and syncope.
- *Disopyramide* can be used if beta-blockade is unsuccessful, to reduce LV outflow obstruction.
- *Verapamil*

Non-pharmacologic treatment of symptoms due to LV outflow obstruction

Several non-pharmacologic approaches are used for symptoms intractable to medical therapy:

(a) *Septal myotomy–myectomy*, in which muscle is removed from the interventricular septum has a mortality of <1%. Complete heart block and ventricular septal defects are possible complications.

(b) *Percutaneous transcoronary alcohol septal ablation* – in this technique, via cardiac catheterization, alcohol is injected into a septal perforator vessel to induce a localized area of myocardial necrosis. Complete heart block and coronary artery dissection are possible complications.

(c) *Atrio-ventricular sequential pacing* from the right ventricular apex can reduce LV outflow gradients.

(2) *Detect and avoid complications*
The main complications of HCM are sudden death <1% per year), atrial fibrillation, infective endocarditis, and heart failure.

Sudden cardiac death (SCD)

- Ventricular arrhythmias are the predominant cause.
- Patients with >3% risk of SCD should receive an ICD.

Atrial fibrillation

Patients with atrial fibrillation should be anticoagulated and cardioverted to sinus rhythm.

Infective endocarditis (IE)

Patients with obstructive HCM should receive antibiotic prophylaxis against IE.

(3) *Counseling, which includes genotyping, family screening, and patient information.*
First-degree relatives should be screened by ECG and echocardiography every 5 years.

Outcome

The overall risk of complications of HCM, including end-stage heart failure, sudden death, and fatal stroke, is about 1%–2% per year.

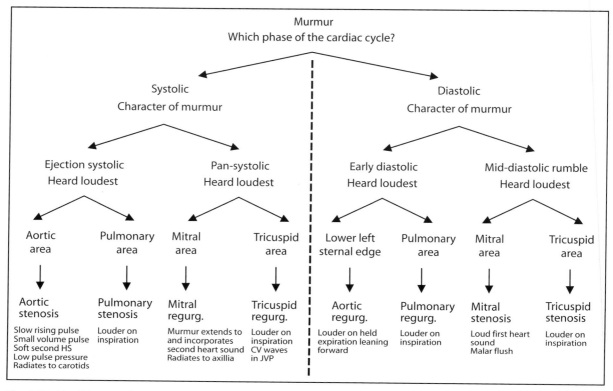

Fig. 5.25. Identifying a cardiac murmur.

Valvular disease

Can present with dyspnea, often exertional, due to pulmonary venous hypertension. Turbulent blood flow across a diseased valve manifests clinically as an audible murmur or a palpable thrill. In Fig. 5.25, there is an algorithm for identifying the common pathologic murmurs.

Aortic stenosis

The most common cause is degenerative calcification resulting from normal mechanical stress on the valve ("wear and tear"). Diabetes mellitus and hyperlipidemia are risk factors.

Etiology of aortic stenosis

Congenital	Unicuspid aortic valve
	Bicuspid aortic valve
Acquired	Degenerative calcification
	Atherosclerotic aortic stenosis
	Rheumatic fever

Clinical features

History Many adults with aortic stenosis are asymptomatic but symptoms include:

- *Dizzy spells*
- *Syncope* often exertional
- *Chest pain*
- *Dyspnea*
- *Heart failure*
- *Sudden cardiac death*

The development of these symptoms in a patient with severe aortic stenosis is generally an indication for urgent surgical intervention, as after the onset of symptoms the average survival is 2–3 years.

Examination

- *Blood pressure* Narrow pulse pressure in severe aortic stenosis
- *Pulse character* Slow-rising, small volume
- *Carotid pulse* Delay in pulsation felt between apex and carotid arteries
- *Chest wall* Systolic thrill over aortic area
- *Heart sounds* Soft second heart sound (due to immobility of the aortic valve)

Table 5.4. Echocardiographic findings in aortic stenosis

	Mild	Moderate	Severe
Aortic valve area	1.5–3.0 cm²	>1.0–1.5 cm²	≤1.0 cm²
Mean pressure gradient across valve	20–30 mmHg	31–49 mmHg	≥50 mmHg
Flow velocity through valve	2.2–3.0 m/s	3.0–4.0 m/s	≥4.0 m/s

- *Added sounds*   Ejection systolic murmur loudest in the aortic area that radiates to the carotid arteries and often to the apex

Epidemiology

The commonest cause of aortic stenosis in patients older than 70 years old is degenerative calcification (50% of cases), whereas under 70 years old, bicuspid aortic valve accounts for about 50% of cases of aortic stenosis.

Investigations
ECG
- Left ventricular hypertrophy in 85% of severe aortic stenosis.
- Calcific infiltration extending from the aortic valve into the conduction system may cause AV conduction defects.

CXR
- Calcification of the aortic valves may be seen as well as post-stenotic dilatation of the ascending aorta.

Echocardiography
- The estimated aortic valve area, the pressure gradient across the valve, and the degree of LVH can be used to assess severity of aortic stenosis (Table 5.4).

Coronary angiography
- Coronary angiography is recommended for patients at risk of IHD, in preparation for aortic valve replacement.
- It can also be used to measure the gradient across the aortic valve, in cases where the severity of the stenosis is in doubt.

Management

All patients with AS should receive antibiotic prophylaxis to reduce the risk of endocarditis during surgical and perhaps dental procedures. Aggressive lipid lowering with high dose statins slows the progression of aortic stenosis. Urgent review and echocardiogram are indicated if chest pain, dyspnea, dizziness, or syncope develop. *Severe AS* should be assessed for surgical replacement of the aortic valve. Other indications for aortic valve replacement are detailed below.

Indications for aortic valve replacement in patients with aortic stenosis:
Symptomatic patients with severe aortic stenosis
Asymptomatic severe AS at high risk of death:
    LV systolic dysfunction
    Abnormal response to exercise such as hypotension
    Ventricular tachycardia
    Marked LVH (>15 mm)
    Aortic valve area <0.6 cm²
Patients with moderate or severe AS undergoing cardiac surgery for other reasons, e.g. CABG or surgery on the aorta or other valves.

Outcome
- On average the aortic valve area decreases by 0.12 cm² and the systolic pressure gradient across the aortic valve increases by 10–15 mmHg per year.
- In symptomatic severe aortic stenosis average survival is 2–3 years.
- Patients with asymptomatic severe aortic stenosis have a more benign course with <1% risk of sudden death per year.

Aortic regurgitation
Aortic regurgitation may be caused by either a primary valvular problem, disease of the aortic root, or both.

Etiology of aortic regurgitation

	Valvular disease	**Aortic root disease**
Congenital	Bicuspid aortic valve	Degenerative aortic dilation
	Associated ventricular septal defect	Systemic hypertension Cystic medial necrosis of aorta
Acquired	Calcification and degeneration Infective endocarditis Rheumatic fever	Marfan or Marfan-like Aortic root dissection or laceration Osteogenesis imperfecta

Myxomatous proliferation of valve	Syphilitic aortitis
Crohn's disease	Relapsing polychondritis
Ankylosing spondylitis	Ankylosing spondylitis
Takayasu's disease	Giant cell arteritis

Clinical features

- Aortic regurgitation can present suddenly or slowly.
  - (1) Acute: caused most commonly by aortic dissection, infective endocarditis, or trauma. It results in a large regurgitant volume load on a normal size left ventricle (LV) which results in cardiovascular collapse, tachycardia, and pulmonary congestion.
  - (2) Chronic: the left ventricle has the opportunity to adapt to the increased load.

Clinical features of chronic aortic regurgitation

History Asymptomatic for a prolonged period of time as the volume overloaded LV undergoes compensatory hypertrophy to maintain a normal ejection fraction. However, with time (usually in the fourth to fifth decades) this compensatory mechanism becomes inadequate to maintain LV systolic function and the LV dilates and the patient develops dyspnea, orthopnea and impaired exercise tolerance, in response to a decline in LV systolic function and increased LV filling pressures.

Examination

Head	De Musset's sign (head nodding with each heart beat)
Pulse character	Collapsing or "water hammer" large volume
Neck	Corrigan's sign (visible carotid pulsation in neck)
Hands	Quincke's sign (capillary pulsations in finger-tips)
Blood pressure	Wide pulse pressure
Femoral pulse	"Pistol shot femorals" (booming sounds over femoral artery in systole and diastole)
Apex beat	Laterally displaced and hyperdynamic
Murmurs	High-pitched early diastolic murmur loudest at lower left sternal edge at the end of expiration

Table 5.5. Echocardiographic classification of aortic regurgitation

	Mild	Moderate	Severe
Width of regurgitant jet as % of outflow tract width	<30%	30–60%	>60%
Pressure half-time	>600 m/s	401–599 m/s	<400 m/s
Left ventricle function	Normal	Mild overload	Marked overload
Flow-reversal in descending aorta	Small/ transient	Increased	Major

Low pitched mid-diastolic murmur of mitral stenosis due to obstruction of mitral valve opening from the jet of aortic regurgitation (Austin–Flint murmur)

Pathology

- In rheumatic aortic regurgitation, fibrosis and retraction give rise to incomplete apposition of the valve leaflets during diastole.
- Fusion of the commissures may prevent complete opening of the valve, resulting in concomitant aortic stenosis.
- Dilatation of the aortic root preventing aortic leaflet apposition in diastole causes functional AR.

Investigations

ECG Left ventricular hypertrophy, left axis deviation or AV conduction defects may be present.

CXR Evidence of cardiomegaly and a dilated aortic root may be present.

Echocardiography

- May indicate the etiology (valve morphology, and aortic root size and morphology).
- Diastolic regurgitant jet across the aortic valve can be analyzed and with the pressure half-time, an assessment of the severity of the aortic regurgitation determined (Table 5.5).

Coronary angiography Coronary angiography is recommended for patients at risk of IHD in preparation for aortic valve replacement.

Management

All patients with aortic regurgitation should receive antibiotic prophylaxis to reduce the risk of endocarditis during invasive surgical and perhaps dental procedures.

Asymptomatic patients

- With aortic regurgitation and normal LV dimensions and systolic function can be followed with regular echocardiography.
- In severe aortic regurgitation and dilatation of the LV and/or impairment of LV function the aortic valve should be replaced.
- In patients with AR and aortic root dilatation, combined aortic valve and root replacement should be considered when the aortic root diameter is ≥5.5 cm.

Symptomatic patients Patients with severe aortic regurgitation who have >NYHA II symptoms should be considered for surgical replacement of the aortic valve.

Indications for aortic valve replacement in patients with chronic severe aortic regurgitation:

Symptomatic patients (NYHA II/III/IV) and normal LV systolic function (EF >50%)

Asymptomatic or symptomatic patients with LV dysfunction and ejection fraction (EF) <50%

Asymptomatic patients with normal LV systolic function and LV dilatation with left ventricular end systole (LVES) >55 mm

Patients undergoing coronary artery bypass grafting (CABG) or surgery on the aorta or other valves

Outcome

- 75% of patients with chronic aortic regurgitation survive for 5 years and 50% for 10 years after diagnosis.
- 25% death within 2–4 years after onset of symptoms.

Mitral stenosis

The main cause of mitral stenosis is rheumatic fever. Other rarer causes are listed below. Symptoms usually appear in the third or fourth decade.

Etiology of mitral stenosis

Congenital	Mitral stenosis
Acquired	Rheumatic fever
	Malignant carcinoid
	Methysergide therapy

Clinical features

History Patients with mild mitral stenosis are asymptomatic at rest, only developing symptoms on exertion, or when there is an increase in heart rate due to exercise, infection, the onset of atrial fibrillation, emotional stress, or pregnancy.

Exertional dyspnea

This is due to pulmonary venous congestion from increased left atrial pressure, which can worsen with either tachycardia or atrial fibrillation.

Lethargy and decreased exercise tolerance

Hemoptysis

This may be due to pulmonary edema, chest infections or the rupture of dilated bronchial veins.

Embolization

Thrombus within the dilated left atrium (particularly in the presence of atrial fibrillation) can embolize to the cerebral or peripheral circulation.

Face	Malar flush
Pulse	Atrial fibrillation is often present
JVP	Prominent "a" waves (if in sinus rhythm)
Apex beat	Tapping, undisplaced
Heart sounds	Loud first heart sound
	Loud second heart sound if pulmonary hypertension
	Opening snap
	Murmur: Mid-diastolic low frequency murmur loudest at apex during expiration

Pathology

In rheumatic mitral stenosis there is fusion of the valve commissures, cusps (at the edges resulting in a "fish mouth" shaped orifice), and chordae (resulting in thickening and shortening of these structures). Left atrial dilatation, fibrosis of the atrial wall, and disorganization of the atrial muscle bundles occurs, usually resulting in atrial fibrillation.

Investigations

ECG Left atrial hypertrophy followed by dilatation may be present, indicated by "P mitrale" i.e. a broad (>120 ms) bifid P wave, most easily seen in lead II, and the P wave is biphasic in V1.

CXR Evidence of pulmonary venous congestion and a "double cardiac silhouette" on the left heart border caused by left atrial dilatation may be visible (Fig. 5.26).

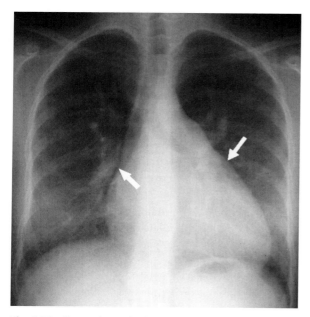

Fig. 5.26. Chest radiograph of patient with mitral stenosis demonstrating pulmonary venous congestion, "a double cardiac silhouette" due to left atrial dilatation (see arrow).

Table 5.6. Echocardiographic classification of mitral stenosis

	Mild	**Moderate**	**Severe**
Mitral valve area	1.5–2.0 cm^2	1.0–1.5 cm^2	<1.0 cm^2
Pressure half-time	<50 m/s	150–200 m/s	>200 m/s
Pressure gradient	<5 mmHg	5–20 mmHg	>20 mmHg
Tricuspid regurgitation velocity	<2.7 m/s	Variable	>3.0 m/s

Echocardiography

- The severity of mitral stenosis can be assessed by measuring the mean transmitral valvular gradient, mitral valve area and pulmonary arterial pressure.
- Mitral valve morphology (leaflet mobility, thickness and calcification) will guide suitability for intervention by percutaneous mitral valvuloplasty.
- Transesophageal echocardiogram will exclude presence of thrombus in the left atrium or atrial appendage (Table 5.6).

Cardiac catheterization

- Coronary angiography is recommended for patients at risk of IHD, in preparation for mitral valve replacement.

- Left and right cardiac catheterization may be required to ascertain pulmonary arterial pressure, pulmonary artery wedge pressure (which correlates with left atrial pressure), and left ventricular end diastolic pressure.

Management

All patients should receive antibiotic prophylaxis to reduce the risk of endocarditis during surgical and perhaps dental procedures.

Asymptomatic patients

- Mild mitral stenosis requires annual review.
- Moderate to severe mitral stenosis with evidence of moderate pulmonary hypertension (PAP >50 mmHg) may benefit from intervention.

Symptomatic patients Patients with moderate to severe mitral stenosis should undergo either:

(1) *Percutaneous mitral balloon valvuloplasty*

- Recommended if valve pliable with little subvalvular fusion and no calcification.
- Relative contraindications include left atrial thrombus and mitral regurgitation.
- The balloon is delivered to the left atrium by puncturing the interatrial septum, and the balloon is then inflated across the stenosed MV.
- Mitral stenosis usually recurs over time, but valvuloplasty may be used to "buy time" particularly in young women who wish to avoid the need for anticoagulation with a mitral prosthesis, for example, if planning a family.

(2) *Open mitral valvuloplasty*

- Recommended for patients with mitral valve morphology unsuitable for percutaneous mitral valvotomy or the presence of left atrial thrombus despite 3 months' anticoagulation.

(3) *Mitral valve replacement*

- Recommended for severe MS if unsuitable for either percutaneous mitral valvuloplasty or open mitral valve repair.

Outcome

10-year survival rate of untreated patients is 50%–60%, but >80% in asymptomatic patients. Patients with mitral stenosis die from progressive heart failure (60%–70%), thromboembolism (20%–30%), pulmonary embolism (10%), and infection (1%–5%).

Mitral regurgitation

Clinical features

Mitral regurgitation can present either suddenly or slowly.

- Acute: caused most commonly by papillary muscle dysfunction due to IHD, rupture of chordae tendinae, infective endocarditis, and trauma (e.g. following mitral balloon valvuloplasty). This results in acute volume overload of the left ventricle reducing cardiac output, causing tachycardia and pulmonary edema. It requires urgent surgical intervention.
- Chronic: expansion of left ventricular end diastolic volume allows increase of total stroke volume maintaining cardiac output.

Mitral regurgitation can be caused by abnormalities of the mitral annulus, the mitral leaflets themselves, the papillary muscles, or the chordae tendinae.

Etiology of mitral regurgitation

Congenital

Mitral valve clefts

Mitral valve abnormalities in association with other congenital defects

Abnormal chordae tendinae

Acquired

Myxomatous degeneration of leaflets (Mitral valve prolapse, Marfan's syndrome, Ehlers-Danlos, pseudoxanthoma elasticum)

Dilation of mitral valve annulus and left ventricular cavity in heart failure and cardiomyopathies

Rheumatic heart disease

Calcification of the mitral valve annulus

Infective endocarditis

Rupture of chordae tendinae or papillary muscle (spontaneous, myocardial infarction, trauma, mitral valve prolapse, infective endocarditis)

Hypertrophic cardiomyopathy

Chronic mitral regurgitation

History

- Patients may be asymptomatic for many years as the left ventricle dilates and hypertrophies to compensate for the mitral regurgitation.
- The left atrium accommodates the regurgitant volume by dilating, thereby initially protecting the pulmonary venous circulation. Eventually LA pressure rises, with subsequent pulmonary venous

Table 5.7. Echocardiography classification of mitral regurgitation

	Mild	Moderate	Severe
Character of regurgitant jet	Thin jet		Dense jet throughout systole to back of left atrium
Area of central jet as % of left atrial area	<20%	20%–40%	>40%
Effect on pulmonary venous flow	None	Blunting of systolic flow	Reversal of systolic flow

hypertension resulting in dyspnea and pulmonary edema.
- When the left ventricle begins to fail, symptoms such as weakness, fatigue, anorexia, and weight loss appear.

Examination

Apex beat	Displaced
Heart sounds	Third heart sound
Murmur	Pan-systolic murmur loudest at the apex which may radiate to the axilla

Epidemiology

- In the West, the commonest causes of chronic mitral regurgitation are mitral valve annular dilatation due to congestive cardiac failure or mitral valve prolapse.
- In countries where rheumatic fever is prevalent, it remains the leading cause.

Investigations

ECG Left atrial hypertrophy followed by dilatation may develop and is indicated by a broad P wave in lead II longer than 120 ms.

CXR Evidence of cardiomegaly, left atrial dilatation, and pulmonary edema may be present.

Echocardiography

- The etiology of mitral regurgitation (valve morphology, papillary muscle function, and chordae tendinae) and its severity can be assessed by analyzing the regurgitant jet (Table 5.7).
- It is important to assess LV function and dimension, and LA size.
- Transesophageal echocardiography may provide additional information.

Cardiac catheterization Coronary angiography is recommended for patients at risk of IHD, in preparation for mitral valve replacement. Left and right cardiac catheterization may also be required to ascertain pressures as a guide to severity of the mitral regurgitation.

Management
All patients with mitral regurgitation should receive antibiotic prophylaxis to reduce the risk of endocarditis during invasive surgical and perhaps dental procedures.

Asymptomatic patients
- Mild to moderate mitral regurgitation and normal LV dimensions and systolic function can be followed in outpatients with regular echocardiography.
- Severe mitral regurgitation should undergo surgical intervention.

Symptomatic patients Once patients become symptomatic (NYHA >II) they should undergo mitral valve surgery, even if the LV systolic function is normal.

Three surgical approaches:
(1) Mitral valve repair avoids need for a prosthetic valve and is the treatment of choice for non-rheumatic posterior leaflet prolapse.
(2) Mitral valve replacement with preservation of part or all of the mitral apparatus.
(3) Replacement with removal of the mitral apparatus. This is performed if the native valve and apparatus are severely distorted by the underlying disease.

Outcome
- 80% with chronic mitral regurgitation survive 5 years and 60% for 10 years after diagnosis.
- Patients with mixed mitral valve disease have 5- and 10-year survival rates of 67% and 30%, respectively.

Mitral valve prolapse
Mitral valve prolapse (MVP) describes a "floppy" mitral valve that billows back into the left atrium in systole, causing mitral regurgitation. It can result from a disorder of the mitral valve leaflet, chordae tendinae, or papillary muscle.

Etiology of mitral valve prolapse
Primary
Most cases are primary

Associations
Ischemic heart disease
Marfan's syndrome
Ehlers-Danlos syndrome
Pseudoxanthoma elasticum
Osteogenesis imperfecta
Myotonic dystrophy
Von Willebrand's disease
Hyperthyroidism
Ebstein's anomaly of the tricuspid valve
Secundum type atrial septal defect
Asthenic habitus
Pectus excavatum
Shallow chest

Clinical features
Most patients are asymptomatic but a proportion will complain of a diverse array of non-specific symptoms that may include chest pain, palpitations, or fatigue.

Low body weight	
Blood pressure	Normal or low
	Orthostatic hypotension
Added sounds	Mid-systolic click after the beginning of the carotid upstroke.
	Mid–late systolic crescendo murmur loudest at the apex and radiating into the axilla.
	The duration of the murmur corresponds to the severity of mitral regurgitation.

Epidemiology
- Most common valvular abnormality, affecting 2%–6% of the population.
- Twice as common in women.
- Strong hereditary component, inherited as autosomal dominant trait, with variable penetrance.

Pathology
- Myxomatous proliferation of the mitral valve leading to redundant, abnormally structured valves. The extent of the prolapse determines the severity of the associated mitral regurgitation.

Investigations
ECG This is often normal, although there may be ST–T abnormalities in patients with papillary muscle ischemia or underlying cardiomyopathy.

Echocardiography The cardinal features of MVP include systolic displacement of one or more leaflets, thickening of the mitral leaflets >5 mm, and late mitral regurgitation.

Management

- Mild MVP and no evidence of MR needs reassurance.
- Mild MR and normal LV dimensions can be followed with regular echocardiography.
- Asymptomatic MVP with severe MR and LV systolic dysfunction, or symptomatic patients with severe MR, should undergo surgical repair/replacement of the mitral valve.
- MVP patients with clinical or echocardiographic MR should receive antibiotic prophylaxis during invasive procedures.

Outcome

In most patients the prognosis is benign, although in a selected group of patients, MVP can progress, requiring surgical repair. Sudden death is a rare complication (<1% per year).

Pulmonary stenosis

- Most cases congenital, although rarer acquired causes include rheumatic fever and carcinoid syndrome.
- Presents with dyspnea, pre-syncope, syncope, and fatigue and progresses to right heart failure.
- Patients with more than mild pulmonary stenosis should receive antibiotic prophylaxis during invasive surgical and dental procedures.
- Asymptomatic patients with mild pulmonary stenosis (<29 mmHg gradient) can be followed up with regular echocardiography.
- Percutaneous balloon pulmonary valvuloplasty is recommended for patients with pliable valves and a valve gradient >30 mmHg at rest and for those with symptoms.
- Open pulmonary valvotomy is required if the valve is calcified or dysplastic.

Pulmonary regurgitation

- Most are due to dilatation of the pulmonary valve ring secondary to pulmonary hypertension. Other causes are mitral valve disease, left ventricular failure, infective endocarditis, rheumatic fever, and carcinoid syndrome.
- Patients are usually asymptomatic until right heart failure develops.

- Patients with pulmonary regurgitation should receive antibiotic prophylaxis.
- Treatment is usually directed at the primary cause of the pulmonary regurgitation. In cases of intractable right ventricular failure due to severe pulmonary regurgitation, valve replacement should be considered.

Tricuspid stenosis

- Most are due to rheumatic fever, although rarer causes include congenital tricuspid atresia and carcinoid syndrome.
- Presents with signs of right heart failure.
- Antibiotic prophylaxis during invasive surgical and perhaps dental procedures.
- A low sodium diet and oral diuretics can often improve the symptoms of systemic venous congestion.
- Patients with severe tricuspid stenosis should undergo tricuspid balloon valvuloplasty, open tricuspid valvotomy, or tricuspid valve replacement.

Tricuspid regurgitation

Causes of tricuspid regurgitation

Congenital

Isolated tricuspid regurgitation

Ebstein's anomaly

Acquired

Dilation of tricuspid valve annulus and right ventricular cavity (usually secondary to right ventricular infarction or long-standing pulmonary hypertension)

Rheumatic heart disease

Infective endocarditis (especially *Staphylococcus aureus* infection in intravenous drug abusers)

Carcinoid syndrome

Papillary muscle dysfunction

Trauma

Connective tissue disease (including Marfan's syndrome)

Radiation injury

Clinical features

History

- Asymptomatic for a prolonged period of time providing that pulmonary hypertension does not develop.
- Eventually, features of right ventricular failure and systemic venous congestion develop.

- *Hepatic tenderness/swelling of abdomen/ fluttering feeling in neck/leg swelling*
- *Fatigue* due to low cardiac output state

Examination

Pulse	Atrial fibrillation is common
JVP	Prominent c-v wave
	Venous systolic thrill/murmur in severe tricuspid regurgitation
Heart sounds	Right ventricular third heart sound
	Loud second heart sound if pulmonary hypertension
Murmurs	Pan-systolic murmur loudest at the lower left sternal edge
	Loudest in inspiration
Others	Pulsatile tender hepatomegaly
	Splenomegaly/ascites/peripheral edema

Investigations

ECG Incomplete right bundle branch block and Q waves in lead V1 may be present.

CXR Evidence of cardiomegaly and right atrial dilatation may be seen.

Echocardiography Can assess the severity of tricuspid regurgitation (see below).

Management

Antibiotic prophylaxis against endocarditis during surgical and dental procedures.

Symptomatic patients should receive diuretic therapy to reduce systemic venous congestion.

Patients with severe tricuspid regurgitation and pulmonary hypertension should be considered for tricuspid annuloplasty or valve replacement.

Prosthetic valves

Diseased valves were first replaced in the 1960s. There are two major types of prosthetic valves:

(1) Bioprosthetic, of which there are three main types:
  (a) Porcine heterografts such as Hancock and Carpentier-Edwards valves
  (b) Homograft aortic valves
  (c) Pericardial valves
(2) Mechanical, of which there are two main types:
  (a) Ball and cage such as Starr-Edwards valve
  (b) Tilting-disk such as Bjork-Shiley, St. Jude, Carbomedics

Recommendations for mechanical vs bioprosthetic valves
Valve replacement with a mechanical prosthesis
- with expected long lifespan
- already possessing a mechanical valve in a different position
- in renal failure or on dialysis
- already requiring warfarin therapy
- <65 years for AVR and <70 years for MVR

Valve replacement with bioprosthetic valve
- at risk of hemorrhage or women of child-bearing age who will not take warfarin
- >65 years old for AVR or patients >70 years old for MVR with no risk factors for thromboembolism*
- undergoing valve replacement for thrombosed mechanical valve

If the valve becomes incompetent, symptoms of congestive cardiac failure may develop.

In addition, patients should be alerted to seek medical attention if persistent fever or symptoms and signs of infective endocarditis develop, especially following invasive surgical or dental procedures or in the presence of systemic sepsis.

Investigations
Echocardiography
- It is important to obtain a baseline echocardiogram post-surgery and later to investigate complications such as thrombosis, infective endocarditis, and valve dysfunction or dehiscence of the valve sewing ring.

Management
Asymptomatic patients
- Annual review/echocardiogram or more urgent review if a new murmur or change in symptoms is noticed.
- Patients with mechanical prosthetic valves require lifelong anticoagulation with warfarin.
- Patients with bioprosthetic valves only require anticoagulation with warfarin for the first 3 months unless there is atrial fibrillation, an embolic event, or poor left ventricular function.
- All patients should receive antibiotic prophylaxis against endocarditis.

---

* Atrial fibrillation, severe LV dysfunction, previous thromboembolism, hypercoagulable condition

Outcome

Mechanical prosthetic valves last up to 35 years in the case of the Starr-Edwards valve. Bioprosthetic valves have an average lifespan of 10–15 years and because of this are not recommended for patients <40 years old.

Infective endocarditis

Infective endocarditis (IE) describes an infection of the heart valves, endocardium, or other structures within the heart. The bacteremia may result from either a focal infection elsewhere (such as of the urinary tract or lung) or it may follow invasive dental or surgical procedures.

Clinical features

History

- Patients can either present insidiously with fever, lethargy, malaise, weight loss or can present as an emergency with acute cardiac failure
- Intravenous drug abuse
- Predisposing valvular disease
- Prosthetic heart valves
- Congenital heart disease
- Previous IE
- Recent dental or surgical procedure
- Hypertrophic cardiomyopathy
- Intra-cardiac shunts

Examination

- Fever
- Hands/feet   Splinter hemorrhage
  Finger clubbing
  Osler's nodes (tender erythematous lesions of finger pads or in palms due to infected microemboli)
  Janeway lesions (slightly raised non-tender hemorrhagic lesions in the palms)
  Nail bed infarcts
- Eyes   Conjunctival hemorrhage
  Roth's spots
- Cardiac   New or changing murmur
  Signs of congestive heart failure
- Abdomen   Splenomegaly
- Renal   Microscopic hematuria

Diagnostic criteria

According to the modified Duke Clinical Criteria for the diagnosis of IE, patients with suspected IE can be assigned to three groups depending on the presence or absence of major and minor diagnostic criteria as outlined below. However, a high index of suspicion should be maintained for patients presenting with non-specific atypical symptoms and signs, especially intravenous drug abusers.

Modified Duke's Clinical Criteria for the diagnosis of IE

Definite IE

Pathologic criteria

Clinical criteria

2 major criteria

or 1 major and 3 minor criteria

or 5 minor criteria

Possible IE

1 major criterion

or 3 minor criteria

Unlikely IE

Alternative diagnosis for features

Resolution of features within 4 days of antimicrobial therapy

No evidence of IE found at surgery or autopsy, after ≤4 days of antimicrobial therapy

Definitions of terms used in Duke's Criteria for the diagnosis of IE

Major Criteria

(1) *Positive blood culture for IE*

  (A) Typical microorganism in two separate blood cultures

    (i) *Streptococcus viridans* or *bovis* or *Hemophilis, Actinobacillus, Cardiobacterium, Eikenella, Kingella* (HACEK) group

    (ii) Community acquired *Staph. aureus* or *Enterococcus* in the absence of a primary focus

(2) *Evidence of endocardial involvement*

  (A) Positive echocardiogram for IE

    (i) mobile echodense intracardiac mass attached to valvular leaflets or mural endocardium or

    (ii) periannular abscess or

    (iii) new dehiscence of prosthetic valve

  (B) New valvular regurgitation

Minor criteria

(1) *Predisposing* heart condition or **intravenous drug abuse**

(2) *Fever*: temperature $\geq 38.0\,^{\circ}\mathrm{C}$

(3) *Vascular involvement* such as arterial emboli, septic pulmonary infarcts, mycotic aneurysm, intracranial hemorrhage, conjunctival hemorrhages, and Janeway lesions

(4) *Immunologic involvement* such as glomerulonephritis (microscopic hematuria), Osler's nodes, Roth spots, and rheumatoid factor

(5) *Microbiologic evidence*: positive blood culture which does not meet major criteria or only serologic evidence of infection with typical microorganism

(6) *Echocardiographic findings* consistent with IE which do not meet major criteria

(7) *Elevated ESR or C-reactive protein*

(8) Newly diagnosed *finger-clubbing*

(9) *Splenomegaly*

(10) *Microscopic hematuria*

Epidemiology
Causative microorganisms in IE

Micro-organisms	Prevalence	Predisposing factors
Streptococcus viridans	50% ——	Native valve IE Prosthetic valve IE (>2 months after surgery)
Staphylococcus aureus	20% ——	Native valve IE Prosthetic valve IE (>2 months after surgery) Intravenous drug abusers (right-sided IE)
Staphylococcus epidermidis	——	Prosthetic valve IE (within 2 months of surgery)
Enterococcus faecalis or *faecium*		Malignancy and manipulation of genitourinary or gastro-intestinal tracts
HACEK	——	Native valve IE
Candida and other fungi	——	Prosthetic valve IE Immuno-compromised Intravenous drug abusers

Investigations
Blood tests

FBC	To detect anemia in subacute IE.
ESR/CRP	Raised inflammatory markers in IE.
Blood cultures	At least three different sets taken under strictly aseptic conditions at different times and from three different sites. The importance of sending multiple blood cultures prior to initiating antimicrobial treatment cannot be over-emphasized. Prolonged incubation on special media may be required to detect unusual organisms which can cause culture-negative IE.

CXR Congestive cardiac failure may be present if significant valvular dysfunction is present.

ECG The presence of new AV block may indicate the development of an aortic root abscess in a patient with IE of the aortic valve.

Echocardiography Transthoracic and transesphageal echocardiography may display the features outlined above and in Fig. 5.27.

Management

Patients require prolonged antibiotics and monitoring for vegetations >10 mm, significant valvular dysfunction, or perivalvular extension indicating a need for surgery.

Endocarditis prophylaxis

Antibiotic prophylaxis is recommended for patients at high or moderate risk, who have underlying structural cardiac abnormalities or prosthetic valves, when they undergo invasive surgical and dental procedures (Table 5.8). It is not necessary for patients at low risk.

Outcome
Complications of IE

(1) *Congestive heart failure*

Caused by: perforation of the valve
rupture of infected chordae tendinae,
valve obstruction from large vegetations,
prosthetic valve dehiscence,
the development of fistulae,
progressive valvular dysfunction, and
ventricular dysfunction.

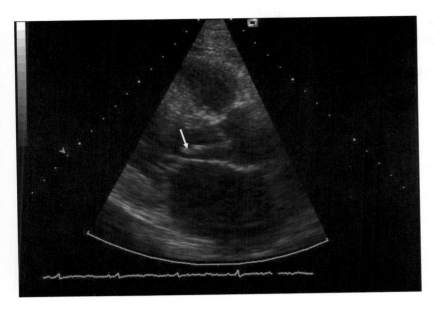

Fig. 5.27. Transesophageal echocardiogram demonstrating a vegetation on the mitral valve (arrow).

Table 5.8. Risk of infective endocarditis according to underlying cardiac abnormality

High Risk	Moderate Risk	Low Risk
Prosthetic valves	Other congenital malformations	Secundum ASD
Previous IE	Acquired valvular dysfunction	Surgically repaired
Complex cyanotic congenital heart disease	HCM	ASD/VSD
	MVP with clinical MR or thickened redundant leaflets	MVP without clinical MR
		ICD
		PPM

(2) Embolization

Embolization of vegetations usually occurs in the first 2–4 weeks of antimicrobial therapy. The greatest risk of embolization is from the anterior mitral valve leaflet.

(3) Periannular abscesses

More common in IE affecting the native aortic valve or prosthetic valves. A periannular abscess in aortic valve IE, near the membranous septum and atrioventricular node, may cause heart block.

(4) Splenic infarction and abscess

(5) Mycotic aneurysms

Mycotic aneurysms (MAs) result from the invasion of the vessel wall by infected embolized vegetation, and usually develop in the cerebral circulation.

Pericardial effusion and cardiac tamponade

A pericardial effusion may complicate acute pericarditis of any etiology. Provided the effusion accumulates slowly, even moderately large effusions can be asymptomatic. If the effusion accumulates rapidly or there is maximal pericardial distension the effusion compresses the ventricles and impairs ventricular filling with reduction in cardiac output and marked elevation of pulmonary and systemic venous pressures, a status known as cardiac tamponade.

Clinical features

History A pericardial effusion which does not compromise cardiac function may be asymptomatic. Large pericardial effusions may cause compression of surrounding structures resulting in dyspnea, cough, or dysphagia. Tamponade presents with dyspnea, tachycardia, and hypotension and even pulseless electrical activity (PEA) cardiac arrest.

Examination

- Tachypnea
- Blood pressure   Hypotension
  Pulsus paradoxus (fall in systolic blood pressure >10 mmHg on inspiration)
- Pulse   Sinus tachycardia
- JVP   Raised, and rises on inspiration (Kussmaul's sign)

- Heart sounds   Quiet
- Lungs   Bibasal crepitations (due to pulmonary edema)
- Other   Poor peripheral perfusion

Epidemiology

The most frequent causes of cardiac tamponade are neoplasm, idiopathic and viral pericarditis, uremia, myocardial infarction, hypothyroidism, invasive cardiac catheterization, bacterial infection, rheumatoid arthritis, and tuberculosis.

Investigations

Investigation of pericardial effusions

ECG

The ECG usually reveals a sinus tachycardia, with reduction in the QRS voltage and T wave flattening. In patients with cardiac tamponade there may be features of electrical alternans (alternating QRS complexes of different size thought to be attributable to the pendular action of the heart within the pericardial effusion).

Chest X-ray

Enlargement of the cardiac silhouette is only seen when there is more than 250 ml of pericardial fluid. The heart may appear globular in shape.

Echocardiography

Echocardiography is the best investigation for detecting and evaluating pericardial fluid. As little as 20 ml may be detected and identification of local effusions can guide drainage. Echocardiography allows the identification of tamponade, by revealing ventricular compression.

Management

Pericardial effusion with no cardiac compromise As long as the pericardial effusion does not compromise cardiac function, pericardiocentesis is not indicated, unless analysis of pericardial fluid is required for diagnosis.

Pericardial effusion persisting for more than 6 months may be due to a previous episode of acute pericarditis, hypothyroidism, chronic heart failure, liver failure, or nephrotic syndrome. It rarely causes symptoms and treatment is directed at the underlying cause.

Cardiac tamponade Patients with clinical and echocardiographic evidence of tamponade should undergo urgent pericardiocentesis.

In pericardiocentesis the drain is most commonly inserted under local anesthesia from a subxiphoid approach under fluoroscopic or echocardiographic guidance.

Constrictive pericarditis

Due to a fibrotic, thickened, and adherent pericardium restricting diastolic filling of the heart. It is a chronic process usually precipitated by an episode of acute pericarditis. The causes are listed below.

Etiology of constrictive pericarditis

Viral 42% (due to a previous episode of viral pericarditis)

Tuberculosis 15%

Rheumatoid arthritis

Post cardiac surgery

Mediastinal radiation therapy

Uremia

Connective tissue disease (rheumatoid arthritis, Systemic Lupus erythematosus)

Neoplasm

Clinical features

History

- *Congestion*
- *Ascites and peripheral edema, larger liver*
- *Exertional dyspnea/orthopnea*
- *Platypnea*
  Dyspnea in the upright position
- *Vague abdominal symptoms*
  Postprandial fullness, dyspepsia, flatulence, and anorexia.

Examination

- JVP   Prominent X and Y descent
  Raised with Kussmaul's sign (an inspiratory increase in systemic venous pressure)
- Blood pressure   Reduced pulse pressure
  Rarely pulsus paradoxus (compare to cardiac tamponade)
- Heart sounds   Diastolic pericardial knock at lower left sternal edge
- Abdomen   Pulsatile hepatomegaly
  Ascites
- Peripheral edema may be absent in young patients with competent venous valves

Investigations

ECG Low voltage, P-wave mitrale, and generalized T-wave inversion.

CXR Calcification of the pericardium in 50% especially in tuberculous pericarditis.

Echocardiography Pericardial thickening/calcification, left atrial enlargement, dilatation of hepatic veins and the inferior vena cava, variation in mitral and tricuspid flow velocities.

CT and MRI These imaging techniques can detect pericardial thickening/calcification and dilatation of hepatic veins and the inferior vena cava.

Management

Treatment is complete resection of pericardium (pericardiectomy).

Dizziness (pre-syncope) and blackouts (syncope)

Dizziness (pre-syncope) or blackouts (syncope) are cardinal symptoms of cardiovascular disease, and are due to transient cerebral hypoperfusion. A thorough history and examination is essential to elucidate the various causes of pre-syncope and syncope and to distinguish cardiac from neurologic causes. The major causes include:

Vascular causes (most common cause of syncope)
- Orthostatic hypotension (Chapter 18) Reflex-mediated syncope (including vaso-vagal syncope and carotid sinus hypersensitivity)

Cardiac causes (10%–20% of cases of syncope)

- Bradyarrhythmias — Sinus node dysfunction/bradycardia Conduction defects
- Tachyarrhythmias — Supraventricular and ventricular tachycardias
- Obstruction to left ventricular outflow — Aortic stenosis, hypertrophic cardiomyopathy

Neurologic causes (10% of cases of syncope) see *Neurologic Disease*
- Epilepsy
- Vertebro-basilar artery ischemia
- Vestibular disorders

Other causes
- Metabolic (hypoglycemia, hypoxemia, drugs, and alcohol)
- Others (hyperventilation, hysteria)

Evaluating the etiology of syncope

History
- ***Quantify the number and frequency of the episodes***
- ***Personal or family history of cardiac disease or syncope***
- ***Medications which may have contributed*** (for example, vasodilators and antihypertensive medications)
- ***Eye-witness account*** (to witness the tonic–clonic movements of an epileptic fit or the facial pallor of a cardiac cause of syncope)
- ***Preceding events or symptoms***
  Was the syncope preceded by:
  (1) anxiety, diaphoresis, confusion and tremor? (hypoglycemia).
  (2) change in posture, such as standing up? (postural hypotension).
  (3) movement of the head or neck, such as shaving? (carotid sinus hypersensitivity).
  (4) exertion? (severe aortic stenosis or hypertrophic cardiomyopathy).
  (5) an aura? (epileptic fit).
  (6) feeling of dizziness? (vasovagal syncope).
  (7) chest pain? (ischemic ventricular arrhythmia).
  (8) palpitations? (arrhythmia).
- ***Duration of syncope***
  For patients with cardiac syncope, the duration of the blackout is usually brief, lasting several seconds only. However, patients with a vaso-vagal episode may be syncopal for longer, and typically, patients with a neurologic cause for syncope may be unconscious for more than 5 minutes.
- ***Associated features of syncope***
  Typically patients with syncope due to a neurologic cause such as epilepsy will experience convulsions, tongue-biting, trauma, and urinary and/or fecal incontinence. Patients with syncope due to hyperventilation or hysteria may report symptoms of anxiety, panic, paresthesiae, tachypnea.
- ***Recovery from syncope***
  Patients experiencing syncope due to cardiac causes recover consciousness rapidly. Patients with Stokes-Adams attacks (transient asystole in patients with atrioventricular conduction block) often appear flushed following the syncopal episode, whereas patients with vaso-vagal syncope are often pale and sweaty. Those with syncope due to

a neurologic cause such as epilepsy may be expected to be drowsy and confused (the post-ictal period) for several hours following the episode.

Investigations

ECG The resting ECG may show the following abnormalities:

QT prolongation (long QT syndrome)

Short PR interval, delta wave
(Wolff-Parkinson-White syndrome)

AV conduction block (especially high-grade)

Bi- or tri-fascicular block

Bundle branch block

RBBB and persistent ST elevation in leads V1–V3
(Brugada syndrome, a familial cause of idiopathic ventricular fibrillation)

Ventricular ectopy

Ventricular hypertrophy

T wave inversion in the right precordial leads with incomplete right bundle branch block (arrhythmogenic right ventricular cardiomyopathy, ARVC)

Holter recording This is useful if the patient is experiencing frequent symptoms (such as several times a week), and it is essential to correlate any arrhythmia seen on the Holter recording with the patient's symptoms.

Event recorders These are useful when the symptoms occur less frequently (for example, a couple of times a month) but last a few minutes or more, since the device usually needs to be activated by the patient to record an event.

Implantable event recorders For patients with very infrequent episodes of syncope (a couple of times a year), this investigation may be helpful in unmasking or excluding an arrhythmic cause.

Echocardiography This can exclude structural heart disease such as hypertrophic cardiomyopathy, aortic stenosis, or mitral valve prolapse.

Carotid sinus massage This is used to identify carotid sinus hypersensitivity. After excluding the presence of carotid bruits by auscultation, pressure is applied and gentle rubbing over the carotid sinus is performed for 5 seconds, one side at a time, with continuous ECG monitoring.

Tilt-table testing This is a test for vaso-vagal syncope (see Reflex-mediated syncope). It involves monitoring during head-up tilting the patient at 70° for 45 minutes, in order to reproduce symptoms of pre-syncope and syncope.

Electrophysiologic testing Diagnostic electrophysiologic (EP) testing should be performed in patients with suspected structural heart disease and unexplained syncope.

Bradyarrhythmias

Bradyarrhythmias are defined as a heart rate <60 bpm, and can be due to disease of any part of the intrinsic conducting pathway of the heart including the sinoatrial node (SAN), atrioventricular node (AVN), the His bundle, and the left and right bundle branches. Bradycardias can present with dizziness, pre-syncope, syncope, exertional dyspnea, or general fatigue. Fig. 5.28 depicts an algorithm for diagnosing the cause of a bradycardia.

Sinus bradycardia

Sinus bradycardia is characterized by the sinus node discharging at a rate of less than 60 bpm.

Etiology of sinus bradycardia

Athletic heart

Acute myocardial infarction (more commonly with inferior MI)

Hypothyroidism

Vomiting

Vaso-vagal syncope

Drugs (amiodarone, AV blockers, atropine, calcium blockers)

During sleep

Eye surgery

Increased intracranial pressure

Intracranial, cervical, and mediastinal tumors

Hypothermia

Gram-negative sepsis

Depression

Anorexia nervosa

Clinical features

Features will depend on the underlying cause and investigations should be directed at identifying reversible causes.

Management

If no underlying cause can be found, treatment is only indicated if there are symptoms or hemodynamic compromise, IV atropine can be given as a temporary

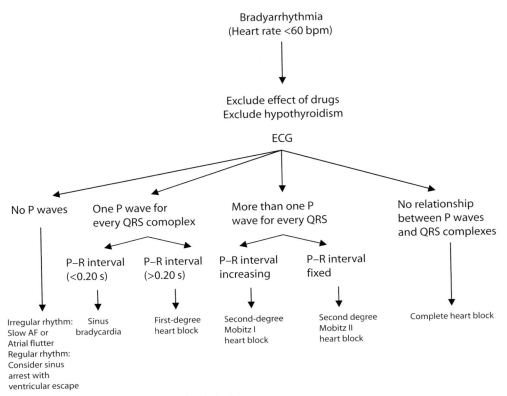

Fig. 5.28. Algorithm for identifying bradyarrhythmia.

measure. A permanent pacemaker may be required for chronic sinus bradycardia.

Sinus node dysfunction

Dysfunction of the heart's intrinsic pacemaker can result in bradyarrhythmia. The different types of sinus node dysfunction are listed below:

(1) *Sinus pause or sinus arrest*

A pause in sinus rhythm, due to slowing or cessation of sinus node automaticity.

(2) *Sinoatrial exit block*

A pause in sinus rhythm, due to conduction delay or block of the atrial impulse from the sinus node to the atrial muscle.

(3) *Sick sinus syndrome*

This condition may be characterized by any or a combination of the following:

- Bradycardia
- Sinus arrest or sinoatrial exit block
- SA or AV node conduction abnormalities
- Atrial fibrillation
  (so-called "tachy-brady" syndrome).

Management

Sinus pause/sinus arrest/sinoatrial block

If symptomatic, treatment is IV atropine acutely or a permanent pacemaker.

Sick sinus syndrome For symptomatic patients, permanent pacemaker implantation is recommended (preferably dual chamber pacemaker). For tachy-brady syndrome, a combination of pacing and anti-arrhythmic therapy may be required.

Conduction blocks

Conduction delays or blocks of the intrinsic intraventricular conducting system of the heart (comprising the His bundle, and left main bundle branch, which divides into the left anterior and posterior fascicles, and right main bundle branches), may present with pre-syncope or syncope.

Fascicular blocks

Delayed fascicular conduction (fascicular block) results in an abnormal early activation of the left ventricle as the fascicular sites are activated out of sequence as outlined below.

165

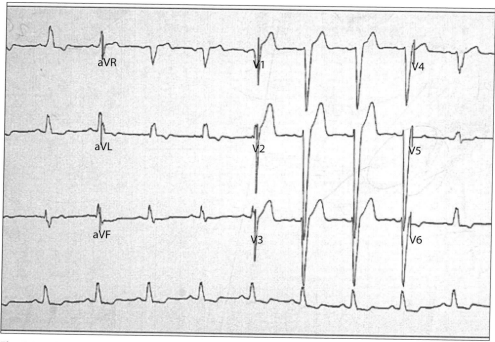

Fig. 5.29. Electrocardiogram demonstrating left bundle branch block.

Classification of fascicular blocks

(1) **Left anterior fascicular block (LAFB)** can be a normal finding, although it may also be associated with myocardial infarction, LVH, hypertrophic and dilated cardiomyopathy.

    ECG   Left axis deviation (mean QRS axis $-45°$ to $-90°$)

          QRS duration less than 120 ms

(2) **Left posterior fascicular block (LPFB)** is usually associated with cardiac abnormalities.

    ECG   Right axis deviation (mean QRS axis $> 120°$)

          QRS duration less than 120 ms

(3) **Left bundle branch block (LBBB)** (Fig. 5.29) usually indicates underlying heart disease, such as ischemic heart disease. The ECG changes of LBBB can obscure the expected ECG findings of an acute myocardial infarction. LBBB is associated with a 10-year survival rate of 50%.

Complete LBBB

    ECG   QRS duration more than 120 ms

          Broad notched R waves (RsR' pattern) in V5, V6, I and aVL with discordant ST–T wave segments

          Absent septal Q waves in left sided leads

Incomplete or partial LBBB

    ECG   QRS duration between 100 and 120 ms

          Absent septal Q waves in left sided leads

          Slurring and notching of the up-stroke of the R waves

(4) **Right bundle branch block (RBBB)** (Fig. 5.30) is a common finding and does not necessarily indicate the presence of cardiac disease, although the new onset of RBBB may indicate pulmonary embolus, ischemic heart disease or congestive heart failure.

Complete RBBB

    ECG   QRS duration more than 120 ms

          Broad notched R (rSr' pattern) waves in right precordial leads V1 and V2, with discordant ST-T wave segments.

          Wide and deep S (SrS' pattern) waves in V5 and V6

Incomplete or partial RBBB

    ECG   QRS duration between 100 and 120 ms

          rSr' pattern in lead V1

(5) **Bi- and tri-fascicular block**

    Bi-fascicular block indicates conduction delay or block in any two fascicles (for example

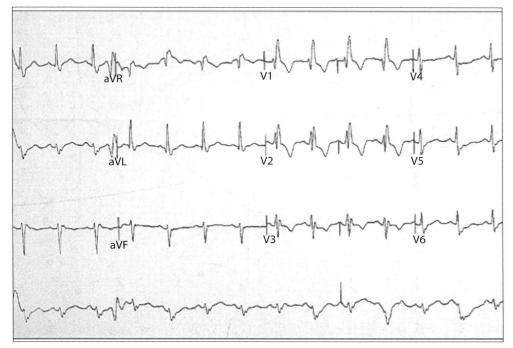

Fig. 5.30. Electrocardiogram demonstrating right bundle branch block.

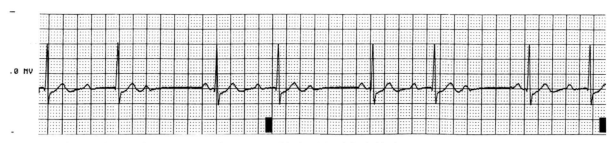

.0 MV

Fig. 5.31. Electrocardiogram demonstrating Mobitz type I AV block or Wenckebach block.

RBBB+LAFB or RBBB+LPFB), which does not affect AV conduction time.

Tri-fascicular block is bi-fascicular block with additional first-degree heart block. The presence of trifascicular block indicates underlying myocardial disease and a risk of higher degree heart block (see next section).

Atrioventricular (AV) block
Atrioventricular block is characterized by an atrial impulse which is either not conducted or conducted with delay to the ventricle, due to underlying intraventricular conduction delays. There are three types of AV block:

(1) First-degree AV block
Delay in the time taken for the atrial pulse to be conducted to the ventricle, P-R interval >0.20 seconds.

(2) Second-degree AV block
Some atrial impulses not conducted to the ventricle. There are two types:

(a) *Mobitz type I (or Wenckebach block)* (Fig. 5.31)
Progressive prolongation of the PR interval until a P wave is non-conducted. This is generally benign and tends not to progress to complete heart block.

(b) *Mobitz type II* (Fig. 5.32)
The PR interval remains constant prior to the non-conducted P wave, and can be quantified as the ratio of P waves to conducted QRS complexes (e.g. 2 : 1, 3 : 1). This type can often deteriorate to complete heart block (see next section).

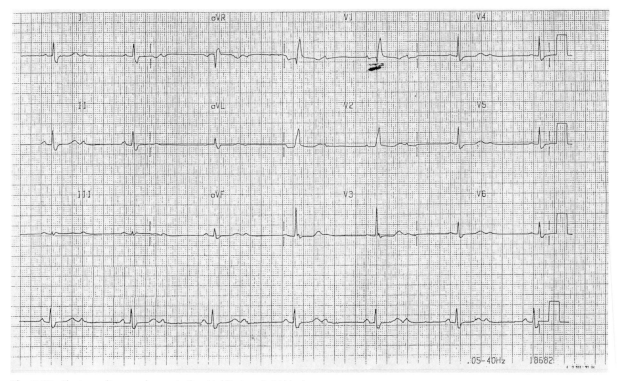

Fig. 5.32. Electrocardiogram demonstrating Mobitz type II AV block.

(3) **Third-degree AV block** (or complete AV/heart block) (Fig. 5.33)

There is complete AV dissociation, with the atria and ventricle contracting independently of each other. The ventricular rate is usually less than 40 bpm.

Causes of AV block

Congenital

Acquired

Degenerative processes

Ischemic heart disease (tri-fascicular block)

Electrolyte disturbances

Drug toxicity

Cardiac surgery

Myocarditis

Intra-cardiac tumors

Infiltrative processes (amyloid, sarcoid, or scleroderma)

Rheumatoid nodules

Calcific aortic stenosis

Hypothyroidism

Management

- Identify and treat reversible causes due to drugs and electrolyte imbalance.
- For emergency treatment of heart block causing hemodynamic compromise, IV atropine boluses may be given but the effect is short lived (<5 minutes). Insertion of a temporary pacemaker or infusion of isoprenaline may "buy time" in situations where bradycardia is likely to resolve spontaneously.
- If hemodynamically significant bradycardia persists, implantation of a permanent pacemaker is required.
- It is useful to recognize that AV block complicating inferior myocardial infarction, where the culprit artery supplies the atrioventricular node, tends to resolve within 2–3 days.
- Heart block in anterior myocardial infarction represents extensive infarction and usually requires a permanent pacemaker.

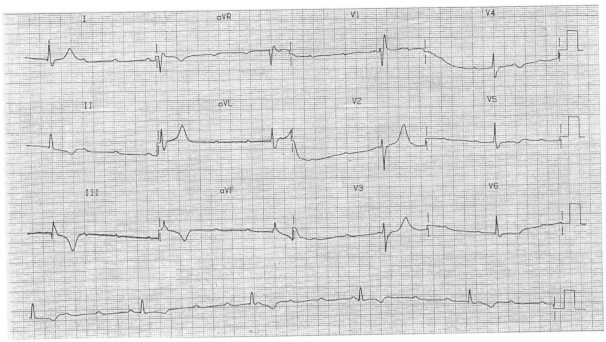

Fig. 5.33. Electrocardiogram demonstrating complete AV block.

- Symptomatic second- or third-degree AV block should be treated with insertion of a permanent pacemaker.

Reflex-mediated syncope

Reflex-mediated syncope comprises a trigger (the afferent limb of the reflex) and the effector (the efferent limb of the reflex). The two most important types are:

(1) vaso-vagal syncope (neurally mediated syncope) and

(2) carotid sinus hypersensitivity.

The effector response of the limb is similar, and involves increased vagal tone and reduced peripheral sympathetic tone, which causes bradycardia, vasodilatation, hypotension, pre-syncope, and syncope. It is the nature of the trigger which distinguishes the different types of reflex-mediated syncope:

Clinical features

Vaso-vagal syncope (neurally mediated syncope)

- Abrupt onset of hypotension with or without bradycardia. Associated with reduced ventricular filling and increased sympathetic tone.
- Triggers include the sight of blood, pain, prolonged standing, a warm environment and stress.

- Light-headedness may occur prior to syncope.
- Diagnosis from the history and confirmed by tilt-table testing (see below).

Carotid sinus hypersensitivity

- Stimulation of carotid sinus baroreceptors in susceptible individuals, by pressure on the neck or movements of the head, mediates a paradoxical withdrawal of sympathetic tone and an increase in vagal tone, causing vasodilatation and bradycardia.
- This may cause falls in the elderly, and is diagnosed by performing carotid sinus massage.

Investigations

Tilt-table testing

- Best test for vaso-vagal syncope.
- A positive test is the development of symptoms in association with hypotension and/or bradycardia, and can be classified into the categories outlined.

Carotid sinus massage

- Diagnostic test for carotid sinus hypersensitivity; a positive test is the development of pre-syncope or syncope on carotid sinus massage and is assigned to the categories of carotid sinus hypersensitivity listed below.

Type 1: Cardio-inhibitory

Heart rate falls with a pause of more than 3 seconds.

Type 2: Vasodepressor

Systolic blood pressure falls by more than 50 mmHg in the absence of bradycardia or falls more than 30 mmHg when symptoms reproduced.

Type 3: Mixed

A combination of the above two responses.

Management

Vaso-vagal syncope (neurally mediated syncope)

- Avoid situations which provoke syncope.
- Increase salt (>3 g day) and fluid intake (2–3 liters per day).
- Beta-blocker for recurrent syncope, especially if syncope preceded by tachycardia.
- Fludrocortisone, serotonin uptake inhibitors (such as paroxetine), or midodrine.
- Permanent pacemaker for failed medical therapy and patients that have a predominantly cardio-inhibitory response during syncope (type 2A).

Carotid sinus hypersensitivity

- Symptomatic patients with a predominantly cardio-inhibitory response require a permanent pacemaker.
- Symptomatic patients with a predominantly vasodepressor response may benefit from elastic support stockings or a sodium-retaining drug (fludrocortisone).

Ankle swelling

Ankle swelling can be a symptom of cardiovascular disease, although it may also be due to hypoalbuminemia from liver or renal disease. Major causes:

- Heart failure
- Deep vein thrombosis (DVT)/cellulitis/chronic venous insufficiency
- Hypoalbuminemia
- Drugs

The history, examination, and investigations are critical in differentiating between various causes of ankle swelling.

Cardiovascular causes of ankle swelling

- Right ventricular failure, tricuspid regurgitation, constrictive pericarditis, or pulmonary hypertension usually cause ankle edema due to increased systemic venous pressure, but in severe cases, mesenteric edema may give rise to malabsorption and hypoalbuminemia, which may contribute to ankle swelling.
- Ankle swelling due to right heart failure is characterized by bilateral pitting ankle edema, sacral edema in the bed-bound patient, raised JVP, hepatomegaly, and ascites.
- Ankle swelling is more marked at the end of the day.

Liver failure

Ankle swelling from hepatic failure is usually bilateral, and may be associated with ascites, hepatomegaly (if acute congestion), and signs of chronic liver disease.

Renal failure

Ankle swelling from renal failure is usually bilateral and pitting, and may be associated with periorbital edema.

Venous causes

Deep vein thrombosis (DVT) may be associated with unilateral pitting edema. Chronic venous insufficiency may follow varicose vein surgery and previous DVT. Ankle swelling from this condition may be associated with bilateral non-pitting edema, venous ulceration, and skin pigmentation.

Drug side effects

The most common drugs are calcium channel blockers, NSAIDs, and steroids.

Deep vein thrombosis (DVT)

Thrombosis of the deep veins of the leg can present as painful leg and ankle swelling. Early detection and treatment of DVT prevent the potentially fatal complication of pulmonary embolism.

Clinical features

History Patients may present with a swollen tender warm leg, restricted to either the calf or involving the whole leg, but may have no symptoms. Determine risk factors for developing DVT. These determine the pre-test probability (see later). Other conditions which are similar are rupture/leak of a knee joint Baker's cyst, lymphedema, venous obstruction, and cellulitis. Enquire about dyspnea, pleuritic chest pain, or hemoptysis. These may indicate pulmonary embolism.

Risk factors for development of DVT

Thrombophilia	Increased relative risk
Antithrombin deficiency	25
Protein C or S deficiency	5

Factor V Leiden mutation:

	Heterozygous	5
	Homozygous	50

Dysfibrinogenemia	18

Antiphospholipid syndrome:

	Anticardiolipin	2
	Lupus anticoagulant	10

Hyperhomocysteinemia	3
Elevated levels of factor VIII, IX, XI	2–3

Acquired

Major surgery or trauma	5–200
History of venous thromboembolism	50
Cancer	5
Hospitalization due to major medical illness	5
Age >50 years	5
>70 years	10
Pregnancy	7
Oral contraceptives	5
Hormone-replacement therapy	2
Estrogen modulators Tamoxifen	5
Raloxifen	3
Obesity	1–3

Examination
- Swollen, warm, tender leg or calf.
- Deep vein thromboses distal to the popliteal veins are called distal DVTs, whereas those proximal to the popliteal vein are termed proximal DVTs.
- Proximal DVTs are associated with a higher risk of pulmonary embolism.
- Lack of signs does not exclude DVT.

Epidemiology
The annual incidence of DVT is about 1 in 1000, with the risk increasing with age.

Pathology
- Development of DVT depends on three factors known as Virchow's triad:
  (1) venous stasis (such as from immobility or venous obstruction),
  (2) damage to the vessel wall, and
  (3) hypercoagulability (such as thrombophilias).

- DVT formation usually begins in the venous sinus of the calf, but proximal migration within the first week is common (about 25%).
- Rarely, massive DVT can compromise the vascular supply to the leg (i.e. phlegmasia cerulea dolens).

Investigations
Blood tests Routine full blood count, clotting screen and renal function should be measured prior to starting anticoagulation therapy.

Thrombophilia screen Should be done for patients <45 years old, a family history of thromboembolism, recurrent DVT or in unusual sites (mesenteric, renal, or hepatic veins), and idiopathic DVT.

D-dimer assays and pretest probability DVT formation is associated with a rise in plasma D-dimer levels, and using this test, combined with the pretest probability of having a DVT, allows patients to be assigned to different risk categories. Patients with a low or a moderate probability and negative D-dimers need no further investigation. Those with moderate or high risk and positive D-dimers should have duplex ultrasound of the leg. D-dimers are also raised in other conditions.

Determining pretest probability for DVT (Wells' criteria)

Active cancer (treatment within 6 months)	1
Paralysis or plaster cast	1
Bed rest >3 days or surgery within 4 weeks	1
Tenderness along veins	1
Entire leg swollen	1
Calf swollen >3 cm	1
Pitting edema	1
Collateral veins	1
Alternative diagnosis likely	−2

Pretest probability

Low	0 or less
Moderate	1–2
High	>3

Ultrasound duplex scanning With a high degree of suspicion and a negative scan, follow-up scanning in 1 week is recommended to exclude proximal migration of DVT.

Management
Aims are to control symptoms, treat the DVT, and prevent distal embolization. All can be undertaken as an outpatient.

Anticoagulation therapy Anticoagulation is initiated with low-molecular weight heparin and then warfarin. Warfarin is given for 3 months for DVT due to a transient risk factor. For idiopathic DVT or DVT due to malignancy, warfarin should be given for 6 months or longer. For patients with thrombophilia, life-long anticoagulation is recommended. The annual risk of bleeding while on warfarin (INR 2–3) is 3%.

Outcome

The risk of pulmonary embolism from untreated proximal DVT is about 50%.

Leg pain

Leg pain can be a symptom of cardiovascular disease. Cardiovascular causes of leg pain include peripheral arterial disease and venous disease, including chronic venous insufficiency, DVT, and post-thrombotic syndrome.

- Peripheral arterial disease (PAD)
- Venous disease
    - Chronic venous insufficiency
    - Deep vein thrombosis (DVT)
    - Post-thrombotic syndrome
- Non-vascular causes
    - Lumbosacral radiculopathy
    - Spinal stenosis
    - Arthritis of hip or knee

Exertional leg pain is characteristic of PAD but chronic venous insufficiency may also cause exertional leg pain. The associated features of skin pigmentation, leg edema, and venous ulceration should distinguish them.

Peripheral arterial disease

Peripheral arterial disease (PAD) refers to the atherosclerotic obstruction of arterial blood supply to the upper and lower limbs. Risk factors for the development of ischemic heart disease also apply to PAD.

Clinical features

History The cardinal symptoms of peripheral arterial disease are intermittent claudication and pain at rest.

Intermittent claudication is characterized by a pain, ache, or discomfort in the affected leg during exercise and relieved at rest. The distance at which the intermittent claudication begins and speed of walking should be noted. It occurs when muscle oxygen requirement exceeds that provided by the arterial supply.

Rest pain A manifestation of critical limb ischemia. Pain and parasthesia are felt in the calf, feet or toes. Elevation of the leg accentuates pain and lowering it or "hanging the feet over the edge of the bed" relieves the pain.

Examination The color (pallor or cyanosis), skin tone (smooth and shiny in ischemia), temperature, capillary refill time, and peripheral pulses should be examined. The major arteries should be auscultated to identify any bruits. Any ulcers, gangrene, or ankle edema should be noted.

Epidemiology

PAD affects <3% of people below the age of 60 years old but 20% of those 75 years or older. Atherosclerotic risk factors increase the risk of PAD.

Pathology

The process of atherosclerosis has been reviewed earlier (Fig. 5.1).

Investigations

Systemic blood pressure measurement This is the simplest method of assessing peripheral arterial stenoses. Systolic blood pressure is measured over selected segments of each limb, and a difference of more than 20 mmHg in the lower limbs or more than 10 mmHg between the upper limbs indicates a stenosis.

Ankle–brachial index The ankle–brachial index (ABI) is the ratio of the systolic blood pressure measured at the ankle to that measured at the brachial artery. An ABI ratio less than 0.9 is abnormal and below 0.5 indicates critical limb ischemia.

Doppler ultrasound and Duplex ultrasound Doppler ultrasound probe placed at 60° over an artery allows changes in the shape of the waveform to be recorded. Flow velocities can be measured and in the presence of a stenosis, systolic peak flow velocity is increased.

Treadmill exercise testing Used to provide objective evidence of intermittent claudication and assess the clinical significance of known peripheral arterial stenoses.

Angiography Magnetic resonance angiography (MRA) is non-invasive and with contrast allows visualization of location and severity of stenoses. Angiography is invasive and contrast may induce an allergic reaction or contrast nephropathy.

Management

Goals include: control of symptoms, preserving limb viability, and halting the progression of disease.

Risk factors for PAD Stopping smoking, aggressive control of diabetes, lipid lowering, anti-platelet therapy, and blood pressure control should all be instituted.

Symptom control

Pharmacologic agents Avoid beta-blockers. Pentoxifylline may improve symptoms of intermittent claudication by reducing blood viscosity, and Naftidrofuryl may improve those with moderate PAD.

Exercise Walking through the point of pain opens collateral vessels and improves walking distance.

Percutaneous transluminal angioplasty (PTA) and stents Used to treat PAD in patients with disabling symptoms or critical ischemia.

Peripheral arterial surgery Revascularization by surgery is undertaken for disabling symptoms refractory to medical therapy, to bypass chronic total occlusions unsuitable for percutaneous intervention, and to preserve limb viability in critical ischemia.

Outcome

The annual mortality of PAD is 4.5% with a sixfold increase risk of cardiac death. About 25% with critical ischemia (ABI <0.5) die within 1 year, and 1 year mortality after amputation is 45%. Diabetes mellitus and smoking predict progression of disease.

References

www.acc.org/clinical/statements.htm American College of Cardiology website with guidelines and statements relevant to the practice of cardiology.

www.heartstats.org A comprehensive resource for epidemiologic data pertaining to cardiovascular disease in the UK.

www.nice.org.uk The website of the National Institute of Clinical Excellence which issues guidelines and technology appraisals relevant to cardiovascular medicine.

Braunwald's Heart Disease: A Textbook of Cardiovascular Medicine 2004

A comprehensive and definitive reference textbook of cardiology.

The Cardiac Insufficiency Bisoprolol Study II: a randomised trial. *Lancet* 1999; **353**, 9–13. (CIBIS-II)

The effect of digoxin on morbidity and mortality in patients with heart failure. The Digitalis Investigation Group. *N Engl J Med* 1997; **336**, 525–533. (DIG)

Effect of losartan compared with captopril on mortality in patients with symptomatic heart failure: randomised trial-the Losartan Heart Failure Survival Study. *Lancet* 2000; **355**, 1582–1587. (ELITE II)

The effect of spironolactone on morbidity and mortality in patients with severe heart failure. Randomized Aldactone Evaluation Study Investigators. *N Engl J Med* 1999; **341**, 709–717. (RALES)

Effect of enalapril on survival in patients with reduced left ventricular ejection fractions and congestive heart failure. The SOLVD Investigators. *N Engl J Med* 1991; **325**, 293–302. (SOLVD)

Lung

John Rees

Contents

Shortness of breath

Shortness of breath is a symptom familiar to everybody from the effects of exercise. In disease states it usually means that the ventilatory response delivered by the lungs is less than expected from the signal sent out from the respiratory center. This inefficiency occurs most often when the work of breathing is increased by narrowing of the airways or by stiffness of the lungs or chest wall. Although breathlessness is most often associated with disorders of the lungs or heart, the origin of the problem may be in other conditions such as anemia or thyrotoxicosis. In addition, there is an element of the sensation of breathlessness related to consciousness. Breathlessness also occurs when the respiratory centres are stimulated through acidosis so that breathing is greater than needed for the degree of exercise being done (Fig. 6.1).

Acute shortness of breath

In this section "acute" will be taken as shortness of breath coming on over hours or a day or two rather than weeks or months. Within this time scale, the speed of onset may be a helpful feature in differential diagnosis (Table 6.1) as may be a number of associated features (Table 6.2). Severe shortness of breath coming on over minutes is most likely to be caused by occlusion of a pulmonary artery by an embolus or acute loss of lung volume in a pneumothorax. The commonest causes of breathlessness coming on over a slightly slower period of minutes or hours would be airflow obstruction in asthma or chronic obstructive pulmonary disease and pulmonary edema in left heart failure where the lungs become stiff and then alveoli flood with edema fluid interfering with gas exchange.

Acute shortness of breath may be the onset of a new medical problem such as a pulmonary embolus (p. 182) or an inhaled foreign body. Alternatively, it may be a repeated problem in exacerbations of an underlying problem such as asthma or an increased level of breathlessness in a chronic condition such as chronic obstructive pulmonary disease (COPD, p. 190).

Conditions which will be considered in detail in this section on acute shortness of breath are:

- Asthma
- Pulmonary embolus
- Pneumothorax
- Pneumonia
- Anxiety/panic attacks

The investigations required to establish the diagnosis and to guide treatment depend on the clinical

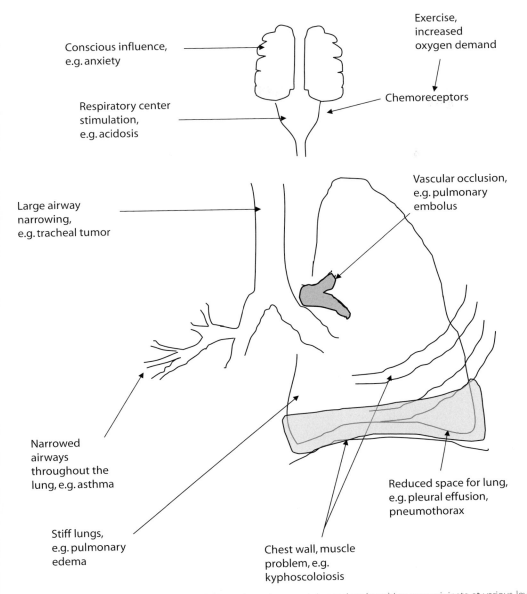

Conscious influence,
e.g. anxiety

Exercise,
increased
oxygen demand

Respiratory center
stimulation,
e.g. acidosis

Chemoreceptors

Vascular occlusion,
e.g. pulmonary
embolus

Large airway
narrowing,
e.g. tracheal tumor

Narrowed
airways
throughout the
lung, e.g. asthma

Reduced space for lung,
e.g. pleural effusion,
pneumothorax

Stiff lungs,
e.g. pulmonary
edema

Chest wall, muscle
problem, e.g.
kyphoscoloiosis

Fig. 6.1. Causes of shortness of breath. The stimulus to increased demand on breathing may originate at various levels in the lungs, brain, and chemoreceptors.

picture. It will usually be possible to limit the differential diagnosis considerably on the basis of the presenting features and the investigations can be targeted at the likely diagnoses (Table 6.3). In practice, one of the difficult features may be differentiating a cardiac from a respiratory problem. The previous history is likely to be very helpful in the differentiation but some of the signs and symptoms may overlap. Wheezing may be heard from the edema around the airways in left heart failure as well as its usual finding in asthma and COPD. Crackles at the lung bases are common in left heart failure, pulmonary fibrosis, and COPD, although they are heard late in the inspiratory phase of breathing in the former two conditions where small airways have closed during expiration and need to snap open again as the lung expands. In chronic airflow obstruction larger airways are involved and the crackles occur towards the beginning of inspiration.

Table 6.1. Time relationships of common causes of acute shortness of breath

Diagnosis	Minutes	Hours	Days	Weeks	Months
Foreign body	⟷				
Laryngeal obstruction (epiglottitis, anaphylaxis)	⟷				
Pneumothorax	⟷				
Pulmonary embolus	⟷				
Anxiety	⟷				
Acute asthma	⟷			⟷	
Extrinsic allergic alveolitis		⟷		⟷	
Acidosis		⟷			
Pulmonary edema		⟷			
Acute exacerbation of chronic obstructive pulmonary disease		⟷			
Pneumonia		⟷			

Table 6.2. Associated features helpful in the differential diagnosis of acute shortness of breath

Associated feature	Likely diagnosis	Other common features
Severe and sudden onset	Pulmonary embolus Pneumothorax	Pleuritic pain, shock Pleuritic pain, chest signs
Worse on lying down	Pulmonary edema (left heart failure) COPD	Cardiac problems Smoking, history
Problems at night	Pulmonary edema Asthma	Cardiac problems, relieved on sitting/getting up Wheeze, relieved by bronchodilators
Inspiratory stridor	Anaphylaxis, laryngeal edema Epiglottitis Foreign body	Tongue swelling, urticaria Child Child
Expiratory wheeze	Asthma Chronic obstructive pulmonary disease	History Smoker, cough, history of COPD
Pleuritic pain	Pneumothorax Pulmonary embolus Pneumonia	Chest signs Predisposing factors Fever, cough
Hemoptysis	Pulmonary embolus Pulmonary edema (frothy pink sputum)	Predisposing factors Cardiac problem (pain, arrhythmia)
Central chest pain	Ischemic heart disease	Risk factors, history
Hyperventilation	Anxiety Acidosis	Feeling of inability to take a full breath Carpopedal spasm Renal failure, hyperglycemia
Fever	Pneumonia Asthma COPD exacerbation Acute extrinsic allergic alveolitis	Chest signs, fever Wheeze, history Smoking, history Cough, fever, relevant exposure (hay, birds, etc.)
Decreased conscious level	Diabetic keto-acidosis	Dehydration

Approach to a patient with acute breathlessness

Assess the severity of the problem with breathing
⇩
If severe, summon help immediately
⇩
Is respiration adequate?
This depends on an assessment of the degree of difficulty the patient is having, and the adequacy of oxygenation and carbon dioxide retention.
⇩
Take a history (focused on major issues initially if symptoms are severe)
⇩
Examine the chest
⇩
Record vital signs (temperature, pulse, respiratory rate, blood pressure, oxygen saturation with a pulse oximeter, peak flow or spirometry)
Consider further investigations such as chest X-ray, arterial blood gases for information on pH and P_aCO_2 (remember the oximeter gives information on oxygen levels but not carbon dioxide), electrocardiogram
⇩
Consider other investigations such as:

- Full blood count to rule out anemia and measure the white count
- Renal function
- Blood culture if pneumonia is suspected
- D-dimers, CT pulmonary angiogram if pulmonary embolus is possible

⇩
Give oxygen treatment (with care in older patients with COPD)
Consider ventilatory assistance if the patient is tired or the CO_2 rising.

Asthma

Definition

Typically, asthma is defined as narrowing of the intrathoracic airways which shows reversibility with time or treatment. Newer definitions have emphasized the inflammatory nature of asthma involving numerous cells including CD4 lymphocytes, mast cells, and eosinophils.

Epidemiology

Asthma appears to have increased in prevalence in most countries of the world. Some countries, such as Australia and New Zealand, have a higher prevalence. In the Far East and in many developing countries the

Table 6.3. Important investigations used in the diagnosis and assessment of patients with acute shortness of breath

Suspected diagnosis	Investigation
Pneumothorax	
Pulmonary embolus	
Pneumonia	
Pulmonary edema	Chest X-ray
COPD	
Foreign body (may need expiratory film also)	
Ischemic heart disease	Electrocardiogram
Asthma	Peak flow
COPD (or use spirometry)	
Pulmonary embolus	
Asthma	
COPD	Arterial blood gases
Pneumonia	
Acidosis (diabetic, renal failure)	

rates are lower, but migration to a developed country or change to that lifestyle is associated with a higher level.

There is a strong genetic component which seems to be linked to a number of different genetic loci. The inheritance may be for atopy, the tendency to develop IgE on exposure to common allergens, which is present in 30%–40% of the population. The increase in prevalence is related to changes in environmental conditions which interact with the genetic predisposition. The most popular explanations of the changes in prevalence are related to maturation of the immune system. In the hygiene hypothesis a smaller number of early viral infections, because of social changes, smaller family size and immunization, may delay the normal maturation of the immune system and the normal switch in infancy from Th1 to Th2 lymphocytes. Maternal smoking is another factor.

The onset of asthma is most often in childhood between 2 and 7 years but it can come on at any age. In children it is twice as common in boys but through teenage years boys are more likely to lose their asthma making the prevalence equal by the end of the teenage years. Estimates of prevalence vary with the precise definition but are around 10%–20% in children, dropping a little in adults.

Mechanisms

The airways in asthma are inflamed. A degree of this inflammation remains even when the asthma

177

Table 6.4. Precipitating factors in asthma

Common precipitating factors
- Pollens (grass, trees, molds)
- Animal dander (cats, dogs, rabbits, rodents)
- House dust mite (*Dermatophagoides pteronyssinus*)
- Infections (rhinovirus, etc.)
- Exercise
- Irritants (atmospheric pollution, cigarette smoke, perfumes)
- Emotion, stress

Less common precipitating factors
- Foods (nuts, dairy products)
- Drugs (aspirin, NSAIDs, ß-blockers
- Occupational agents (see Table 6.5)

Table 6.5. Some occupational agents involved in asthma

Agent	Occupation
Isocyanates	Polyurethane foam makers, adhesive, paint workers
Flour, grain	Bakers, millers
Laboratory animals and insects	Scientific laboratory workers
Platinum salts	Metal refiners
Proteolytic enzymes	Biological detergent manufacture
Acid anhydrides, hardening agents, epoxy-resins	Manufacturing, coating, adhesives
Azodicarbonamide	Plastic blowing
Colophony fumes	Electronic soldering
Wood dusts	Carpenters, wood workers
Cotton, flax, hemp dust	Processing materials
Latex	Health professionals, laboratory workers
Hair sprays	Hairdressers
Drug manufacture (antibiotics, ispaghula)	Pharmaceutical workers

is in remission and this helps to explain the tendency to relapse. The initial inflammation may be induced by a specific allergic response but the inflamed airway is then sensitive to numerous other specific allergens and non-specific triggers such as dust, cold air, or exercise. This hyperresponsiveness of the airways to various stimuli can be measured by challenge with inhalation of histamine or methacholine.

In younger patients there are more likely to be identifiable extrinsic causes for asthma. Most of these causes are inhaled allergens, but there is a wide range of precipitating factors (Table 6.4). Patients with an atopic predisposition have a tendency to produce specific IgE in response to common allergens. They often are sensitive to multiple factors. The presence of specific IgE can be shown by skin prick testing or, more expensively, by measurement in the blood of specific IgE antibodies.

In older patients similar inflammatory changes exist in the airways but there may be less day to day variation and less evidence of specific precipitating factors other than infections. These infections are most often viral.

Many hundreds of substances have been implicated in occupational asthma (Table 6.5). This probably makes up around 2%–5% of adult asthma but is an important subgroup since early detection and avoidance may change the natural history of the asthma in a way not possible with other triggers.

Samples from the airway wall show the inflammatory nature of asthma (Fig. 6.2). There is an inflammatory infiltrate of eosinophils, mast cells, and neutrophils. Macrophages and lymphocytes are involved in control of the process. There is associated edema of the airway wall with shedding of the epithelium. The smooth muscle hypertrophies, mucus

secretion changes, and the lumen may be blocked by thick mucus plugs in acute episodes.

A number of cytokines and mediators are important in the inflammatory process, controlling cell migration and tissue damage (Fig. 6.3). Persistent inflammation seems to lead to fibrosis which permanently limits airway caliber.

Clinical features

The major clinical feature of asthma is shortness of breath with expiratory wheezing. However, cough may be a prominent symptom and may be the only manifestation in some cases (see page 200). The pattern is of variability in the degree of airway narrowing and shortness of breath. The variation may be spontaneous or in response to identifiable triggers such as those in Table 6.4. A typical pattern is of a diurnal variation in the airway calibre with the most severe obstruction in the early hours (2–4 am) of the morning and greatest calibre in the afternoon. The precise reason for this rhythm is uncertain. Patients may wake in the night with wheeze and cough, and questions about sleeping are an important part of the history in asthma.

Questions in the history should cover:
- Pattern of symptoms
- Precipitating factors

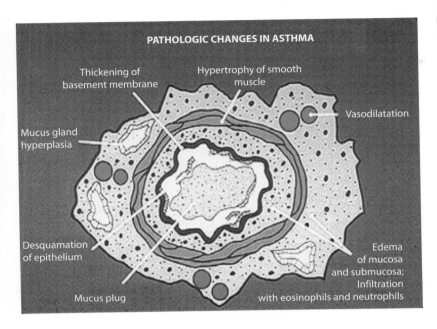

Fig. 6.2. Changes in the airway wall in asthma.

PATHOLOGIC CHANGES IN ASTHMA

Thickening of basement membrane

Hypertrophy of smooth muscle

Vasodilatation

Mucus gland hyperplasia

Desquamation of epithelium

Edema of mucosa and submucosa; Infiltration with eosinophils and neutrophils

Mucus plug

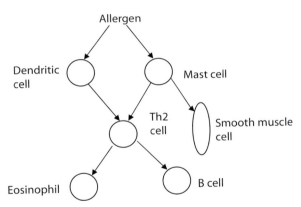

Allergen

Dendritic cell

Mast cell

Th2 cell

Smooth muscle cell

Eosinophil

B cell

Fig. 6.3. Cells involved in the pathology of asthma.

- Relevant exposure (pets, work, hobbies, etc.)
- Disturbance at night
- Cough
- Effectiveness of treatment
- Experience of acute attacks
- Understanding of management of chronic problems and exacerbations
- Smoking history
- Family history

Another typical feature is precipitation by exercise. This may come on during exercise or in the minutes after stopping. It is more pronounced with exercise in cold, dry air and more noticeable in children. Exercise induced asthma does not provoke hyperresponsiveness and sensitivity to other agents as seen with exacerbations induced by allergens. Exercise should be encouraged, covered by appropriate medication.

The clinical pattern of asthma may be one of occasional mild symptoms, persistent breathlessness, or severe exacerbations. Exacerbations should always be taken seriously since they can be life-threatening. Most severe attacks are preceded by a few days of worsening symptoms or increased diurnal variation. This gives the opportunity to adjust treatment and reverse the decline. Severe attacks and death are usually associated with lack of appreciation of the seriousness of asthma. Patients need to be helped to understand the pattern of their asthma and its management.

Table 6.6 shows levels of severity of acute asthma exacerbations.

In acute exacerbations of asthma certain signs and symptoms are used to evaluate the severity of an attack (Fig. 6.10).

Investigations

The most important investigation in asthma is measurement of the degree of airflow obstruction. This is achieved most simply by measuring the peak expiratory flow (PEF). This can be done with a cheap portable peak flow meter which asthmatics can keep at home to monitor their condition (Fig. 6.4). The

Table 6.6. Levels of severity of acute asthma exacerbations (British Thoracic Guidelines)

Near fatal asthma	Raised $PaCO_2$ and/or requiring mechanical ventilation with raised inflation pressures
Life-threatening asthma	Any one of the following in a patient with severe asthma:
	– PEF <33% best or predicted – bradycardia
	– SpO_2 <92% – dysrhythmia
	– PaO_2 <8 kPa – hypotension
	– normal $PaCO_2$ (4.6–6.0 kPa) – exhaustion
	– silent chest – confusion
	– cyanosis – coma
	– feeble respiratory effort
Acute severe asthma	Any one of:
	– PEF 33–50% best or predicted
	– Respiratory rate ≥25/min
	– Heart rate ≥110/min
	– Inability to complete sentences in one breath
Moderate asthma exacerbation	– Increasing symptoms
	– PEF >50–75% best or predicted
	– No features of acute severe asthma

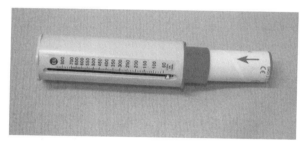

Fig. 6.4. Peak flow meter.

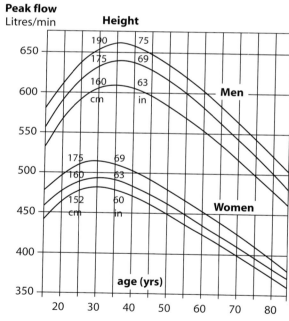

Fig. 6.5. Predicted peak flow values with age and sex. From Gregg I and Nunn A.J. BMJ 1989; **298**, 1068–70, with permission.

predicted values depend on age, sex, height and race (Fig. 6.5). Typical patterns in asthma are the diurnal variation with dips in the early hours of the morning (Fig. 6.6) and the progressive deterioration seen before a severe exacerbation (Fig. 6.7). In certain situations such as suspected occupational asthma more regular monitoring of peak flow through days on and off work may be needed to establish links.

The obstruction to airflow will also be evident in a spirometry trace (Fig. 6.8) where forced expiratory volume in one second (FEV1) is reduced proportionately more than forced vital capacity (FVC) to give a ratio between the two (forced expiratory ratio) of less than the normal 70%–80%.

Hyperresponsiveness of the airways is a characteristic of asthma. This can be demonstrated by measuring changes during and after exercise when the cooling and drying of the mucosa stimulates airway narrowing. A quantitative measure of hyperresponsiveness can be

established through the inhalation of increasing concentrations of histamine or methacholine.

Skin tests introduce tiny amounts of antigen into the upper layers of the epidermis. A wheal 15 minutes later shows the presence of specific IgE. Skin prick tests should be interpreted in the context of the clinical asthma. A positive response does not necessarily

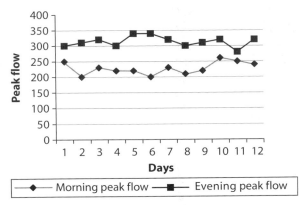

Fig. 6.6. Peak flow pattern of diurnal variation.

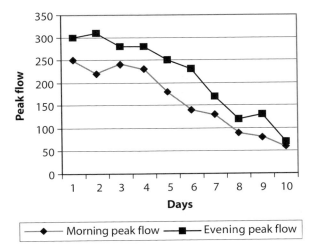

Fig. 6.7. Deterioration in peak flow in the days before an exacerbation.

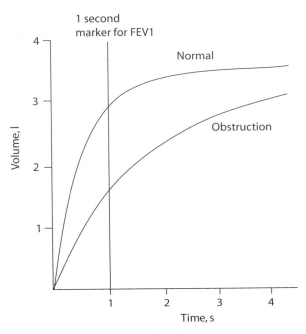

Fig. 6.8. Spirometry trace in airflow obstruction.

mean that the agent is clinically important in the asthma. Estimations of specific IgE in the blood give similar information.

Other investigations are used when complicated forms of asthma are suspected. A rare condition called Churg–Strauss syndrome or allergic granulomatosis consists of asthma with arteritis and eosinophilic infiltration of organs such as the lungs, skin, heart, nervous system. It is associated with a high ESR and very high eosinophil count. Churg–Strauss syndrome requires prolonged treatment with corticosteroids and immunosuppressants.

In allergic bronchopulmonary aspergillosis (ABPA) there is an IgE response to the fungus *Aspergillus fumigatus* which can be found in eosinophil laden plugs in the airways. *Aspergillus* is a widely distributed fungus found in the earth and in rotting vegetation. These plugs obstruct bronchi and lead to local damage to the walls with proximal bronchiectasis (see p. 204). Characteristic findings are a raised blood eosinophil count and an early and late response to *Aspergillus* on skin prick testing.

Management

A very important part of the management is to involve the patient in an understanding of asthma and its treatment. Joint management by patient and doctor or nurse is helpful to control a variable disease with precipitating factors, some of which may be identifiable. Patients should be involved in the production of their own written management plan, which should then be reviewed regularly.

Asthma is a disease which cannot usually be cured unless there is a single identifiable trigger such as a drug or occupational cause. Identifiable causes should be removed whenever possible but this may not be possible with widespread agents such as pollen or house dust mite. Management then relies on control with medication which needs to be continued even when symptoms are absent. Desensitization can have a minor effect but it may become more useful with the development of new safer and more effective techniques.

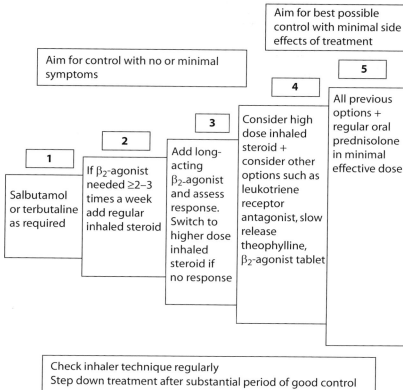

Aim for best possible control with minimal side effects of treatment

Fig. 6.9. Guidelines for treatment of chronic asthma (taken from BTS/SIGN guidelines). Treatment can start at any step. The aim is to establish good control. Treatment should be reviewed at least at 3- to 6-month intervals. (Adapted from: British Guideline on the Management of Asthma. A national clinical guideline. British Thoracic Society and Scottish Intercollegiate Guidelines Network, May 2008 with permission).

Aim for control with no or minimal symptoms

5

All previous options + regular oral prednisolone in minimal effective dose

4

Consider high dose inhaled steroid + consider other options such as leukotriene receptor antagonist, slow release theophylline, β₂-agonist tablet

3

Add long-acting β₂-agonist and assess response. Switch to higher dose inhaled steroid if no response

2

If β₂-agonist needed ≥2–3 times a week add regular inhaled steroid

1

Salbutamol or terbutaline as required

Check inhaler technique regularly
Step down treatment after substantial period of good control

Many of the drugs available for asthma treatment can be given by inhalation, reducing the side effects since a small quantity of the drug is delivered to the appropriate site in the airways. Many different devices are available and most patients can be taught to take their drugs by inhalation but it requires careful and regular attention to inhaler technique and compliance.

The drugs available for asthma treatment are:

Bronchodilators
(1) ß-agonists
(2) Anticholinergics (ipratropium bromide)
(3) Theophylline

Beta-agonists are the main bronchodilator used in the management of asthma. They are used almost always by inhalation. Short acting agents such as salbutamol and terbutaline act within minutes and last for a few hours. They are used as needed to reverse airway narrowing or before exercise and frequency of use can be used as a guide to control. Long-acting agents such as salmeterol and formoterol work for 12 hours and regular use often provides very

effective symptom control. Formoterol has a faster onset of bronchodilatation than salmeterol and can be used on an as required basis in some management plans. It can be used in a combined inhaler with budesonide as the single agent for regular treatment and relief.

Anti-inflammatory drugs
(1) Corticosteroids
(2) Leukotriene receptor antagonists
(3) Mast cell stabilizers (sodium cromoglycate)

When more than occasional inhalations of ß-agonists are required, a regular suppressive agent should be considered. The most effective agents are usually an inhaled corticosteroid such as beclomethasone dipropionate, budesonide, or fluticasone. These need to be used regularly. At the doses needed in asthma-inhaled corticosteroids have few side effects other than occasional oral candidiasis, dysphonia, or bruising in older patients. Most of the steroid benefit comes at low dose although larger doses are needed in some patients. Leukotriene receptor antagonists such as

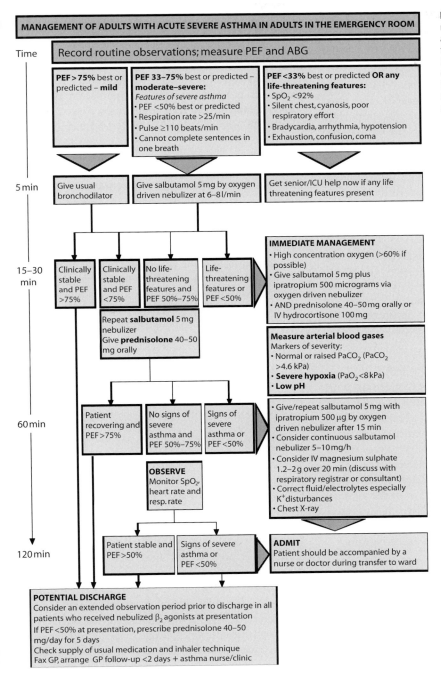

Fig. 6.10. Guidelines for the management of acute exacerbations of asthma in the acute setting. (Adapted from: British Guideline on the Management of Asthma. A national clinical guideline. British Thoracic Society and Scottish Intercollegiate Guidelines Network, May 2008 with permission.)

montelukast or zafirlukast provide an alternative or additional agent. They are taken orally and are less effective than inhaled corticosteroids, but may produce an alternative or additional effect. Sodium cromoglycate is less effective and is not often used now except in children.

The treatment of chronic asthma depends on the severity of symptoms and airflow obstruction. It is often represented as a series of steps as in those from the British Thoracic Society guidelines (Figs. 6.9, 6.10).

Over the next few years newer agents acting on IgE, eosinophils, cytokines and lymphocyte maturation will become available. Omalizumab is a humanized monoclonal antiIgE antibody which has been shown to be effective but requires regular injection.

Acute exacerbations In acute exacerbations of asthma a careful assessment of severity and close monitoring of progress are essential. The important elements of treatment are high inspired oxygen and high doses of bronchodilators and corticosteroids. In exacerbations ß-agonists are often given by nebulizer to deliver a high dose and overcome difficulties in coordination with inhalers. Corticosteroids are given orally or intravenously. The other important modalities are oxygen and bronchodilators as set out in the treatment guidelines shown (Fig. 6.10). Fluid and electrolytes need to be monitored and replaced as necessary. Intravenous magnesium is used in severe attacks. Antibiotics might be used if there is fever, purulent sputum, or chest X-ray changes, but they are not used routinely as, even when infection is the trigger, the organisms are usually viruses.

Outcome

A common question of parents is whether children will grow out of their asthma. This is more likely in boys and in milder disease. If asthma is severe and continuous as a child, it is likely to continue to be a problem. Even if it remits, the predisposition may remain given a sufficient trigger. Asthma which appears later in life tends to be more persistent.

One of the hopes of adequate treatment is that it may suppress damaging inflammation in the airways and prevent irreversible obstruction from structural damage to the airway wall. There is certainly evidence that adequate treatment will reduce exacerbations.

Pulmonary embolus

Definition

In pulmonary embolism material freed from some part of the venous system is detached and lodges in the pulmonary arterial tree. The most common material is thrombus detached from a clot in a peripheral leg vein, but emboli may also be portions of tumor, fat from bone trauma, or air.

Epidemiology

The reasons for the thrombus forming in the peripheral vein are classically an alteration in the vessel wall (such as compression), in the blood flow (reduced muscle pump with inactivity), or in the constituents such as an excessive number of platelets, increased fibrinogen and platelet stickiness after an operation, or an inherited problem such as protein C or S deficiency.

Mechanisms

The occlusion of a branch of a pulmonary vein interferes with gas exchange through ventilation–perfusion mismatching in the lung and causes passive congestion of an area of lung which may lead to infarction.

Clinical features

Classical features of a pulmonary embolism are shortness of breath, hypoxia, pleuritic chest pain if there is an associated pulmonary infarction causing irritation of the pleura. Cough and reflex airway narrowing causing a wheeze may occur, and hemoptysis may be a feature. Fever may develop from the pleural inflammation and the pleural involvement may lead to pleural effusion which may be blood stained. A large pulmonary embolus which occludes a large proximal pulmonary artery may cause a reduction in cardiac output with hypotension.

The jugular venous pressure tends to be high and cyanosis may occur with a large embolus. Fever, tachycardia, and tachypnea are common.

Occasionally, repeated small pulmonary emboli produce little or no acute problems but the gradual development of pulmonary hypertension.

Investigations

These divide into investigations to establish the diagnosis and to investigate the cause. The degree of clinical suspicion of deep vein thrombosis and pulmonary embolism will determine the course of investigation for diagnosis. One initial approach is to measure D-dimers from the breakdown of fibrin. Although a positive test may have many causes, a negative test makes recent thromboembolism unlikely and further investigation is not usually indicated unless the degree of clinical suspicion is high.

Plain chest X-ray is often unhelpful, although it may show a pleural effusion, a wedge shaped area of consolidation, linear atelectasis, or an area of decreased vascular markings. None of these is specific and the chest X-ray is often normal. Similarly, the ECG can show findings of right heart strain with an S wave in lead 1 and Q wave and inverted T wave in lead 3 (S1Q3T3 pattern), but is more likely to show just a tachycardia.

One other approach is to try to find evidence of deep vein thrombosis through Doppler ultrasound of the legs. More invasive is venography of the leg veins. These techniques do not diagnose the pulmonary embolism but the potential for embolism. However, they may be normal even with an embolus since the whole clot may have detached or the source may be elsewhere such as the arm veins.

The other alternative is to look for evidence of the embolus itself through a ventilation–perfusion lung scan to show an area that is ventilated but not perfused. This is effective with previously normal lungs but difficult to interpret with underlying lung disease. Pulmonary arteriography has been the gold standard investigation in the past. However, CT pulmonary angiography with contrast injection timed to delineate the pulmonary arteries now provides good imaging of the proximal vessels and is used widely in diagnosing significant pulmonary emboli.

If there is no obvious reason for a pulmonary embolus, such as recent surgery, then a predisposition to clot, thrombophilia, should be considered. Most of the relevant tests for protein C and protein S deficiency, and factor V Leiden need to be sent off before starting oral anticoagulants which interfere with the measurements.

Management

The management depends on the degree of circulatory compromise produced by the embolus. If this is substantial, producing a low cardiac output and low blood pressure, then the treatment would be thrombolysis providing there are no contraindications, such as recent surgery. Otherwise the mainstay of treatment is anticoagulation to reduce the chances of any further embolism. The original pulmonary embolus will usually lyse or recannulate providing the extent of the obstruction is not too great. Anticoagulation is usually started with low molecular weight heparin subcutaneously. Oral warfarin is then started for long term control but takes some days to develop its full effect. It is controlled by regular measurements of the International Normalized Ratio (INR) which compares the patient's clotting against a standard reference value. Treatment is for 3–6 months if there was an obvious precipitant but may be longer after spontaneous thromboembolism and lifelong after recurrent embolism or with thrombophilia.

Outcome

Pulmonary embolism produces a significant mortality particularly post-operatively or post-trauma. However, most cases recover well. Pulmonary hypertension from repeated emboli is more difficult to treat except by anticoagulation to reduce the chance of further emboli.

Pneumothorax

Definition

In pneumothorax there is escape of air from the lung into the pleural space breaking the pleural seal and allowing the lung to deflate separating visceral and parietal pleura. The lung collapses down from the chest wall and the lay description of a pneumothorax would usually be collapse of the lung, although this term is more often used medically for absorption collapse where air is absorbed from the lung after obstruction of the airway.

Epidemiology

Primary pneumothorax can occur spontaneously with no known underlying lung disease. Certain lung diseases are more likely to be complicated by pneumothorax. Smokers are much more likely to develop pneumothoraces.

Respiratory conditions associated with an increased risk of pneumothorax

COPD

Asthma

Cystic fibrosis

Idiopathic pulmonary fibrosis and other fibrosing lung conditions

Pneumocystis carinii pneumonia

Tuberous sclerosis, lymphangioleiomyomatosis

Lung biopsy

Mechanisms

Air leaks from the lung into the pleural space. In primary pneumothorax the leak is from subpleural blebs or bullae which are otherwise asymptomatic. As the lung deflates the leak in the visceral pleura may seal limiting the size of the pneumothorax. Size is defined by the distance of the lung edge from the ribcage. If this distance is greater than 2 cm then the pneumothorax is classified as large since this two-dimensional measure equates to a lung volume change of around 50%.

In a secondary pneumothorax the disease process usually involves the lung up to the visceral pleura and causes the leak.

Clinical features

Symptoms of a peumothorax are typically acute pleuritic chest pain and breathlessness as the air leak occurs and the lung deflates.

Rarely, the leak in the pleura acts like a flap valve allowing a positive pressure to build up in the pleural space. This creates a tension pneumothorax which begins to interfere with the function of the other lung

185

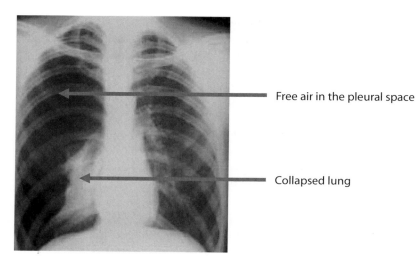

Fig. 6.11. In pneumothorax plain chest radiography is the key diagnostic test, showing a lung edge of the visceral pleura surrounded by a space with no lung markings.

Free air in the pleural space

Collapsed lung

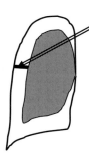

A distance of 2 cm on the X-ray represents a volume loss of around 50%

and with cardiac filling and output. This is a medical emergency that needs immediate action to release the pressure in the pleural space.

Investigations

Plain chest radiography is the key diagnostic test, showing a lung edge of the visceral pleura surrounded by a space with no lung markings (Fig. 6.11).

Management

Intervention is needed for symptomatic pneumothoraces and for asymptomatic primary pneumothoracs larger than 2 cm and secondary pneumothoraces larger than 1 cm. Smaller asymptomatic pneumothoraces can be left to resorb, which they do at the rate of about 1.8% of the hemithorax volume per day, so that a 25% pneumothorax would take about 2 weeks to resorb.

In primary pneumothoraces and small secondary pneumothoraces the initial intervention is simple aspiration or insertion of a small catheter with a one-way valve. Aspiration is done with a needle and syringe usually through the second rib space anteriorly. This is successful 60%–70% of the time, but is less helpful in older patients, secondary and larger pneumothoraces.

In larger pneumothoraces or when aspiration or catheter drainage is unsuccessful an intercostal drain is inserted and connected to an underwater seal. Where there is a persistent air leak or the lung fails to expand, thoracic surgery may be needed, usually through a video-assisted technique.

Outcome

Pneumothoraces recur in around 20% of cases. Chances are reduced by stopping smoking. After two pneumothoraces, the chances of recurrence are around 50% and pleurodesis to stick the pleural layers together and prevent the lung from collapsing should be considered.

Pneumonia

Definition

Pneumonia is acute inflammation of the lung in which air in the alveoli is replaced by an inflammatory exudate. It can be classified according to its

Table 6.7. Organisms causing community acquired pneumonia

Organism	Typical features
Streptococcus pneumoniae	Acute onset, lobar distribution, herpes simplex on the lip may occur
Mycoplasma pneumoniae	Increased in outbreaks every 3–4 years
Legionella pneumophila	Outbreaks related to contamination of water systems
Chlamydophila psittaci and *pneumoniae*	*Chlamydophila psittaci* often caught from birds
Viral pneumonia	Influenza, chickenpox, respiratory syncytial virus (RSV)
Staphylococcus aureus	Cavitates, may complicate influenza
Mycobacterium tuberculosis	Upper lobe predominance, often slower onset with weight loss, night sweats, hemoptysis, extrapulmonary sites may be involved
Pneumocystis carinii	Fungus affecting immunocompromised, especially HIV-infected, individuals

distribution in the lung: lobar where it is anatomically limited and bronchopneumonia with diffuse spread. However, a more useful division is in to community acquired and hospital acquired pneumonia, qualified by whether the patient is immunocompromised, since these situations are associated with a different range of organisms.

Epidemiology
Pneumonia is fourth in the leading causes of death in Europe, partly because it is the final problem in a number of unrelated conditions. It is a common complication in intensive care units and in patients debilitated by cancer or malnutrition.

In community acquired pneumonia *Streptococcus pneumoniae* is the commonest organism. Other common community acquired pathogens are listed in Table 6.7.

In hospital acquired pneumonia the microbiology is quite different. Many are caused by Gram-negative organisms or by methicillin resistant *Staphylococcus aureus* (MRSA).

Mechanisms
Spread is by inhalation from person to person (viruses, mycoplasma) or from birds (psittacosis) or water droplets (*Legionella*). Bacteria in the lung invoke an inflammatory reaction in which alveoli are consolidated by an exudate containing fibrin and red blood cells. The inflammation may spread from underlying lung to the pleura, producing pleuritic pain or a pleural effusion, which may itself become infected producing an empyema.

In hospital acquired pneumonia, severity of underlying disease and antibiotic therapy may leave the patient susceptible, accompanied by risks of aspiration and organisms prevalent in hospital environments such as MRSA.

Clinical features
In most cases there is a short illness with cough, fever, and possibly pleuritic chest pain. As the pneumonia develops, the sputum may become purulent and may contain red blood cells giving a "rusty" appearance. In mycoplasma, legionella and chlamydia infections the preceding illness tends to be longer with a dry cough, muscle aches, and malaise.

Examination of the chest will show the signs of consolidation (dullness to percussion, increased tactile vocal fremitus, and bronchial breathing) in lobar pneumonia.

A number of scoring systems have been produced to grade the severity of community acquired pneumonia and recommend safe places for treatment. The CURB65 score recommended by the British Thoracic Society is shown below.

CURB65 score used to grade community acquired pneumonia
Any of:
- **Confusion** (mental test score of 8 or less or new disorientation in person, place or time)
- **Urea** >7 mmol/l
- **Respiratory** rate ≥30/min
- **Blood** pressure (SBP <90 mmHg or DBP ≤60 mmHg)
- **Age** ≥65 years

Score 1 point for each feature present
0–1 = probably suitable for home treatment
2 = consider hospital referral
3–5 = urgent hospital admission

Investigations
A chest X-ray is the investigation which establishes the presence of lung parenchymal involvement and gives information about the distribution (Fig. 6.12).

Full blood picture, electrolytes, renal and liver function should be measured. Hyponatremia, impaired renal and liver function can occur in any severe pneumonia but are most likely with *Legionella* infection. C reactive protein can be a useful guide to severity and progress. Cold agglutinins are found in

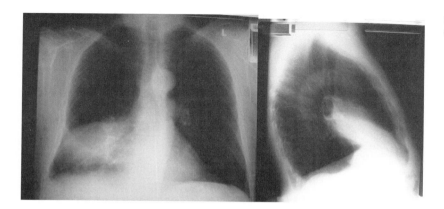

Fig. 6.12. Right middle lobe consolidation on PA and lateral view.

50% of *Mycoplasma* infections. Oxygen saturation should be checked and arterial blood gases if saturation is low.

Blood cultures are positive in around 25% of patients and should be performed in patients admitted to hospital. Sputum culture is worth doing in those who have not started antibiotics and in severe pneumonia. In severe or difficult cases it may be worth looking for pneumococcal and legionella antigen in the urine. Antibody rises against *Legionella*, *Mycoplasma* and *Chlamydia* may provide retrospective confirmation of the cause of pneumonia.

If tuberculosis is suspected, sputum will need to be sent for specific staining and culture. *Pneumocystis* will usually require more invasive methods such as bronchoscopy and alveolar lavage.

Management

Adequate hydration, oxygenation, and pain relief are important parts of the management. Antibiotic therapy should be started as soon as the diagnosis is made and this is usually before any conclusive microbiologic evidence is available. *Streptococcus pneumoniae* can be treated with benzylpenicillin or amoxicillin unless the illness arose in an area with a high prevalence of penicillin resistant pneumococci. *Legionella*, *Mycoplasma*, and *Chlamydia* (atypical organisms) lack a normal bacterial cell wall and are, therefore, not sensitive to penicillins and cephalosporins. They respond to macrolides, tetracyclines, and fluoroquinolones. In severe pneumonia antibiotics should cover pneumococcus and atypical organisms, combining a cephalosporin or penicillin and a macrolide (e.g. cefuroxime and clarithromycin). Outside hospital for milder pneumonia a macrolide, doxycycline, or a fluoroquinolone provide appropriate coverage.

For hospital acquired pneumonia antibiotic cover for Gram-negative organisms is needed and local microbiologic advice should be sought to take account of local prevalence and resistance.

Outcome

In most cases community acquired pneumonia responds to antibiotic treatment and there is complete resolution of the lung changes. In older patients and those with underlying disease there may be more problems and organisms such as staphylococci produce a significant mortality. Hospital acquired pneumonia carries a high mortality related to associated disease and the more virulent organisms involved.

Complications of pneumonia are empyema, lung abscess, and fibrosis of the involved lung. When the consolidation does not clear, an underlying obstructing lesion such as a tumor or a foreign body should be excluded.

Anxiety/panic attacks/hyperventilation

Definition

An acute or chronic feeling of shortness of breath brought about by hyperventilation beyond physiologic needs. Acute episodes merge into panic attacks.

Epidemiology

Hyperventilation is commoner in relation to anxiety and may be more common in obsessional personalities and in association with stimuli such as bereavement or worry about illness. It may be associated with respiratory problems such as asthma.

Mechanisms

Hyperventilation reduces arterial $PaCO_2$ causing a respiratory alkalosis which produces peripheral and circumoral paraesthesiae, muscle pains and feelings of faintness.

Clinical features

Tingling in the fingers and around the lips is characteristic of acute hyperventilation. In chronic hyperventilation there may be sensations of breathlessness, particularly a need to take deep inspirations, and a feeling that deep breaths are insufficient. These symptoms often occur at rest, may be transient, and are associated with a lack of any abnormal signs.

Investigations

To some extent hyperventilation is a diagnosis of exclusion, ruling out other respiratory problems particularly intermittent conditions such as asthma. The diagnosis is confirmed by finding normoxia with hypocapnia persistently or prolonged hypocapnia after a period of voluntary hyperventilation. Reproducing the symptoms with voluntary hyperventilation may help explain the problem to the patient.

Management

Management is difficult unless the patient is convinced of the nature of the problem and then undergoes breathing control exercises with an experienced physiotherapist.

Outcome

Hyperventilation has no long-term sequelae but may be distressing to the sufferer who may remain convinced that there is an underlying problem.

Chronic shortness of breath

When shortness of breath is persistent for many weeks or months, then the differential diagnosis changes. Respiratory conditions are likely to be either those that limit airflow through airway narrowing such as asthma or COPD or those that restrict the ability to expand the lungs because of stiffness of the lungs themselves or the chest wall and muscles. Conditions such as cardiac failure with pulmonary edema can produce acute or chronic breathlessness. Other problems such as thyrotoxicosis or anemia may sometimes present as shortness of breath.

One of the important considerations in the assessment and diagnosis of a patient complaining of shortness of breath is to explore any element of variability of the breathlessnes (Table 6.8). If there is variability, then exacerbating and relieving factors need to be considered. Other important features are quantification

Table 6.8. Variability of chronic shortness of breath, exacerbating and relieving factors

Shortness of breath varies with:	Association
Time	Asthma, pulmonary edema (both may be nocturnal)
Season	Asthma, hypersensitivity pneumonitis
Activity	Most breathlessness is worsened by exercise, but provocation particularly in asthma, anxiety
Position	Pulmonary edema, muscle weakness both worse lying flat (rarely worse standing in liver failure)
Environment	Asthma, COPD, extrinsic allergic alveolitis
Emotion	Anxiety
Treatment	Bronchodilators in short term

Table 6.9. New York Heart Association criteria

Class	Patient symptoms
Class I (Mild)	No limitation of physical activity. Ordinary physical activity does not cause undue shortness of breath.
Class II (Mild)	Slight limitation of physical activity. Comfortable at rest, but ordinary physical activity results in dyspnea.
Class III (Moderate)	Marked limitation of physical activity. Comfortable at rest, but less than ordinary activity causes dyspnea.
Class IV (Severe)	Unable to carry out any physical activity without discomfort.

of breathlessness and the elucidation of any associated symptoms (Table 6.10).

Limitation

In order to assess the effect of shortness of breath on quality of life and to evaluate change with time it is useful to have a simple measure of the severity of shortness of breath. It is conventional to do this in terms of everyday tasks. This can prove difficult because the degree of breathlessness that an individual will tolerate will vary and patients are not always good at estimating distances. These can be quantified in scales for grading dyspnea in terms of everyday tasks and standardized walking tests to see how far patients can walk in set times under standardized conditions such as the 6 or 12 minute walking tests.

The New York Heart Association criteria are used to grade symptoms of dyspnea with particular reference to heart failure (Table 6.9).

Table 6.10. Associated symptoms may help in the assessment of chronic shortness of breath

Symptom	Associated condition
Cough	Asthma, COPD, heart failure, pulmonary fibrosis
Palpitations	Heart failure, thyrotoxicosis
Wheeze	Asthma, COPD
Weakness	Muscle problems
History of relevant drug use	Chemotherapy, beta-blockers, aspirin
Typical skin or other system changes	Sarcoid

Chronic shortness of breath conditions
- COPD
- Sarcoidosis
- Pulmonary fibrosis
- Occupational lung diseases
- Drug effects
- Pleural effusion
- Muscle/chest wall problems

Chronic obstructive pulmonary disease (COPD)

Definition
A chronic, slowly progressive disorder characterized by airflow obstruction (reduced FEV1 and FEV1/FVC ratio) that does not change markedly over several months. Most of the lung function impairment is fixed, although some reversibility can be produced by bronchodilator (or other) therapy.

Epidemiology
By far the most important cause of COPD is cigarette smoking. Although cough and sputum production is very common in smokers, only 15%–20% will develop significant COPD but this accounts for 85%–90% of COPD worldwide. There is presumably a genetic link to susceptibility but the precise mechanisms are unknown. 1%–2% of COPD is related to a homozygous deficiency of the major anti-protease alpha-1-antitrypsin. A small minority of cases relate to indoor and industrial pollution. Smoking marihuana also produces chronic airflow obstruction.

COPD causes 6% of deaths in men in the UK, 4% in women, and is the fifth most common cause of death in UK. It also causes a considerable morbidity accounting for 9% of sickness absence in UK. Its significance is increasing and it will be the fourth commonest cause of death in Western Europe by 2010.

Mechanisms
Hereditary deficiency of alpha-1-antitrypsin accounts for just 1%–2% of cases of COPD but was important in developing the concept of imbalance in the protease–antiprotease system causing lung damage in COPD. In alpha-1-antitrypsin deficiency there is no protection from the proteases released from neutrophils attracted to the lung by cigarette smoke. In normal COPD the amount of proteases may overwhelm the normal anti-protease protection.

There are three major abnormalities in the lung: chronic bronchitis caused by mucus gland enlargement and hypersecretion, inflammatory bronchiolitis damaging and obstructing small airways, and emphysema in which the alveolar walls are broken down. By the time COPD is clinically evident, considerable irreversible damage will have occurred in the small airways and alveoli.

Clinical features
The major clinical features of COPD are cough and sputum production and shortness of breath. Sputum may be purulent, particularly in infective exacerbations. Small, streaky hemoptysis is not uncommon, but should raise the question of other problems such as carcinoma of the bronchus. The symptoms are slowly progressive with loss of lung function at two to three times the normal rate of decline. Acute exacerbations of COPD are common and are usually infective, caused by viruses and three main bacteria: *Streptococcus pneumoniae*, *Haemophilus influenzae*, and *Moraxella cattarrhalis*.

On examination, there may be signs of overinflation of the lungs with early inspiratory crackles at the lung bases and, possibly, expiratory wheeze. In severe cases there may be central cyanosis.

Long-standing COPD with chronic hypoxia may lead to cor pulmonale. The chronic hypoxia causes pulmonary vasoconstriction, increasing the load on the right heart and leading to raised jugular venous pressure and ankle edema in cor pulmonale. Patients who develop these features are sometimes referred to as "blue bloaters" as opposed to "pink puffers" who maintain better blood gases and avoid cor pulmonale at the expense of being more breathless.

Investigations
Respiratory function tests are an essential part of investigation and monitoring. A practical approach

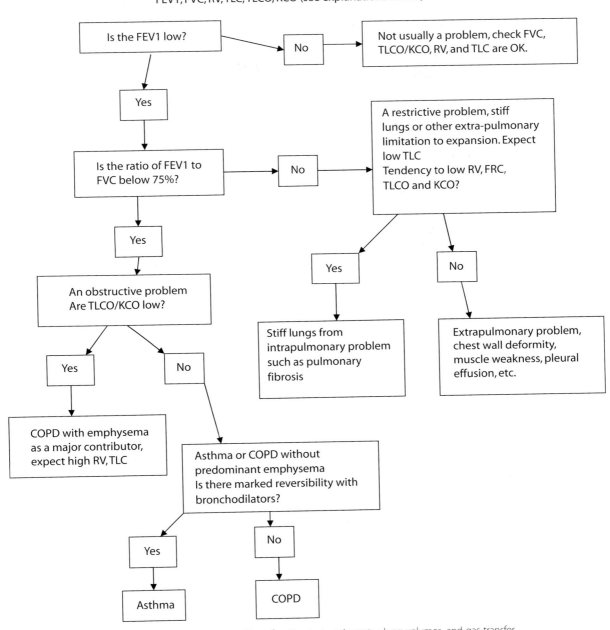

FEV1, FVC, RV, TLC, TLCO, KCO (see explanations below)

Fig. 6.13. A simple approach to the interpretation of lung function tests: spirometry, lung volumes, and gas transfer.

to the interpretation of respiratory function tests in common conditions is shown in Fig. 6.13. Spirometry giving a volume–time trace is most important, showing a reduction in the ratio of forced expiratory volume in the first second (FEV1) to forced vital capacity (FVC) (Fig. 6.14). The FEV1 level as % predicted is related to survival and is used to classify

the severity of COPD. The criteria used in the NICE COPD guidelines are shown in Table 6.11.

Chest X-ray shows overinflation but, often, little else unless emphysema is severe. In severe emphysema lung volume is increased, lung markings are decreased, and the walls of bullae may be visible. CT scan can help to show the distribution and extent of

FEV1 = forced expiratory volume in the first second of a forced expiration

FVC = forced expiratory capacity, the maximum volume that can be expelled from the lungs in a forced maneuver

Lung volume measurements require a body plethysmograph or helium dilution to measure the total volume of air in the lungs

RV = residual volume, the air remaining in the lungs after full expiration

TLC = total lung capacity, the sum of the residual volume and the vital capacity

FRC = functional residual capacity, the resting volume of the lungs at the end of a relaxed expiration, without any respiratory muscle action

Transfer factor measurements, measured by breathing a gas containing a small amount of carbon monoxide and helium and looking at the changes between inspired and expired levels. It is a measure of the quantity of carbon monoxide which is transported across the alveolar–capillary membrane for each kPa of alveolar carbon monoxide pressure (PCO). The helium is used to assess alveolar volume.

TLCO (or DLCO) = transfer factor of the lung for carbon monoxide, the value for the whole lung.

KCO = diffusion coefficient, the TLCO divided by the alveolar volume to which the gas has access. TLCO is affected by the surface area and thickness of the alveolar capillary membrane as well as many other things. Even in the absence of lung disease, small lungs inevitably have a small alveolar–capillary membrane surface area, so division by the alveolar lung volume in the KCO allows for this and can aid interpretation. It makes the abnormality more obvious in emphysema where the lung volume is large and less marked in fibrosis where the volumes are small. Where the lung volume reduction is caused by a problem outside the lungs, e.g. muscle weakness, the KCO may well be raised a little.

emphysema, but is not a practical technique for screening or follow-up.

Arterial blood gases show hypoxia. Hypercapnia may occur through marked ventilation–perfusion mismatching. One important practical consequence is that those who have a raised $PaCO_2$ may have reduced responsiveness to a raised CO_2 level and be partially

Table 6.11. Grades of severity of COPD according to FEV1

Grade	FEV1 level
Mild	50%–80% predicted
Moderate	30%–49% predicted
Severe	<30% predicted

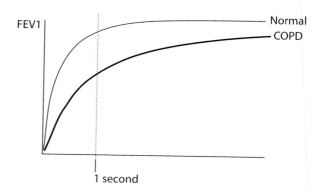

Fig. 6.14. Volume–time trace in COPD compared to normal.

dependent on hypoxic ventilatory drive. If they are given treatment with additional inspired oxygen, particularly during exacerbations, this drive may be removed, resulting in a reduction in minute ventilation and a rise in CO_2. Oxygen therapy needs to be controlled carefully in COPD. Figure 6.15 shows a practical approach to the interpretation of arterial blood gas measurements.

Figure 6.15 is a simple scheme showing the relationships of pH, PaO_2 and $PaCO_2$ and HCO_3^-. In real clinical life a great deal of helpful information comes from the clinical history and the clinical context. More than one problem may be present to complicate the interpretation. In addition, you should always know the inspired oxygen concentration to interpret the gases.

In acute exacerbations of COPD the important treatments are shown in Table 6.13.

Outcome

Life expectancy is considerably reduced when the patient has severe COPD, with median survival of 2–3 years by the time the criteria for LTOT are reached. The key to improving survival is stopping smoking early. This reduces the rate of decline of lung function, measured as FEV1, back to that of a non-smoker or non-susceptible smoker (Fig. 6.16). In late COPD attention needs to be given to palliative care for breathlessness and decisions about end of life treatment and the approach to intubation in the case of severe exacerbation.

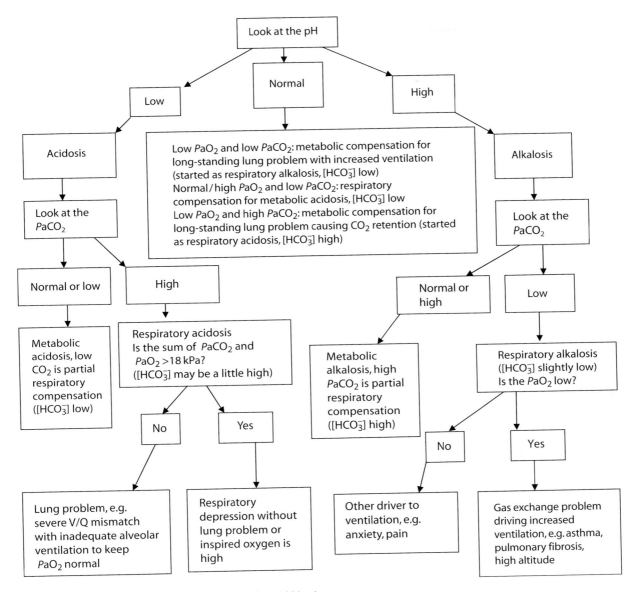

Fig. 6.15. A simple approach to the interpretation of arterial blood gases.

Sarcoidosis

Definition
A systemic disease of unknown cause producing granulomatous infiltration in a variety of organs, most commonly lymph nodes, lungs, and skin.

Epidemiology
Sarcoidosis can occur at any age but onset is most common between 20 and 40 years. It is commoner in African-Americans (eight times the white population) and Scandinavians and the manifestations vary between racial groups.

Mechanisms
Sarcoidosis is likely to be an immunologic response to an infective or environmental agent but the precipitating agent has not been identified. Affected organs are infiltrated with non-caseating granulomas containing multinucleate giant cells. $CD4^+$ lymphocytes are decreased in the blood and increased in affected tissues.

Table 6.12. Management of COPD

Treatment	Comments
Stopping smoking	Stopping smoking at any stage is helpful. It reduces the rate of loss of lung function to that of a non-smoker or non-susceptible smoker. Repeated attempts may be necessary. Simple advice at every medical contact with a smoker is the least that can be done and has a small response rate. Higher success is produced by the use of appropriate support, nicotine replacement therapy, bupropion, and varenicline.
Bronchodilators	**Short acting:** although reversibility is limited bronchodilators form an important part of treatment. Their purpose is to relieve symptoms not affect the natural history. Inhaled anticholinergics (ipratropium bromide) and β-agonists (e.g. salbutamol) are most useful. Oral theophyllines are also used but have more side effects.
	Long acting: beta-agonists, salmeterol and formoterol (twice daily), and the long acting anticholinergic tiotropium (once daily) have been shown to produce sustained bronchodilatation, improve symptoms, and reduce exacerbations.
Antibiotics	Used in exacerbations but have no place in chronic stable COPD.
Corticosteroids	**Inhaled corticosteroids** have been shown to reduce exacerbations and improve quality of life although they do not significantly change the loss of lung function and an effect on mortality in COPD is debated. Recommended with FEV_1 <50% predicted and exacerbations >1/year. Long-term **oral steroids** have considerable side effects and are not generally used in COPD.
Vaccination	Influenza vaccination annually is recommended, although the effectiveness is less than in young people. Pneumococcal vaccination is also recommended but only needs to be given once.
Oxygen	Oxygen is the only treatment known to improve the prognosis in COPD, other than stopping smoking. Long-term domiciliary oxygen therapy (LTOT) can be provided by an oxygen concentrator at home and used for a minimum of 15 hours each day to be effective. The main criterion for LTOT is a PaO_2 <7.3 kPa when stable (or <8 kPa and cor pulmonale).
Ventilation	Non-invasive ventilatory support is useful in acute exacerbations and some patients benefit from continued use at home.
Rehabilitation	Exercises to increase the efficiency of non-respiratory muscles can reduce the work of breathing needed for a given task and increase exercise tolerance and quality of life. It is usually combined with advice on nutrition and other factors.
Surgery	Lung transplantation is used in emphysema, but limited by the shortage of organs. In lung reduction surgery removal of some lung volume in both lungs allows the diaphragm to recover its domed shape and increases its efficiency as an inspiratory muscle.

Table 6.13. Important treatments in acute exacerbations of COPD

Bronchodilators	Usually given by nebulizer in acute exacerbations. Salbutamol 2.5–5 mg with ipratropium bromide 500 mcg in addition for severe exacerbations.
Antibiotics	Antibiotics make a small difference in rate of recovery especially in more severe attacks. Simple oral antibiotics such as amoxicillin and doxycycline are appropriate.
Corticosteroids	Oral steroids improve the rate of recovery and are usually given for 7–14 days in moderately severe exacerbations.
Oxygen	Acute exacerbations are the time when uncontrolled oxygen may be dangerous. Treatment should start with 24% or 28% oxygen through a high flow, high volume mask, with monitoring of blood gases.
Ventilation	Non-invasive ventilation is useful in preventing deterioration and avoiding intubation in severe exacerbations where the pH is 7.25 to 7.35. This is now widely available in hospitals admitting patients with COPD and has reduced the need for intensive care and invasive ventilation.

Clinical features

Clinical features depend on the organs affected. The common manifestations are shown in Table 6.14.

Investigations

The chest X-ray may show typical changes of bilateral hilar lymphadenopathy (BHL) with or without pulmonary infiltration (Fig. 6.17). Inflammatory markers such as the erythrocyte sedimentation rate may be raised and the level of angiotensin-converting enzyme is raised in most active cases. However, definitive diagnosis usually relies on clinical features with the finding of the typical granulomas on biopsy of affected tissues such as skin, lymph node, or lung tissue. Investigations such as serum calcium and electrocardiogram should be performed routinely in sarcoidosis. Hypercalcemia occurs through activation of vitamin D by cells in sarcoid granulomas. Granulomas occur in other conditions. Often the major differential diagnosis of the biopsy findings is tuberculosis, where the granulomas are often caseating and organisms may be found on smear or culture.

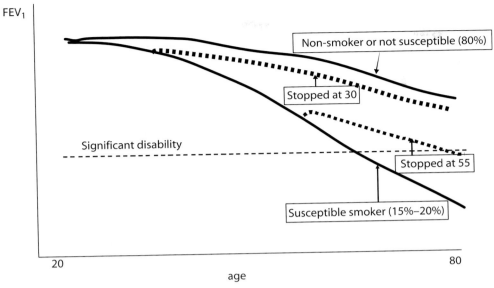

Fig. 6.16. Age-related FEV1 changes in non-smokers and smokers not susceptible to COPD, and in smokers susceptible to COPD continuing smoking or stopping aged 30 or 55.

Management

BHL may require no treatment, resolving spontaneously over 2 to 3 years in two thirds of cases. However, 10% progress to pulmonary fibrosis. Corticosteroid treatment reduces the sarcoid infiltrate and is used for problematic disease (see below). Steroids often need to be continued for 1 to 2 years once started for pulmonary sarcoidosis. Mild musculoskeletal symptoms may respond to NSAIDS and hydroxychloroquine provides an alternative treatment for skin manifestations.

Indications for the use of oral corticosteroids in sarcoidosis

- Posterior uveitis
- Progressive lung involvement
- Cardiac sarcoidosis
- Severe disfiguring skin disease
- Hypercalcemia
- Neurologic involvement
- Symptomatic muscle or bone involvement

Outcome

Spontaneous remission occurs in 60%–80% BHL but only in 30% stage 3 pulmonary disease (pulmonary fibrosis). Some of the non-pulmonary manifestations tend to be more chronic. Once remission has occurred, spontaneously relapse is uncommon, around 10% of patients.

Pulmonary fibrosis

Definition

The term pulmonary fibrosis is used to describe localized lung fibrosis which occurs when inflammatory conditions such as tuberculosis or pneumonia heal by scarring rather than resolution. This causes asymmetric contraction of part of the lung. In this section we deal with widespread symmetric pulmonary fibrosis known as idiopathic pulmonary fibrosis (IPF) or cryptogenic fibrosing alveolitis (CFA). A similar end result of diffuse fibrosis can occur after drug induced lung damage, after extrinsic allergic alveolitis from known allergens (e.g. farmer's lung), in association with connective tissue disorders such as rheumatoid arthritis, and after exposure to dusts such as silica or asbestos.

Epidemiology

Idiopathic pulmonary fibrosis is an uncommon condition with an incidence around 1 per 10 000 adults per year. It is more common in men and presents most often in the 50–80 age range. Apart from the specific causative factors, such as rheumatoid or specific dust disease, exposure to wood or metal dust is more common in the occupational history, and familial cases occur.

Table 6.14. Common manifestations of sarcoidosis

Organ	Frequency %	Manifestations
Lungs	95	Stage 0 no X-ray changes Stage 1 Bilateral hilar lymphadenopathy (BHL) Stage 2A BHL and lung infiltration Stage 2B lung infiltration Stage 3 lung fibrosis
Skin	25	Erythema nodosum, papules, plaques Lupus pernio = involvement of the skin of the nose Löfgren's syndrome = fever, BHL, erythema nodosum, arthralgia
Lymph nodes	15	Any nodes, spleen
Liver	12	Abnormalities of liver enzymes common but clinical problems unusual
Eyes	12	Anterior or posterior uveitis, lacrimal gland enlargement
Salivary glands	4	Heerfordt's syndrome = parotid gland enlargement, fever, VII cranial nerve palsy
Nervous system	4	Cranial nerve palsies, meningitis, mass lesions
Endocrine	4	Hypercalcemia Hypercalciuria Diabetes insipidus
Heart	2	Conduction abnormalities, muscle infiltration
Musculo-skeletal system	1	Arthralgia, myalgia

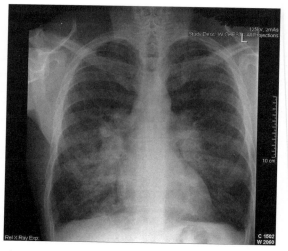

Fig. 6.17. Chest X-ray in sarcoidosis with bilateral hilar lymphadenopathy and parenchymal involvement.

Hypersensitivity pneumonitis or extrinsic allergic alveolitis

This is a distinct condition that occurs in response to a wide range of identifiable organic antigens such as molds on wet hay (farmer's lung) or avian protein (bird fancier's lung). Acute episodes with cough and fever occur 4–6 hours after exposure. Prolonged or repeated exposure can result in irreversible fibrosis. Antibodies can be found in the blood and the condition responds to removal of the antigen and/or corticosteroids.

Mechanisms

Idiopathic pulmonary fibrosis has been classified according to the radiographic and histologic findings. The subdivisions of IPF relate to prognosis in that a more persistent cellular element to the lung involvement may be associated with a greater chance of response to therapy. The commonest form is usual interstitial pneumonia (UIP) which has a typical subpleural distribution of fibrosis with cyst formation and enlargement of bronchi (traction bronchiectasis) identified from the CT scan and which has a very poor response to treatment. The fibrosis associated with connective tissue diseases has a more patchy distribution, is known as non-specific interstitial pneumonitis (NSIP), and is more likely to respond to treatment.

Clinical features

Shortness of breath is the dominant symptom and may be associated with a dry cough. Clubbing of the fingers is common and, on examination, there are fine, late inspiratory crackles at the lung bases.

Investigations

Respiratory function tests show a restrictive pattern with reduction in FEV1 and FVC but a normal or high ratio of the two. Gas transfer is reduced with progressive hypoxia. The chest X-ray most commonly shows a diffuse small nodular infiltrate in the lower zones, but changes are more readily identified on high resolution CT scanning where the degree of fibrosis and of inflammatory alveolar infiltrate (ground-glass shadowing) can be identified. The distribution can help in identifying the sort of fibrosis. Ground-glass shadowing suggests an active cellular alveolitis and greater likelihood of response to treatment (Fig. 6.18).

Transbronchial biopsies taken at fibreoptic bronchoscopy are too small to be useful except in the

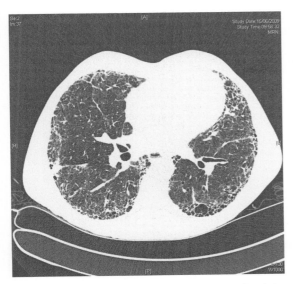

Fig. 6.18. CT scan in usual interstitial pneumonia with subpleural distribution of fibrosis, cyst formation and traction bronchiectasis.

diagnosis of alternative conditions such as sarcoidosis. If tissue is required it is usually obtained by a video-assisted thoracoscopic biopsy under general anaesthetic. Often a presumptive diagnosis is made from high resolution CT and respiratory function tests.

Management
Treatment is disappointing in UIP although other forms of idiopathic pulmonary fibrosis such as NSIP may respond to corticosteroids, perhaps with an immunosuppressive agent as a steroid sparing drug. If disabling breathlessness develops oxygen may be a helpful adjunct. Other agents are under trial and N-acetyl cysteine has shown some promise.

Outcome
Prognosis is poor with a median survival of 2–3 years, but some forms have prolonged survival or remission.

Occupational lung disease
Definition
Occupational lung disease covers a wide variety of conditions from occupational asthma to pulmonary fibrosis.

Epidemiology
Outside of occupational asthma the most important conditions are coal workers' pneumoconiosis, asbestosis, and silicosis.

Mechanisms
The problems in occupational dust disease are caused by the fibrotic reaction to the dust, causing stiff lungs. Asbestos exposure is associated with four lung conditions which develop 20–40 years after exposure:
- diffuse fibrosis (asbestosis)
- pleural plaques
- mesothelioma of the pleura
- bronchial carcinoma

Clinical features
The clinical features of diffuse fibrotic occupational lung disease such as asbestosis are the same as idiopathic pulmonary fibrosis. A detailed occupational history is necessary since the relevant exposure may have been years earlier. Pleural plaques do not usually cause any physiologic or clinical disturbance but serve as a marker of significant previous asbestos exposure.

Investigations
Chest X-rays show diffuse lung involvement and may show characteristic features such as larger nodules in coal worker's pneumoconiosis, a rim of calcification in the lymph nodes in silicosis, or associated pleural plaques after asbestos exposure. Respiratory function tests show a restrictive defect (Fig. 6.19).

Management and outcome
Prevention by control of exposure is the key to management. No other treatment affects the progress of the disease.

Drug-induced lung disease
Epidemiology
Drugs such as beta-blockers can provoke asthma. Sensitivity reactions to aspirin can produce asthma and pulmonary eosinophilia. Diffuse pulmonary fibrosis is most commonly seen with amiodarone and with cytotoxic agents such as bleomycin or methotrexate. Mechanisms vary, methotrexate and nitrofurantoin produce a hypersensitivity response, whereas amiodarone builds up a metabolite in alveolar cells and causes direct damage, especially in lungs with underlying disease.

Clinical features
With lung damage from exposure to cytotoxic agents, radiation therapy and hypoxia may increase the damage. Clinical features are progressive breathlessness and diffuse damage on X-ray and CT. Lung function tests show a restrictive defect.

197

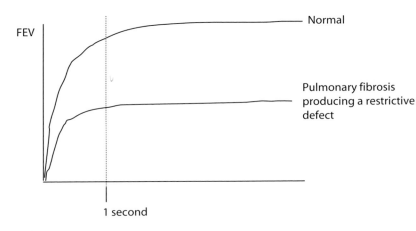

Fig. 6.19. Volume–time trace in idiopathic pulmonary fibrosis compared to normal.

Management

Management depends on being aware of the potential problems, differentiating the problem from other conditions such as heart failure in patients treated with amiodarone or from opportunistic infections in those on cytotoxics. The likely drug is withdrawn and corticosteroids added, if necessary, to speed up resolution. In amiodarone damage the problem may recur after resolution with steroids because of the long half-life of amiodarone metabolites which continue to have their effect for several months.

Pleural effusion

Definition

A collection of fluid between the visceral and parietal pleurae.

Epidemiology

Pleural effusions are divided conventionally, and usefully, in to transudates and exudates (Table 6.15). They are differentiated by the level of protein in the fluid and the lactic dehydrogenase level. Transudates are produced when fluid leaks out of the vessels because of increased hydrostatic pressure or reduced oncotic pressure, whereas exudates are produced when there is an abnormality of the pleura itself. Common causes are shown in Table 6.16.

Mechanisms

There is a small amount of fluid in the normal pleural space. This turns over quickly, absorbed by the parietal pleural lymphatics. Pleural effusions develop when this normal absorption mechanism is overloaded.

Clinical features

Pleural effusions cause shortness of breath. When there is associated inflammation of the pleural surfaces, pleuritic pain may also be present.

Table 6.15. Pleural effusion: differentiation of transudates and exudates

	Transudate	Exudate
Pleural/serum protein ratio	<0.5	>0.5
Pleural/serum LDH	<0.6	>0.6
Pleural protein (inaccurate if serum protein is low)	<3 g/dl	>3 g/dl

Table 6.16. Common causes of pleural effusion

Transudates	Left heart failure
	Hypoalbuminemia
	Nephrotic syndrome
	Liver disease
	Malnutrition
	Ascitic fluid passing through diaphragm
Exudates	Malignancy
	Primary lung cancer
	Mesothelioma
	Infection
	Tuberculosis
	Empyema
	Parapneumonia
	Pulmonary embolism
	Connective tissue disease
	Rheumatoid arthritis
	Systemic lupus erythematosus
	Trauma
	Pancreatitis
	Hypothyroidism
	Meig's syndrome (ovarian fibroma)
	Chylothorax

On examination, there is dullness to percussion with reduced breath sounds and air entry over the site of the effusion, and the mediastinum may be pushed away from large effusions.

Investigations

When there is more than 250 ml of pleural fluid it becomes visible on the chest X-ray blunting the

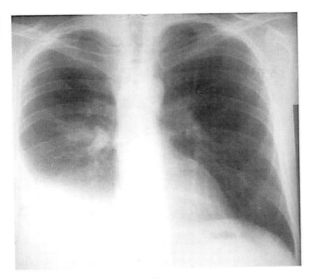

Fig. 6.20. Right-sided pleural effusion.

costophrenic angle. Larger effusions fill up the pleural space (Fig. 6.20) and move with position and gravity. When effusions are small or loculated through pleural adhesions, it is safer to identify the site for aspiration with transcutaneous ultrasound.

Aspiration of the effusion allows analysis of the fluid for protein, glucose, pH, cytology, and culture. It is possible to biopsy the pleura at the same time with a special needle or under direct vision at thoracoscopy looking directly into the pleural space.

Management

The important element of management is to find the underlying cause and deal with it. The effusion may need to be drained for symptomatic relief. In circumstances when an effusion is prolonged and troublesome and the underlying cause cannot be relieved it may be appropriate to perform a pleurodesis where the visceral and parietal pleura are deliberately inflamed with an irritant such as talc to stick them together and remove the space for future effusions to accumulate.

When the fluid in the pleural space is pus (empyema) or blood (hemothorax) this should be fully removed if possible since empyemas will not respond to antibiotics alone and blood may lead to dense adhesions, calcification, and subsequent restriction of lung expansion.

Muscle/chest wall problems (Chest pain, see Chapter 5)

Definition

Deformity of the chest wall by kyphoscoliosis or weakness of the respiratory muscles in motor neurone disease or diaphragmatic paralysis can lead to a restrictive defect and shortness of breath.

Epidemiology

There are a number of possible causes most of which are uncommon. Muscle weakness may result from inherited muscular dystrophy or acquired motor neuron disease. These will cause progressive weakness. Abnormalities of the thoracic cage such as kyphoscoliosis, trauma, or surgery will restrict chest expansion, exacerbated by lung conditions or obesity. In the past poliomyelitis was the most frequent problem.

Mechanisms

The limitation of lung expansion leads to areas of atelectasis and intrapulmonary shunting worsening hypoxia.

Clinical features

Breathlessness on exertion and eventually at rest is the main feature. Cough and sputum clearance may be impaired. There may be associated features in other muscles.

Respiratory function tests show a restrictive pattern without marked reduction in gas transfer unlike the findings in diffuse pulmonary fibrosis (Fig. 6.13). There may be other features particular to specific diagnoses such as bilateral diaphragm palsy where breathlessness is worsened on lying flat when the abdominal contents press up on the lungs. Vital capacity worsens when supine and breathlessness is worse in water such as when bathing or swimming. When lying flat, the abdominal wall moves inwards paradoxically on inspiration.

Investigations

X-rays and respiratory function tests are helpful. Tests of overall respiratory muscle power can be done from maximal inspiratory and expiratory pressures generated at the mouth. More detailed assessment requires esophageal and gastric balloons. Gas exchange problems are often worse at night when ventilation drops slightly and overnight oximetry with measurement of $PaCO_2$ is helpful.

Management

Often little can be done for the underlying process but non-invasive ventilation is likely to be helpful to reduce respiratory work. Initially, or in milder problems, the ventilatory support may only be needed overnight. However, the likely progress of the underlying problem and the level to which treatment will be increased must be considered.

Outcome

With the advent of non-invasive ventilatory support (positive pressure at the mouth without intubation), the respiratory insufficiency can be overcome and the outlook depends on the progress of the underlying problem and issues such as aspiration, sputum clearance, and respiratory infections.

Cough

Cough is a symptom experienced by everyone at some time. Most often it is associated with a viral upper respiratory tract infection and settles spontaneously within a week or so. Such viral infections may damage the airway epithelium and result in post-viral hyperresponsiveness with a cough that lasts for weeks. A cough may also be the first symptom of serious underlying disease such as carcinoma of the bronchus. The history is very important in planning any investigations and establishing the cause of a cough (Table 6.17).

One of the important features is to ask about sputum production (Table 6.18) since examination of sputum may help in establishing the diagnosis.

When patients cough up blood it is important to establish the amount of blood and the source (Table 6.19). A careful history can usually distinguish hemoptysis from hematemesis but this may be difficult with large bleeds. It is important to distinguish bleeding from the mouth or nose.

Further investigation should be considered in a cough that lasts longer than 3–4 weeks. A scheme for investigation is shown in Table 6.17, but a careful history and examination are the most important part of the scheme and may point to a more relevant approach to investigation and diagnosis. The chest X-ray is a key early investigation which may disclose an underlying lesion such as a carcinoma of the bronchus or tuberculosis.

A common problem in general practice and chest clinics is the patient with a persistent dry cough and a normal chest X-ray. In the absence of smoking as a cause the most likely diagnoses are asthma (or "cough variant asthma"), upper airway problems with post nasal drip, or gastro esophageal reflux. There may be little in the history and examination to point definitively to one diagnosis and further investigation is often appropriate (see below). An alternative approach is an empirical trial of treatment but vigorous prolonged treatment of the underlying problem may be needed to suppress the associated cough. If the cough is productive of purulent sputum persistently or intermittently then bronchiectasis is possible even in the presence of a normal chest

Table 6.17. Important questions in the clinical history in a patient with a cough

Questions	Possible relevance
Length of history	Acute viral infections usually resolve in 2–3 weeks
Sputum production	See Table 6.18
Smoking history	Previous or current smoking increase risk of COPD and carcinoma
Precipitating factors • Cold air • Dust • Exercise • Perfumes, sprays	May point to asthma, although many coughs are precipitated by smoky atmospheres or change in temperature
Specific triggers	Asthma
Relieving factors	May help to establish underlying cause
Time of day • Nighttime • Early morning	Esophageal reflux, pulmonary edema Asthma, bronchiectasis
Position • Lying flat	Esophageal reflux, pulmonary edema
Frequency	Frequency and severity are often difficult to quantify in a symptom such as cough, a witness may be helpful
Associated symptoms • Dizziness, loss of consciousness • Vomiting • Shortness of breath • Inspiratory whoops	 Cough syncope more common in older patients Any profuse cough, particularly whooping cough Asthma, foreign body, tumor, COPD Whooping cough

Table 6.18. Characteristics of sputum

Color	Blood, purulence
Amount	Difficult to quantify, traditionally done in terms of teaspoon, eggcup, or teacup, >100 ml = bronchorrhea
Tenacity	
Frothy	Pulmonary edema
Presence of blood	See Table 6.19
Plugs	Allergic broncho-pulmonary aspergillosis

X-ray, and high resolution CT scanning will be the best investigation to detect this.

Investigations appropriate for a persistent (>3 months) dry cough (Fig. 6.21)

- Chest X-ray
- Respiratory function and reversibility

Table 6.19. Causes of hemoptysis

Cause	Typical features
Acute exacerbation of chronic bronchitis	Streaks of blood in purulent sputum
Pneumonia	Rusty sputum
Pulmonary edema	Frothy pink sputum
Pulmonary embolus	Pleuritic chest pain, shortness of breath
Bronchiectasis	Recurrent episodes of purulent sputum
Tuberculosis	Fever, night sweats, weight loss
Bronchial carcinoma	Associated features, chest X-ray
Arteritis (e.g. Wegener's granulomatosis)	High ESR. Upper airway and renal lesions
Goodpasture's syndrome	Hematuria, basement membrane antibodies
Arterio-venous malformation	Hereditary haemorrhagic telangiectasia

- Histamine challenge
- Sinus X-rays/CT
- 24-hour esophageal pH monitoring

When there is persistent sputum production, the differential diagnosis changes. Purulent sputum is caused by degenerating white cells in the sputum. Although asthma may be associated with purulent sputum from eosinophils other diagnoses become more likely (Table 6.20).

Carcinoma of the lung

Definition
Most malignant tumors of the lung arise in the bronchial epithelium. Occasional tumors such as bronchoalveolar cell carcinoma arise more peripherally. Benign lung tumors (adenomas, hamartomas) are less common accounting for 5%–10% of lung tumors. In addition, the lung can be the site of metastases.

Epidemiology
Carcinoma of the lung is the commonest cause of death from cancer in the UK, causing around 27% of cancer deaths (40 000 per year). More than 90% of cases of primary lung cancer are related to cigarette smoking, and the risk increases with the length and intensity of exposure. Passive smoking carries a small risk. Occupational exposure such as asbestos, uranium, arsenic, and radiation are occasionally relevant.

Malignant tumors of the pleura (mesotheliomas) usually have an occupational history of exposure to asbestos, although this may have been 30 or 40 years earlier and may require a detailed occupational history (Fig. 6.22).

Mechanisms
The important differentiation in the pathology is into small cell (20%–25%) and non-small cell types. Non-small cell carcinoma can be further subdivided into squamous cell (30%), adenocarcinoma (30%), and large cell (15%) types.

Clinical features
Carcinoma of the lung can present in a variety of ways:
- Incidental finding on a chest X-ray
- Local symptoms
- General features of malignancy
- Local invasion
- Metastases
- Non-metastatic distant manifestations

Local symptoms are the commonest form of presentation. The origin in the bronchial mucosa leads to cough, hemoptysis, or shortness of breath caused by local airway obstruction.

General features of malignancy such as anorexia, weight loss, and malaise are common as the disease progresses.

As tumors enlarge **local invasion** can occur into:
- pleura and chest wall (pain)
- pericardium (pericarditis, arrhythmias, pericardial effusion, and tamponade)
- superior vena cava (facial swelling, headache, fixed raised JVP)
- esophagus (dysphagia)
- nerves such as:
  - phrenic (raised hemidiaphragm)
  - recurrent laryngeal ("hoarse" weak voice and cough)
  - brachial plexus (arm pain, hand weakness)

The importance of these features is that they usually indicate that the tumor is technically unresectable.

Metastases occur most often to lymph nodes in the hila, mediastinum and neck, liver, bone, brain, and adrenal glands.

Distant non-metastatic or paraneoplastic complications are:
- clubbing and hypertrophic pulmonary osteoarthropathy (tenderness with periosteal elevation at the end of the long bones) – all types except small cell

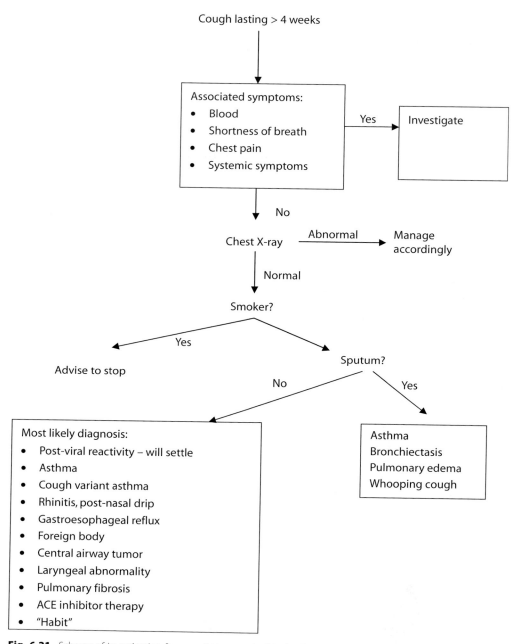

Fig. 6.21. Scheme of investigation for a persistent cough: this should always be guided carefully by a detailed clinical history and examination.

- anemia
- thrombophlebitis
- hormone secretion by the tumor
  - ACTH and ADH from small cell tumors
  - parathyroid hormone-like substance from squamous cell
- neurological problems (most often small cell)

- Eaton–Lambert or myasthenic syndrome
- cerebellar degeneration
- peripheral neuropathy

Investigations
Chest X-ray is the initial investigation in most cases and 98% of tumors will be visible on a plain chest

Table 6.20. Causes of cough with sputum production

Diagnosis	Associated features
COPD/chronic bronchitis	Smoking history
Asthma	Wheezing, reduced peak flow
URTI	Temporary
Carcinoma	Abnormal chest X-ray, smoking history
Bronchiectasis	Repeated episodes
Abscess	Abnormal chest X-ray
Tuberculosis	Abnormal chest X-ray, sweats, fever, weight loss
Sinus disease	Upper airway symptoms
Foreign body	History, chest X-ray

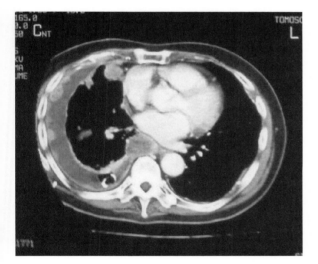

Fig. 6.22. Mesothelioma with right-sided pleural thickening and pleural fluid on CT scanning.

X-ray at presentation. CT scanning and, if available, PET scans help in staging. Blood picture, electrolytes, liver function, and calcium help assess complications (Fig. 6.23).

Respiratory function is important in assessing operability related to associated COPD. Sputum cytology may be positive but the definitive diagnosis is by biopsy, usually at fibreoptic bronchoscopy.

The investigations allow staging according to the TNM classification (Table 6.21).

Management

The first consideration must be assessment for surgical resection since the best results come from surgery with or without chemotherapy or radiotherapy. In limited disease 5-year survival after surgery is around 50%. However, only about 20% of tumors are operable at presentation. Radiotherapy to limited disease can be curable and chemotherapy often produces a response but rarely a cure. Small cell carcinomas are rarely operable and behave more aggressively. They do have a better response rate to chemotherapy, although cure is rare.

Mesotheliomas respond poorly to treatment. They can be treated aggressively by resection, radiotherapy and chemotherapy but, overall, few patients respond well to any treatment.

Palliative therapy is an important part of the care of carcinoma of the lung and mesothelioma. Palliative radiotherapy for hemoptysis or bone lesions, pain relief, and intervention such as drainage of pleural effusions or pleurodesis may be very helpful.

Outcome

The outcome related to staging is shown in Table 6.21.

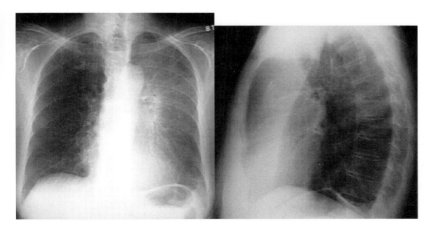

Fig. 6.23. Left upper lobe collapse on PA and lateral chest X-ray caused by a carcinoma obstructing the left upper lobe bronchus.

203

Table 6.21. International TNM staging system for lung cancer

- Primary tumor (T)
  - T1 – Tumor diameter ≤3 cm without invasion more proximal than lobar bronchus
  - T2 – Diameter >3 cm or any size with any of:
    - invasion of visceral pleura
    - atelectasis involving less than entire lung
    - proximal extent more than 2 cm from carina
  - T3 – Tumor of any size with any of:
    - invasion of chest wall
    - total atelectasis of one lung
    - within 2 cm of the carina but not invading it
    - involvement of diaphragm, mediastinal pleura, or pericardium
  - T4 – Tumor of any size with any of:
    - invasion of the mediastinum
    - invasion of esophagus, trachea, or carina
    - invasion of heart or great vessels
    - involvement of a vertebral body
    - malignant pleural or pericardial effusion
    - satellite nodules within the same lobe as the primary tumor
- Regional lymph node involvement
  - N0 – No regional lymph nodes involved
  - N1 – Ipsilateral peribronchial or hilar nodes involved
  - N2 – Ipsilateral mediastinal or subcarinal nodes
  - N3 – contralateral mediastinal or hilar nodes involved or any scalene or supraclavicular nodes
- Metastatic involvement
  - M0 – No metastases
  - M1 – Metastases present

Stage groupings are as follows:
- IA – T1N0M0
- IB – T2N0M0
- IIA – T1N1M0
- IIB – T2N1M0 or T3N0M0
- IIIA – T1–3N2M0 or T3N1M0
- IIIB – Any T4 or any N3M0
- IV – Any M1

For each stage, the prognoses, or estimated 5-year survival rates, in Europe are as follows:
Stage IA – 60%
- Stage IB – 38%
- Stage IIA – 34%
- Stage IIB – 24%
- Stage IIIA – 13% (Stage IIIA lesions have a poor prognosis, but they are technically resectable)
- Stage IIIB – 5% (Stage IIIB lesions are non-resectable)
- Stage IV – Less than 1%

Bronchiectasis and lung abscess

Definition
Bronchiectasis is abnormal and persistent dilatation of bronchi resulting from damage to the airway wall. It may be local or generalized. It interferes with mucociliary clearance and allows recurrent infections.

Table 6.22. Causes of bronchiectasis

Condition	Problem	Associated features
Generalized conditions		
Cystic fibrosis	Viscid secretions	Autonomic recessive inheritance, pancreatic insufficiency, diabetes mellitus, sinus disease, liver disease, male infertility
Immotile cilia syndrome (Kartagener's)	Ineffective mucociliary clearance	Situs inversus, infertility in males, sinus disease, ectopic pregnancy in females
Hypogammaglobulinemia	Recurrent infections	Infections at other sites
Local conditions		
Measles, whooping cough	Childhood pneumonias	Much less common now
Foreign body	Local airway damage	
Tuberculosis	Localized damage	Often upper lobe
Allergic broncho-pulmonary aspergillosis	Proximal bronchiectasis	Asthma

Epidemiology
Bronchiectasis may be caused by a generalized process that interferes with lung protection or a localized airway problem (Table 6.22).

Mechanisms
In some cases the airway damage in bronchiectasis may be worsened by repeated infections producing a vicious circle requiring vigorous treatment with antibiotics and postural drainage.

Clinical features
Cough with purulent sputum, permanently or in exacerbations, is the main feature of bronchiectasis. Persistent purulent secretions in the dilated airways may lead to fetor which can be distressing for the patient. Hemoptysis can occur from dilated vessels in the walls of the damaged airways. Abscesses may form in the lung or occasionally in other organs such as the brain.

Lung abscesses are areas of damaged lung containing purulect secretions. They may form as part of bronchiectasis, from septic emboli, or from the

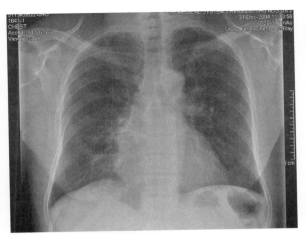

Fig. 6.24. Lung abscess with a horizontal fluid level in the right lower zone.

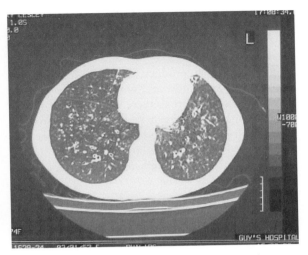

Fig. 6.26. Bronchiectasis: dilated and thick-walled bronchi on HRCT.

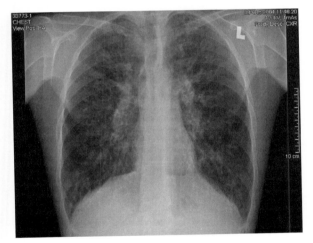

Fig. 6.25. Chest X-ray in cystic fibrosis showing overinflated lung fields, and tramline and cystic shadows from bronchiectasis. The concentration of the changes in the upper lobes is typical of cystic fibrosis.

breakdown of consolidated lung in pneumonia in tuberculosis, staphylococcal or *Klebsiella* infection. Intravenous drug users are at particular risk from infection at injection sites or from right sided endocarditis.

Investigations
The chest X-ray will show round lesions in lung abscess, often with a fluid level (Fig. 6.24). In bronchiectasis there may be changes such as tramline and cystic shadows from the thickened, dilated airways (Fig. 6.25) but subtler changes are much more easily seen on high resolution CT scanning (Fig. 6.26).

Cystic fibrosis is diagnosed on the clinical picture and abnormal sweat chloride concentrations and genetic analysis. Gammaglobulins, including subclasses, should be measured to rule out hypogammaglobulinemia, and cilial motility can be assessed from sperm analysis in males or studies of nasal cilia.

Microbiology of the sputum helps to direct antibiotic therapy. In cystic fibrosis typical organisms are *Staphylococcus aureus* early on, followed by *Haemophilus influenzae* and then persistent *Pseudomonas aeruginosa*.

Management
The important parts of the treatment of bronchiectasis are control and prevention of infection. This is achieved by regular, usually twice daily, physiotherapy and postural drainage of the affected area of lung, and by prompt appropriate antibiotic therapy for infections. Nebulized bronchodilators in between episodes may be helpful in reducing the frequency of exacerbations. Bronchodilators may help shortness of breath and, in cystic fibrosis, nebulized DNase decreases sputum viscosity. In cystic fibrosis nutritional support is an important feature because of the pancreatic dysfunction. Gene therapy offers hope for future treatment in cystic fibrosis.

In localized bronchiectasis resection of part or all of a lobe may occasionally be appropriate, if no other areas of lung are involved. In cystic fibrosis lung transplantation for end stage disease offers the only surgical option.

If hemoptysis is a problem then bronchial artery embolization may be needed to block dilated vessels.

However, they tend to recur if the underlying problem is not controlled.

Outcome

Bronchiectasis may produce repeated infections over many years with little accelerated decline in lung function. In cystic fibrosis there is progressive decline in lung function although survival is improved by vigorous airway hygiene and nutritional support with median survival now in the 30s.

Amyloid is a rare complication of chronic infection in bronchiectasis (Fig 6.24).

Tuberculosis

Definition

Tuberculosis is caused by infection with *Mycobacterium tuberculosis*. Other mycobacteria can be pathogenic but are much less common than tuberculosis.

Epidemiology

Worldwide tuberculosis is a massive problem, with 3 million deaths per year and 1.9 billion people affected. Ninety percent of these are in sub-Saharan Africa, South East Asia, India and China. Many of them have little access to appropriate management. In the UK tuberculosis cases decreased throughout the twentieth century but began to increase again in urban areas in the late 1980s. Cases are most common in immigrants from endemic areas and those with alcohol, nutritional, and social problems.

Mechanisms

Tuberculosis is most often acquired in childhood, primary tuberculosis, by droplet spread but most cases heal spontaneously within 6 months leaving often a small calcified lesion in the lung (Ghon focus) sometimes with calcification in the draining lymph nodes. Spread may occur early in primary tuberculosis to give pleural disease with effusions or blood-borne dissemination giving miliary tuberculosis with small foci spread through the lungs and many other organs.

Tuberculosis may be reactivated later, post-primary tuberculosis, and the likelihood is increased by immunosuppression, particularly HIV, or malnutrition. Diabetes, steroid treatment, chemotherapy, and immunosuppressive drugs also increase the risk of reactivation of tuberculosis. Of those who are infected with tuberculosis around 5% will develop clinical disease within the first 2 years, 5% later in life, but untreated HIV infection increases the relapse rate to around 10% per year and accounts for many cases in the developing world.

Table 6.23. Extrapulmonary manifestations of tuberculosis

Site	Manifestations
Miliary	Blood-borne spread, small nodules in lung and other organs, may be seen in the retina
Nervous system	Subacute meningitis, cranial nerve palsies
Bones	Vertebral collapse and paravertebral abscess
Skin	"Lupus vulgaris" especially face and neck
Genitourinary	Renal involvement, epididymis, Fallopian tubes
Gastro-intestinal	Peritonitis, abdominal pain with ascites and nodular peritoneal involvement
Heart	Pericarditis, acute and leading on to constriction

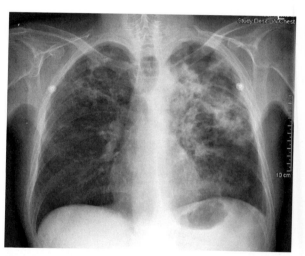

Fig. 6.27. Infiltration and cavitation, predominantly in the upper lobes, in active tuberculosis.

Clinical features

General clinical features of tuberculosis are anorexia, weight loss, fevers, and night sweats. Other features depend on the area involved. Pulmonary tuberculosis is most common and causes cough, sputum, and hemoptysis but in 15%–20% of cases tuberculosis presents outside the lungs, extrapulmonary tuberculosis (Table 6.23).

Investigations

The commonest site for post-primary pulmonary tuberculosis is in the upper lobes (Fig. 6.27). Cavitation is common and healing often leaves upper lobe fibrosis and calcification. Key to the diagnosis is finding acid-fast mycobacteria in suitable specimens, usually sputum. An initial auramine or Ziehl–Nielsen stain may identify mycobacteria, confirmed by

Table 6.24. Antituberculous drugs and their common adverse effects

Drug	Major adverse effects
Rifampicin	Rise in liver enzymes, hepatitis, orange/red discoloration of urine, tears, enzyme induction reducing the effect of oral contraceptives, prednisolone, anticonvulsants, etc., thrombocytopenia, flu-like syndrome with intermittent use
Isoniazid	Hepatitis, peripheral neuropathy (prevented by co-therapy with pyridoxine), psychosis
Pyrazinamide	Gastro-intestinal upset, hepatitis, hyperuricemia
Ethambutol	Optic neuritis, color vision disturbance (vision should be checked at onset and patient counseled about effects)

culture which takes up to 6 weeks. Culture is important to identify atypical mycobacteria and to test drug sensitivities. Biopsy of affected organs will show caseating granulomata and may also stain or culture positive for mycobacteria.

The tuberculin skin test is positive in those who have had primary tuberculosis or BCG vaccination. A strongly positive test may be a pointer to active disease but is not diagnostic. Serologic tests are becoming available to help in the diagnosis of tuberculosis.

Management

Antituberculous treatment will cure nearly all cases of tuberculosis, providing the right drugs are taken for a sufficient period. If there is any doubt about adherence to therapy then directly observed therapy (DOT) should be used with the patient taking the tablets under direct supervision three times a week. Treatment is with a combination of either three or four drugs (Table 6.24) for 2 months with two drugs (rifampicin and isoniazid) continued for another 4 months.

Outcome

If a full course of treatment is taken, chances of relapse are very small. The situation is much more difficult with **multiple drug resistant tuberculosis** (MDRTB), defined as resistance to at least rifampicin and isoniazid. Patients in hospital should be kept in negative pressure rooms and treatment includes second-line antituberculous drugs for a prolonged period until the sputum can be shown to be repeatedly negative on culture. Extensively resistant *Mycobacterium tuberculosis* (EDRTB) is resistant to second-line drugs and poses a possible future threat.

Hypersomnolence

Daytime sleepiness may be a manifestation of a social, respiratory, or neurological problem. Sleep is an important area to explore in the medical history. It is a common symptom that needs to be differentiated from general tiredness. It is subjective and various scales have been used to try to quantify sleepiness. Most common is the Epworth sleepiness scale (Table 6.25). A value of 10 or more fits with excessive sleepiness. A sleep diary producing a record of time in bed and asleep over a period of 1–2 weeks may also be very helpful in making the diagnosis.

The identification of the likely cause of sleepiness requires a careful history and examination of the patient and from anybody able to give information about their sleep. The important features are shown in Table 6.26.

Obstructive sleep apnea

Definition

Apneas are interruptions to breathing lasting at least 10 seconds. They are either central where there is no drive to the respiratory muscles, or obstructive where the respiratory muscles contract but collapse of the upper pharyngeal airway prevents inspiration. Hypopneas are defined as a 50% reduction in breath volume, obstructive hypopneas have the same consequence as apneas. In obstructive events there is paradoxical inward movement of the rib cage with inspiratory effort. Severity is defined by the apnea/hypopnea index (AHI), the number of events per hour of sleep. An AHI above 5 is often regarded as abnormal but associated problems are usually associated with an AHI above 15 and levels of over 60 (i.e. one per minute) occur in severe OSA. The term obstructive sleep apnea syndrome (OSAS) is used for the combination of OSA and daytime hypersomnolence. Central apneas are less common, they occur in Cheyne–Stokes periodic breathing, common in heart failure, and other mechanisms interfering with central respiratory drive.

Epidemiology

OSA is more common in men. The majority are middle aged and overweight, particularly with a thick neck. Upper airway abnormalities such as tonsillar enlargement, acromegaly, short mandible and hypothyroidism are associated, as are various muscle problems. Significant OSA occurs in around 2%–4%

207

Table 6.25. Epworth Sleepiness Scale

For each of eight situations the likelihood of falling asleep should be given a score of 0–3 according to the scale:
0 = would never doze or sleep.
1 = slight chance of dozing or sleeping
2 = moderate chance of dozing or sleeping
3 = high chance of dozing or sleeping

Situation	Score 0–3
Sitting and reading	
Watching TV	
Sitting inactive in a public place	
Being a passenger in a motor vehicle for an hour or more	
Lying down in the afternoon	
Sitting and talking to someone	
Sitting quietly after lunch (no alcohol)	
Stopped for a few minutes in traffic while driving	

Table 6.26. Conditions causing daytime somnolence

Condition	Important features
Inadequate sleep opportunity	Late to bed, up early, shift work, television in bedroom. Sleep diary useful
General medical problem disturbing sleep (pain, nocturia, etc.)	Pain at night, obtain history of cause of waking, poor sleep (NB nocturia is also a symptom of OSA)
Insomnia	Anxiety, difficulty initiating sleep, poor habits at sleep onset (caffeine, exercise/ stimulation just before bed, reading in bed, watching television in bed)
Obstructive sleep apnea	Snoring, obesity, often male, alcohol consumption, observed apneas terminated by snorting
Depression	Early morning waking
Narcolepsy	Cataplexy, onset in teens/20s, HIA type, hypnagogic hallucinations, sleep paralysis
Periodic leg movement disorder	Restless legs in evening, restless night

of the middle aged male population and half that number of women.

Mechanisms

The mechanism of obstruction seems to be related to lack of motor output to the upper airway muscles which then allow the pharynx to collapse under the negative intra-airways pressure induced by diaphragmatic contraction. The apnea terminates when the brain senses the obstruction and sends a message to the pharyngeal muscles to open the airway. However, this is at the expense of a disturbance of sleep, not usually enough to wake the patient, but sufficient to disturb the quality of sleep. Occasionally the patient wakes with a feeling of choking. Apneas are more likely in the supine position and after alcohol or sedatives.

Clinical features

The main symptom is hypersomnolence as a result of disturbed sleep. The other common presentation is through the noise of the snoring or anxiety about apnea from a bed partner. The vascular and metabolic consequences are an increased prevalence of hypertension, cardiovascular and cerebrovascular events, and glucose intolerance.

Investigations

The most important part of the investigation is to ask the right questions about sleep and snoring to suspect the diagnosis. Investigations vary from simple oximetry through the night to detect repeated oxygen desaturations to full poysomnography monitoring oxygen, airflow, ECG, EOG, eye movements, and leg movements (Fig. 6.28).

Management

Simple measures include weight reduction, reducing alcohol consumption, and avoiding the supine position at night. A mandibular positioning device fits over upper and lower teeth holding the mandible forward by 6–7 mm and increasing the posterior pharyngeal space and is effective in mild to moderate OSA.

The gold standard treatment is continuous positive airway pressure at 8 to 15 cm water pressure applied through a close fitting nasal or full face mask. This stops the pharynx from collapsing during inspiration. These treatments prevent the obstructive apneas while they are used. Surgery to produce a more permanent cure is useful with problems such as large tonsils but is unreliable in the majority of cases of OSA.

Outcome

The daytime hypersomnolence produces problems with social functioning, work, and driving. Patients must be told to report significant obstructive sleep apnea or daytime hypersomnolence from any other cause to the Driving Vehicle Licensing Authority.

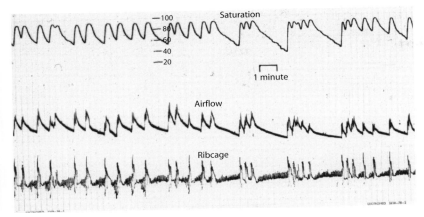

Fig. 6.28. Repeated desaturations in severe obstructive sleep apnea.

The other issues are the increased risk of hypertension and vascular disease. The relative risk is approximately doubled and interacts with other risk factors.

Narcolepsy

Definition
Narcolepsy is a disturbance of the sleep–wake cycle in which there is pathologic daytime sleepiness with the tendency to episodes of rapid eye movement (REM) sleep soon after sleep onset. In around 25% of cases it is associated with cataplexy in which temporary partial or complete loss of muscle tone occurs in association with stress or emotion such as laughing.

Epidemiology
The prevalence of narcolepsy is around 1 in 2000, considerably less than OSA. Onset of symptoms is between the ages of 10 and 25 although diagnosis is usually delayed by 10–15 years. There is a close association with certain HLA types.

Mechanisms
There is a reduction of hypocretin secreting neurones in the brains of narcoleptics which may be related to an increase in obesity in narcolepsy.

Diagnosis
The diagnosis is made from the typical story of profound sleepiness without another cause often with associated cataplexy, sleep paralysis or hypnagogic hallucinations. A multiple sleep latency test in which a patient lies down in a darkened room every two hours through the day shows reduced sleep latency and the presence of REM sleep soon after sleep onset rather than the normal delay for 90–120 minutes.

Clinical features
Apart from daytime sleepiness and cataplexy, other common features are hallucinations at sleep onset or wakening and muscular paralysis at sleep onset.

Investigations
The diagnostic test is the multiple sleep latency test. HLA typing usually shows positive for DQB1*0602 and/or DRB1*1. These are common HLA types and the main use is that a negative test makes narcolepsy less likely.

Management
Short naps at the onset of tiredness may help. Amphetamines have been largely replaced by modafinil. This is a central alpha agonist and also stimulates hypocretin neurones. Antidepressants can be helpful in preventing cataplexy.

Outcome
With treatment sleepiness can often be reduced to a reasonable level and there is often some improvement after middle age.

Further reading

British Thoracic Society Guidelines. http://www.brit-thora cic.org.uk/page235.html.

Gibson J, Geddes D, Costabel U, Sterk P, Corrin B. *Respiratory Medicine*, 3rd edn, Saunders, 2002.

NICE respiratory guidelines. http://guidance.nice.org.uk/ topic/respiratory.

The Global Initiative for Chronic Obstructive Lung Disease (GOLD). http://www.goldcopd.com/.

Ear, nose, and throat

Rachael Hornigold, Simon Hogan and Michael Gleeson

Contents

Hearing loss

Disturbance of hearing is distressing. Understanding how the ear functions assists management (Fig. 7.1).

It can be divided into sensorineural or conductive. The former implies a disorder of the inner ear (cochlea), cochlear nerve, or the auditory system of the brain, the latter a problem of the external or middle ear. The two can be differentiated on clinical testing and by audiography. An audiogram charts hearing in each ear. Hearing is measured by presenting the patient with sounds of different frequency at increasing amplitude until the patient hears the sound. It is charted on a logarithmic decibel scale, compared to normal hearing.

Conductive hearing is measured using direct application of vibration to the skull.

Sensorineural hearing loss
Presbyacusis
Clinical features
Develops gradually and is symmetric. Examination is normal. Age-related hearing loss is the most common cause of sensorineural loss.

Epidemiology and pathology
More than 50% of people age >75 yrs have presbyacusis. It is thought to be due to degeneration of cochlear hair cells, reduction of blood flow to the inner ear and degeneration of central auditory pathways in the brain.

Investigation
An audiogram usually reveals a sloping high-frequency hearing loss. If hearing loss is asymmetric or the patient has other symptoms, another diagnosis should be considered.

Management
Provision of hearing aids and other accessories.

Outcome
Usually progressive.

Noise induced hearing loss
Clinical features
Another common cause of gradual hearing loss, often in a younger population. Examination is normal.

Epidemiology and pathology
Noise levels of >90 dB cause pathologic change of the inner ear. Initial damage may be temporary but permanent with increasing and repeated exposure.

Management
Prevention of noise exposure and hearing aid provision.

Outcome
Usually progressive.

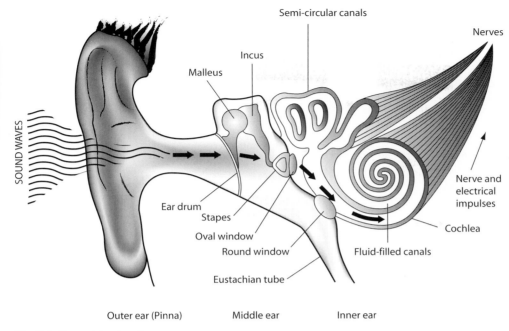

SOUND WAVES

Semi-circular canals

Nerves

Incus

Malleus

Nerve and electrical impulses

Ear drum

Stapes

Oval window

Round window

Eustachian tube

Cochlea

Fluid-filled canals

Outer ear (Pinna)   Middle ear   Inner ear

Fig. 7.1. The peripheral auditory system.

Congenital causes of hearing loss (hereditary: syndromic/non-syndromic; in utero)

This is a rarer cause of hearing loss, the incidence is 1 in 1000 live births. Congenital hearing loss may be conductive and sensorineural, and sometimes mixed. All neonates in the UK are screened for it may present as part of a syndrome, and babies with congenital deafness should be carefully screened for other abnormalities. There are many treatment strategies available, including cochlear implantation.

Infective (labyrinthitis/viral) (see Vertigo)

Vestibular Schwannoma and tumors of the cerebello-pontine angle (CPA)

Vestibular Schwannoma, also known as acoustic neuroma, is a benign tumor of Schwann cells of the vestibular nerve. It is rare, incidence 1 in 100 000 per year, but should be excluded in asymmetrical sensorineural hearing loss. Other symptoms are unilateral tinnitus and vertigo. Investigation is MRI scanning. Other tumors at the cerebello-pontine angle are uncommon and include meningiomas, bony tumors, and other rarities.

Ototoxicity

Two hundred substances cause cochlear or vestibular damage but few drugs in common use are ototoxic. Thus a drug history is pivotal in new onset hearing loss, tinnitus and vertigo. Some individuals are genetically susceptible to ototoxic drugs which include aminoglycosides, loop diuretics, aspirin, beta-blockers, anti-epileptic drugs, and cisplatin. Alternative non-ototoxic drugs should be substituted if possible or a risk–benefit analysis performed. For example, should hearing be sacrificed during treatment of toxic shock?

Traumatic

Skull base fracture may occur following head injury. It should be suspected in patients with characteristic bruising patterns: raccoon eyes and Battle sign (post-auricular bruising) and leaking of CSF from the nose or ears. The fracture line may damage the inner or middle ear and cause both conductive and sensorineural hearing loss.

Conductive

Wax/foreign body

Clinical features

Most common cause is wax impaction. It is easily diagnosed on otoscopy.

Epidemiology and pathology

The skin of the external auditory meatus ordinarily migrates from the center of the tympanic membrane outwards, down the canal, carrying wax and keratin

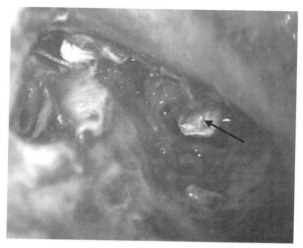

Fig. 7.2. Operative view of the middle ear demonstrating cholesteatoma (arrowed) with its characteristic skin-like appearance.

debris with it. In this way the ear is self-cleaning but wax can impact due to anatomically narrow or unusually shaped canals, skin conditions, and the use of cotton buds.

Management
Wax softeners, such as olive oil or sodium bicarbonate eardrops, and microsuction of the wax under direct vision. Although most common in children, foreign bodies may be found in the external auditory canals of adults. Exotic insects in holidaymakers, plant matter in gardeners, and a cornucopia of objects in the psychiatric patient may be retrieved.

Chronic suppurative otitis media
Suspected in patients who present with recurring middle ear infection and a long history of ear problems starting in childhood. Occasionally a cholesteatoma develops (Fig. 7.2). This is a collection of abnormal skin in the middle ear which may erode ossicles and other structures causing hearing loss and occasionally facial nerve damage. Management is aggressive treatment of infection, regular review and imaging with fine-cut CT with removal of cholesteatoma if discovered.

Otitis media with effusion
Common in childhood but fluid behind the tympanic membrane of adults is rare. Examination of the post-nasal space is required to identify lesions blocking the Eustachian tube. Management is short-term topical nasal decongestants, trial of antibiotics, and

occasionally insertion of a ventilation tube (grommet) to ventilate the middle ear.

Otosclerosis
An autosomal dominant disease affecting 1% of population due to abnormal bone growth in the ossicles leading to conductive hearing loss. It may be unilateral or bilateral. Treatment is a hearing aid, and sometimes removal of the stapes and prosthetic replacement.

Painful ear (otalgia)
If sudden, short lived, and associated with other symptoms it is likely to be due to local infection. Severe pain may rarely be due to malignancy of the auditory canal. Every patient with persistent otalgia should undergo ENT examination to exclude referred pain.

Local causes
- *Otitis externa*
- *Acute otitis media*
- *Malignancy of auditory canal/middle ear*

Referred pain
Common due to the extensive sensory supply to the ear and close proximity to other structures. Pain can be referred to the ear via the trigeminal, facial, and glossopharyngeal nerves and also via the second and third cervical spinal nerves. A common cause of referred pain to the ear is temporomandibular joint dysfunction but may also be due to cancer of the head or neck.

Tinnitus
Sensation of sound which is not related to external acoustic or electrical stimuli. Everybody suffers on occasion. Persistent or recurrent tinnitus can indicate otologic diseases. It is described as ringing, buzzing or pulsatile. True tinnitus does not include vascular bruits or palatal "clicking" (palatal myoclonus) which are real sounds.

Any otologic disease may produce tinnitus. It is common in hearing loss, particularly noise induced, in Menière's disease, and ototoxicity.

The mechanism of tinnitus is unknown. It is agreed that a potential generated within the auditory system is processed to produce the perception of sound. If no otologic cause can be found it may be due to systemic disease: hypertension, heart failure, neuropathy, multiple sclerosis, and drugs.

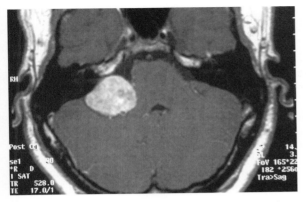

Fig. 7.3. MRI scan of the brain revealing a right sided vestibular Schwannoma at the cerebellar-pontine angle.

Investigation includes otoscopy, and pure tone audiogram. Unilateral tinnitus should be further investigated with MRI to exclude vestibular Schwannoma (Fig. 7.3).

Management

Exclusion of treatable underlying cause and control of symptoms. Aids, such as white noise producers, and visits to a tinnitus clinic for counseling on how to manage often disabling symptoms are effective. Tinnitus is usually short lived but may persist.

Vertigo

True vertigo is the hallucination of movement. Patients perceive the environment moves about them. The term vertigo does not describe the sensation of dizziness or faintness.

An understanding of the vestibular system is helpful. The semicircular canals are situated in the petrous temporal bone and are fluid-filled membranous tubes lined with cilia. These bend as the fluid moves within the tubes, firing signals down the vestibular nerve to the brain. The three semi-circular canals are at right angles to one another and therefore detect movement of the head (angular acceleration). The utricle and saccule are dilations of the membranous tube that have gel "cushions" lying on the cilia with tiny crystals (otoconia) lying within them. These detect linear acceleration. The nerve impulses from the vestibular organs pass via the vestibular nerve to the vestibular nuclei situated in the brainstem. The vestibular system contributes approximately 15% to balance, another 15% coming from proprioception and 70% from vision. All three inputs are processed and balance is maintained by the brainstem and cerebellum.

It can therefore be seen that vertigo can be divided into peripheral causes: affecting the semi-circular canals and vestibular nerve, and central: affecting the brainstem and cerebellum. It is important to examine the ears carefully, as middle ear disease such as cholesteatoma can extend to the vestibular system.

Peripheral causes
Vestibular neuronitis and labyrinthitis
Clinical features
These conditions represent the commonest causes of vertigo and are probably synonymous. They are characterized by an acute and disabling onset of vertigo.

Epidemiology
They may occur following an upper respiratory tract infection, and are thought to represent viral infection of the peripheral vestibular system.

Investigation
An MRI may be performed if the condition fails to resolve or is recurrent.

Management
Symptomatic, with the use of vestibular sedatives, such as cinnarazine.

Outcome
The vertigo resolves after several days.

Benign paroxysmal positional vertigo (BPPV)
Clinical features
This common condition accounts for approximately 20% of vertigo. Patients present with intermittent vertigo on moving the head, often in a particular direction. There are no otologic abnormalities on examination.

Epidemiology and pathology
It may be caused by displacement of otoconia from the utricle into the semi-circular canals, formation of calcium crystals within the semi-circular system, or recurrent vestibular neuronitis. It may occur following head injury.

Investigation
The diagnosis of BPPV can be confirmed by performing the Halpike maneuver. The patient is positioned sitting on the bed with head held firmly by the examiner and turned to 45° to the right or left. The patient is then allowed to lie down rapidly with the head 30° below the horizontal. Nystagmus may be seen and the symptoms may be reproduced. This is then repeated on the other side.

Management

Vestibular rehabilitation can help, including treatment with the Epley maneuver. This involves a series of head positions, with the aim of repositioning any vestibular debris/otoconia.

Menière's disease
Clinical features

Menière's disease is characterized by episodic vertigo, usually unilateral deafness, and tinnitus. Patients may also complain of aural fullness. Symptoms may last for up to 24 hours at a time and are often associated with nausea, vomiting, and nystagmus. It is most common in middle age. Examination is normal. Menière's disease accounts for 15% of cases of vertigo.

Epidemiology and pathology

The cause is still unknown, but it may be an autoimmune response following viral infection or labyrinthine ischemia. The primary pathology is expansion of the endolymphatic compartment within the bony labyrinth. This increased pressure leads to distortion of the sensory components of the cochlea and semi-circular canal leading to hearing loss, tinnitus, and vertigo.

Investigation

An audiogram may reveal a sensorineural hearing loss, the diagnosis is usually made on the characteristic history.

Management

Reduction of salt and fluid intake; betahistine, a labyrinthine vasodilator and vestibular sedatives during the attacks. Surgery can be used in severe cases to decompress the endolymphatic sac or to selectively damage or destroy the labyrinth.

Outcome

Progressive disease may lead to hearing loss.

Ototoxicity

There are a number of ototoxic drugs that can cause both peripheral and central vertigo. These include the aminoglycosides, diuretics, co-trimoazole, and metronidazole. Other causes of vertigo are vestibular Schwannoma and tumors of the cerebello-pontine angle (CPA) (see Hearing loss).

Central causes

Cerebrovascular disease (see Chapter 9)
Migraine (see Chapter 9)
Multiple sclerosis (see Chapter 9)
Cerebellar tumor (see Chapter 9)

Facial weakness

Facial weakness may be part of a generalized neuromuscular condition or it may be isolated. The nerve supply to the muscles of facial movement is via the seventh cranial nerve. When due to an upper motor neurone lesion, the frontalis muscle is relatively spared due to bilateral innervation.

The course of the infranuclear (lower motor neuron) facial nerve is convoluted, and passes through a variety of areas at which it can become damaged. It arises at the pontine facial nucleus and passes into the petrous temporal bone via the internal auditory meatus with the vestibular and cochlear nerves. It then passes through the temporal bone within the facial canal, through the geniculate ganglion giving off branches within the middle ear to stapedius and the chorda tympani supplying taste to the anterior two-thirds of the tongue and secretomotor function to the lacrimal and submandibular glands. It passes out of the temporal bone via the stylomastoid foramen and enters the substance of the parotid gland where it divides into its terminal branches to supply the muscles of facial expression.

When dealing with facial nerve palsy, it is important to attempt to pinpoint the area of the facial nerve involved as this will guide further investigation and management. Examination should include otoscopy, assessment of vertigo, and pure tone audiography (Table 7.1).

Bell's palsy
Clinical features

Bell's palsy describes an acute onset of lower motor neurone facial nerve palsy. It is the most common cause of facial nerve palsy and is a diagnosis of exclusion following appropriate investigation to rule out other causes.

Epidemiology

It is thought to be viral in origin and is often temporary in nature.

Investigation

An MRI scan is usually performed to rule out other causes.

Management

Prednisolone 40 mg daily for at least 1 week improves the chance of recovery.

Outcome

Around half of patients will fully recover within months, another 35% will be back to near normal after a year.

Table 7.1. Facial nerve palsy

Cause	Typical history	Otalgia	Hearing loss	Forehead sparing	Clinical findings/Otoscopy
Bell's palsy	Rapid onset, previous episode	Often	Unusual	No	Normal
Ramsey–Hunt	History of varicella, rapid onset, tinnitus, vertigo	Severe	CHL or SNHL	No	Vesicles around and within ear canal. Edematous ear canal with crusting
Central cause	Often sudden onset, may have hemiparesis	No	No	Yes	May have other findings on neurologic examination
Suppurative otitis media	Acute otitis media or chronic symptoms such as recurrent infection, discharge, and cholesteatoma	Severe	CHL	No	Acute – tense red drum or perforation with purulent discharge Chronic – perforation, discharge cholesteatoma, polyps, or granulations
Trauma	History of head injury or facial laceration	If temporal bone fracture	If temporal bone fracture	No	If temporal bone fracture may have hemotympanum or perforation Facial laceration over parotid gland
CPA tumor	Slow onset, may have vertigo, tinnitus, sensory loss	Rare	Often SNHL	No	May have none
Parotid tumor	Gradual onset, facial pain		No	No	Parotid swelling, cervical lymphadenopathy

Ramsay–Hunt syndrome (herpes zoster oticus)

Clinical features

The patient usually presents with a sudden onset facial palsy and a painful ear, tinnitus, and occasionally vertigo. Crusting vesicles involving the external ear and within the ear canal are pathognomic for this condition (Fig. 7.4).

Epidemiology

Facial nerve infection with the herpes zoster virus.

Management

High dose acyclovir and oral steroids are used for at least 1 week to improve the chance of recovery.

Outcome

Around half of the patients obtain recovery of normal facial function.

Central neurologic causes (see Chapter 9)

Cerebrovascular disease

Multiple sclerosis

Intracerebral tumor

Infection (acute or chronic suppurative otitis media)

The facial nerve can be damaged as it traverses the middle ear within the facial canal. This may be due to pressure or direct toxic effects of suppurative infection. Middle ear disease may cause bony destruction of the canal to expose the facial nerve; however the

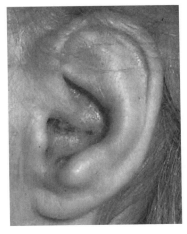

Fig. 7.4. Vesicles of the pinna characteristic of Ramsey–Hunt syndrome.

facial nerve is congenitally dehiscent through the canal in up to 6% of the population.

Trauma (surgical or other, temporal or parotid)

Facial nerve damage may occur during operative procedures such as excision of a tumor at the cerebello-pontine angle, excision of the parotid gland, or fractures of the temporal bone.

Tumor (at CPA or parotid)

Common sites for tumors causing facial nerve palsy are at the cerebello-pontine angle (CPA) and within the parotid gland. Tumors of the facial nerve itself are extremely rare.

Table 7.2. Facial pain

Condition	Age	Unilateral/bilateral	Associated symptoms	Associated signs
Sinusitis	Any	Often bilateral	Nasal congestion, facial swelling, post-nasal drip	Facial swelling, pus draining from sinus
TMJ dysfunction	Any	Unilateral	Pain on eating	Popping/clicking of joint, pain reproduced on joint palpation
Referred pain	Any	May be unilateral in cluster headache or bilateral in tension headache	Visual symptoms in migraine, headache, nasal congestion and sweating in cluster headache	Rarely
Giant cell arteritis (Temporal arteritis)	>60	Unilateral	Muscle girdle pain, visual symptoms	Thickened, tender temporal artery
Trigeminal neuralgia	Any	Unilateral	Rarely, trigger point	Rarely
Herpes zoster	Any	Unilateral	Paresthesia, itching	Vesicles in trigeminal nerve distribution

The most common tumor to affect the cerebello-pontine angle is the vestibular Schwannoma (see Hearing loss). MRI is helpful in diagnosis. Management may include conservative management with serial scanning, surgical excision, or radiotherapy.

Facial pain

Neurologic, maxillofacial, and rheumatologic disorders may cause facial pain (Table 7.2).

Sinusitis

Clinical features

Symptoms include facial pain, swelling and tenderness over the infected sinus, nasal congestion and general malaise. Chronic sinusitis usually follows on from acute sinusitis, with symptoms of nasal congestion, facial pain, and rhinorrhea persisting for weeks or months.

Epidemiology and pathology

There are paired air-filled sinuses in the face: the frontal, maxillary, and ethmoid sinuses, draining into the middle meatus of the nose, and the unpaired sphenoid sinus. Acute infection may develop in any, leading to a pansinusitis when all become involved. The most common route of infection is nasal, any narrowing of the drainage pathways into the nose leads to accumulation of secretions, poor ventilation, and development of infection. The maxillary sinus is the most common to be infected. The majority occur following a viral upper respiratory tract infection. Static secretions become secondarily infected, most usually by *Pneumococcus* or *Hemophilus* species. Fungal infection should be suspected in the immunocompromised.

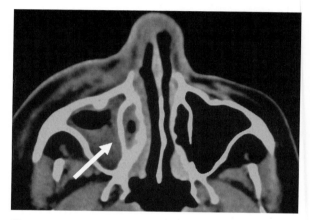

Fig. 7.5. CT scan through the nose showing opacification of the right maxillary sinus (arrowed). The left side is full of air, which is normal.

Investigation

It may be possible to visualize pus drainage into the meatus on endoscopic examination of the nose. CT scan will reveal degree of sinus involvement and complications (Fig. 7.5).

Management

Management of acute sinusitis includes analgesia, broad spectrum antibiotics, and nasal decongestants. Acute surgical drainage may rarely be necessary.

Management of chronic sinusitis includes a course of antibiotics and the use of topical nasal steroids or antihistamines to reduce nasal congestion. If medical methods fail, endoscopic sinus surgery can be performed to clear the drainage pathways of the sinuses.

Outcome

The vast majority of cases will resolve with the above management. Complications of acute sinusitis are rare but can be life-threatening and include orbital complications, such as orbital cellulitis and abscess formation, osteomyelitis and intracranial complications, such as meningitis, abscess, or venous sinus thrombosis.

Temporomandibular joint dysfunction

Temporomandibular joint (TMJ) dysfunction is a common cause of chronic facial pain. Anatomic disturbance of the joint may occur and can lead to unilateral facial pain or otalgia. It is often possible to discover focal symptoms and signs on taking a full history, including pain on eating, trismus, popping, locking, and clicking within the joint, and teeth grinding. The diagnosis may be confirmed on MR imaging of the joint.

Referred pain (including migraine)

A number of other conditions can lead to the perception of facial pain, and a careful history of other symptoms often leads to the diagnosis. These may include other causes of headache, such as migraine and tension headache. Cluster headaches can present with characteristic unilateral pain, often centered upon the face and often associated with sweating, nasal congestion, and swollen conjunctiva.

Giant cell arteritis (temporal arteritis)

This is an inflammatory condition affecting the medium-sized arteries that supply the head, orbit, and optic nerves. It usually affects the elderly who may present with a tender, thickened temporal artery. The main concern is the potential for visual loss, and management with high dose steroids is often commenced prior to confirmation of diagnosis by temporal artery biopsy.

Trigeminal neuralgia
Clinical features

It is characterised by pain in one or more regions supplied by the three main divisions of the trigeminal nerve. The pain is usually described as a short, intense knife-like (lancinating) sensation, triggered by an innocuous stimulus of a "trigger zone," for example brushing the hair. It is almost always unilateral and the most common division to be affected is the mandibular (Vc), followed by the maxillary (Vb), and then ophthalmic (Va) divisions.

Epidemiology and pathology

Trigeminal neuralgia is a severe pain syndrome, thought to be due to local demyelination of the trigeminal nerve within the cranial cavity. It may be related to compression by a vascular loop and typically occurs in the middle aged and elderly. Before treatment methods were discovered, it was associated with suicide in sufferers.

Investigation

MRI of the skull base, to rule out other causes and identify any vascular anomaly that may be compressing the nerve.

Management

If a vascular loop is discovered, operative decompression of the nerve may provide relief. Other methods of management include the use of anticonvulsant drugs such as carbamazepine and gabapentin; and chemical or thermal ablation of the nerve.

Acute herpes zoster and post-herpetic neuralgia
Clinical features

Presents with pain, itching, and paresthesia along the course of the affected nerve, and is followed a few days later by the development of cutaneous vesicles. The ophthalmic division (Va) is the most commonly affected.

Epidemiology and pathology

Herpes zoster may lie dormant in the trigeminal ganglion following childhood infection (chicken pox) and reactivate at times of immunocompromise, particularly in the elderly. This leads to the condition of shingles.

Management

Analgesia and antiviral agents such as acyclovir. It is thought that early use of these agents, and also tricyclic antidepressants, may reduce the incidence of post-herpetic neuralgia.

Outcome

Post-herpetic neuralgia may occur in up to 50% of people following herpes zoster and is characterized by a burning pain over the nerve distribution. It may be treated with tricyclic antidepressants.

Nose bleed (epistaxis)

Epistaxis is an underrated condition, both in terms of potential seriousness and as an indicator for underlying disease. The majority will be managed by the patient at home, or by a general practitioner.

Table 7.3. Nasal obstruction

Condition	Age	Usually bilateral	Rhinorrhea	Epistaxis	Loss of smell	Associations
Rhinitis and turbinate hypertrophy	Any	Yes	Yes	Rarely	Occasionally	Asthma, hayfever
Septal deformity	Any	No	No	No	No	Trauma
Nasal polyps	Any	Yes	Yes	Rarely	Yes	Asthma, hayfever, CF
Nasal tumor	Older	No	No	Yes	Rarely	Hardwood dust, EBV
Foreign body	Any	No	Offensive	Rarely	No	Learning disabilities
Choanal atresia	Young	Varies	No	No	No	Syndromes

The cases that make it to the attention of ENT surgeons are often those that cannot be stopped by simple methods, that are recurrent in nature, and that are associated with other symptoms. The causes of epistaxis can be divided into local, general or systemic.

Local causes
Idiopathic / environmental
The anterior mucosa is constantly exposed to the external environment, leading to dryness, potential ulceration, and bleeding on the anterior nasal septum at Little's area. This area is the point of anastomosis of vessels from the internal and external carotid arteries (Kiesselbach's plexus).

Traumatic
The most common cause is nose-picking. Other causes include fracture and foreign bodies, particularly in children or adults with learning difficulties.

Inflammatory
Iatrogenic
Steroid sprays used in rhinitis can lead to thinning and dryness of the nasal mucosa – making it more likely to ulcerate and bleed.

Neoplastic (tumors of nose, sinuses, nasopharynx)
Basal cell and squamous cell carcinoma and rarely malignant melanoma may arise on the surface and bleed. Sinonasal tumors account for 10% of head and neck cancers and occur more commonly in the Arab, Japanese, and African populations. Fifty percent are squamous but anaplastic, lymphomas, and adenocarcinomas may occur. Predisposing factors include chronic inflammatory nasal conditions and smoking. Sinonasal tumors tend to present late, and can extend locally to involve the orbit, other sinuses, and the cranial cavity. Management includes careful staging and surgical excision where possible.

General causes (hypertension, clotting dyscrasia, Rendu–Osler–Weber)
Patients with Rendu–Osler–Weber, or hereditary hemorrhagic telangiectasia, have multiple telangiectasia affecting their skin, mucosa, lung, and gastrointestinal tract. They are difficult to manage and associated epistaxis may be fatal.

Nasal obstruction
Nasal obstruction is common and is usually due to a common cold. When persistent, it may rarely indicate potentially lethal conditions.

Air enters the nostrils (nares) and passes into the nasopharynx, larynx, trachea, and lungs. The nose performs several important functions during this process. Stiff hairs within the nasal vestibule act as filters for particles to stop them passing into the respiratory tract. The air is warmed and humidified as it passes over the highly vascular secretory epithelium, the surface area of which is increased by the lateral turbinates or concha. High up in the nasal cavity lie the receptors of the olfactory nerve, responsible for the detection of odors and contributing to taste perception.

Patients with nasal obstruction may present with other nasal symptoms, which give a clue to the diagnosis (Table 7.3). Every patient complaining of nasal obstruction should undergo careful examination of the nose and nasopharynx to rule out a potentially serious cause. A simple test for obstruction is breathing onto a mirrored surface if there is obstruction there will be no misting.

Rhinitis and turbinate hypertrophy
Clinical features
Rhinitis is a common complaint, affecting 30% of the population. The main symptom is of nasal obstruction or stuffiness, accompanied by rhinorrhea and irritative symptoms such as sneezing and itching.

When the nose is examined, the mucosa appears pale, swollen and watery, with enlarged turbinates.

Epidemiology and pathology

Rhinitis can be broadly divided into two forms: allergic rhinitis and intrinsic (non-allergic) rhinitis. Allergic rhinitis is often seasonal and is also associated with eye symptoms such as watering and itching. The cause is a hypersensitivity reaction within the nasal mucosa to allergens such as pollen. Increased levels of the immunoglobulin IgE lead to edema of the nasal mucosa. Intrinsic rhinitis is an inflammatory condition of the nose, not due to an external allergen. It tends to be familial and may follow infection.

Investigation

The diagnosis is usually clinical; however the allergen causing the symptoms can be found using skin or blood tests radio allergo-sorbent test (RAST). This will detect different amounts of IgE from a patients blood reacting with specific antigens.

Management

Management of allergic rhinitis can be conservative, surgical or medical. If practical the allergen can be avoided. Most patients are managed with a combination of oral antihistamines (e.g. cetirizine) and topical nasal steroid sprays. Desensitization, when the patient undergoes injection of the allergen, can be effective, but there is the risk of anaphylaxis. If the main symptom is that of obstruction and medical treatment is ineffective, the nasal airway may be optimized surgically by reduction of the inferior turbinates, usually by cautery.

Septal deformity

The nasal septum is a cartilaginous structure that divides the right and left sides of the nasal cavity. It may be displaced, leading to unilateral nasal obstruction. Treatment should only be commenced if the patient is troubled by symptoms, the septum can be straightened by a septoplasty.

Nasal polyps

Occasionally when the nasal mucosa becomes edematous and inflamed, such as in rhinitis, nasal polyps can occur. It is thought that increasing swelling in the tissues leads to polyp formation from underlying connective tissue in some individuals. The main symptoms are of nasal obstruction. Nasal polyps are usually bilateral. If unilateral, painful or bleeding, the patient should undergo urgent investigation to rule out a malignancy. The treatment of nasal polyps is usually a combination of medical and surgical. Steroid nasal spray or drops can be used, as can oral antihistamines, or the polyps can be excised.

Nasal tumors

Malignant tumors tend to occur in the older age group and present with unilateral nasal obstruction, bleeding, and discharge. Diagnosis is made on clinical examination, tissue biopsy, and CT scan which can assess degree of tumor invasion. Prognosis is generally poor. Surgical excision of the tumor, if possible, is the mainstay of treatment, often with adjuvant chemo- or radiotherapy.

Foreign body

Nasal foreign bodies are much more common in children but can occasionally occur in adults, particularly those with learning difficulties or psychiatric problems.

Choanal atresia

This occurs when the posterior membrane blocking off the back of the nose fails to atrophy before birth. Treatment is surgical – the bone or membrane is removed.

Sore throat

Sore throats are common, and are most often due to a self-limiting viral upper respiratory tract infection, but rarely a life-threatening condition may be present (Table 7.4).

Pharyngitis

Pharyngitis is generally part of an upper respiratory tract infection, and can be viral, bacterial, or even fungal in nature. It is generally self limiting and requires no active treatment other than symptomatic relief, but if symptoms persist further investigations may be required to rule out a more sinister cause.

Tonsillitis
Clinical features

Tonsillitis is common and characterized by swelling and redness of the palatine tonsils resolving in days. There is often an associated cervical lymphadenopathy.

Epidemiology and pathology

Tonsillitis is a relatively common disease, but it is still not fully understood. It is caused by either viral or combined viral and bacterial infection.

Table 7.4. Sore throat

Condition	Age	Associated symptoms	Signs	Investigation
Pharyngitis	Any	Upper respiratory tract infection (URTI)	Erythema of throat	Throat swab may show *strep.*
Tonsillitis	Young adults	Dysphagia, voice change	Tonsillar hypertrophy, lymphadenopathy	Throat swab may show *strep.*
Glandular fever	Young adults	Systemic malaise	Tonsillar hypertrophy, grey tonsillar slough, lymphadenopathy, hepatosplenomegaly (rare)	Monospot test for Estein–Barr virus (EBV) LFTs may be deranged
Quinsy	Young adults	Dysphagia, voice change, unilateral symptoms	Unilateral paratonsillar swelling, displaced uvula, trismus	Pus for micro-organisms and sensitivities (MC&S)
Oropharyngeal ulceration	Any	Halitosis, hemoptysis, weight loss	Single or multiple areas of ulceration	Biopsy may reveal carcinoma
Parapharyngeal/ Retropharyngeal abscess	Any	Systemic malaise, voice change, dysphagia, stridor, dyspnea	Often no signs, occasional bulging into pharynx	CT delineates abscess
Epiglottitis	Children but ↑ in adults	Drooling, SOB, systemic malaise, voice change, dysphagia, stridor	If suspected <u>do not</u> examine	<u>No</u> investigation, direct visualization of larynx performed at intubation

Investigation

Blood tests include the monospot test to assess for the presence of Epstein-Barr virus (EBV) (see below). In cases of unilateral tonsillitis, further investigation should rule out lymphoma or squamous cell carcinoma.

Management

If severe, may require hospital admission, intravenous antibiotics and analgesia. Recurrent tonsillitis (usually five episodes a year for at least 2 years) can be managed by tonsillectomy.

Outcome

Occasionally a collection of pus may develop in the areolar tissue surrounding the tonsil forming a quinsy. This will need to be drained. Tonsils may become extremely large and the airway may be compromised.

Glandular fever

Infection with EBV leads to the development of infective mononucleosis. Young patients often present with tonsillitis, their tonsils tend to be covered in a grey slough (Fig. 7.6), and there is marked lymphadenopathy. The diagnosis may be confirmed with the monospot blood test. Liver function should be checked and the patient advised to avoid contact sports for at least 6 weeks as some patients may develop hepatosplenomegaly.

Oropharyngeal ulceration (inc. neoplasia)

Ulceration of the oral cavity may involve the pharynx, leading to a sore throat. Most painful ulceration is

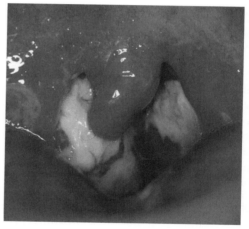

Fig. 7.6. Infected tonsils covered in slough – characteristic of glandular fever.

aphthous ulceration. These are typically small, may be multiple, and heal within a few days. Widespread oropharyngeal ulceration can indicate systemic diseases. Ulcers that are atypical, do not resolve, or are present in a smoker should be biopsied as they may represent neoplastic disease.

Parapharyngeal/retropharyngeal abscess

Pus from several sources can collect within the fascial sheaths of the neck. There is limited space so this can rapidly lead to sore throat, dysphagia, and breathing difficulties. Initial management may be intravenous antibiotics but it may warrant surgical drainage.

Table 7.5. Hoarseness and voice change

Condition	Age	Duration	Painful	Dysphagia	Associated features
Laryngitis	Any	Usually self-limiting, can be chronic	☑	Rarely	May have associated URTI
Benign vocal cord lesion	Any	Often static, can improve	☒	Rarely	Voice abuse, respiratory papillomatosis as child
Laryngeal carcinoma	Older	Progressive	As disease progresses	Progressive	Smoking
Vocal cord palsy	Any	Often static	☒	Rarely	Trauma/tracheostomy/intubation, thyroid surgery, lung cancer

Epiglottitis

The incidence of epiglottitis decreased with the introduction of vaccine against *Haemophilus influenza* type B (HIB). Only rarely are other bacteria involved. Typical presentation is of a stridulous patient, leaning forward and drooling. If epiglottitis is suspected surgeon and anesthetist should be contacted and the patient examined under anesthetic with appropriate equipment for intubation and tracheostomy nearby.

Hoarseness and voice change

Hoarseness and voice change are common symptoms and usually due to voice abuse, but other causes include hypothyroidism and laryngeal carcinoma (Table 7.5).

Laryngitis
Clinical features
Acute laryngitis is common. The majority suffer from it at some stage. It is characterized by loss of voice, often associated with a sore throat.

Epidemiology and pathology
In many it is a combination of viral illness weakening the integrity of the laryngeal mucosa and external factors such as cigarette smoke or dusty environments. Chronic laryngitis can be representative of an underlying sinister pathology or it may simply be due to over-use or abuse of the larynx.

Investigation
Laryngoscopy to rule out sinister pathology.

Management
The mainstay of treatment is symptomatic relief with analgesia, voice rest, and steam inhalation. Other causes of chronic laryngitis include chronic acid reflux or fungal infection, particularly in the immunocompromised patient. In these cases, treatment of the underlying disease will allow the laryngeal inflammation to settle.

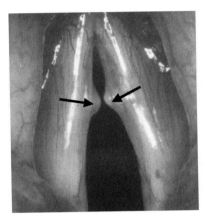

Fig. 7.7. Vocal cord nodules (arrowed).

Outcome
Symptoms can persist from a few days up to 2 weeks; any hoarseness of voice lasting longer than 21 days must be investigated thoroughly.

Benign vocal cord lesions (nodules/polyps/papillomatosis)
Vocal cord nodules commonly occur in those who exert their voices. They appear as smooth bilateral swellings at the border of the middle and anterior thirds of the vocal cords (Fig. 7.7). They typically resolve with rest and voice therapy, though can become "organized" and persistent, when surgical removal may be considered. Vocal cord polyps occur unilaterally from the medial edge of the cord and occur as a result of "hemorrhage" in the submucosal layer. Treatment is the same as for vocal cord nodules.

Vocal cord papillomas decrease with increasing age. No treatment is curative and many undergo surgical ablation with laser or excision to preserve the gross structure of the vocal cords and restore airway patency and voice.

Laryngeal carcinoma
Clinical features
Initially hoarseness though it may present with dysphagia, weight loss, otalgia, halitosis, and neck

221

Table 7.6. Salivary gland swelling

Cause	History	Painful?	Examination findings	Age	Associations
Infection	Short	Yes	Tender, hot, red	Any	Dehydration
Calculi formation	Intermittent	Yes	Tender	Any	Swelling on eating
Neoplastic	Long	Rarely	Firm, fixed, if malignant may be palpable lymph nodes	>50 yrs	Facial nerve palsy
Sjogrens Syndrome	Long	Rarely	Firm, decreased secretions	Any	Rheumatoid arthritis, connective tissue diseases

swelling (either due to cervical lymphadenopathy or the tumor itself).

Epidemiology and pathology

The most common head and neck cancer in the Western world. Rare cancers affecting the larynx include fibrosarcoma and adenocarcinoma. It occurs mainly in those who drink alcohol and smoke. Laryngeal carcinoma is uncommon in those who do not smoke.

The larynx is divided into three areas, supraglottis, glottis, and infra-glottis. The commonest site of tumor is in the glottic region (70%).

Investigation

Biopsy, MRI, or CT scans are performed to aid in diagnosis and allow staging of the tumor by the TNM system.

Management

Early stage tumors may be amenable to radiotherapy or laser excision but larger or recurrent tumors may require more radical surgery such as laryngectomy.

Outcome

Dependent on TNM staging, prognosis is good in early tumors.

Vocal cord palsy

Clinical features

Patients usually present with a hoarse voice, though if the cord palsy is bilateral the patient may be stridulous.

Epidemiology and pathology

The larynx is innervated by branches of the vagus nerve including the recurrent and superior laryngeal nerves. These are responsible for abducting (opening) and adducting (closing) the vocal cords. Common causes of palsy include malignant invasion or compression of the nerves in the neck or the chest (bronchial carcinoma) or direct invasion of the larynx. Iatrogenic causes account for approximately 20%–25% of vocal cord palsies, particularly following thyroid, pharyngeal, or thoracic surgery. Trauma, either to the neck or penetrating to deeper structures, accounts for some.

Investigation

Laryngoscopy to visualize the palsy and CT scans to investigate the cause.

Management

Depending on the nature of the palsy, treatment can vary from conservative to thyroplasty or tracheostomy.

Head and neck swelling

There are many causes of head and neck swelling. In this section, swelling of salivary glands and cervical swellings will be discussed (Table 7.6).

Salivary glands

There are two main pairs of salivary glands: the parotids and submandibular, and many minor salivary glands of the upper respiratory tract. Diseases usually present with swelling. The cause can be often be determined by history, especially pain and chronicity.

Infection (viral/bacterial)

Salivary gland swelling can be due to viral or bacterial infection. Viral infection is most commonly due to mumps virus. Bacterial salivary gland infection may occur following dehydration and systemic illness and can be treated with antibiotics. Infective swelling of salivary glands is often painful, may be bilateral and is short lived.

Calculi formation

Calculi present with intermittent swelling and pain on eating. This may progress to persistent swelling, duct stricture, and stenosis. If duct occlusion by calculi occurs, the stones may be retrieved by duct manipulation or incision. The diseased gland may need excision.

Table 7.7. Causes of neck swelling

Cause	History	Painful?	Examination findings	Age	Associations
Reactive/Infective	Short	Yes	Tender nodes throughout neck	Any	URTI, head and neck infection
Thyroid	Long	No	Midline swelling	Any	Hyper/hypothyroid
Neoplastic	Long	Rarely	Firm, fixed	>50 yrs	Smoking
Neck space infection	Short	Yes	Tender, diffuse swelling	Any	Stridor, sepsis
Pharyngeal pouch	Long	No	Lateral swelling	>60 yrs	Esophageal dismotility
Branchial cyst	Long	No	Lateral swelling	Any	May be infected
Laryngocele	Long	No	Swelling on Valsalva	>60 yrs	Brass musicians
Vascular	Long	No	Pulsatile lateral swelling	Any	Familial

Neoplastic

Neoplastic lesions are generally firm, persistent, and painless swellings. The majority (80%) of salivary gland tumors occur in the parotid gland (Fig. 7.8). Neoplastic lesions of the salivary glands may be benign or malignant. Eighty percent of parotid lesions are benign, as are two-thirds of submandibular gland and one in two minor salivary gland tumors. Of the benign parotid gland tumors, 80% are pleomorphic adenomas. They are managed by surgical excision with a wide margin to prevent capsule rupture and recurrence. An example of a malignant salivary gland tumor is the adenoid cystic carcinoma, a slow growing tumor which may spread down nerve sheaths and may lead to facial pain and palsy.

Inflammatory (Sjogren's, see Chapter 11)

Neck swellings

Neck swellings may be single or multiple, focal or diffuse. They may be midline, in which case a thyroid swelling should be suspected, unilateral, or bilateral. Although the majority of causes of neck swelling are reactive or benign, a malignant cause should always be excluded (Table 7.7).

Reactive/infective cervical lymphadenopathy

The most common cause of cervical lymphadenopathy is reactive or infective due to a viral cause. Cervical lymphadenopathy is common following tonsillitis or URTI, it is important to rule out TB in at-risk groups. Persistent lymphadenopathy must be fully investigated.

Thyroid and thyroglossal cyst (see Chapter 12)

Neoplastic

The majority of tumors within the head and neck may spread to lymph nodes of the neck. A malignant

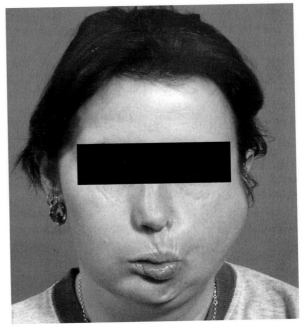

Fig. 7.8. Left parotid swelling with associated facial asymmetry due to facial nerve weakness.

deposit must be considered with any persistent lymph node swelling. Lymphoma must be excluded especially if multiple neck nodes enlarge in a young person. Lymph nodes containing metastatic deposits are hard and often fixed to skin or underlying structures. Fine needle aspiration cytology, lymph node excision, imaging including CT from the skull base to diaphragm and endoscopic examination of the pharynx and larynx may reveal a primary lesion.

Neck space infection (see Sore throat)

Pharyngeal pouch

A pharyngeal pouch is a posterior herniation of pharyngeal mucosa through a weak area of the posterior

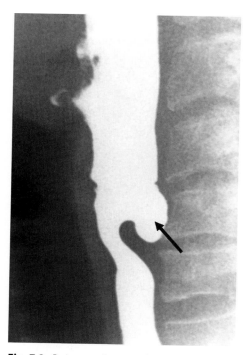

Fig. 7.9. Barium swallow revealing pharyngeal pouch (arrowed).

pharyngeal wall. Patients tend to be elderly and may present with dysphagia, neck swelling, regurgitation of food, halitosis, and chest infection due to aspiration. Diagnosis can be made by barium swallow, which reveals the pouch (Fig. 7.9). Treatment may be conservative or may involve open excision or endoscopic stapling of the pouch.

Branchial cyst

Rare swellings that usually arise deep to the anterior border of sternocleidomastoid at the junction of its upper third and lower two-thirds. Diagnosis requires fine needle aspiration cytology, a malignant lymph node needs exclusion. Treatment is surgical excision.

Laryngocele

These are rare neck swellings arising from the laryngeal saccule. They are intermittent, often becoming apparent on performing the Valsalva maneuver. A laryngocele may be visible on plain X-rays of the neck, as an air-filled sac. Treatment is surgical excision.

Vascular

Vascular causes of neck swellings are rare. They include carotid artery aneurysms and vascular malformations. Carotid body tumors may present as pulsatile neck swellings. These are tumors of paraganglion tissue and are often hereditary in nature.

Further reading

Gleeson M, Clarke R, Jones NS, *Scott-Browns Otorhinolaryngology: Head and Neck Surgery*. Oxford University Press, 2008.

Ludman H, Bradley P, *ABC of Ear, Nose and Throat*. BMJ Publishing, 2007. http://www.entuk.org

Teifion Davies

Contents

Assessing psychiatric problems

The symptoms of psychiatric disorder are common: several surveys have found that, at any time, as many as a third of the adult population report suffering from worry, tension, sleep disturbance, or pessimism. As is the case in all branches of medicine, many of these symptoms lie on a continuum from occasional and transient experiences of everyday life, through those that are understandable consequences of specific circumstances, to those occurring only as part of a recognized syndrome or disorder. This can be understood by analogy with one of the commonest presenting features of physical illness: pain. Aches and pains might be an irritating but trivial experience for a healthy person, and acute or intense pain might result from a specific and demarcated injury, while persistent pain might signal a clinically significant underlying illness. To pursue this analogy further, pain is a percept, that is a psychological phenomenon for which there is no reliable objective test nor laboratory investigation. The evaluation of the pain reported by a patient is, therefore, a clinical skill in which every doctor would regard himself or herself as competent. This evaluation will depend on a careful and detailed elucidation of the development of the pain, its characteristics and localization in time and space, its associations with the activities of the patient's life, and its effects on the patient's functioning. Where the source of the pain is an underlying physical disorder, the evaluation will be informed by knowledge of the pathophysiology of the affected structures.

Evaluation of psychiatric symptoms must follow a similar course.

Psychiatric problems

- Presenting complaint
- Medical history
- Psychiatric history
- Mental state examination
- Physical examination
- Tests and investigations
- Differential diagnosis

A common cause of difficulty for the student seeking to understand psychiatric symptoms is that many of them arise from dysfunction in other psychologic, or mental, processes whose structural pathology has yet to be elucidated scientifically. The solution to this difficulty is surprisingly simple: it is to extend the clinical investigation in breadth and depth to cover all *relevant* aspects of the patient's life. The result, the psychiatric history, is merely an extension of the general medical history that takes full account of the patient's background and upbringing, culture and social circumstances, expectations and attributions. The seemingly limitless extent of such history-taking can appear daunting but, with practice and experience, those features *relevant* to a diagnosis can be focused upon quickly (although further details might be relevant to consideration of, and response to, treatment). The analogy here is with the review of systems and the aim, as in medicine generally, is to distinguish a pattern of symptoms that matches the configuration found in recognized disorder.

The signs of psychiatric disorder are sought during the systematic psychiatric examination (called the mental state examination), which is performed usually after a full history has been obtained. Another cause of difficulty for the student concerns the apparent lack of objectivity of the mental state examination when compared with the physical examination. Again, this distinction is more apparent than real. For instance, when palpating the abdomen, a student might report detecting a liver edge, ballotting a kidney, or sensing the pulsations of the abdominal aorta. Confidence in these findings does not come from visualization of, or direct contact with, these structures but from clinical inference based on a comparison of the pattern of palpation to what is known of the normal and pathologic appearances of abdominal organs, gained from prior anatomic and imaging studies. Similarly, normality or abnormality of a patient's mood, thought, and perception is inferred from comparing what is observed of the patient's appearance and behaviour, and his or her responses to systematic direct questioning, to what is known of the normal pattern of these phenomena in someone of similar age, sex, and social and cultural background.

The physical examination and careful selection of tests and investigations are core components of the psychiatric assessment of any patient, but are frequently overlooked. Patients with psychiatric disorders have a high prevalence of co-morbid physical illness, and consequently the standardized mortality ratio from all causes is raised. A general physical examination should be performed as for any medical patient. This should focus on signs of primary physical disorder that might present with psychiatric symptoms (e.g. thyroid disease presenting as mood disorder), or co-morbid physical illness that might complicate the diagnosis, course, or treatment of a primary psychiatric disorder (e.g. renal or hepatic disease that might affect choice of treatment for mania or psychosis). Laboratory tests and other investigations should be selected to exclude suspected physical disease or to clarify its progression.

How are the symptoms and signs of psychiatric disorder, obtained from the psychiatric history and mental state examination, to be organized to reach a diagnosis? Psychiatric disorders may be classified into groups and arranged to form a diagnostic hierarchy (Fig. 8.1). In this hierarchy, disorders at each level may contain any of the features of disorders at lower levels, but they are characterized by the occurrence of features that are not found in disorders at lower levels. Use of this hierarchy helps to make sense of the potentially bewildering overlap of symptoms between different disorders. Thus, hallucinations and delusions are characteristic features of levels from "functional psychoses" upwards, but only the highest levels (drug induced and organic disorders) are characterized by findings of visual hallucinations or fluctuating consciousness. Similarly, a variety of anxiety features may occur at any level, but typically they emerge and are the predominant cause of disability at the level of "neuroses." The first step in forming a diagnosis is to work up from the bottom of the hierarchy, to establish at which diagnostic level this patient's predominant symptoms are first encountered. The second step in diagnosis is to compare the patient's symptoms and signs with those of the group of disorders within this diagnostic level and establish the best fit, which suggests the most likely diagnosis. As all the disorders at a similar level will share many features, this step involves careful delineation of the pattern of symptoms and signs. The third and final step is to determine whether the patient has additional, perhaps secondary, symptoms that do not fit the likely diagnosis but might suggest a more severe variant found at a higher diagnostic level. For example, a patient may suffer from symptoms and signs of depression characteristically found in the level of mood disorders, but experience occasional auditory hallucinations and delusional beliefs suggestive of the functional psychosis, psychotic depression.

The relations between presenting problems, their characteristic timing and the underlying diagnosis are shown in Table 8.1.

The clinical features stressed in this chapter will be those required to make a diagnosis according to the criteria of the *World Health Organization's International Classification of Diseases*, 10th edition (ICD-10).

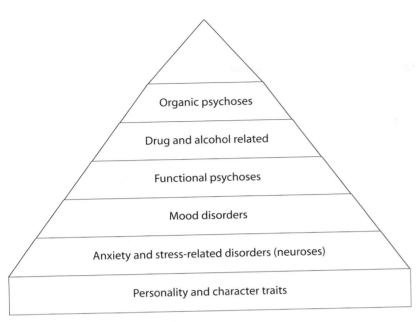

Fig. 8.1. Diagnostic hierarchy of psychiatric disorders.

Organic psychoses

Drug and alcohol related

Functional psychoses

Mood disorders

Anxiety and stress-related disorders (neuroses)

Personality and character traits

Each level *includes* all symptoms of all lower levels.
Each level *excludes* symptoms typical of higher levels.

Anxiety

Anxiety is a common emotion and most people will have experienced transient, situational anxiety as a normal concomitant of their everyday activities. In these normal circumstances, anxiety may be recognized as a state of psychologic and somatic preparation for unpleasant or testing situations such as examinations, public performances, or risky sports – the well-known "fight-or-flight" reaction – where a degree of arousal serves to increase the chances of success or survival.

Components of anxiety

Psychologic
Emotional: apprehension, fear of impending death or doom; tension, irritability, restlessness, fatigue; loss of libido.

Cognitive: reduced concentration.

Perceptual: increased sensory acuity and intolerance of stimulation; illusions (misinterpretations of real stimuli), pseudo-hallucinations.

Somatic (mainly secondary to autonomic overactivity)
Cardiorespiratory: tachypnea (over-breathing, hyperventilation), dyspnea, palpitations, chest pain, pallor, cold periphery.

Gastro-intestinal: loss of appetite, dry mouth, lump in the throat (globus); nausea, vomiting, loose stool.

Neurologic: dizziness, blurred vision, paresthesia, numbness, sweating; muscle tension and tremor, carpopedal spasm; increased urinary frequency.

Circadian
Worsens during day; initial and middle insomnia.

However, when the components of anxiety occur repeatedly, or are disproportionate to the task in hand, they may be troublesome and are potentially disabling. Extensive community surveys in the UK and USA have found that about 30% of the general population have at least one anxiety symptom at any time, while some individual symptoms are particularly common.

Prevalence of some anxiety symptoms in the general population
- Fatigue: 27%
- Sleep problems: 25%
- Irritability: 22%
- Worry: 20%
- Panic: 10%

Table 8.1. Relationship between presenting symptoms, periodicity, or other features and the differential diagnosis

Presenting problem	Characteristics	Differential diagnosis
Anxiety	Unprovoked, continuous	Generalized anxiety disorder Obsessive-compulsive disorder
	Unprovoked, intermittent	Panic disorder Post-traumatic stress disorder
	Provoked, persistent	Substance misuse *Endocrinopathy*
	Provoked, intermittent	Simple phobias Social phobia Agoraphobia
Mood disturbance: depression	Recurrent, periodic	Dysthymia Bipolar affective disorder Cyclothymia
	Recurrent, episodic	Depressive episode Recurrent depressive disorder *Brief recurrent depression*
	Continuous, persistent	Depression of chronic illness *Anemia* *Endocrinopathy* *Renal failure* *Post-concussional syndrome* *Post-schizophrenic depression*
Mood disturbance: mania	Recurrent, periodic Episodic Continuous	Bipolar affective disorder Manic episode Substance misuse (amphetamines) Acute brain syndrome *Huntington's disease* *Endocrinopathy (hypothyroidism)*
Sleep disturbance	Increased sleep, hypersomnia	Depression Obstructive sleep apnea *Narcolepsy* *Kleine–Levin syndrome* Anxiety
	Decreased sleep, insomnia	Depression Non-organic insomnia Mania Drug or alcohol withdrawal Insomnia of chronic illness Restless legs syndrome
Behavior disturbance: energy and drive	Continuous fatigue	Depression
	Intermittent fatigue	Anxiety Dysthymia Chronic fatigue syndrome
	Continuous increased energy	Mania
Appetite disturbance	Increased appetite	Mania Bulimia nervosa *Kleine–Levin syndrome*
	Decreased appetite	Depression Anxiety Anorexia nervosa Acute physical illness Chronic physical illness

Table 8.1. (cont.)

Presenting problem	Characteristics	Differential diagnosis
Libido disturbance	Increased libido	Mania Paraphilia *Excessive sex drive* *Erotomania*
	Decreased libido	Depression Anxiety Schizophrenia *Acute physical illness* *Chronic physical illness*
Behavior disturbance: motor activity	Increased behavioral activity: agitation, restlessness	Mania Anxiety Extrapyramidal side effects of medication
	Increased behavioral activity: bizarre	Schizophrenia Acute brain syndrome Frontal space-occupying lesion
	Decreased behavioral activity	Depression *Acute or chronic physical illness*
Behavior disturbance: speech	Increased quantity of speech	Mania Anxiety
	Decreased quantity of speech	Depression Schizophrenia Elective mutism
	Disrupted or disorganized flow of speech	Schizophrenia Amnesic syndrome
Memory loss	Sudden onset	Organic amnesic syndrome (post-traumatic amnesia)
	Gradual onset	Dementia *Depressive pseudo-dementia*
	Auditory hallucinations	Schizophrenia Mania Depression *Drug-induced psychosis*
	Visual hallucinations	Delirium Acute intoxication Withdrawal (delirium tremens)
Perceptual disturbance	Somatic and visceral (tactile) hallucinations	Schizophrenia Alcohol withdrawal (delirium tremens) Acute intoxication
	Olfactory hallucinations	*Complex partial seizures*
	Perceptual illusions	Anxiety
	Perceptual distortions	Mania Delirium *Hyperthyroidism* *Drug withdrawal (benzodiazepines)* *Complex partial seizures*
	Pseudo-hallucinations	Anxiety Post-traumatic stress disorder
Disordered thinking	Intrusive unwanted thoughts	Anxiety Post-traumatic stress disorder Obsessive-compulsive disorder

Table 8.1. (cont.)

Presenting problem	Characteristics	Differential diagnosis
	Increased quantity of thought	Mania Anxiety Substance misuse
	Decreased quantity of thought	Depression Schizophrenia
	Loss of control of thinking	Schizophrenia
	Persecutory content of thought	Schizophrenia Persistent delusional disorder Depression
	Grandiose content of thought	Mania Schizophrenia Substance misuse
	Nihilistic content of thought	Depression *Dementia*
Disturbance of consciousness	Acute confusion	Delirium *Dementia* *Withdrawal (delirium tremens)* *Acute intoxication*

Table 8.2. *Demography of the anxiety and stress disorders*

	GAD	Phobias	Panic disorder	PTSD	OCD
Prevalence	5%	10%	1%	2%	1.5%
Female : male	3 : 2	2 : 1 (social phobia 1 : 1)	2 : 1	2 : 1	3 : 2
Age of onset	Early adulthood	Childhood or adolescence	Adolescence or early adulthood	Any age; 1–6 months after trigger event	Adolescence or early adulthood
Duration for ICD–10 diagnosis	4–6 months	1 month	1 month	Weeks	2 weeks
Course	Continuous, fluctuating	Intermittent	Intermittent	Persistent	Continuous
Outcome	Without treatment, 80% still symptomatic after 3 years	The longer the duration of symptoms, the worse the prognosis	The longer the duration of symptoms, the worse the prognosis	Most improve over 1 year	60% improve in 1 year; 40% incomplete remission

Anxiety and stress-related disorders (neuroses)

Although anxiety is the principal symptom of all the neuroses (anxiety disorders and disorders associated with exposure to extreme stress) their other clinical features overlap so that making a specific diagnosis depends on the mode of onset, course, and development of a cluster of core symptoms (Tables 8.2, 8.3, and 8.4). Anxiety *per se* might not be the presenting complaint as many patients will experience discomfort in one or more bodily systems and might be more concerned about physical than psychologic causes. Therefore it is important to take a full medical history and perform relevant physical examination in addition to the psychiatric history and mental state examination. Appropriate laboratory investigations should focus on eliminating potentially significant physical pathology, and specific treatment might need to be delayed until critical results are to hand. Differentiating these disorders is important as their

Table 8.3. Usual age of onset of the anxiety and stress disorders

Childhood	Adolescence	Early adulthood	Middle age	Old age
Phobias				
	Panic disorder			
	Obsessive-compulsive disorder			
		GAD		
		Post-traumatic stress disorder		

Table 8.4. Clusters of core clinical features of the anxiety and stress disorders

	GAD	Phobias	Panic disorder	PTSD	OCD
Spontaneous panic			X		
Cued panic and avoidance		X	X	X	X
Anticipatory worry	X	X	X	X	X
Irritability	X		X	X	X
Hyperarousal hypervigilance	X		X	X	
Depersonalization–derealization			X	X	X
Intrusive thoughts	X			X	X

Notes:
Depressive symptoms may emerge at any time in each of these disorders.
In 8% of the population these are sufficiently severe to diagnose a mood disorder, or mixed anxiety and depressive disorder.

management and prognosis varies to some extent. The common outcome of all severe or untreated anxiety disorders is depression, and this should be sought and treated actively.

Conditions considered in this section on anxiety and stress disorders are:

- Generalized anxiety disorder (GAD)
- Phobic anxiety disorders (simple phobia, social phobia, agoraphobia)
- Panic disorder
- Post-traumatic stress disorder (PTSD)
- Obsessive-compulsive disorder (OCD)

Generalized anxiety disorder

Generalized anxiety disorder is the most common of the anxiety disorders and in many ways the most difficult to characterize. The patient often presents late, having experienced an ever-changing series of anxiety symptoms, fluctuating in intensity over several months or even years. By this late stage, depression or panic attacks might also be present. Attempts to self-medicate with alcohol or illicit drugs are common, and the patient may have visited several general practitioners in search of a simple medical treatment. Where short-term treatment with an anxiolytic has been given, the recurrence of symptoms when the treatment ceases tends to increase the patient's anxiety by setting up a vicious cycle of worry that he or she will never recover fully.

Clinical features

- Any number of features from those listed might be present, although the patient might not complain of feeling anxious as such. The onset of symptoms is frequently linked to a stressful life event.
- The major psychologic complaint is of worrying thoughts, often related to real concerns but out of proportion to the problem, that build up during the day and prevent the onset of sleep.
- There may be significant physical symptoms resulting from inappropriate overactivity of the autonomic nervous system (both sympathetic and parasympathetic branches). These compound the patient's worries as he or she will interpret them as signaling serious physical illness. In some cases, the patient will have been treated unsuccessfully for a presumed physical cause and failure of treatment will exacerbate the anxiety.
- Overbreathing has the paradoxical effect of producing a subjective sense of dyspnea,

choking, tight chest, and sometimes chest pain. Prolonged overbreathing causes paresthesiae, numbness, or carpopedal spasm.

- As noted in Table 8.4, patients with generalized anxiety do not usually show spontaneous panic, and the absence of this feature is a good pointer to the diagnosis. However, in severe or longstanding illness both panic attacks and depersonalization–derealization might appear after months of other symptoms.

- The combination of irrational fears, perceptual abnormalities (illusions and pseudo-hallucinations), and agitation may result in misdiagnosis as psychosis or mania.

- Attempts to control the symptoms with alcohol or drugs (including anxiolytics) may result in dependence, and this will complicate both diagnosis and treatment.

- The prolonged build up and course of the disorder, its disabling effects on the patient's life and relationships, and the pessimism this produces, predispose to development of a depressive disorder. The clinical history should take account of the time-course of these symptoms to establish whether the depression is primary or secondary.

Investigation

Only sufficient laboratory investigations to exclude potential physical causes of anxiety should be undertaken: principally metabolic or endocrine abnormalities such as hyperthyroidism, hypoglycemia, and pheochromocytoma. Over-investigation, or lack of a clear plan of investigation, will exacerbate the anxiety.

Epidemiology

Generalized anxiety disorder has a point prevalence of about 5% of the adult population, and is slightly more common in women than men. It is also more common in urban than rural communities, but there is little difference in prevalence between racial groups. Its prevalence approaches 10% in those attending primary care, and is higher still in general hospital inpatient units.

Family and adoption studies have found an increased risk of anxiety disorders in the families of probands with generalized anxiety: the risk is greater in monozygotic twins than dizygotic twins or other siblings, suggesting a clear genetic component. Psychologic development is also of importance as the key

psychologic feature of anxiety, the inability to control worrying thoughts, appears to be acquired in childhood. Separations and other relationship breakdowns, personal ill health or loss of a loved one, whether in childhood or adulthood appear to be significant social stressors that increase vulnerability or precipitate the disorder.

Etiology and pathogenesis

Norepinephric neurons in the locus ceruleus normally increase their firing in response to novel sensory stimuli, and influence the autonomic nervous system via connections with the hypothalamus and midbrain. Experimental and neuroimaging studies suggest that overactivity of norepinephric transmission is involved in production of anxiety. However, both gamma-aminobutyric acid (GABA) and serotonin pathways appear to be involved as GABA agonists (benzodiazepines) and serotonin $5HT_{1A}$ agonists (buspirone) are anxiolytic; the GABA antagonist flumazenil can provoke anxiety. Both psychologic and neural factors that provoke overbreathing, that is hyperventilation in excess of metabolic need, appear to be involved in precipitating some of the somatic symptoms. The mechanism involves reducing arterial P_{CO_2} which causes uptake of calcium $[Ca^{2+}]$ ions from nerve and muscle membranes by plasma protein anions, and this results in aberrant electrical activity in nerves and muscles that is experienced as paresthesia, numbness, or carpopedal spasm.

Management

The mainstay of management is psychological treatment. It is important to acknowledge the reality of the distress experienced by the patient, who may have postponed seeking advice for fear of "wasting the doctor's time." For mild or recent onset cases (before the 6-month threshold for definite diagnosis has been reached), reassurance and problem-solving approaches supported with "bibliotherapy" (i.e. use of one of the many excellent self-help manuals publicly available) may be adequate. If there is overbreathing, then breathing control techniques or rebreathing in a paper bag (an old but reliable treatment) should be taught. The treatment plan should include clear guidance about when to return for further advice, and reassurance that any physical illness will be investigated and treated. Some patients with mild symptoms are unable to support themselves through use of a self-help manual, and these should be offered anxiety management or relaxation training.

Moderate or longstanding cases will benefit from cognitive behavior therapy (CBT), usually delivered by a clinical psychologist or other specially trained healthcare worker.

More severe or complicated cases, such as those with depressive symptoms or features of alcohol or drug misuse, are likely to require medication in addition to psychologic treatment. An antidepressant drug, most likely a selective serotonin reuptake inhibitor (SSRI) should be used as first line treatment: there is little to choose between these drugs on the basis of efficacy, and all require about 2–4 weeks to take effect. However, as all SSRIs may produce a transient worsening of some anxiety symptoms, it is helpful to provide a few days supply of a long-acting benzodiazepine to pre-empt unwanted effects. The serotonergic $5HT_{1A}$ agonist buspirone is also effective in some cases but takes about 2 weeks to give beneficial effects. Tricyclic antidepressants offer the advantage of blocking reuptake of both serotonin and norepinephrine, but their anticholinergic side effects may be troublesome. There is evidence from clinical trials that a combination of medication (any of those mentioned above, including benzodiazepines) and CBT is more effective than either alone.

Other drugs Antihistamines produce useful mild sedation without the risk of dependence. Low-dose antipsychotics have been used extensively in the short-term treatment of anxiety, both for their sedative actions and for tranquilization (a calming effect associated with a reduction in anxious thoughts that occurs without sedation). Although they do not induce dependence, their long-term use is limited by the risk of significant side effects. Pregabalin, a GABA agonist that binds to neuronal calcium channels, is a relatively new treatment for generalized anxiety disorder.

Phobic anxiety disorders

Phobic anxiety is a disproportionate and irrational fear provoked by the thought or presence of a specific object (such as a creature), situation (e.g. public transport), or phenomenon (e.g. thunder). It is usual to distinguish between simple phobias where a single object or situation is the source of anxiety, and complex phobias such as social phobia and agoraphobia. Simple phobias are thought to be extremely common in the general population but as many sufferers do not regard them as clinical problems, estimates of prevalence based on community samples are unreliable.

Simple phobia
Clinical features
- Intense anxiety generated by the presence of the phobic object or situation, or by thinking about that object.
- Core diagnostic features, as shown in Table 8.4, are cued or situational panic, anticipatory worry and apprehension, and avoidance of the phobic object or situation.
- In most cases of phobic anxiety, the cued anxiety may be accompanied by any number of features listed above. However, in phobias of blood, viscera, or bodily injury the usual sympathetic nervous overactivity is replaced by a powerful vaso-vagal (parasympathetic) outflow leading to fainting.
- The source of the anxiety is usually well known to the patient who will rarely be concerned that his or her symptoms are due to physical illness. However, the first time a patient faints because of his or her blood phobia, he or she might require reassurance over physical health.
- Most simple phobias do not cause major disruption of the patient's life, although in some cases avoidance behavior will have led to radical changes in lifestyle. A patient may fear embarrassment if he or she encounters the phobic object in public.

Investigation
Investigations may be considered as for generalized anxiety. However, where there is a clearly demarcated reaction to a single phobic object investigation is unlikely to add to management. Repeated fainting, as in blood phobia, warrants an ECG and in the rare cases where fainting is accompanied by signs of generalized seizure an EEG might be indicated.

Epidemiology
Most simple phobias emerge in childhood and extinguish as the child grows to adulthood. As noted above, estimates of prevalence in adults are unreliable as few sufferers report them or seek medical treatment: estimates vary from 8%–10%, being greater in women. As with other anxiety disorders, simple phobias cluster in families and are likely to have both genetic and social-psychologic contributions.

Etiology and pathogenesis
There is sociobiologic evidence of inherent fears of novel or potentially threatening objects as a widespread human evolutionary characteristic.

Management

The principal treatment is the behavioral technique of exposure, beginning *in vitro* (that is, thinking about the phobic object) and then *in vivo* (i.e. exposure to the actual causative object or situation) to desensitize the patient. This may be combined with relaxation or cognitive therapy to deal with accompanying symptoms. Drug treatment is rarely helpful long term, and is restricted to very short courses of anxiolytics or beta-blockers to reduce the symptoms of anxiety in specific unavoidable situations (for instance, an aeroplane flight in someone with fear of flying).

Social phobia

Clinical features

- Excessive anxiety arising repeatedly in situations where the patient believes he or she may be scrutinized by others, even by strangers.
- The key features are anticipatory worries of being criticized or of appearing "stupid," fear of embarrassment, and resulting avoidance of provoking situations.
- Patients often report blushing, stammering, clumsiness, or trembling in any public place but particularly when in confined spaces or in close contact with others such as on buses or trains.
- Symptoms may be worse when far from home, or the patient feels unable to escape. In these situations panic attacks are more likely.
- Any of the non-specific features of anxiety may be present.
- Alcohol is often used to reduce the symptoms of social phobia and alcohol misuse is more common in this than other phobias.
- Secondary depressive symptoms emerge in about 40% of cases and might complicate the initial presentation and management.

Investigation

As for generalized anxiety.

Epidemiology

The prevalence rate is 2.5%, and unlike other phobias it is equally prevalent in men and women. The severely disabling nature of this phobia means that most sufferers come to medical attention.

Etiology and pathogenesis

The familial clustering of cases suggests that both genetic and environmental factors contribute. Social phobia often manifests itself first in adolescence and it

is likely that this period of heightened vulnerability to social pressures might provide the trigger in a predisposed individual.

Management

Psychologic treatment with CBT uses graded exposure to feared social situations to desensitize and reduce avoidance and cognitive strategies to challenge the patient's anticipatory worries. Anxiolytic drugs may be used to provide short-term control of symptoms so that the patient can perform some unavoidable acts in public. Monoamine oxidase inhibitors (MAOIs) such as phenelzine or moclobemide and SSRIs have some efficacy and improve long-term outcome when combined with CBT.

Agoraphobia

Clinical features

- The core feature is excessive irrational anxiety of being away from a safe place, usually the controlled and confined circumstances of home.
- Avoidance of leaving the familiar home setting is particularly severe and disabling. Many sufferers are totally housebound.
- A specific fear of open spaces is less common but might form part of a more general fear of being outdoors. Patients are just as likely to fear social events or gatherings.
- The first episode occurs characteristically in a public place away from home and is completely unexpected and bewildering. Further episodes occurring in similar circumstances lead to development of anticipatory worry and avoidance.
- Panic attacks are more common in this than other phobias. Any of the non-specific features of anxiety may be present.
- The most severe of the phobic disorders, its course is chronic and continuous with fluctuating severity.

Investigation

As for generalized anxiety, only those necessary to exclude contributory physical illness.

Epidemiology

Onset is usually during early adult life and up to 75% of sufferers are women; the overall prevalence is about 3%. Twin studies suggest a significant genetic component.

Etiology and pathogenesis

As the onset usually follows a spontaneous panic attack, agoraphobia is often regarded as a variant of panic disorder. Following the initial attack, anxiety generalizes to all situations in which the patient is away from home. As for panic disorder, the mechanism of symptom generation is excessive autonomic overactivity in response to situations the patient has previously found stressful; fear of precipitating this reaction causes avoidance.

Management

The aim of treatment is to break down the patient's avoidance and encourage a return to those situations the patient anticipated as stressful. This is achieved by relaxation training followed by very gradual behavioral exposure. Depressive symptoms are common and will require specific antidepressant treatment. The greater the frequency of panic attacks before treatment, or their intensification during exposure, the poorer the likely outcome.

Panic disorder

Panic attacks occur sporadically in 10% of adults and are a variable feature of all the anxiety disorders. However, panic disorder differs in that it is the only disorder that is characterized by the occurrence of spontaneous, unprovoked, and unpredictable panic attacks. As there is no identifiable phobic stimulus, the patient comes to dread the panic itself but is unable to find a way to avoid it. This leads to development of a disabling secondary phenomenon termed phobophobia, "fear of fear." Panic disorder is the most disabling of the anxiety disorders.

Clinical features

- Sudden and paroxysmal onset occurring in the absence of a specific stimulus. Symptoms escalate rapidly to a crescendo of overwhelming anxiety.
- An unshakable conviction that the attack will end in catastrophe or death is common. The fear of catastrophe may be so great that the patient will risk death, or assault others, to escape.
- Panic attacks may commence during sleep or periods of relaxation.
- Anticipatory worry is intense but focuses on the panic attack itself rather than on stressful or anxiety-provoking situations.
- The onset of an attack is so rapid that some patients do not report experiencing anxiety as such. Instead, they may report choking, chest pain, dyspnoea, disorientation, a sense of unreality (depersonalization–derealization), blackout, or collapse.

- An attack is often followed by a period of disorientation, fatigue, or exhaustion.
- Although no specific situation can be identified as provoking panic, patients will avoid any situation in which panic might have perilous consequences, such as driving, climbing ladders, taking a bath. The result is a rapidly growing list of avoided situations until all activities, even sleep, seem impossibly dangerous.
- Between attacks the patient may show an exaggerated concern about minor physical symptoms, some of which will be accountable to autonomic nervous activity.

Investigation

Many will present to medical services and undergo investigation for a range of potential conditions. It is important to have a clear plan of investigation to exclude the small number of cardiorespiratory (heart attack, asthma), neurologic (seizures), and metabolic or endocrine (hypoglycemia, thyrotoxicosis) conditions that might present in this manner. Pressure to pursue further investigations without good cause should be resisted.

Epidemiology

Panic disorder has a prevalence of 2% and is twice as common in women as men. Prevalence is raised in the relatives of probands but there have been too few twin studies to confirm a predominantly genetic component. Early childhood experience of trauma including serious medical illness contributes to vulnerability.

Etiology and pathogenesis

A biochemical abnormality of central norepinephric neurotransmission has been proposed, and is seen as setting off a "fight-or-flight" reaction in the absence of threatening stimuli. The cognitive theory proposes that an undue conscious preoccupation with bodily sensations leads to an automatic and non-conscious triggering of autonomic activity. Either or both of these mechanisms may cause an abrupt but unnoticed increase in respiratory rate, with the consequences noted under generalized anxiety.

Management

Explanation of the nature of the attacks is crucial. Symptoms can be controlled with benzodiazepines (usually diazepam) but the high doses necessary, long duration of treatment, risk of dependence and high rate of relapse on ceasing treatment count against this

235

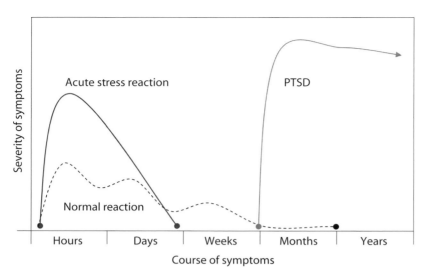

Fig. 8.2. Onset, severity and course of symptoms in response to trauma.

regimen. The tricyclic antidepressant imipramine and the SSRIs have proven efficacy but the delay of several weeks before they take effect can be difficult for patients to tolerate. CBT focusing on redressing the misinterpretation of bodily sensations is as effective as drug treatment in the short term and is superior in the long term. A practical strategy is to commence diazepam and an antidepressant simultaneously but taper the diazepam over a few weeks and commence CBT as the patient begins to show a response to medication.

Post-traumatic stress disorder

Human beings show a range of responses to stressful events and an individual's reaction will depend on his or her vulnerability and resilience, pre-existing psychiatric morbidity, preparedness and the nature of the event. It is normal to experience an immediate reaction to acutely stressful events: where the stressor is relatively mild the reaction involves a brief period of being dazed or disoriented, gradually developing symptoms of autonomic activity, and a desire to avoid or forget about the provoking events. These experiences are proportionate to the events. An acute stress reaction is a more severe and abnormal response in which the patient is immediately dissociated from his or her surroundings and might wander into further danger (Fig. 8.2). This is followed by a period of labile and varied emotions, changing from anxiety to anger to despair or from withdrawal to overactivity, lasting several hours. There may be sleep disturbance but symptoms usually remit rapidly, always

within 2–3 days. A delayed but severe and long-lasting response is called post-traumatic stress disorder (PTSD).

Clinical features

- Onset of symptoms is delayed but occurs typically between a few weeks and 6 months following the trauma.
- History of a clear traumatic event of exceptional severity; rarely, a series of lesser traumas may be sufficient.
- Key features are recurring, intrusive memories of the traumatic event often accompanied by intense visual imagery (flashbacks), amounting to reliving the event.
- Memories provoke autonomic overactivity with many features of anxiety, but hypervigilance, hyperarousal and startle responses are especially prominent.
- Irritability, insomnia, and nightmares of dreadful events (not necessarily the provoking trauma) are common.
- Between acute symptoms, the patient may show emotional numbness or detachment.
- "Human agency" (e.g. rape, armed assault) and personal responsibility increase the severity of symptoms. Survivors of natural disasters may experience "survivor guilt."
- Presentation may follow self harm or a suicide attempt, and the risk of further attempts remains high until symptoms begin to resolve.

- Course may be perpetuated by presence of physical injury sustained during the provoking traumatic event.
- Secondary features are common and include excessive use of drugs or alcohol, breakdown of established relationships, and avoidance of situations associated with the trauma. This might prevent a return to work. About 80% with PTSD develop other psychiatric disorders especially depression.

Investigation

It is important to detect and treat physical injuries sustained in the original trauma. Apart from this, investigation should be selective and aimed to reassure the patient that there are no undetected physical sequelae.

Epidemiology

At least 10% of adults who experience an extreme stressful event will develop PTSD; the point prevalence in the general population is 1.2% of men and 2.7% of women. Children, elderly people, and those with pre-existing psychiatric disorders may be more vulnerable (see below). Some events are more likely than others to cause PTSD: witnessing the death of another person causes PTSD in less than 20% of cases; being the victim of rape or armed assault causes PTSD in more than 20%. Twin studies of victims of war or natural disaster suggest that at least 30% of the variance in propensity to develop PTSD is genetic. Recent systematic reviews show that occurrence of PTSD is more likely in those who receive immediate post-trauma debriefing.

Etiology and pathogenesis

Early descriptions emphasized the importance of pre-existing mental disorder. Recent studies have found these to be less important and shifted focus to the characteristics of the trauma rather than the victim. Neuroimaging has shown structural (reduced hippocampal volume) and functional changes (prolonged overactivity of amygdala and arousal systems) in the brain. It has been suggested that the balance between excitatory glutaminergic and inhibitory GABAergic neurotransmission is impaired leading to dysfunctional memory formation. Psychologically, this results in failure to process the memory normally, so it is recalled in vivid emotional and visual detail rather than the more usual verbal form.

Management

Initial management of uncomplicated cases consists of sympathetic and practical support in minimizing secondary disability by enabling patients to talk through their experiences and emotions. Short-term use of anxiolytic or hypnotic medication can help but longer term treatment carries a high risk of dependence in these patients. More specific treatment is required to prevent chronicity when resolution is not occurring . This usually involves CBT techniques to recall, confront and desensitize the trauma while challenging dysfunctional thought patterns such as "survivor guilt." The response to medication is variable: there is evidence of SSRI efficacy but not of norepinephrine reuptake inhibitors. In the most severe or chronic cases, combinations of antidepressant and antipsychotic agents my be required.

Obsessive-compulsive disorder

Obsessive-compulsive disorder (OCD) is characterized by the recurrence of irrational and distressing thoughts, worries or doubts (obsessions) or the impulse to perform pointless actions (compulsions) in a stereotyped manner, and anxiety if they are resisted.

Clinical features

- The thoughts are intrusive, repetitive and stereotyped; they are usually unpleasant or repugnant to the patient. They involve doubts, disgusting images or fears about performing illegal or shocking acts. Patients may ruminate on these obsessions for long periods.
- The compulsive behaviors may take the form of simple checking or counting, or may involve complex sequences of actions that must be performed in stereotyped fashion (rituals). Patients derive no pleasure but might experience temporary relief of anxiety. If a compulsive act is interrupted it must be repeated and this sequence may continue indefinitely to the exclusion of all normal activity.
- Patients recognize these thoughts and actions as their own and not due to an external agency (as distinct from thought insertion of schizophrenia).
- They acknowledge that their thoughts and actions are excessive, irrational or pointless and might complain of "going mad."
- Obsessions and compulsions are resisted initially, although this produces secondary anxiety and so resistance diminishes if the disorder becomes

chronic. Conversely, reduction of anxiety provides negative reinforcement which perpetuates the symptoms.

- Secondary disability sets in rapidly with inability to carry out daily routine, such as getting to work on time. A substantial proportion of patients present late, when the illness has been present for several years and has become chronic with significant depressive features.

Investigation

As for generalized anxiety, investigation should be minimal and focused on specific concerns. For instance, a patient with obsessional doubts about contracting a sexually transmitted infection may require serologic testing before he or she can commence psychologic treatment.

Epidemiology

Unitary obsessional or perfectionistic traits are common in the general population and are valued in certain occupations (e.g. medicine). An obsessional (anankastic) personality disorder in which these traits overshadow other aspects of character has a prevalence of about 2% in the general population. However, relatively few of those with any form of obsessional personality go on to develop OCD; only about 25% of patients with OCD have a history of obsessional traits. Peak onset is in the third decade (men younger than women) and there is a slight female excess in prevalence. There is a markedly increased incidence of OCD in the families of sufferers but the relative importance of genetic and environmental factors has not been elucidated.

Etiology and pathogenesis

Neuroimaging studies of patients have found tantalizing indications of reduced size and yet increased activity in the caudate nucleus with increased metabolism in the anterior cingulate gyrus and functionally linked frontal and subcortical structures. Neurotransmitter pathways involving serotonin, dopamine and norepinephrine have been implicated, none conclusively.

Management

OCD presents difficulties in treatment, partly because of the tendency to present late by which time behavioral patterns have become set and depressive features may be prominent. Although both medication and psychologic treatments have some efficacy, neither is effective in preventing progression to chronicity in all cases. Most will require specialist psychologic treatment but as there is likely to be a waiting time for this treatment, initial advice should be given to resist intrusive thoughts and rituals and medication commenced. Both SSRIs (especially fluoxetine) and the tricyclic clomipramine have proven efficacy but only in relatively high doses which will take several weeks to achieve. A short course of an anxiolytic may help.

The cognitive and behavioral techniques used include: thought stopping, response prevention, permitting rumination only for a set period each day which is then gradually reduced, and exposure and desensitization to anxiety-provoking situations such as dirt or contamination. Recurrence is common, especially on cessation of medication, so the patient must be well trained in behavioral techniques before gradual withdrawal of medication is contemplated.

Mood disorders

Normal mood is constantly fluctuating: in a normal lifetime most people will experience periods of happiness, even great happiness or elation, and at other times feel sad or miserable. These emotional experiences can be understood as an interaction between the person's personality or character and the situations or events they encounter. What differentiates these normal variations in mood from features of disorder is that the former are generally understandable both to the affected person and to others who share the same culture, proportionate to the circumstances, and do not obliterate completely the activities of daily living. By contrast, mood disorder requires that the variation is, at best, partially understandable, disproportionate and pervasive so that even if circumstances return to normal, the patient's mood does not.

Terms applied to mood states
Abnormally elevated
Euphoria → elation → ecstasy

Normal
Euthymia

Abnormally depressed
Dysthymia → dysphoria → melancholia

Mood disorders constitute a major public health problem. According to World Health Organization estimates, depressive disorders are the major cause of disability worldwide, affecting over 50 million people (over 10% of the world adult population) at any time. A further 14 million (3%) suffer bipolar affective disorder. These totals are increasing year-on-year, with women and people in developing countries being affected disproportionately.

Conditions considered in this section on mood disorders are:

- dysthymia
- mixed anxiety and depressive disorder
- depressive disorders
- bipolar affective disorder and mania

Dysthymia

Dysthymia lies on the continuum from normal intermittent experience of unhappiness to the well-defined but infrequent episodes of incapacitating depression. It is characterized by a long-standing periodicity of mood in which short periods (weeks) of mild depression alternate with similar periods of near normality of mood.

Clinical features

- The patient usually presents after several years of symptoms, often at the instigation of family or friends, and may not believe that his or her experiences represent illness.
- The periods of depressed mood rarely last more than 2–3 weeks but recur spontaneously after a period of normality of similar duration.
- The core features are mildly depressed mood, a sense that life is an effort and nothing is enjoyable, and associated feelings of worthlessness and low self-esteem.
- Each period of symptoms remits spontaneously.
- The symptoms are rarely so severe as to interfere with activities of daily living, and are insufficient to meet criteria for any other mood disorder.
- Periodic occurrence of symptoms over a period of at least 2 years is required for a formal diagnosis.

Investigation

It may be advisable to eliminate other potential causes of intermittent or periodic ill-health, such as those related to menstruation in women, especially if medical treatment is contemplated.

Epidemiology

Depending on the criteria used, community studies in Europe and the USA estimate prevalence from 1.3%–6%, with a slight female excess (up to 8% of women in some studies). Onset is usually in early adolescence,

and over 70% of cases go on to develop other psychiatric morbidity, usually depressive episodes.

Etiology and pathogenesis

Although there is a higher incidence in the families of people with depressive disorders, the genetic contribution is unclear. The early onset, lifelong course, and relapse on cessation of treatment (see below) are suggestive of a depressive personality trait, possibly as the result of early developmental experiences.

Management

Cognitive therapy focuses on confronting low self-esteem and ideas of worthlessness: patients may learn to control their symptoms for several years, but there is gradual deterioration with the passage of time. Medical treatment with an SSRI antidepressant (e.g. fluoxetine 20 mg daily) is effective but, as relapse is inevitable on cessation of treatment, this should be continued indefinitely. As such, it should not be embarked upon lightly and only after full explanation.

Mixed anxiety and depressive disorder

Mood symptoms are common in the general population: most community studies of people who are not receiving treatment find point prevalence to be 16%–20%. When this is combined with the high prevalence of anxiety symptoms (about 30%, see above), it is not surprising that many people present to general practitioners with a mixture of symptoms in which neither diagnostic group is predominant.

Clinical features

- A mixed and variable presentation of anxiety and depressive symptoms sufficient to cause ongoing distress.
- This is largely a diagnosis of exclusion: symptoms must not be present in sufficient quantity nor severity to justify diagnosis of a specific anxiety nor mood disorder.
- Features of inappropriate autonomic activity *must* be present.
- There must be no evidence of a clear precipitating stressful event.
- The exact mixture of symptoms may vary in a single patient over time. The emergence of new symptoms may precipitate presentation.

Investigation

Exclusion of physical illness that might present with mixed, non-specific symptoms should be considered.

Epidemiology

In community studies, about 8% of people meet diagnostic criteria for this disorder but not for any other. Untreated cases may resolve over time or go on to develop more severe psychiatric morbidity, especially in response to stressful life events.

Etiology and pathogenesis

There have been no specific etiologic studies and the likely pathogenesis is as for the depressive disorders (see below).

Management

Reassurance, problem-solving, and self-help (bibliotherapy) are most important; specific cognitive therapy or anxiety management training may be necessary in persistent cases. Medical treatment is usually unnecessary: anxiolytics risk dependence and SSRIs may exacerbate these mild symptoms.

Depressive disorders

Depressive disorders are a major cause of distress and disability worldwide and constitute a disproportionate burden on the socio-economic systems of many countries, particularly in the developing world. They are associated with high rates of physical and psychiatric comorbidity, and elevated standardized mortality ratio from all causes. A depressive episode occurring without mania is often termed "unipolar depression" in contrast to the bipolar disorders to be discussed later. Such an episode may arise spontaneously or in the course of any chronic physical or psychiatric disorder; when a second episode occurs it is termed recurrent depressive disorder. In this section these terms are used synonymously.

Clinical features

- A depressive episode might be preceded by a prodromal period of variable length during which the mood is persistently suboptimal but other features are not present. This prodrome might include the depressive phase of dysthymia (see above).
- Formal diagnosis requires the presence of at least two core features (depressed mood, anhedonia, or anergia) plus at least three of the associated psychologic or somatic features, for most of each day for at least 14 days.
- Severity is assessed from the number of features present in excess of the minimum necessary for diagnosis. Psychotic features are present in the most severe episodes (melancholia).

- As severity increases, the overall mood becomes fixed and unresponsive to external stimuli: a paradoxical state in which bad news elicits no response.
- Suicidal thoughts are common and do not usually require specific action unless distressing, intrusive, and persistent, or if specific plans and intentions are evolving.
- "Atypical" features such as over-eating (hyperphagia) and excessive sleeping (hypersomnia) are uncommon and may obscure the diagnosis.
- "Double depression" is the occurrence of a depressive episode in someone with pre-existing dysthymia.
- Some groups show particular presentations: irritability and dysphoria (hostile mood) in younger men; indecisiveness and inability to cope at work in middle aged men; cognitive impairment ("pseudodementia") and agitation in old age; pain or other bodily complaints predominate in some cultures.
- The symptoms of a depressive episode may not emerge simultaneously, nor recover at the same rate (Figs. 8.3, 8.4). Particularly during the recovery phase, this may produce a distressing mismatch between the patient's energy level and his or her mood and is associated with increased risk of suicide (Table 8.6).

Investigation

While there are no specific diagnostic laboratory tests for depression, a plan of investigation should be considered that takes account of: the many organic factors that might give rise to depression (see Table 8.7); the fact that severely depressed patients neglect or ignore physical illness; the possibility that antidepressant drugs may exacerbate some disorders (cardiac disease, epilepsy) or interact with other medication. In addition, some presentations merit special consideration: presence of "atypical" features; patients who have suffered several relapses; first presentations in older patients; or if electroconvulsive therapy (ECT) is contemplated. Finally, the plan of investigation should be reviewed and repeated in patients who have not responded to first- and second-line treatments.

Epidemiology

Data from the UK give the population prevalence as about 2%, although the rate in people consulting a general practitioner for any reason is nearer 10%,

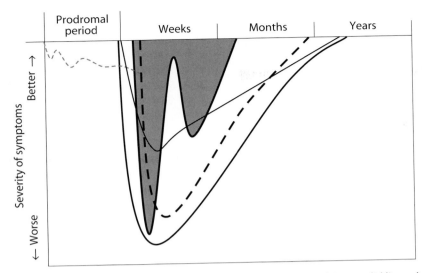

In this figure the "mood envelope" of depression is shown as a fainter solid line arising from a prodromal period of low-grade mood disturbance (dashed line). Core features are present from the onset (e.g. anergia, broken line) but others (such as psychotic symptoms, shaded area) may be intermittent; sex drive (solid black line) is often the last to recover.

Fig. 8.3. The mood envelope of an untreated depressive episode.

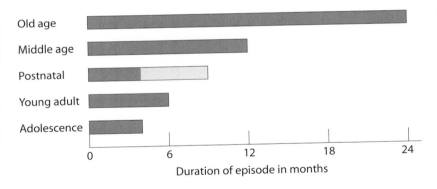

Fig. 8.4. Typical duration of an untreated episode of depression at different ages.

and up to 20% in general hospital inpatients. Incidence is relatively low in childhood (although it may be rising), and the peak age of onset is 30–40 years. The female–male ratio is 2:1 until middle age after which it approaches equality; in both men and women the duration of an untreated episode increases markedly with age (Fig. 8.4). Postnatal depression has a peak onset about 6 weeks post-partum and affects 10–15% of women; these episodes are typically relatively short but may be prolonged in 10% of cases.

Etiology and pathogenesis
The etiology of depression is clearly multifactorial with contributions from both inherited and acquired factors. Siblings of patients with depression have a 10%–15% lifetime risk of suffering the same illness, dizygotic twins a 25% risk, and monozygotic twins about a 50% chance. The current consensus from family and twin studies is as follows:

- Genetic factors are much more potent than environmental factors in the etiology of unipolar depression;
- What is inherited is a *liability* to develop depression not a *vulnerability*, i.e. a person's chance of becoming depressed is all-or-none rather than continuously graded as would be predicted by a stress-diathesis model;

Table 8.5. Symptoms and signs of depressive disorder

Core features (at least 2 must be present for diagnosis)	Depressed mood Anhedonia (loss of ability to experience interest and enjoyment) Anergia (reduced energy and increased fatigue)
Psychologic features may be present in mild, moderate, or severe episodes	Reduced self-esteem (worthlessness) Ideas of guilt or blame, especially regarding past events Pessimism about future (hopelessness) Ideas of self-harm or suicide Indecisiveness (helplessness)
Somatic ("biologic") features are present in moderate or severe episodes (somatic syndrome)	Sleep disturbance: early morning waking (>2 hours early) Marked loss of appetite; weight loss (>5% body weight) Diurnal variation in mood, worse in morning Amenorrhea Psychomotor retardation: slowed thinking (bradyphrenia), speech, and movement Reduced sex drive
Psychotic symptoms occur in severe episodes	Delusions: sin, guilt, poverty, nihilism. Incurable illness Auditory hallucinations (second person): accusing, blaming, defaming Olfactory hallucinations: filth, decomposition Stupor

Table 8.7. Some of the more common organic causes of depressive symptoms

Cardiac and vascular	Myocardial infarction, cerebral ischemia
Endocrinopathies	Thyroid disease (especially hypothyroid), Addison's disease, Cushing's disease, diabetes
Hematological	Anemias, leukemias
Infections	Classically glandular fever, HIV/AIDS, influenza
Neurologic	Parkinson's disease, stroke, multiple sclerosis, head trauma
Nutritional deficiencies	B_{12}, folic acid
Oncologic	Primary carcinoma (classically occult tumors of pancreas and lung)
Other	Chronic or life-threatening physical illness of any kind

Table 8.6. Impact of depressive episodes of different severity

Mild	Can get by	May be able to continue working and other activities, but coping with novel situations will be limited
Moderate ± somatic syndrome	Cannot work	Might put self or others at risk due to lack of concentration even in familiar settings
Severe ± psychotic symptoms	Cannot live	At high risk of suicide or of death through inanition

- Lifetime risk of depression is greatest in the first-degree relatives of probands (patients) with more severe depression.

Environmental factors including social and emotional experiences during development play an important part in determining *vulnerability*. For instance, experience of adversity during early childhood (e.g. death of a parent) or later (financial difficulties, unsupportive relationships) will contribute to the type and severity of a subsequent depressive disorder. Significant or threatening life events in adolescence or adulthood are the major precipitants of a first depressive episode but are less important in later episodes. Some social factors are protective: presence of a confiding adult relationship (a confidante) appears to reduce the incidence of depression in women at increased vulnerability.

Both biologic and psychologic factors mediate the features of depression. The monoamine theory proposes that depression results from a reduction in the production or synaptic effectiveness of the monoamine neurotransmitters serotonin (5HT) and norepinephrine. In summary: drugs that deplete central monoamines (e.g. reserpine) cause depression; drugs that increase central monoamines (e.g. MAOIs) reduce depression; reduced monoamine metabolites (particularly 5-hydroxyindoleacetic acid, 5-HIAA) are found in CSF in severely depressed patients; recent functional neuroimaging studies have shown extensive down-regulation of 5HT receptors in brains of depressed patients. Most effective antidepressants increase synaptic availability of serotonin, norepinephrine, or both, either by reducing their metabolism in the synaptic cleft (MAOIs) or by blocking presynaptic autoreceptors and preventing reuptake into the presynaptic cell (tricyclics, SSRIs). There is also evidence of reduced dopaminergic transmission in depression, and the putative contributions of these individual and combined

Table 8.8. Dysfunctional neurotransmitter systems interact to produce the symptoms and signs of depression

	Single	In combination		All
		Dopamine	**Noradrenaline**	
Serotonin	Tension, irritability sleep disturbance	Lack of appetite (anorexia)	Anxiety	Depressed mood and thinking
Norepinephrine	Lack of interest (apathy)	Lack of energy (anergia)		
Dopamine	Lack of drive (anhedonia)			

Table 8.9. Most frequently reported neuroendocrine findings in depression

Corticotrophin releasing hormone (CRH)	Hypothalamo-pituitary axis overactivity in response to stress
	Hypercortisolemia
	Non-suppression by dexamethasone
	Decreased cellular immunity
Thyrotropin releasing hormone (TRH) and thyroid stimulating hormone (TSH)	Raised basal TSH and blunted response to TRH Sub-clinical hypothyroidism
Growth hormone (GH) Somatostatin	Increased daytime GH Decreased nocturnal GH Reduced somatostatin
Luteinizing hormone (LH) follicle stimulating hormone (FSH)	Menstrual irregularity Amenorrhea

deficits to the clinical picture is shown in Table 8.8. Finally, there is increased activity in central cholinergic neurons resulting in sleep disturbance (increased REM, nightmares) and memory impairment.

Some of these neurotransmitter defects may be mediated by neuroendocrine pathways, as serotonergic and dopaminergic neurones are important in modulation of hypothalamic–pituitary function . In turn, some effects may be secondary to dysregulation of sleep as maximal release of growth hormone and FSH–LH takes place during slow-wave sleep, and this is disrupted and replaced by REM sleep in depression. The neuroendocrine findings most frequently reported in depression are listed in Table 8.9.

The major psychologic mechanism is called cognitive shift, characterized by: a tendency to experience automatic negative thoughts in everyday life (the well-known triad of worthlessness, hopelessness, and helplessness); and cognitive distortions. The latter are typified by selective abstraction (focusing on minor negative events), underestimation of positive events,

generalization (viewing isolated negative experiences as the norm), and personal responsibility. These cognitive distortions are self-fulfilling and mutually reinforcing. Risk of relapse is related to frequency of previous episodes (Fig. 8.5).

Management (Table 8.10)

It is an important principle of treatment that, regardless of the severity of the episode or the treatment modality chosen, the patient should be seen and reviewed frequently. The doctor should be pro-active in arranging a series of appointments spread over several weeks and not leave it to patient to "turn up": negative cognitions of wasting the doctor's time will prevent this with the result that the episode is prolonged or exacerbated. The management of milder cases of depression is similar to that of mixed anxiety and depression (above): the emphasis is on psychologic support and problem solving as the episode is likely to resolve spontaneously. Older patients, those who have suffered previous episodes, and those whose symptoms worsen or fail to resolve will require antidepressant medication, and might benefit from cognitive behavioral therapy (CBT).

In moderate depression, CBT and antidepressants are of about equal efficacy and both should be considered; choice may depend on availability or the patient's preference. CBT is a specific and structured intervention that aims to facilitate the patient in identifying and challenging automatic and negative thought patterns. CBT is effective when used alone, and there is evidence that it is more so when combined with antidepressant medication. Most mild to moderate cases of depression are treated in primary care, and here the first-line medication is an SSRI. Due to the latency of weeks before benefits appear, medication should be commenced immediately unless there are clear reasons for not doing so (practical points on the use of these drugs are given in the section on Anxiety disorders). The need for specialist

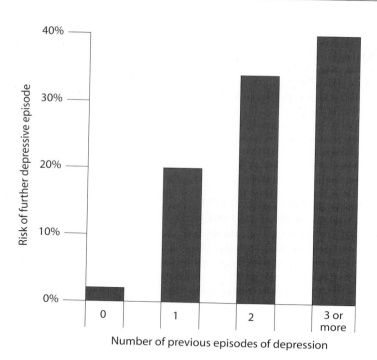

Fig. 8.5. Risk of relapse in depression increases with the number of previous episodes ("kindling").

Table 8.10. Management of depression

	Psychologic	Pharmacologic	Physical
Mild	Support and reassurance; problem solving; anxiety management; (CBT)	(Antidepressants)	
Moderate	CBT	Antidepressants	
Severe		Antidepressants	ECT
		Antipsychotics	
Refractory	CBT	Antidepressants in combination	
		Antipsychotics	
		Lithium	
		Thyroid hormone	

advice should be considered at this point, especially if first onset in old age, significant physical or psychiatric comorbidity, intrusive and persistent suicidal thoughts. The patient needs to be seen regularly for support, encouragement, and to ensure concordance (compliance) with treatment. Initial medication should not be changed unless there has been no response after a minimum of 6 weeks' treatment with a therapeutic dose (equivalent to fluoxetine 20 mg daily). About one-third of patients will show little response at 6 weeks, and in these the diagnosis should be reviewed before increasing the medication to its maximal dose. Regular review should continue, and the antidepressant should be changed to another group if the patient experiences intolerable side effects or shows no improvement at 10 weeks. Specialist advice might be useful in further management.

Severe depression can be life threatening because the presence of psychotic phenomena will increase risk of suicide and retardation may cause the patient to cease all voluntary activity including eating and drinking. In these circumstances, emergency admission is necessary and this might need to be compulsory (under the Mental Health Act in the UK 2007) if the patient cannot or will not consent. Immediate treatment will include attention to any injuries acquired in a suicide attempt, general supportive measures to treat cachexia, dehydration, or hypothermia, and specific treatment of psychotic depression. A combination of a suitable antipsychotic drug and an antidepressant should be commenced (antipsychotics are dealt with in the section on Psychotic disorders, below). ECT should be considered if the patient refuses food and drink: this is an effective treatment in severe depression and, as with other potentially life-saving measures, has few contraindications (recent hemorrhagic stroke or heart attack).

A seizure is induced by unilateral or bilateral administration of a measured electrical charge to the head under general anesthesia and neuromuscular blockade. Response is often rapid, even after a single administration, but a full course will usually involve 4–6 administrations at intervals of a few days.

However severe the episode, treatment should continue until the patient has been symptom-free for some months. If treatment ceases too soon symptoms will recur and may become chronic; older patients require treatment for longer periods, for 2 years or more for a single episode over the age of 70 years. The risk of further episodes increases greatly each time the patient becomes depressed, causing cumulative disruption to the patient's life, so long-term prophylaxis ("maintenance") should be considered. For patients seen in secondary care this often means continuing antidepressant treatment indefinitely; in primary care this might be less acceptable, but should be discussed with the patient.

Treatment-resistance is failure to respond to two separate classes of antidepressant in full dosage for at least 6 weeks each; an episode that shows persistent treatment resistance is often termed refractory depression. In these cases, a full review should be performed of the patient's physical health, psychiatric diagnosis, and social and cultural context including his or her beliefs about illness. Any necessary tests and investigations should be performed, and brain imaging may be considered. If the diagnosis is confirmed, several combination or augmentation regimens may be considered, but their use is limited to secondary care. The most likely to be successful is addition of the mood-stabilizing drug lithium to full-dose antidepressant treatment (effective in about 50% of "resistant" cases). Alternatives are: addition of a second antidepressant from a different chemical group (but this risks precipitating a serotonergic syndrome); addition of the serotonin precursor tryptophan, a calcium antagonist, or the $5HT_{1A}$ agonist buspirone; augmentation with thyroxine or tri-iodothyronine, especially if tests show low-normal T_4 and high-normal TSH. There is some evidence for each of these measures but little to suggest which patients are most likely to benefit from which treatment.

Bipolar affective disorder (including mania)

Bipolar affective disorder (manic-depression, bipolar disorder) is a severe mood disorder characterized by the phasic occurrence of two distinct mood states, elation and depression, either serially or separated by a period of normal mood. An isolated episode of elation with psychotic features is termed mania (the term hypomania is used sometimes to denote a condition with less intense elation and no psychotic features). For a formal diagnosis of bipolar disorder, at least two mood episodes must have occurred, one of which must be mania. It is useful clinically to distinguish between classical bipolar disorder (termed bipolar I) in which episodes of mania predominate and depression is less frequent, bipolar II in which depressive episodes are more common but the elation is less marked, and bipolar III in which mania is triggered by antidepressant treatment of a unipolar depressive episode. Other recognized variants are rapid cycling bipolar where four or more mood episodes of either kind occur in the space of one year, and mixed states in which features of both depression and mania appear within a single episode. Cyclothymia is the long-term alternation of mild elation and mild depression (cf. dysthymia).

Clinical features

- Mania is characterized by elevated mood ranging from inappropriately cheerful and optimistic to impatient, irritable, excited, and aggressive. This is a subjectively unpleasant state that should not be confused with normal happiness.

- Behavior is overly energetic, erratic, and socially disinhibited with wild excesses, particularly of spending or traveling. The patient is distractible and unable to concentrate on any issue for more than a few minutes.

- Speech is rapid, pressured, and flits from topic to topic. This reflects the patient's thinking which flows uncontrollably from one grandiose notion to the next (flight of ideas). These grandiose thoughts are often delusional, and involve personal status (e.g. being the King), ability (superhuman powers), or invulnerability, the latter leading to dangerous risk-taking.

- Sleep is greatly reduced, and appetite might be excessive or completely lacking.

- Psychotic features such as delusions or hallucinations are present in mania but not hypomania.

- Median duration of an untreated manic episode is 4 months during which the patient risks exhaustion, dehydration, or injury.

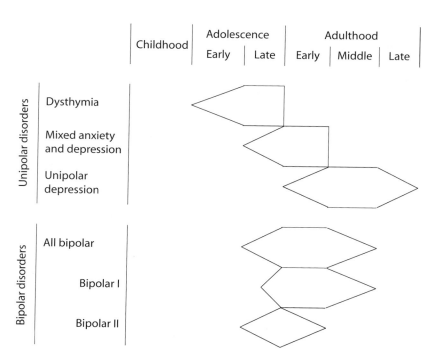

Fig. 8.6. Typical age of onset of the major mood disorders.

- Mania may be mimicked by intense anxiety, agitated schizophrenia, frontal lobe disease, or stimulant drug misuse. Cushing's disease, hyperthyroidism, and rarely severe hypothyroidism ("myxedema madness") may precipitate a manic episode.
- Depressive phases are similar in most respects to episodes of unipolar depression; a typical untreated episode lasts about 6 months. The risk of suicide is greater than during unipolar depression.
- Rapid fluctuations in mood, "mood swings," recurring erratically on most days for several months suggests a personality disorder rather than a primary mood disorder.

Investigation

Investigation should focus on eliminating potential physical causes of mania or depression, assessing the physical effects of a manic or depressive episode, and screening liver, renal, thyroid, and cardiac (ECG) function if treatment with lithium is contemplated.

Epidemiology

The overall prevalence of bipolar disorder (i.e. bipolar I and bipolar II combined) varies from country to country but averages about 1.2% with men and women affected equally. It is rare in childhood but age of onset is typically in late adolescence or early adulthood (Fig. 8.6). However, bipolar II disorder differs in some respects from this average: its prevalence appears higher, its onset younger, and women are affected disproportionately. Thus it differs from both classical bipolar disorder and depression, and it has been suggested that it represents a separate disease entity.

Etiology and pathogenesis

Concordance between monozygotic twins is 70%, and for dizygotic twins 15%, compared with 10% in other siblings. Therefore, genetic factors, most likely polygenic, account for almost all the susceptibility to bipolar disorder, leaving little room for environmental factors. A first episode of mania may be precipitated by a significant life event but later episodes lack this trigger. One such life event is childbirth as the post-partum psychosis that follows within about 3 weeks of delivery in 1 in 500 births is usually manic. However, certain patterns of behavior including excessive use of illicit drugs or alcohol, irregular sleep, and sometimes shift work, can increase the likelihood of relapse. Pathogenesis of mania is viewed as the converse of depression: elevated monoaminergic activity including dopamine, and disordered activity in the hypothalamic–pituitary pathways involved in adrenal and thyroid regulation. The key question, as yet unanswered, is: what provides the switching mechanism? Structural and functional brain imaging have drawn attention to changes in several regulatory nuclei, but it is too soon to postulate a clear mechanism.

Management

Acute mania will usually require emergency treatment, including compulsory admission. Traditionally, antipsychotic agents have been used both for their tranquilizing and antipsychotic effects, and the so-called atypical antipsychotics are just as effective but with fewer side effects. Lithium is also effective but requires pre-treatment screening tests and rapid escalation of dose to achieve a plasma concentration of about 1 mmol/l, which must then be monitored frequently. Sedation might be necessary and the partial GABA-agonist clonazepam is favored above sedative antipsychotics as it has mood stabilizing properties. ECT has a place in management of severe and intractable mania.

The devastating effects of manic episodes, coupled with the effectiveness of mood stabilizing drugs in preventing relapse in 60%–70% of cases, strongly indicates commencing a mood stabilizer after a first manic episode. However this is rarely acceptable to a young patient who might have difficulty accepting the illness let alone its long-term treatment. Lithium is highly effective in classical bipolar I disease; an alternative is sodium valproate and this may also be effective in some variants (rapid cycling and mixed states). Carbamazepine is licenced in the UK for use in rapid cycling disease, but its induction of hepatic enzymes and binding to plasma proteins make it complex to manage in conjunction with other medication. Other anti-seizure agents (e.g. topiramate) have been used with some success when the patient cannot tolerate lithium or valproate. There is accumulating evidence of efficacy of atypical antipsychotics (olanzapine and quetiapine) as mood stabilizers. CBT also has an important role as it can be used to identify dysfunctional behavior patterns (triggers) and early mood changes, so that the patient can put in place a contingency plan to minimize their effect.

Treatment of bipolar depression (as in bipolar II) is more troublesome: all antidepressants carry a risk of "switching" to mania (so-called bipolar III), and should be used only in conjunction with an anti-manic agent. For maintenance, lithium reduces the risk of depressive relapse by about 25% and other mood stabilizers appear less effective. Recently, both the anti-seizure drug lamotrigine and the atypical antipsychotic quetiapine have been used to treat the acute depressive phase and reduce the risk of depressive relapse.

Psychotic disorders

Psychosis is the term applied to a mental state in which thought, perception, behavior, and sometimes mood, are disturbed and distorted in such a way that the patient is out of touch with objective reality (Fig. 8.7). The critical feature is that the sufferer is unable to test or challenge the mismatch between his or her subjective state and reality in the outside world. Indeed, the patient may interpret the disparity as indicating that the world, rather than the patient, has changed in some irrational or threatening manner. The characteristic symptoms of psychosis are delusions and hallucinations.

Delusions are fixed, incorrigible (i.e. not amenable to rational argument or evidence) ideas and beliefs that are incongruent with the patient's cultural or

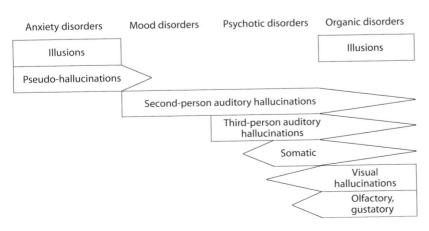

Fig. 8.7. Spectrum of perceptual disorder.

Table 8.11. Some of the more common physical causes of psychotic symptoms

Autoimmune	SLE
Cardio-respiratory	Hypoxemia (especially in elderly or post–operative)
Drugs	Both acute intoxication and withdrawal: alcohol, amphetamines (ecstasy, MDMA), cannabis, cocaine, LSD, steroids
Endocrinopathies	Thyroid disease, Cushing's disease, diabetes mellitus, post-partum
Infections	Classically neurosyphilis, HIV/AIDS, hyperpyrexia of any cause (especially in children or the elderly)
Neurologic	CVA, Creutzfeld–Jacob disease, dementia, epilepsies (classically temporal lobe), head trauma, Huntington's disease, cerebral tumors

social group. The important distinction is with over-valued ideas, such as some political or religious beliefs, that are held in the face of evidence to the contrary but are acceptable within a recognized society or culture. Hallucinations are perceptions that arise in the absence of actual sensory stimuli; to the patient they have all the defining properties of normal perceptions, and the absence of a stimulus is seen as perplexing rather than contradictory.

Psychotic experiences may occur in any condition that impairs the patient's ability to monitor and appraise exteroceptive or interoceptive stimuli, or to integrate current thoughts and beliefs with knowledge of the social and physical world. Thus many medical and neurologic disorders, both acute and chronic, may precipitate psychotic symptoms at some time during their course (Table 8.11); some presentations, such as visual or olfactory hallucinations occurring in combination with disorientation and impaired level of consciousness (delirium) are suggestive of physical illness. The more abrupt and severe the onset of the physical disorder the more likely it is to produce psychotic symptoms and diagnosis of a primary psychiatric illness should not be made until physical causation can be eliminated.

Psychotic symptoms appearing acutely in the course of a physical illness may be managed success-fully with low-dose antipsychotic medication. Medication should be introduced cautiously and increased slowly especially in older people because of side effects or masking features of the primary disease.

The principal psychotic psychiatric disorders are schizophrenia, schizoaffective disorder, transient psychotic disorders, and persistent delusional disorders. Schizophrenia is the major disorder in this group and will be discussed in detail below. Schizoaffective disorder is diagnosed when both schizophrenic and mood symptoms, sufficient for diagnosis of both of these disorders, occur simultaneously. By definition, this simultaneity precludes diagnosis of either disorder separately.

Transient psychotic disorders are characterized by abrupt transition from normality to psychosis usually following a severe stressful experience (e.g. imprisonment, forced migration). The clinical picture is pleomorphic (rapidly changing) with both florid schizophrenic and affective (mood-related) features. Young people and women are most affected, and symptoms resolve spontaneously within a few days or weeks often without treatment.

The persistent delusional disorders are a heterogeneous group in which the common finding is of a single fixed but encapsulated delusion (i.e. concerning only a limited component of the patient's life) in the absence of all other features of psychosis, especially of schizophrenia. This delusional belief may be carried for many years and may cause remarkably little interference with the patient's functioning. A range of named syndromes is included: delusional jealousy (Othello syndrome); erotomania (de Clérambault syndrome); delusional dysmorphophobia (delusions concerning body shape or appearance); delusional misidentification (Capgras and Fregoli syndromes); delusional infestation (Ekbom syndrome). Onset is usually in middle age and may follow a traumatic experience; symptoms must persist for at least 3 months for diagnosis; treatment is as for schizophrenia, but outcome is often poor.

Schizophrenia

According to World Health Organization figures, schizophrenia ranks in the top ten causes of disability, affecting over 12 million people worldwide. The predominant form of schizophrenia encountered in urban settings in the developed world is acute paranoid schizophrenia. Some of the classical subtypes are rarely seen except in developing countries (e.g. catatonic schizophrenia, Table 8.12).

Clinical features
- The typical patient is a young man whose symptoms have developed acutely over a relatively short period. Positive symptoms (abnormal phenomena a normal individual does not

Table 8.12. Clinical subtypes of schizophrenia

Paranoid	Acute onset, prominent persecutory delusions, auditory or somatic hallucinations, thought interference
Simple	Gradual onset, odd behaviors, social isolation, overriding preoccupations, but few clear delusions or hallucinations
Hebephrenic	Gradual onset often in mid-teenage, disorganized and unpredictable ("childlike") thought and behavior, labile mood, fleeting delusions or hallucinations
Catatonic	Rapid onset, prominent motor features (bizarre postures or movements, brief periods of intense excitement), uncommunicative so difficult to elicit delusions or hallucinations, stupor

Table 8.13. Diagnostic features of schizophrenia

Group A	
Core diagnostic features, one of which must be present for 1 month for diagnosis. All are "first rank" symptoms except persistent delusions	• Thought interference: insertion, withdrawal or broadcasting (mind being read)
	• Thought echo (thoughts spoken out loud by another)
	• Delusions of control or passivity (feelings or actions being controlled externally)
	• Delusional perception (a new delusion arising from a normal perception)
	• Persistent delusions that are impossible or culturally incongruent
	• Hallucinatory voices in third person giving commentary on patient's actions
	• Somatic or tactile hallucinations

Group B	
Associated features, at least two of which must be present for 1 month if features of Group A are not present	• Thought block resulting in disrupted speech
	• Persistent hallucinations in any modality
	• Catatonic motor phenomena
	• "Negative" features (lack of normal attributes), including apathy, paucity of speech or thoughts, blunted or incongruous emotions
	• Significant deterioration in personal attributes and behaviors, resulting in social withdrawal

experience) predominate, particularly intensely held paranoid delusions.

- The form of thought is disordered, with disruption of the process of thinking (insertion, withdrawal, block, slow thinking, illogical thinking) manifesting as odd speech patterns. Content of thought is characterized by paranoid delusions, usually of persecution, grandiosity (persecuted because he is important), special reference (events having great personal significance), or control (by external or "alien" agency).

- The characteristic disorder of perception is the third-person auditory hallucination giving a running commentary on the patient's every action. The patient may perceive these phenomena as arising at great distance (extracampine hallucinations). Somatic (both visceral and tactile) hallucinations cause particular distress; visual, olfactory, and gustatory hallucinations are less common.

- Mood may be delusional (something is going on, or the world has changed in a strange way), blunted (unvarying or indifferent to circumstances), or incongruous (out of keeping with thoughts and behavior).

- Behavior may be odd or inappropriate to the circumstances; the patient may be withdrawn or preoccupied (for instance, with hallucinatory experiences). Aggressive behavior is uncommon except when the patient feels threatened by his or her experiences.

- These phenomena must arise in clear consciousness, and in the absence of central or peripheral neurologic dysfunction, including drug misuse, that would account for them.

- For a formal diagnosis, core features (some of which are referred to as "first rank" symptoms, see Table 8.13) must be present for at least one month.

- A prodromal syndrome of perplexed mood, disorganized thinking, and reclusive or bizarre behaviors may extend over weeks or months before acute presentation.

- Isolated features might be present in childhood (e.g. self-absorption, social isolation) but the full disorder is not apparent until at least mid-teenage.

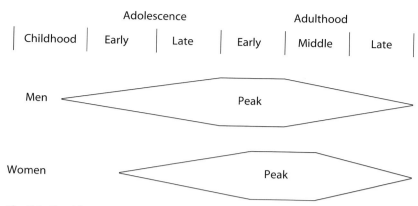

Fig. 8.8. Sex differences in age of onset of schizophrenia.

If many symptoms are present in childhood, a specific diagnosis such as autistic disorder or Asperger's syndrome should be considered.

- Abrupt onset of psychotic symptoms in the absence of physical illness may follow a severe and disorientating experience. Such psychogenic episodes usually show florid affective (mood-related) features, and resolve spontaneously within a few days or weeks often without treatment. Only persistence beyond 1 month suggests schizophrenia.
- Secondary disability is the major burden in chronic schizophrenia as there is further deterioration with each episode. This may be cognitive (impaired performance), social (disrupted education, employment, and relationships), or physical (standardized mortality ratios for all causes, cardiovascular disease, and cancers are elevated in schizophrenia).

Investigation

Many putative biologic markers have been reported but none provides the basis of a diagnostic test. Therefore, the plan of investigation should aim to: exclude physical causes that mimic schizophrenia; establish the extent of secondary conditions that might result from the patient's schizophrenic behavior; give a baseline for future medical treatment.

Epidemiology

Major international studies have established that the prevalence of schizophrenia is remarkably similar in all cultures: the lifetime risk is about 1% and the point prevalence is 0.5% worldwide (except in Ireland and Sweden where it is higher). There are indications that the disease is evolving (the catatonic subtype is now rare in industrialized societies) and the incidence is falling, but this might be due to changes in diagnostic criteria. Important sex differences exist: men are affected on average about 5 years younger (from late childhood; peak onset mid-twenties) than women (from mid-teens; peak onset late twenties); the incidence in men is higher than in women until middle age after which the sex ratio reverses; and the course is more severe in men (Fig. 8.8). There is a socioeconomic class bias with higher prevalence in deprived areas of inner cities, lower socioeconomic groups, and recent immigrants. It is unclear whether this is because being brought up in deprived circumstances causes schizophrenia (the "breeder" hypothesis), or because sufferers become economically deprived (the "drift" hypothesis).

Etiology and pathogenesis

Evidence of a genetic basis for schizophrenia is compelling: concordance between monozygotic twins is 40%, compared with 15% for dizygotic twins, 10% for other first-degree relatives, and 1% in the general population. The mode of inheritance of schizophrenia is polygenic and, in contrast to depression, the inherited susceptibility to develop schizophrenia may be seen as a degree of *vulnerability* (rather than all-or-none liability). Thus, the occurrence of schizophrenia in an individual conforms to a multifactorial stress–diathesis model (see Fig. 8.9) which proposes that sufficient environmental stress will produce symptoms even in those at low genetic risk. This raises the intriguing question of the relative contributions of developmental and social factors to pathogenesis.

Recent interest has focused on neurodevelopmental mechanisms of pathogenesis: the biologic

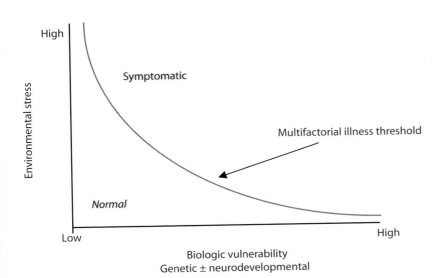

Fig. 8.9. Multifactorial stress–diathesis model of schizophrenia.

Table 8.14. Structural and functional imaging findings in brains of non-medicated schizophrenics

Whole brain	Increased ventricle : brain ratio
Mesial temporal lobe	Disruption of hippocampal pyramidal cells
	Cell loss in amygdala and entorhinal cortex
Prefrontal cortex	Smaller neurons
	Reduced neuron density
Frontal lobe function	Hypofrontality : reduced metabolic activity

vulnerability to schizophrenia is a composite of genetic susceptibility and disordered neuronal development which disrupts normal neurologic and psychologic processes. Post-mortem studies, and *in vivo* structural and functional imaging of never–medicated patients, have provided ample evidence of focal and general abnormalities (see Table 8.14). Some of these abnormalities may arise from intra-uterine or early developmental insult: patients have a high prevalence of abnormal dermatoglyphic (fingerprint) patterns that are formed during the second trimester of pregnancy, the time when the mesial temporal lobe is developing. Children who later develop schizophrenia are often noted to show subclinical ("soft") neurologic signs. Normal brain maturation continues throughout childhood and adolescence, so later insults might also contribute: recent studies suggest that cannabis misuse in early adolescence (before

16 years) may have a causative influence, while later use may precipitate illness or relapse.

The association with low socioeconomic status and deprivation has been noted above. The mechanism by which such factors contribute to etiology is unclear but it is likely to be increased exposure to adverse neurodevelopmental influences. This would explain the falling incidence of catatonic schizophrenia in industrialized societies, while it remains common in developing countries where intra-partum and childhood morbidity is high.

Several neurotransmitter systems have been implicated in the pathogenesis of schizophrenic (and other psychotic) symptoms. The classical hypothesis is that overactivity in mesolimbic and mesocortical dopaminergic pathways causes psychosis. This is based on observations that dopamine-releasing agents (e.g. amphetamines) produce schizophrenia-like symptoms in normal individuals, there is up-regulation of dopamine D_2 receptors in the brains of schizophrenics, and all effective antipsychotic drugs are (at least partially) dopamine D_2 blockers. However, while dysregulation of dopaminergic transmission may account for the hallucinations and delusions, it does not explain the so-called "negative" features. Other neurotransmitters (serotonin, norepinephrine) and excitatory amino acids (glutamate, aspartate) may play a part, and this suggestion has been supported by the fact that the recent generation of antipsychotic drugs are "atypical" in that they bind only weakly to dopamine D_1 and D_2 receptors but also show affinity for serotonergic receptors.

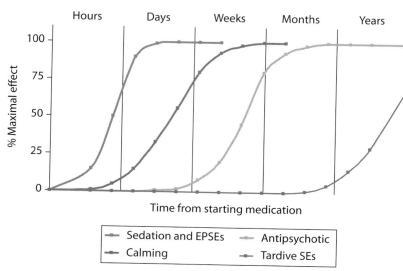

Fig. 8.10. Time course of antipsychotic drug effects.

Diagram based on data from older typical antipsychotics.
Newer atypicals produce fewer early effects (sedation and EPSEs).
EPSEs: extrapyramidal side effects including acute dystonia and akathisia.
Tardive SEs: late onset side effects such as tardive dyskinesia.

The structural and functional abnormalities result in cognitive deficits, principally impaired reception of sensory information and dysfunctional cognitive processing. There is systematic misinterpretation of others' speech and facial expression and of the patient's own proprioceptive sensations, an inability to manipulate conceptual information, and failure to filter out irrelevant information. As a result, normal sensations, including those arising in the patient's own body, are perceived as strange and the patient's own thoughts appear alien and threatening.

Management

Management of acute schizophrenia is largely pharmacologic, although psychologic (CBT, family therapy) and social (rehabilitation) therapies are valuable in preventing relapse and promoting return to normal functioning. Specific antipsychotic medication should be commenced as soon as possible as there is strong evidence that the most important factor in reducing long-term morbidity is reducing the duration of untreated psychosis.

Antipsychotic drugs are divided into two groups: the older "typicals" (so-called because they exert their antipsychotic effects by potent binding to postsynaptic dopamine D_2 receptors); and the newer "atypicals" (as noted above, these bind weakly to D_2 receptors). All are about equally effective in reducing acute psychotic symptoms, but use of the typicals is limited by their propensity to generate side effects at low dosage. Blocking D_2 receptors in the nigrostriatal pathway causes extrapyramidal (motor) side effects, and in the tubero-infundibular pathway causes hyperprolactinemia. Their muscarinic effects may potentiate motor side effects such as Parkinsonism or occulo-gyric crisis. In contrast, at therapeutic dosage the atypicals block activity in mesolimbic and mesocortical dopaminergic neurons but only affect other pathways at higher doses. Possibly due to their modulation of serotonergic neurotransmission, the atypicals are also effective against some of the "negative" features. For these reasons, they have displaced the older antipsychotics as first-line treatment of newly diagnosed schizophrenia.

Management of the acute episode should aim to reduce distressing psychotic symptoms and control agitation. The typical antipsychotics were often used for their rapid sedative effects but with these came acute dystonia and akathisia (a distressing sense of psychologic and motor restlessness; see Fig. 8.10). As atypical drugs are less sedating, an oral or parenteral benzodiazepine should be used depending on urgency: the choice is between diazepam (10 mg, long half-life) and lorazepam (1–2 mg, short half-life). This should be ceased as soon as the calming effects of the antipsychotic become apparent. Antipsychotics achieve 80% blockade of mesolimbic D_2 receptors in

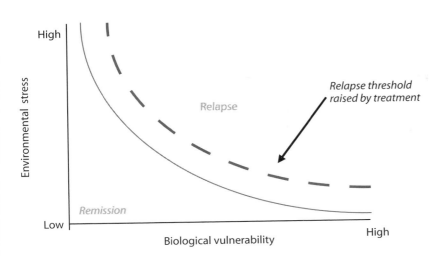

Fig. 8.11. Treatment modifies the vulnerability to relapse of schizophrenia.

hours, and this may account for their calming effects as the full antipsychotic effect requires stabilization of neurotransmission in several interacting pathways and this develops over a period of weeks. If the first antipsychotic fails to control symptoms, then the dose should be increased cautiously; if this is unsuccessful, an alternative atypical should be tried for several weeks. Continued failure to control symptoms indicates the use of clozapine: this highly effective atypical drug is reserved for treatment of refractory cases as it carries a 3% risk of causing a life-threatening neutropenia and weekly full blood count is mandatory.

Although about 20% of patients may recover fully after a single episode of schizophrenia 80% will suffer recurrent episodes or develop chronicity with concomitant social and intellectual decline. Regrettably it is not possible to predict those that would remain well without further treatment, so maintenance medication should be recommended to all. All antipsychotics are effective in reducing the risk of relapse of "positive" symptoms from about 80% to 15% at 1 year; additionally, atypicals appear to be effective in preventing and treating "negative" symptoms. Ideally, the drug used to control the acute symptoms should be continued, although a lower dosage might be adequate and will reduce the risk of developing side effects. For some patients with disorganized lifestyles long-acting intramuscular depot preparations might be advisable, although these are mostly typical antipsychotics with higher rates of side effects. In all cases, antipsychotic treatment is most effective if combined with psychologic or social interventions (see below and Fig. 8.11).

Cognitive therapy treats the hallucinations and delusions of schizophrenia as automatic negative thoughts (cf. depression) and challenges the irrational nature of abnormal beliefs. Clinical trials have demonstrated reduced distress and improved social functioning, and many patients may benefit from attending "voices groups" using cognitive techniques. Family therapy aims to reduce the level of expressed emotion (critical comments, hostility, and emotional over-involvement) found in the families of schizophrenic patients and known to be implicated in causing relapse. Used with antipsychotic medication, family therapy can reduce the high risk of relapse in patients with high expressed emotion families from over 90% to about 50% over 2 years. Other psychologic strategies such as motivational interviewing may be useful in improving adherence to medication regimens. Social programs aim to give structure to the patient's life ("something to get up for"), encourage personal autonomy, improve social functioning, and increase employability.

Outcome is variable, and 5 years following a first episode about 20% of patients will have recovered fully. However, for the majority the illness runs a chronic relapsing course: about 30% suffer recurrent acute episodes; another 30% are chronically ill with varying degrees of progressive deterioration (about half of these in supportive care); about 10% die by suicide. Better outcome is predicted by acute onset following a clear precipitant in an older patient who has already made good academic and social progress, and who accepts and adheres to treatment. Insidious onset without precipitants in a younger

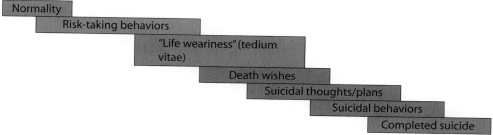

Fig. 8.12. Spectrum of suicidal thoughts and behaviors.

patient with limited social skills who rejects medication bodes ill.

Suicide risk

Suicide rates have increased worldwide by 60% in the last 50 years so it is now the fifth most important cause of life-years lost, with a 1% lifetime risk. Death by suicide may be viewed as the extreme of a behavioral spectrum (see Fig. 8.12), and an individual may move along this continuum in either direction depending on a variety of personal and social factors. A high proportion of individuals who go on to kill themselves make contact with medical services in the month prior to death, often for apparently non-psychiatric reasons. Therefore, it is important for doctors in all branches of medicine to be familiar with the management of suicide risk.

Clinical features
- Fleeting suicidal thoughts are very common in the general population and do not necessarily indicate a psychiatric disorder.
- They are particularly frequent following personally significant upsets in relationships, health, or employment, adolescents being especially affected.
- Most patients are distressed by their suicidal thoughts but feel unable to discuss them with family or friends for fear of causing upset. Equally, they may be reluctant to seek medical advice in case they are ignored or, worse, compulsorily admitted to a psychiatric ward.
- Increasing time spent ruminating on suicide, or attempts to blot out the thoughts with drugs or alcohol, suggest rising risk.
- Individuals from particular backgrounds or with certain characteristics (e.g. psychiatric disorder) are at greater risk.

- A checklist may be used to assist assessment of "suicidality" (planning, intent, and imminence of a suicide attempt), but this remains an essentially clinical judgment.
- Approaching anniversaries of significant adverse events (e.g. bereavement) or "putting one's affairs in order" may be significant in planning suicide.
- Opportunity (home alone) and means (prescribed drugs) might bring forward an attempt.
- Previously, women tended to use less violent means (e.g. overdose) and men more violent (shooting, hanging, jumping) but these distinctions are becoming blurred.
- Some patients hold recurring suicidal ideas of varying intensity for several years.

Common and important risk factors for suicide
Demographic factors
- Male sex
- Increasing age (but see below)
- Low socio-economic status
- Single or socially isolated
- Social or family disruption
- Some occupations (e.g. farming)
- Availability of means (guns, drugs)

Clinical factors
- Deliberate self harm
- Depression
- Schizophrenia
- Personality disorder
- Anxiety disorders
- Drug/alcohol misuse
- Chronic or painful physical illness

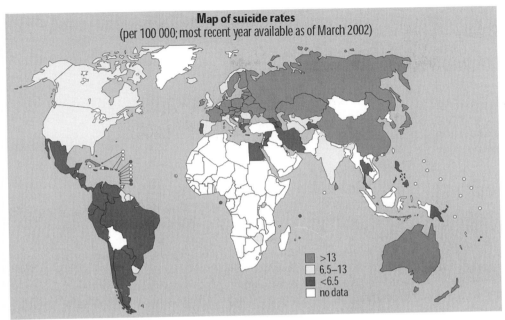

Map of suicide rates
(per 100 000; most recent year available as of March 2002)

>13
6.5–13
<6.5
no data

Fig. 8.13. Worldwide distribution of suicide rates 2002 (WOM WHO http://www.who.int/mental_health/management/en/SUPRE_lyer1.pdf, reproduced with permission).

Checklist for suicide risk screening in clinical practice
Pre-admission
Suicidal thinking
- Rarely, occasional, often/intrusive, constant
- No thought of death, not wishing to be alive, wishing to be dead, intention to kill self

Planning
- None, thought of means, acquired means, plan for event

Intent
- None, variable, definite/specific

Pre-discharge (following suicide attempt)
Suicidal thinking
- As for Pre-admission, plus
- Pleased to be alive, neither pleased nor disappointed, wishes had died
- Regrets attempt, no regrets, regrets failure

Planning
- As for Pre-admission

Intent
- As for Pre-admission, plus
- Try harder next time

Epidemiology

There are wide variations in risk of suicide between countries (Fig. 8.13). In the UK the rate is 8/100 000/ year but falling year-on-year and is amongst the lowest in Europe. In countries of the former Soviet Union rates are ten times higher and rising. This is accounted for to some extent by an inverse relationship between suicide rate and a country's economic prosperity; easy availability of weapons is another factor. Rates vary with age: it is rare in childhood, and uncommon but increasing in adolescents; in the UK, there has been a significant increase in men under 25 years of age where it accounts for over 20% of deaths; the rates in middle and older age are falling. In all countries and at all ages, rates are higher in men than women (Fig. 8.14); in the UK the overall ratio is about 2:1, about 4:1 in the USA, and over 5:1 in some former Soviet countries.

All psychiatric disorders and many chronic or painful physical diseases carry an increased risk of suicide. Standardized mortality ratios for suicide are greatest in patients who have a history of deliberate

255

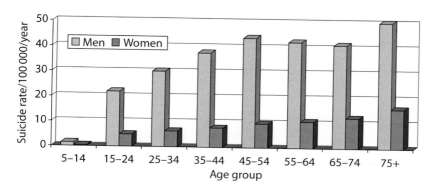

Fig. 8.14. Suicide rates by age and sex worldwide 2000 (WHO data).

self harm (25% increase); mood disorders have a 20% increase and schizophrenia 10%–12%; other psychiatric disorders confer a 10% increased risk.

Management

Given the reluctance of sufferers to talk of their suicidal thoughts, the first step in management is to provide a sympathetic and receptive hearing. Symptoms and signs of psychiatric disorder should be sought cautiously, as this enquiry might deter the many patients who are not suicidal as the result of prior psychiatric morbidity. Enquiry about suicidal thoughts should be routine for all patients with established psychiatric disorder and those with chronic, or newly diagnosed, disabling physical illness.

The aims of management are to prevent harm, treat definite psychiatric disorder, encourage hope and resilience, and give support and assistance in solving practical problems. An imminent suicide attempt may require emergency admission, compulsory if necessary, even if it is uncertain whether there is an underlying psychiatric disorder. Patients with an established history of deliberate self harm or severe psychiatric disorder who experience mounting suicidal intention are at high risk and are likely to require admission. Actively suicidal patients will require constant supervision until the underlying cause can be treated adequately. For those at intermediate risk, full psychiatric assessment should be considered and the patient encouraged to accept: admission may be unnecessary if the patient has a supportive family. Brief focused psychotherapy has been shown to help those without psychiatric disorder, and practical problem solving may help those whose suicidal thoughts were the result of a temporary personal setback.

Further reading

Davies T, Campbell I, Biochemical aspects of psychiatric disorders, "suicide" in Marshall WJ, Bangert SK (eds), *Clinical Biochemistry: Clinical and Metabolic Aspects*, 2nd edn,Elsevier, 2008.

Davies T, Craig T (eds). *ABC of Mental Health*, 2nd edn. Wiley-Blackwell, 2008.

Geider M, Cowen P, Harrison P. *Shorter Oxford Textbook of Psychiatry*, 5th edn. Oxford University Press, 2006.

Gelder M, Mayou R, Geddes J. *Psychiatry: An Oxford Core Text*, 3rd edn. Oxford University Press, 2005.

Marshall WJ, Davies T Biochemical aspects of psychiatric disorders, in Marshall WJ, Bangert SK (eds), *Clinical Biochemistry: Metasolic and Clinical Aspects*, 2nd edn. Churchill Livingstone, 2008.

National Institute for Health and Clinical Excellence. www.nice.org.uk.

Katia Cikurel, Leone Ridsdale and Lina Nashef

Contents

Epilepsy

This is common and has serious physical and social consequences.

Definitions

An epileptic seizure is a transient occurrence of signs and/or symptoms due to abnormal excessive or synchronous neuronal activity in the brain.

Epilepsy is a disorder of the brain characterized by an enduring predisposition to generate epileptic seizures and by the neurobiologic, cognitive, psychologic, and social consequences the diagnosis requires at least one epileptic seizure (International League Against Epilepsy proposals).

Idiopathic epilepsy syndrome: epilepsy, with no underlying structural brain lesion or other neurologic signs or symptoms. It is presumed to be genetic and usually age dependent.

Approaching the history (Table 9.1)

Symptomatic epilepsy syndrome: epileptic seizures are the result of one or more identifiable structural lesions of the brain.

Status epilepticus: defined as a seizure that does not stop within the average period for that type of seizure. An operational definition of more than 5 minutes is appropriate for starting life-saving treatment.

Individualized protocols for chronic epilepsy recommend intervention when the seizure lasts longer than habitual self-terminating events. A patient attending the emergency department still convulsing should be treated immediately.

Aura is a sensory seizure without loss of awareness. It can happen alone (a simple partial seizure) or precede a complex partial seizure (with loss of awareness) or a secondary generalized convulsion. It can also

Table 9.1. Differentiating epilepsy from syncope

	Epilepsy	Syncope
Aura or prodrome	Smell, taste, déjà vu, Depersonalization Rising sensation` Limb jerking	Feeling faint, nausea Distant hearing Tinnitus Weak legs
Appearance	Change in color	Pale and clammy Flushing on recovery
Motor	Rhythmic	None or brief irregular jerking
Automatisms	Sometimes	Unlikely
Tongue biting	Sometimes	Unlikely
Incontinence	Sometimes	Less likely
Return of consciousness		
Observer	Gradual	Short
Patient	In hospital or elsewhere	Same place as collapse
Patterns and triggers	Clustering On awakening or diurnal Hyperventilation Sleep deprivation Menstrual cycle Photic stimulation Alcohol, drugs Stress	Arrhythmias with sleep or exercise Emotion, pain, prolonged standing

provide an indication of where the seizure originated, e.g. a déjà-vu feeling indicates a temporal onset.

Prodrome means the symptoms that precede a blackout. More commonly, the term refers to the feeling before a faint.

Acute symptomatic seizures. Given sufficient provocation, epileptic seizures occur without having epilepsy e.g. after recent head injury, during CNS infections and strokes, or secondary to metabolic derangement.

Febrile seizures (FS): a specific term for seizures occurring without previous afebrile episodes between 6 months and 6 years of age and associated with fever not due to CNS infection. There is a small risk of later epilepsy following FS and this is slightly higher if focal, prolonged, or in a cluster.

Differential diagnosis
Histories from patient and witness are paramount. Not all stiffness or shaking is epileptic. Rigidity, irregular jerking, and incontinence can occur in faints. The common simple faint or vaso-vagal attack occurs either

because of peripheral vasodilation resulting in blood pressure fall and/or increased vagal tone, resulting in bradycardia or brief sinus arrest. It is triggered by fear, sight of blood, tiredness, stress, and prolonged standing.

In Parkinson disease with autonomic dysfunction there may be faints after a heavy meal or a hot bath.

Cardiac arrhythmias causing syncope may be unprovoked, but in long QT syndrome this is more likely during exercise or sleep.

Anterior circulation transient ischemic events affecting one hemisphere cause loss of function rather than of consciousness. The rate of spread of auras is slower in migraine than in epilepsy.

Intermittent loss of consciousness may be due to acute hydrocephalus and ventriculoperitoneal shunt malfunction.

Clinical diagnosis
A detailed and accurate history from patient and witnesses is the most important aspect of diagnosis.

Approaching the history
- Description of events immediately before and after (a) from patient (b) from witnesses (usually the patient is not aware of what occurred)
- Triggers and circumstances: alcohol, sleep deprivation, stress, excitement, menstrual cycle, certain antidepressants, certain antimalarial drugs, photic stimulation, or recreational drugs
- Pattern: diurnal, relation to sleep or menstruation, clustering
- Context: previous febrile seizures, simple or complex, birth trauma, congenital deficit, head injury, CNS infection, alcohol excess, stroke
- Family history
- Previous history of epilepsy: details or presentation including any episodes of status epilepticus or injury, previous investigations including early EEGs, previous treatment, doses, side effects and response
- General medical history, cardiac history and medication, or recreational drugs

Examination
- Color, responsiveness, pulse, and breathing
- Skin: evidence of neurocutaneous syndrome, e.g. neurofibromatosis, tuberous sclerosis, or vascular anomaly
- Cardiac/vascular: any evidence of predisposition to cardiac syncope or vascular disease

- Evidence of new or long-standing neurologic deficit that might indicate focal brain pathology predisposing to epilepsy
- Evidence of raised intracranial pressure.
- Blood sugar/BM stick, if obtunded/ sweaty/comatose
- Temporal evolution of the attack and of the recovery phase
- Limb, face, head, and eye movements/forced deviation; any lateralizing motor features such as unilateral jerking, paucity of movement, tonic or dystonic posturing (contralateral), or limb automatisms (ipsilateral); oro-alimentary automatisms; hyper-motor features, vocalization; responsiveness; plantar responses; post-ictal confusion, paresis or dyphasia, amnesia

Classification

It is not sufficient to make a diagnosis of "epilepsy." A more refined accurate diagnosis aids prognosis and management. Not all types of seizures or epilepsy respond to all antiepileptic drugs. Seizures may be worsened by inappropriate medication. Focal epilepsies with a structural cause may be cured by resective surgery.

The diagnosis is based on the following five levels or axes.

Axis 1: Description of the seizure(s). This is referred to as the ictal phenomenology (semiology). A glossary of terms is available to facilitate communication

Axis 2: Seizure type

Axis 3: Syndrome: a useful concept – "A complex of signs and symptoms that define a unique epilepsy condition." It allows grouping of similar presentations with useful implications for investigations, prognosis, and management. A syndrome may suggest a cause but does not define it. There may be several.

Axis 4: Cause (if known):

- Genetic, peri-, and prenatal acquired disorders (non-progressive pathology) e.g. infective, anoxic or ischemic
- Postnatal acquired disorders: e.g. head injury, CNS infections, stroke, alcohol, tumors
- Malformations of cortical development, hippocampal sclerosis
- Degenerative disorders
- Vascular anomalies e.g. cavernomas, arteriovenous malformations (Fig. 9.1).
- Chromosomal abnormalities e.g. ring chromosome 20
- Mendelian diseases (e.g. Fragile X, Angelman and Rett syndromes)

- Neurocutaneous disorders e.g. Sturge–Weber, neurofibromatosis, and tuberous sclerosis
- Metabolic disorders e.g. pyridoxine dependency, porphyria, mitochondrial diseases.

Axis 5: Impairment

Examples of epileptic seizures:

Generalized:

Generalized tonic clonic seizures, GTCS ("Grand mal")

Tonic seizures

Atonic seizures

Absences ("Petit mal," but the latter term, at least in the UK, has often been misused, covering all ills)

Myoclonus

Focal (Partial):

Previously when the term partial seizure was prefixed with "simple" or "complex" it indicated loss of awareness or not. This is still a helpful distinction, but not always possible to apply. Sometimes a partial seizure is associated with secondary GTCS. The partial onset may be apparent as an olfactory aura or jerking of one limb. Sometimes it is inferred, for example if a clear structural focus for the seizure is found.

Continuous seizure types:

Status epilepticus (generalized and partial)

Epidemiology

Prevalence 5–10/1000. The incidence, 50/100 000, is lower in developed than in developing countries. Incidence in childhood, adolescence, and old age is higher than in adults. Risk of recurrence after first seizure depends on the time the patient is first seen. The majority respond to anti-epileptic drugs but 30% remain uncontrolled due to intractability, life style, non-adherence to treatment, or sub-optimal management. There is increased mortality due to the diseases causing epilepsy and epilepsy itself. Patients may die suddenly and unexpectedly without structural cause largely due to uncontrolled seizures. Accidents, injuries, and drowning are preventable by reducing exposure.

Fertility is reduced. Genetic susceptibility is inherited commonly as a complex trait, with risk higher in generalized epilepsy syndromes (5%–8%) compared with partial (2%–4%).

Pathology

Cortical hyperexcitability may be due to an imbalance between excitatory and inhibitory mechanisms, ion

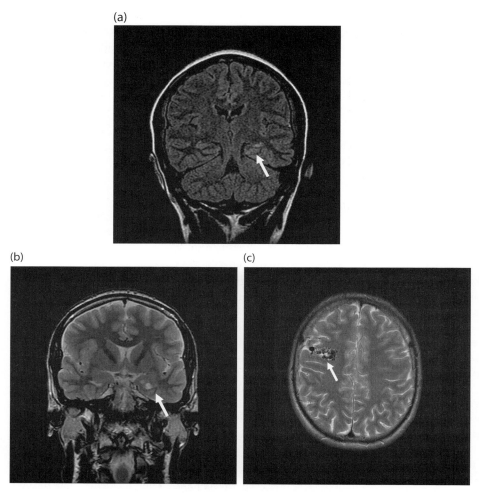

Fig. 9.1. MRI of three brains showing arrowed abnormalities. (a) Left-sided hippocampal sclerosis (mesial temporal sclerosis) – atrophy and high signal in the left temporal lobe (arrow) causing temporal lobe epilepsy. (b) Indolent left amygdalar lesion (arrow) presenting as temporal lobe epilepsy. (c) Right frontal arteriovenous malformation (arrow), presenting with secondary generalized seizures.

channel or receptor disorders. A focal brain lesion or toxic or metabolic causes can also cause epilepsy.

Idiopathic Most often present in childhood, adolescence, and in early adult life, although later presentations occur. Idiopathic epilepsy may be focal or generalized, the latter presenting with absences, myoclonic jerks, and/or generalized tonic clonic seizures. There may be photosensitivity. EEG may be abnormal while imaging and neurologic examination are usually normal. Mendelian idiopathic epilepsies usually have a genetic basis in ion channels control. The underlying basis of the more common inherited complex epilepsies is unknown but may be due to an interaction of genes and environmental factors.

Symptomatic epilepsies Can begin at any age and there are many causes:

- Hippocampal sclerosis (HS) may be secondary to prolonged childhood febrile seizures. The clinical history is that of complex partial seizures (CPS), often with a déjà-vu aura. HS can be demonstrated by MRI.
- Tumors may be long-standing, static, and neurodevelopmental; benign or slowly growing such as meningiomas and oligodendrogliomas or malignant primary tumors or metastases.
  A previously well adult with a first seizure should have early brain imaging to exclude new tumors.
- Alcohol is a trigger for seizures in established epilepsy, especially with sleep deprivation.

Withdrawal seizures and chronic epilepsy may develop due to long-term brain damage secondary to excess alcohol and associated head injuries.

- Remote symptomatic epilepsy secondary to brain injury, e.g. meningitis, encephalitis, traumatic brain injury, stroke can occur at any age. Seizures are also associated with some degenerative disorders or vascular changes in late life.

Investigations

These support the clinical diagnosis, characterize the epilepsy and inform the etiology.

Routine hematology, biochemistry, and ECG. Other specific investigations guided by clinical assessment are:

- Electroencephalography (EEG)
- Neuroimaging
- Neuropsychometry as indicated

EEG is important in characterizing seizures. A first awake EEG is normal between attacks in 50% of patients. It is less helpful in classification of epilepsy presenting in middle age and in the elderly because most are partial. Diffuse slowing of background activity may be due to many causes including medication, chronic brain pathology, encephalopathy, post-ictal state.

Focal slowing is due to local pathology.

Focal (or multifocal) epileptiform discharges (spikes, sharp waves or spike and slow waves) indicates focal epileptiform activity.

Generalised discharges, usually generalized spike and wave, indicate idiopathic or symptomatic generalized epilepsies.

EEG can be carried out between attacks (with the patient awake or asleep), or during attacks, usually with a video or an awake EEG, with a) hyperventilation and b) photic stimulation. Ambulatory EEG can be helpful if discharges occur at certain times e.g. on awakening.

EEG video telemetry is useful for capturing attacks and correlating clinical features with the EEG and is recommended for all with frequent uncontrolled seizures.

High-quality structural imaging is essential for all but those with a confident diagnosis of idiopathic epilepsy, e.g. benign neonatal convulsions, childhood absence epilepsy. MRI is the investigation of choice (Fig 9.1).

Management

- Patient education about safety, seizure triggers, legal obligations, implications for employment and education, and self-management including the importance of adherence to treatment
- Involvement of partner, relative, or carer
- Antiepileptic drug treatment (AED) long term
- Identification of other treatment modalities, such as resective surgery or vagus nerve stimulation (VNS)
- Treatment of the acute attack if prolonged or not self-limiting
- Review of diagnosis and reassessment if response not as predicted
- Advice for special groups, e.g. preconception counseling
- Management of associated disorders, depression or learning difficulty

Drug management Recommended when diagnosis is probable or certain. Treatment with anti-epileptic drugs (AEDs) is offered after more than one unprovoked epileptic seizure. The balance is between the inconvenience and side effects and the risks of uncontrolled seizures. The aim is to achieve seizure control with the lowest number of drugs (one where possible) at the lowest effective doses and minimum adverse effects.

The choice relies on matching epilepsy characteristics with profiles of the drugs and the patient.

Idiopathic generalized epilepsy (IGE)

It is easier to treat IGE in males. Sodium valproate is effective at well-tolerated low to moderate doses for all seizure types. Disadvantages are weight gain and inadvisability for women of reproductive age. Lamotrigine is often used in pregnancy. It is safer but not as effective as valproate in IGE. Levetiracetam, zonisamide and topiramate are also effective but information on safety in pregnancy is limited. Topiramate is not as well tolerated but is effective. Others of value are benzodiazepines and phenobarbital. Benzodiazepines result in habituation, tolerance and loss of efficacy.

Partial epilepsy

Carbamazepine and lamotrigine are first choice. Lamotrigine is better tolerated but carbamazepine more effective. Both cause allergies, and slow introduction is advised. Both are relatively safe in pregnancy. Others are oxcarbazepine, levetiracetam, topiramate, pregabalin, gabapentin, tiagabine, zonisamide, phenobarbital, and phenytoin.

General principles

Monotherapy and if unsuccessful change to another with an overlap period. Do not withdraw first drug until new medication successfully established.

Withdraw gradually. Sometimes more than one medication is needed. A sub-group continue to have seizures despite several drugs. This may be due to inappropriate AED, misdiagnosis, progressive neurologic disease, or intractability.

There are individual and racial differences in drug metabolism. Start on low doses, particularly in the elderly, and titrate up. Titration is easier with frequent seizures. Drug half-life influences dosing frequency, intervals between dose changes, and combined therapy. Withdrawing one enzyme-inducing drug can raise levels of a remaining drug. AED levels can guide dosing, maximize benefit, and reduce toxicity but are not targets. Because of non-linear pharmacokinetics, phenytoin levels are essential. Dose changes should be small when levels are close to the therapeutic range. Interactions occur between AEDs and other drugs.

Early adverse events

- Side effects which are likely to settle: advise slower titration, dose reduction and reassure patient
- Clear allergic side effects, severe blood dyscrasias, liver failure, or severe mood or behavioral disturbances: discontinue medication
- Worse seizures: consider an alternative AED
- Cognitive impairment, despite slow titration, consider an alternative.

Long-term effects

- Acne, coarsening features, hirsutism, gum hypertrophy (phenytoin), weight gain (valproate, gabapentin, pregabalin, carbamazepine), weight loss (topiramate, zonisamide), Dupuytren's contracture and Peyronie's disease (phenobarbitone), hyponatremia (carbamazepine and oxcarbazepine), folate deficiency, liver function dysfunction (many AEDs), low vitamin D levels (enzyme-inducing AEDs), osteoporosis (enzyme-inducing AEDs and valproate) and hormonal effects on menstrual cycle, fertility, and libido.

Drug interactions

- Reduction of efficacy of the oral contraceptive pill and steroids with enzyme-inducing AEDs
- Increased or decreased effects on warfarin
- Enzyme-inducing AEDs reduce half-life, efficacy, and duration of action of other AEDs. Valproate may prolong the half-life of some AEDs.

Women of child-bearing age and pregnancy

- Some AEDs cause congenital abnormalities and relevant women should be warned of risk of neural tube defects, cleft palate

- Sodium valproate and phenobarbital are less safe, carbamezapine and low dose lamotrigine have low risk
- Risks greater with multiple drugs
- Folic acid supplements and fetal screening advisable
- Vitamin K in late pregnancy for enzyme-inducing AEDs

Withdrawal of AEDs

When seizure free for minimum of 2 years but preferably 5 years. Decision to withdraw is made by an informed patient and not by the physician. Relapse is less likely the longer seizure freedom. Risk of relapse is 30%–40%. Withdrawal of combination AEDs should be one at a time and no withdrawal should be abrupt.

Guidance on driving

It is a legal requirement to stop driving and inform the licencing authority after one epileptic event of any type. Patients may hold a group 1 license following a seizure-free period of 1 year or a 3-year period of attacks arising in sleep only. Group 2 driving regulations are stricter. Patients should not drive during withdrawal of medication and for 6 months afterwards.

Status epilepticus

There is risk of brain damage and death in status epilepticus – see Neurologic emergencies.

Outcome

The predisposition to epilepsy tends to endure and has psychologic and social consequences.

Headache
Acute onset, single episode

Sinusitis
Migraine, first attack
Head injury
Subarachnoid hemorrhage
Meningitis/encephalitis

Recurrent headaches

Tension headache
Migraine
Cluster headache
Trigeminal neuralgia

Progressively worsening headaches

Giant cell arteritis
(Temporal arteritis) (over 60s)
'Benign' intracranial hypertension
Brain tumor/space-occupying lesion

Persistent recurrent headaches

Chronic tension headache

Chronic migraine, with or without medication overuse

Secondary headaches, due to organic lesions, require further investigation and distinction from primary headaches like migraine in which the focus is on management.

The history is pivotal and the following mnemonic can help in collecting relevant characteristics: PPQRST + A.

P – provocative factors: stress, bending over, coughing, combing hair

P – palliative factors: lying down in the dark, taking analgesics

Q – quality of the pain, is it aching?

R – region: one sided, over the eye, occipital or temporal area?

S – severity: dull or worst pain ever?

T – timing: first ever, episodic, or present more than 15 days a month?

A – associated features: nausea, vomiting, photophobia, eye watering?

Examination

Should exclude papilledema. This reduces the probability of raised intracranial pressure but it can take days or weeks to develop. The following features raise the possibility of a secondary cause:

- Sudden onset first or worst headache (? subarachnoid hemorrhage)
- Headache made worse by coughing, bending, or straining (? raised intracranial pressure)
- Headache worse on waking, with vomiting (? raised intracranial pressure)
- Loss of consciousness or seizures (? space-occupying lesion)
- Confusion or cognitive impairment (? space-occupying lesion)
- Local tenderness, such as over temporal artery (? giant cell arteritis)
- Fever (? systemic illness)
- Neck stiffness (? meningism)
- Weakness, clumsiness, or numbness (? tumor)

Migraine

Diagnostic criteria for migraine without aura are:

A. At least five attacks fulfilling criteria B–F

B. Headache attacks lasting 4–72 hours (untreated or unsuccessfully treated)

C. Headache has at least two of the following:

Unilateral

Pulsating

Moderate or severe pain intensity

Aggravation by movement

D. During headache at least one of the following:

Nausea or vomiting

Photophobia and phonophobia

E. Normal physical examination

F. Not attributed to another disorder

The diagnostic criteria for a typical aura with migraine are:

A. At least two attacks fulfilling criteria B–E

B. Aura of at least one of the following, but no motor weakness:

Fully reversible flickering lights, spots, or lines and/or loss of vision

Fully reversible pins and needles and/or numbness

Fully reversible dysphasic speech

C. At least two of the following:

Homonymous visual symptoms and/or unilateral sensory symptoms

At least one aura symptom develops gradually over >5 minutes and/or different aura symptoms occur in succession over >5 minutes

Each symptom lasts >5 and <60 minutes

D. Headache fulfilling criteria B–D for migraine without aura (see above) begins during the aura or follows aura within 60 minutes

E. Not attributed to another disorder

Epidemiology

Primary headache is the commonest neurologic symptom, affecting 90% of the population at some time. In one year, tension headaches are reported by 80% women and 60% men, migraine reported by 15% women and 5% men. Headache occurrng on 15 or more days a month is reported by 5% and accounts for 20% work absence and 25% neurology referrals.

Pathology

A neurovascular disorder secondary to neural activation. Episodes probably result from primary dysfunction in brainstem nuclei involved in sensory and nociceptive modulation of craniovascular afferents. Pain arises from (1) pain-sensitive cranial blood vessels, (2) trigeminal nerve fibers that innervate them, and (3) the cranial parasympathetic outflow.

In practice, severe headaches not meeting these criteria are classified as migraine for the purpose of management. Most of these have migraine without aura.

Investigations

Where diagnosis is clear on history, further investigations are not necessary. Where unclear or in an elderly patient or where there is anxiety, a brain scan may reassure both parties.

Management

A challenge in headache management is overuse of analgesics. Dependence, rebound headache, and toxicity need to be explained. If headaches are frequent the relative advantages and side effects of prophylactic medication should be explained.

Aspirin 300–900 mg, paracetamol and non-steroidal anti-inflammatory agents are effective in migraine and tension headache when used intermittently.

First-line treatment when the above have failed is a "triptan" (5HT1B/1D-receptor agonists).

Prophylactic medication Frequent headaches or analgesic overuse are indications for prophylactic treatment. Two thirds obtain 50% reduction of headache frequency especially if analgesic use is reduced. The beta-blocker propranolol or the tricyclic antidepressant, amitriptyline are first line. Other commonly used prophylactics are pizotifen and anti epileptics, sodium valproate, gabapentin, and topiramate.

Behavioral treatments Cognitive behavioral therapy, stress management, and relaxation therapy can be as effective as prophylactic medication.

Outcome

A third have co-morbid symptoms of anxiety or depression. Engaging with patients' ideas and concerns provides reassurance. Repeat examination including blood pressure and occasional brain imaging may be the only way to reduce anxiety. Headache is also a common somatization symptom and can then benefit from cognitive behavior therapy, relaxation, and stress management training.

Headaches are episodic, and may recur and remit throughout life, especially in women, but diminish during pregnancy and after menopause. Frequency is low in the elderly, where new onset headache always requires investigation.

Headache syndromes

Tension headache. Patients describe pain of a boring quality which is bilateral, diffuse, not worsened by head movement, and has no associated features. Probe for psycho-social factors.

Cluster headache. An episode may last 60–90 minutes and is unilateral, beginning without warning, severe, and three times more common in men. The location is particularly around the eye, temple, and forehead. It is associated with eye- and nose-watering and vomiting. It is called cluster headache because it occurs over periods of weeks or months. Sumatriptan self-administered subcutaneously is the most effective remedy.

Paroxysmal hemicrania. This is a much rarer syndrome which affects women twice as often as men. This is strictly unilateral and severe, occurring 15 or more times daily lasting 2–25 minutes. Ipsilateral eye watering, nasal congestion, reddening of the eye, ptosis are usually present. It responds well to indomethacin.

Disorders of speech and swallowing

Disorders of speech and swallowing arise from different levels of the nervous system and can be due to several diseases (Table 9.2). The level is indicated in brackets with the most common conditions listed below.

Sudden onset:
- Stroke (brain)

Sub acute onset:
- Space-occupying lesions (brain)
- Multiple sclerosis (central nervous system – brain and spinal cord)
- Guillain–Barré syndrome (peripheral nerve)
- Polymyositis (muscle)

Gradual onset:
- Parkinson's disease and extrapyramidal disorders (basal ganglia and connections)
- Motor neuron disease (upper motor neuron and anterior horn cell)
- Myopathy (muscle)

Variable onset:
- Myasthenia gravis (neuromuscular junction)

Table 9.3 outlines additional clinical features that will help define the cause of speech or swallowing difficulties.

Definitions
Dysarthria

Disorder of articulation. Speech sounds abnormal and is often slurred.

Table 9.2. Timing of onset of speech and swallowing difficulties

Diagnosis	Minutes	Hours	Days	Weeks	Months	Years	Variable
Stroke	←→						
Space-occupying lesion			←——————→				
Parkinsonism					←————————→		
Multiple sclerosis			←——————→				
Motor neuron disease							←→
Myasthenia gravis					←——→		
Guillain–Barré syndrome		←——————→					
Myopathy					←————————→		
Polymyositis			←——→				
Oropharyngeal lesions			←——————→				

Dysphasia

Disorder of spoken language. There are two components, comprehension (reception) and expression. These can be affected individually or together. Dysphasia occurs with damage to the dominant hemisphere (Fig. 9.2). If Wernicke's area in the parietal cortex is affected there is lack of comprehension of speech. The patient is fluent but speech is full of jargon, paraphrasia (wrong but similar sounding words), and neologisms (made-up words). If Broca's area in the frontal cortex is damaged, there is full comprehension of speech but an inability to recall and vocalize correct words with difficulty naming objects (nominal dysphasia).

Table 9.3. Clinical features to be looked for in speech and swallowing problems

History	Examination
Onset: sudden or gradual	Quality of speech
Age	Receptive/expressive difficulty
Progressive, static, or intermittent	Fatiguability/ptosis
Risk factors for stroke	Hemiparesis/pattern of weakness
Weakness in limbs/pattern	Wasting/fasciculation
Tremor/slowness	Parkinsonian features
Previous neurologic episodes	Cerebellar signs
Alcohol intake	Lesions/masses in mouth/throat

Dysphonia

Disorder of the volume of vocalization.

Dysphagia

Difficulty with swallowing.

Dysarthria, dysphagia, and dysphonia may result from lesions in the motor cortex down to diseases affecting the buccal cavity, oropharynx, and larynx. Relevant sites within the nervous system include cerebral cortex, basal ganglia, cerebellum, brainstem, cranial nerves, and the neuromuscular junction.

Sudden onset

The predominant cause of sudden-onset difficulty with speech and swallowing is a vascular event within the brain (stroke). It may cause dysarthria, with or without dysphagia and/or dysphasia.

They may also be affected in a sub-acute manner by a number of neurologic conditions (Table 9.2). Additional symptoms and signs of these conditions are discussed later in this chapter.

Rapid onset neurologic deficit

Rapid onset neurologic dysfunction (developing over seconds or minutes), whether motor weakness, sensory loss, speech difficulty, or headache, is usually caused by a vascular event or trauma.

The vascular events may be ischemic, either thrombotic, embolic, or hemorrhage. It is difficult to differentiate clinically between an ischemic stroke and an intracerebral bleed. Other types of hemorrhage have characteristic onset, symptoms, signs, and progression.

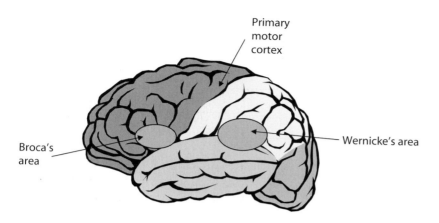

Fig. 9.2. The position of the main areas responsible for speech within the brain.

Primary motor cortex

Broca's area

Wernicke's area

Transient ischemic attack (TIA)

A focal, non-convulsive, neurologic deficit in the brain, caused by a vascular event lasting less than 24 hours. It is usually caused by an embolic phenomenon, commonly due to disruption of an atheromatous plaque or cardiac emboli.

Clinical features

Anterior circulation (carotid arteries):

- Amaurosis fugax (temporary blindness in one eye – ipsilateral to the affected carotid artery)
- Dysphasia
- Contralateral hemiparesis or monoparesis
- Contralateral hemisensory loss
- Contralateral homonymous visual field loss
- Any combination of the above

Posterior circulation (vertebral arteries):

- Diplopia
- Dysarthria/dysphagia
- Vertigo
- Unilateral/bilateral paresis or sensory loss
- Vertigo
- Homonymous hemianopia with macula sparing
- Binocular visual loss
- Ataxia
- Loss of consciousness (rare)
- Any combination of the above

Epidemiology

The incidence is 30 cases per 100 000 population per year. A third develop a stroke within 5 years if the cause is not fully addressed.

The pathology, risk factors, and investigation are the same as for completed stroke.

Investigation

Explore for carotid stenosis, atrial fibrillation, and investigate risk factors: hypertension, hyperlipidemia, and diabetes.

Management

Aspirin as soon as possible unless contraindications. Alternative anti-platelet drugs are dipyridamole or clopidogrel.

Indications for anticoagulation are atrial fibrillation or endocardial thrombosis. If carotid stenosis of greater than 70% on the affected side operative endarterectomy or radiologic stenting is warranted.

Stroke

A focal, non-convulsive, neurologic deficit in the brain, caused by a vascular event lasting more than 24 hours. Ischemic or thromboembolic events account for 85% and hemorrhage, usually secondary to hypertension, for 15%.

The most common presentation is hemiparesis, often with dysarthria, caused by occlusion of the middle cerebral artery or one of its branches. When the dominant hemisphere is affected, there may be dysphasia.

Clinical features

Onset sudden with loss of function.

Middle cerebral artery

- Contralateral hemiparesis/hemiplegia
- Contralateral cortical hemisensory loss
- Dysphasia – if dominant hemisphere (usually left)
- Dysarthria
- Contralateral homonymous hemianopia
- Neglect of contralateral limb/dressing apraxia – if non-dominant hemisphere

Anterior cerebral artery stroke

Occlusion proximal to the anterior communicating artery is often well tolerated due to cross flow, but distal occlusion will cause:

- Contralateral weakness in *lower limb only*
- Contralateral cortical sensory loss in *lower limb only*

Posterior cerebral artery stroke

- Proximal occlusion: (a) midbrain syndrome (Weber's syndrome) with ipsilateral third nerve palsy and contralateral hemiparesis, (b) thalamic syndrome; hemiballism; chorea or hemisensory loss
- Cortical vessel occlusion: homonymous hemianopia with macular sparing (macular area supplied by middle cerebral artery)
- Bilateral occlusion: Anton's syndrome (cortical blindness) – the patient is blind but lacks insight and denies blindness

Specific brainstem syndromes

- Lateral medullary syndrome (Wallenberg's syndrome) – occlusion of posterior inferior cerebellar artery (PICA) causing sudden vertigo, vomiting, ipsilateral ataxia, ipsilateral facial sensory loss with contralateral loss of pain and temperature in the limbs ("Harlequin syndrome"), nystagmus, and ipsilateral Horner's syndrome
- Locked-in syndrome – caused by bilateral infarction, usually at the level of the pons. The patient is mute and paralyzed although fully conscious.
- There are other patterns but the two most notable are above

Epidemiology

Third most common cause of death in the United Kingdom. The incidence is 150–200 cases per 100 000, with 60 000 deaths per year. The incidence increases with age.

Pathology

Ischemia causes impaired brain metabolism and if severe enough, cell death occurs. This may result from narrowing and ultimate occlusion of arteries by atherosclerosis, lipohyalinosis or, rarely, vasculitis; emboli from atherosclerotic plaques, or clots, or rupture of vessels causing bleeds.

Risk factors

- Hypertension – thrombotic, hemorrhagic strokes and lacunar infarcts
- Diabetes mellitus – increases risk of ischemic stroke twofold
- Smoking
- Hyperlipidemia – less significant than in coronary artery disease
- Cardiac disease – coronary artery disease as marker for atherosclerosis. Atrial fibrillation, other arrhythmias, cardiomyopathy, and valve disease
- Family history – close relatives. In young, thrombotic tendencies or homocysteinuria
- Oral contraceptive – may increase the risk of thromboembolic stroke and cerebral venous thrombosis
- Patent foramen ovale

Investigation

Essential to distinguish ischemic and hemorrhagic stroke or an alternative cause, especially in younger patients.

Initial:

CT, or MRI scan to rule out hemorrhage and (Fig. 9.3) less likely, a tumor. This also enables assessment for thrombolysis and excludes arterial dissection in young persons.

Full blood count (polycythemia; thrombocythemia, thrombocytopenia; infection), urea and electrolytes (dehydration; renal failure; liver failure), erythrocyte sedimentation rate (inflammatory disease; vasculitis), clotting screen (bleeding tendency or anticoagulation treatment), blood glucose and urinalysis (diabetes mellitus), fasting lipids (hyperlipidemia), blood cultures if endocarditis suspected.

In a young person a thrombophilia screen (protein S and protein C deficiencies, antithrombin III deficiency, Factor V Leiden, APC resistance, anti-phospholipid antibodies, lupus anticoagulant) and homocysteine level to rule out a thrombophilic tendency or homocysteinuria, and autoantibodies anti-nuclear antibody (ANA), anti-neutrophil cytoplasmic antibody (ANCA), anti-double stranded DNA (*anti*-dsDNA) to rule out a connective tissue disease or vasculitis (see Chapter 11).

Electrocardiography to detect atrial fibrillation or paroxysmal arrhythmia and MI (risk of mural thrombus).

Chest X-ray to explore neoplasia or cardiomegaly.

Blood culture and echocardiogram if endocarditis or valvular disease suspected.

Additional:

Carotid Doppler

(a)

(b)

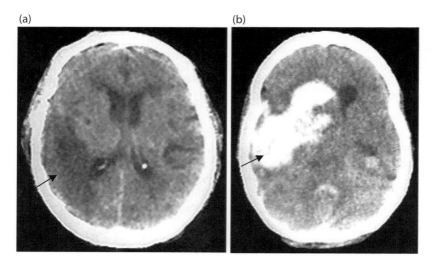

Fig. 9.3. CT scans of the brain from two different patients. (a) A few hours after an ischemic stroke. There is a wedge-shaped area of hypodensity (darker area marked by arrow) showing the area of infarction. (b) A few hours after a hemorrhagic stroke. There is an area of hyperdensity (white area marked by arrow) showing the area occupied by fresh blood. (Fresh blood appears white on a CT scan.)

Angiography (IV, CTA or MRA) for diagnosis and management of intracerebral aneurysms and arteriovenous malformations and for the degree of carotid or vertebral stenosis or dissection.

Management

Rapid diagnosis, admission, and initiation of treatment maximise recovery and prevent recurrence. Intracerebral hemorrhage is treated conservatively unless there is risk of coning or a cerebellar bleed, when surgery may be indicated.

Presentation within 3 hours may allow thrombolysis with intravenous anteplase (tissue plasminogen activator-rtPA) followed by aspirin.

If presentation of ischemic stroke is later than 3 hours and hemorrhage excluded, 300 mg aspirin continued daily or alternative anti-platelet drug.

Monitor blood pressure – treat if systolic >200 mm Hg or diastolic >110 mm Hg. Adequate blood pressure is required to maintain cerebral blood flow. Dropping the blood pressure can extend infarction.

Prevention of early complications:

- Aspiration pneumonia – nasogastric feeding if necessary
- Deep vein thrombosis (DVT) and pulmonary emboli (PE) – thromboembolic stockings (TEDS), subcutaneous heparin, early mobilization if possible
- Cardiac arrhythmia (especially if the cause of the stroke)
- Pressure sores – regular turning if bed-bound
- Cerebral edema – may require crainiectomy (rare)

- Anticoagulation for arrhythmia once bleed has been excluded at least 5 days after ischemic stroke to prevent secondary hemorrhage, antibiotics for endocarditis
- Rehabilitation – physiotherapy, occupational therapy, speech therapy, and psychologic support.

Outcome

A third die within 10 days, a third recover within a month and a third are left with residual disability that may or may not improve. Mortality is higher with intracerebral hemorrhage. The worst prognosis is predicted by reduced consciousness, dense hemiplegia, and conjugate gaze palsy.

There is further 60%–70% mortality within 3 years from chest infection, pulmonary emboli, or other atherosclerotic disease.

Extradural hemorrhage

A consequence of head trauma, causing tearing of the middle meningeal vessels. The bleed may arise from either the veins or arteries or both. There is usually an associated fracture of the skull in the parietal or temporal region.

Epidemiology

1%–3% of all hospital attendances with head injury. In comatose patients (Glasgow Coma Score 8 or less), the incidence is 10% (Table 9.4).

The most common cause is road traffic accidents followed by falls, assaults, sporting injuries, and birth trauma.

Table 9.4. The Glagow Coma Scale (GCS)

Eye Opening (E):	
Nil	1
To pain	2
To speech	3
Spontaneous	4
Best Motor Response (M):	
Nil	1
Abnormal extension	2
Abnormal flexion	3
Withdraws	4
Localizes	5
Obeys command	6
Best Verbal Response (V):	
Nil	1
Incomprehensible sounds	2
Inappropriate words	3
Confused speech	4
Oriented	5
Recorded as E + M + V	
(e.g. E4; M6; V5 = 15) (Minimum = 3/maximum = 15)	
GCS of E2; M4; V2 or less is considered as coma	
Tracheostomy, endotracheal tube, or facial injuries invalidate the verbal response	

It is less common under age 2 and above 60 because of greater adherence of dura mater to the inner calvarial table. Males are affected 4 : 1.

Pathology
A blow to the head sufficient to deform the skull and strip the underlying dura mater from the inner calvarial table.

Clinical Features
Classically, the patient may be unconscious at the time of impact, and then have a variable "lucid interval", before progressing into coma. If not recognized and drained, coning and death ensue.

Investigation
Urgent CT scan. Compression of the underlying brain is characteristic with effacement of the ipsilateral ventricular system and shift of midline structures.

MRI scanning is less useful acutely and lumbar puncture is contraindicated.

Management
Surgical evacuation of the hematoma is indicated usually through a craniotomy, over the point of maximum hematoma thickness.

Management on an intensive care unit is usually required and patients may require neurorehabilitation.

Outcome
An unrecognized extradural hematoma will increase in size and cause coning and death. Favorable outcomes in 55%–94%. Mortality is 5%–41%.

Subdural hemorrhage
Due to rupture of cortical bridging vessels between the dura mater and the brain, usually associated with trauma. Head injury is less severe than in extradural hematomas and without fracture. Patients on anticoagulants and with bleeding tendencies are particularly at risk.

Acute subdural bleeds are clinically evident by 48–72 hours and composed of clot. Chronic subdurals tend to be fluid and present over 20 days. Subacute hematomas detected between 3 days and 3 weeks after trauma usually contain mixed clot and fluid.

Clinical features
Determined by severity of injury at time of impact and rate of hematoma growth.

In acute hemorrhage, altered consciousness, pupillary changes (usually dilatation ipsilateral to the bleed), and focal motor deficits. In a more chronic subdural, there may be indolent, fluctuating confusion, drowsiness, and headache.

Epidemiology
Incidence higher in men. Patients tend to be older than those with other head injuries, average age 40. The frequency is 1%–5% of all head injuries and 5%–22% of severe head injuries. Falls are the most common cause.

Pathology
Usually caused by acceleration–deceleration causing arterial or venous lacerations.

Investigation
CT scan. In chronic cases, the hematoma may be the same density as the brain substance and MRI scan is then invaluable.

Management
Evacuating a thin acute subdural hematoma (less than 3 mm) is rarely indicated but for larger hematomas or worsening neurologic status, evacuation of

hematoma, control of hemorrhage, resection of non-viable brain, and removal of confluent intra-parenchymal hemorrhage are performed.

More chronic lesions may be managed conservatively and often regress spontaneously.

Outcome

Severe brain injury is less common than in extradural hemorrhage.

Mortality with severe head injury with an evacuated subdural hematoma ranges from 42%–65%. The outcome is favorable in chronic subdural bleeding.

Subarachnoid hemorrhage

Caused by spontaneous rupture of an intracranial vessel, usually arterial and most commonly due to saccular ("Berry") aneurysms. A small proportion are caused by bleeding from arteriovenous malformation.

Clinical features

Headache occurs in 85% to 95%. It is sudden and explosive often associated with nausea or vomiting, and classically described as the "worst headache of one's life" and as if one has been "hit over the head with a cricket bat".

Pain may radiate into the occipital or cervical region. Meningism often develops with neck stiffness and positive Kernig's sign. Seizures, photophobia, lethargy, and altered consciousness may occur. Persistent change in the level of consciousness may be due to hydrocephalus, persistently elevated intracranial pressure, or vasospasm.

Focal neurologic signs from the hematoma may include limb weakness, dysarthria, third nerve palsy. Fundoscopy may reveal subhyaloid and vitreous hemorrhages.

Occasionally patients develop a severe headache as described above, which settles. This can be due to a "sentinel bleed," followed by a full subarachnoid hemorrhage within 2–20 days.

Epidemiology

The incidence is 10 to 12 per 100 000, with saccular aneurysms accounting for 75%–80%. The prevalence of aneurysms in the adult population is between 2% and 5%, and the risk of bleeding 1% per year.

A familial relationship may exist, alone via autosomal dominant inheritance, or in association with other disorders such as Marfan's and Ehlers–Danlos syndromes, pseudoxanthoma elasticum, polycystic kidneys, and coarctation of the aorta.

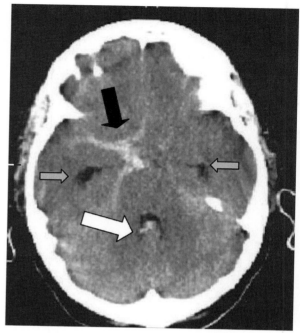

Fig. 9.4. CT scan of the brain showing a subarachnoid hemorrhage. The black arrow indicates blood, which is maximal on the right side. The white arrow indicates blood in the fourth ventricle and the temporal horns are prominent (gray arrows), indicating early hydrocephalus. An angiogram subsequently revealed an aneurysm of the right posterior communicating artery in this patient.

Pathology

Cerebral arteries penetrate the cranial cavity and smaller branches enter the brain. When blood extravasates from a ruptured vessel into the subarachnoid space, it spreads through the CSF. It is irritant and causes meningeal signs, or it may clot and block CSF flow leading to hydrocephalus. The volume effect of the blood can cause raised intracranial pressure. Reduced cerebral perfusion can cause reduced consciousness and death.

Investigation

CT scanning, without contrast, is the investigation of choice (Fig. 9.4) It should detect subarachnoid blood in more than 85% within 48 hours of the bleed. It should also demonstrate magnitude of the bleed, location, and any hydrocephalus.

If CT scan is equivocal or negative or unavailable, a lumbar puncture should be carried out, but only if, patient is alert without signs of raised intracranial pressure or focal signs. The CSF may appear blood stained or xanthochromic (straw colored supernatant). The xanthochromia occurs due to breakdown products of hemoglobin and may take up to 6 hours to develop. MRI scanning is unhelpful.

Most require cerebral angiogram to determine location and size of the aneurysm and degree of vasospasm, usually a few days after the bleed.

Management

- Bed rest and fluid replacement
- Regular neurologic observations
- Analgesia
- Calcium channel blockers – usually nimodipine which reduces vasospasm
- Control of excessive hypertension – with care to avoid hypotension, which can cause neurologic deterioration
- If seizures occur anticonvulsants should be prescribed
- Transfer to a neurosurgical unit when stabilized

Subsequent management

Neuroradiological intervention with coiling or Surgical clipping of the neck of the aneurysm. The timing of intervention is controversial: too early and it can be harmful due to retraction of a swollen non-compliant brain, and a potentially unstable patient; too long and there can be risk of rebleeding and the effects of vasospasm. Most surgeons opt for the earliest possible intervention from about 3 days after the bleed.

Outcome

15% to 20% die prior to reaching hospital. Of the remainder many develop rebleeding from the aneurysm, delayed ischemic neurologic deficit due to vasospasm, hydrocephalus, and seizures.

Incidence of rebleeding is 4% within first 48 hours and 20% within 2 weeks. After 6 months the rebleed rate is 3% per year. Early aneurysmal rebleeding has a mortality rate of 60% to 70%.

Hydrocephalus, acute or delayed, occurs in 20%. Mortality approximates 50%, and 50% of survivors suffer permanent neurologic disability. For non-aneurysmal subarachnoid hemorrhage mortality is less than 3% with only 4% rebleeding during the following 6 months.

Arteriovenous malformations

Represent an aberrant persistence of embryonic vascular connections between arteries and veins. They are rare causes of intracerebral hemorrhage or other vascular events, but are potentially treatable, especially if found prior to bleeding.

Clinical features

Most commonly hemorrhage, but also seizure or focal deficits. Cerebral imaging uncovers many asymptomatic AVMs.

Seizure, the second most common presenting symptom, occurs in 30%.

Epidemiology

Many are asymptomatic so estimates of incidence and prevalence are difficult. However, based on prospective post-mortem examinations of over 3000 brains, the incidence was found to be approximately 0.6%. Risk of hemorrhage in patients with arteriovenous malformations who have not had a previous hemorrhage is 1%–4% annually.

Pathology

Most often congenital anomalies with abnormal connections between arterial and venous circulations.

Investigation

CT scanning but large hematomas may obscure an AVM. Occasionally the serpiginous enlarged feeding vessels may be seen on CT. Cerebral angiogram if treatment is planned.

Management

Three therapeutic options: (1) surgical resection, (2) embolization, (3) stereotactic radiosurgery.

Outcome

AVMs with hemorrhage have mortality of 10% and an annual rebleed rate of 6% to 18%. Over 60% have minimal or no deficit but 3% are severely disabled.

Many are found incidentally or present with seizures or focal deficits. Intervention depends on risk–benefit discussion.

Traumatic spinal injury

Spinal transection is usually due to severe trauma caused by anterior dislocation of a vertebra. There is loss of all motor, sensory, autonomic, and sphincter function below the level of the lesion, either immediately if complete, or within hours as a result of edema if incomplete. The neural supply to the diaphragm via the phrenic nerve (C3, 4 and 5) is also lost in high level compression.

Clinical features

There are two stages:

(1) Spinal shock – loss of all reflex activity below the level of the lesion, flaccid limbs, atonic bladder with overflow incontinence, atonic bowel, gastric

dilatation, loss of vasomotor control and genital reflexes. This stage can last up to 2 weeks.

(2) Heightened reflex activity – occurs after 1–2 weeks, with spasticity of the limbs, hyper-reflexia, extensor plantar responses, spastic bladder (small capacity with urgency, frequency, and automatic emptying), and hyperactive autonomic function (sweating and vasomotor responses).

A similar picture may result from ischemic infarction of the cord (anterior spinal artery syndrome) or hemorrhage into the spinal cord (AVM, epidural or subdural hemorrhage).

Epidemiology

The annual incidence of spinal cord injury (SCI), excluding death at the scene, is 40 per million population. Road traffic accidents account for 37%, ballistic violence 27%, falls 21%, and sports injuries 7%.

Pathology

Spinal cord injury can result from: mechanical insult, biochemical derangement, hemodynamic alteration, or premorbid pathology. This produces initial neural dysfunction. Over a period, the spinal cord becomes swollen and necrotic with changes in the microvasculature and sluggish axoplasmic flow. Progressive gray matter necrosis ensues, with fragmentation of white matter.

Investigation

Prior to investigations, it is essential to immobilize the spine. Anteroposterior and lateral plain radiographs of the entire spine in all trauma cases. Radiologic localization with CT/MRI is essential since multilevel trauma is not uncommon.

Management

Screening of trauma victims for spinal cord injury is routine. Immobilization of the spine continues until instability is ruled out. Intravenous methylprednisolone reduces damage to cellular membranes and inflammation. Indications for surgery include spinal instability, progressive neurologic deficits with extrinsic spinal cord compression, compound spinal injuries with or without neurologic dysfunction.

Outcome

Most upper extremity recovery is expected during 6 months after injury. Eleven percent of patients improve by at least 1 grade, but only 2.8% gain useful motor function. Late conversion (30 days to 2.5 years post-injury) from complete to incomplete spinal cord injury occurs in 4%–10%.

Cardiopulmonary complications are the major cause of death. Mortality is 5%–10% even with advanced life support. Other mortality and morbidity are due to sepsis secondary to urinary tract infection, decubitus ulcers, deep venous thrombosis, pulmonary emboli, and contractures.

Slower onset neurologic deficit

With upper motor neuron signs (central nervous system)

- Space- occupying lesions (brain)
- Multiple sclerosis (brain, brainstem, and spinal cord)
- Motor neuron disease (brain and spinal cord)
- Cord compression/myelopathy (spinal cord)

With lower motor neuron signs

- Radiculopathy (nerve root)
- Plexopathy (brachial and lumbo-sacral plexus)
- Peripheral neuropathy (peripheral nerve)
  - Mononeuropathy
  - Mononeuritis multiplex
  - Polyneuropathy

Neuromuscular junction disorders:

- Myasthenia gravis
- Lambert Eaton myasthenic syndrome (LEMS)
- Botulism/botulinum toxin

Myopathies:

- Inherited
- Acquired

When neurologic deficits present more slowly a combination of history, examination, the distribution and type of deficit, and associated features is used to try to make the diagnosis (Table 9.5).

Distinguishing features:

- Space-occupying lesion – signs of raised intracranial pressure (headache worse in morning), progressive focal neurologic signs
- Multiple sclerosis relapsing–remitting; multifocal neurologic signs
- Motor neuron disease – progressive pure motor syndrome
- Cord compression/myelopathy progressive upper motor neuron signs in both legs or all four limbs, sensory level, bladder, and bowel dysfunction
- Radiculopathy pain radiating in distribution of a nerve root and relevant dermatome, sensory loss, weakness in the relevant myotome. If at the level

Table 9.5. Speed of onset of some neurologic disorders may be characteristic

Diagnosis	Days	Weeks	Months	Years	Variable
Space-occupying lesion			◄———————►	——►	
Multiple sclerosis:					
(1) Acute relapse	◄——————————►				
(2) Secondary progression		◄————————►			
Cord compression	◄————————►				
Motor neuron disease			◄——————►		
Radiculopathy	◄————————►				
Peripheral neuropathy:					
(1) Acute	◄————►				
(2) Chronic		◄——————————►			
Myasthenia gravis					◄——►
Lambert–Eaton syndrome					◄——►
Botulism/Botox	◄———►				
Myopathy			◄———►		
Polymyositis		◄——————————►			

of a tendon reflex, there may be reduction or loss of the reflex

- Plexopathy usually unilateral in one limb
- Peripheral neuropathy, most commonly an ascending "glove and stocking" sensory change in a typical axonal sensory neuropathy; may be distal weakness and wasting in some forms of neuropathy
- Mononeuropathies and entrapment neuropathies; signs in distribution of the single nerve
- Myasthenia gravis: variable muscle weakness especially after exertion, particularly affecting muscles of the eyelid (ptosis), extraocular muscles (diplopia), proximal limb muscles, and bulbar musculature (dysarthria and dysphagia); normal reflexes
- Lambert-Eaton Myasthenic Syndrome (LEMS) – variable muscle weakness, may improve with exertion; mainly proximal muscle, usually associated with occult neoplasia. No sensory symptoms and signs
- Botulism: symmetric, descending flaccid paralysis, with prominent cranial palsies causing diplopia, dysarthria, dysphonia, dysphagia, facial weakness, pupil dilatation
- Myopathy – usually proximal muscles, sometimes inherited, raised creatine kinase (CK).
- Polymyositis with possible skin involvement, raised ESR and CK, typical changes on EMG; inflammatory change on muscle biopsy. No sensory involvement.

Space-occupying lesions

These require exclusion in any slowly progressive neurologic deficit, affecting speech, swallowing, cranial nerve, limb function, or any symptoms or signs of raised intracranial pressure.

The cause may be due to tumors, infections such as tuberculosis, toxoplasmosis, bacterial abscesses, or inflammatory conditions such as sarcoidosis.

Clinical features

Raised intracranial pressure – headache worse on lying down and in the morning, vomiting and papilledema. These features develop slowly. The full picture is more common with posterior fossa tumors. As a result of

273

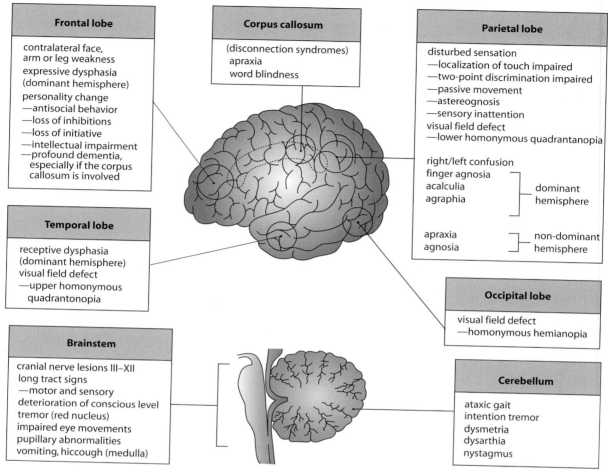

Frontal lobe

contralateral face,
arm or leg weakness
expressive dysphasia
(dominant hemisphere)
personality change
—antisocial behavior
—loss of inhibitions
—loss of initiative
—intellectual impairment
—profound dementia,
especially if the corpus
callosum is involved

Corpus callosum

(disconnection syndromes)
apraxia
word blindness

Parietal lobe

disturbed sensation
—localization of touch impaired
—two-point discrimination impaired
—passive movement
—astereognosis
—sensory inattention
visual field defect
—lower homonymous quadrantanopia

right/left confusion
finger agnosia
acalculia
agraphia

> dominant
hemisphere

apraxia
agnosia

> non-dominant
hemisphere

Temporal lobe

receptive dysphasia
(dominant hemisphere)
visual field defect
—upper homonymous
quadrantonopia

Occipital lobe

visual field defect
—homonymous hemianopia

Brainstem

cranial nerve lesions III–XII
long tract signs
—motor and sensory
deterioration of conscious level
tremor (red nucleus)
impaired eye movements
pupillary abnormalities
vomiting, hiccough (medulla)

Cerebellum

ataxic gait
intention tremor
dysmetria
dysarthia
nystagmus

Fig. 9.5. Focal neurologic signs according to the site of the space-occupying lesion.

raised intracranial pressure the brainstem may be compressed by the cerebellar tonsils being squeezed through the foramen magnum (coning). This is usually fatal. The uncus of the temporal lobe may herniate causing third nerve palsy.

False localizing signs are sixth nerve palsy caused by stretching of the nerve during its long intracranial course and third nerve palsy due to herniation of the temporal lobe. Progressive focal neurologic signs including dysarthria, dysphasia, and hemiparesis are due to compression, infiltration, or edema (Fig. 9.5).

Seizures and slowly progressive focal neurologic signs are the most common presentation of intracerebral tumors.

Epidemiology

Intracranial tumors may be benign e.g. meningiomas or malignant, e.g. gliomas. They can arise within the cranial cavity ("primary") or may be metastatic, e.g. lung, breast. Primary intracranial tumors account for approximately 10% of all neoplasms.

Malignant – gliomas (especially astrocytomas and oligodendrogliomas) 40%; metastases (the older the patient, the more likely it is that an intracerebral lesion is a metastasis) 25%; meningioma 10%; pituitary adenoma 10%; neurofibroma/Schwannoma 5%; others 15%.

Pathology

- Gliomas – malignant, primary, intrinsic arising from neuroglia within the cerebrum. They rarely metastasize outside the central nervous system and spread by direct extension.

Astrocytoma is the commonest.

Oligodendroglioma – slow-growing, sharply defined tumors which may calcify.

Ependymoma – derived from ependymal cells and the choroid plexus arising anywhere throughout the ventricular system or spinal canal.

Glioblastoma multiforme – a highly malignant tumor with poor prognosis.

- Meningiomas – benign, arising from meninges extrinsic to the brain substance. They may grow slowly to a considerable size before symptoms develop. They often calcify.
- Pituitary tumors – are usually benign. They may cause endocrine dysfunction. If sufficiently large, they present with visual dysfunction due to compression of the optic chiasm, resulting in bitemporal hemianopia.
- Neurofibromas and Schwannomas – these arise from Schwann cells. The principal intracranial site is the cerebellopontine angle, arising from the eighth cranial nerve sheath ("acoustic neuroma/Schwannoma"). This is a common finding in neurofibromatosis type 2, but is more commonly sporadic. Typical features include ipsilateral sensory deafness and tinnitus, ipsilateral fifth and lower motor neuron seventh nerve palsies, and ipsilateral cerebellar signs.

Investigation

If suspected, imaging with CT or MRI, preferably with contrast. MRI is the investigation of choice for posterior fossa mass lesions. Small masses and meningeal lesions may be missed on CT scanning.

Electroencephalogram (EEG) is unhelpful. A brain biopsy is often needed.

Management

The area around a tumor becomes edematous and can be reduced with dexamethasone or other steroids.

Seizures may be difficult to control with anticonvulsants in a rapidly growing tumor and after surgery. Benign tumors, such as meningiomas, can often be removed entirely. Malignant tumors, which may not be well circumscribed, are usually debulked if symptomomatic. Some low grade tumors are treated conservatively.

Radiotherapy is usually recommended for gliomas and radiosensitive metastases. It is palliative to reduce size of tumor.

Chemotherapy is adjuvant to debulking surgery and radiotherapy in highly malignant tumors.

Outcome

For malignant high grade primary brain tumors, 1 year survival is less than 50%. Benign tumors, especially meningiomas and neurofibromas, are often cured by excision.

Multiple sclerosis

Particularly affects young adults with high levels of morbidity but low mortality. The disease classically runs a relapsing–remitting course but often becomes secondarily progressive, with a slow decline in function with or without definite acute relapses. A few patients show progression from onset (primary progressive).

Clinical features

No single presentation is diagnostic although some patterns are suggestive.

Clinically a patient must have more than one episode of central nervous system (CNS) or optic nerve involvement to make the diagnosis. The episodes may be separated by many years initially. It is not uncommon to have an episode of optic neuritis in the teens or early 20s and re-present in late 20s or 30s with an episode of CNS neurologic dysfunction.

Many patients complain of "Uhthoff's phenomenon" with worsening of symptoms when hot, e.g. in the bath.

Common presentations

- Optic and retrobulbar neuritis – subacute loss of central vision (central scotoma), usually unilateral and often with pain on ocular movement. Recovery is usual over days or weeks. On examination it is usual to find a relative afferent papillary defect (Marcus-Gunn pupil – Fig. 9.6), defects in color vision, and a pale optic disc on ophthalmoscopy (optic atrophy).

Ophthalmologic findings depend on whether the area of demyelination is at the optic nerve head (optic neuritis/papillitis), when the disc looks pink and swollen, or in the optic nerve behind the eye (retrobulbar neuritis), when the disk looks normal.

Optic neuritis is the forerunner to episodes of demyelination in 70%. It may occur in temporal association with transverse myelopathy and can be bilateral (Devic's syndrome; neuromyelitis optica). This also has other causes.

In many, optic neuritis is asymptomatic and discovered by finding optic atrophy.

- Brainstem presentation – common, particularly of cerebellar connections and the medial longitudinal

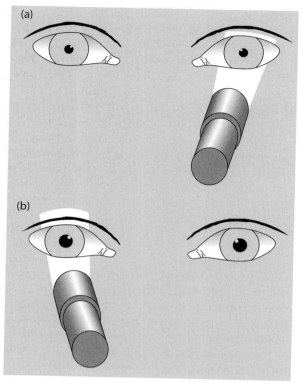

(a)

(b)

Fig. 9.6. Relative afferent pupillary defect (RAPD) in the right eye. The light shone in the normal left eye (a) causes consensual constriction of both pupils, but swinging the light to the abnormal right eye (b) causes the right eye (and to a lesser extent the left eye) to dilate. Less light gets into the afferent arc of the reflex and the transmission is slower due to the right optic neuritis.

fasciculus (MLF), joining 3rd and 6th nerve nuclei from opposite sides to allow conjugate eye movements (internuclear ophthalmoplegia).

Common brainstem clinical features are:

Diplopia – most commonly internuclear ophthalmoplegia from a lesion in the MLF (failure of adduction of the ipsilateral eye, with coarse nystagmus of the opposite eye when looking away from the side of the lesion). More commonly bilateral, when it is pathognomonic of MS.

Nystagmus – affecting both eyes, usually on lateral gaze, indicating involvement of the cerebellar connections.

Dysarthria – usually cerebellar ("scanning dysarthria").

Ataxia – unilateral or bilateral from involvement of the cerebellar connections.

Vertigo – often severe and persistent for days to weeks.

Upper motor neuron signs (pyramidal signs) – with involvement of the corticospinal tracts within the brainstem. The signs will be contralateral to the plaque, if above the decussation of the tracts in the medulla, and ipsilateral if below.

Myelopathy (spinal cord lesion) – spastic paraparesis (affecting both legs) or tetraparesis/quadraparesis (affecting both arms and legs bilaterally) are common with a sensory level, bladder dysfunction, and spasms of the limbs.

Epidemiology

More common in temperate climates, the incidence increasing proportionally with distance from the equator. In the UK it is 90–180 per 100 000, higher in Scotland and lower in southern England. Moving from a high prevalence to a low prevalence area before puberty reduces the risk. Women are more often affected. The peak age of onset is 20–30.

Pathology

Pathogenesis is unknown. Immunologic mechanisms play a major role.

There is destruction of myelin (demyelination) with relative preservation of axons. Areas of demyelination are called "plaques." In an acute lesion, mononuclear cells and lymphocytes are found. Remyelination is rare and the mechanism of functional recovery is uncertain. There is a particular predilection for demyelination to occur in the periventricular region of the brain, the brainstem, cerebellar connections (especially the medial longitudinal fasciculus/MLF), cervical cord, and optic nerves.

Investigations

There is no definitive diagnostic test. Two or more relapsing–remitting CNS or optic nerve episodes and two or more positive tests make diagnosis secure.

MRI may show plaques of demyelination which are typically multifocal, particularly in the periventricular region, the brainstem and spinal cord. The pattern of white matter hyperintensity is suggestive but also occurs in vascular, granulomatous and inflammatory disorders (Fig. 9.7). Once formed the lesions persist, despite complete clinical recovery. The number of lesions on MRI bears no relation to the severity of the clinical picture. In primary progressive MS, which tends to be more severe, there are few MRI lesions.

Routine cerebrospinal fluid (CSF) examination is usually normal even during acute relapse.

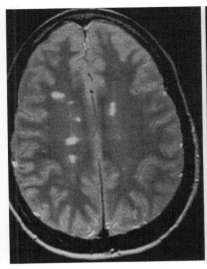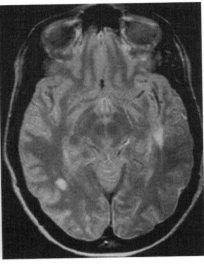

Fig. 9.7. Axial MRI scans of the brain showing hyperintense lesions in multiple sclerosis.

Occasionally, there may be mild pleocytosis (increased white cell count) or raised protein.

Oligoclonal bands in the CSF but not the serum, in the context of an indicative clinical picture, are suggestive but also found in infective and inflammatory conditions involving the CNS.

Evoked potentials are electrophysiologic tests with electrodes on the scalp, recording time taken for impulses to be conveyed along the visual, sensory, and auditory pathways to the brain. These may be delayed but are not specific. Visual evoked potentials (VEPs) are most commonly performed and are delayed in previous optic neuritis.

Management
If acute relapses are mild they usually settle spontaneously and it is better to avoid medication.

If relapse is more severe affecting normal function a short course of high dose oral or IV steroids. This may shorten relapse but not alter the outcome.

Multiple relapses require disease modifying therapy with restriction of steroids for severe relapses. The beta-interferons 1a and 1b and copaxone modulate the immunologic response and reduce the relapse rate by 30%–40%. Other immunosuppressants including mitoxantrone and the monoclonal antibody natalizumab are also used.

Baclofen and tizanidine are anti-spasticity agents and can be helpful. Botulinum toxin is also used where contractures develop.

Anticholinergic drugs may help incontinence in conjunction with intermittent self-catheterization.

Prevention or early treatment of urinary tract infections is essential, because intercurrrent infection causes relapse. Disturbing and painful sensory symptoms may be helped by amitriptyline, gabapentin, carbamazepine, or other anticonvulsives.

Intention tremor due to cerebellar involvement is helped by clonazepam. In severe cases, surgery may be considered with the use of deep brain stimulation.

Outcome
Over 85% present with a relapsing–remitting picture. Some have few and minor relapses separated by years, others have multiple severe relapses each year with additive residual disability.

About 50% progress to the secondary progressive form. After 15 years, 30% are still working and 40% still walking. Mortality is low and life expectancy slightly reduced.

Motor neuron disease (MND)
Progressive degeneration of motor nerve cells in the motor cortex (upper motor neuron), the somatic motor nuclei of the brainstem, and the anterior horn cells of the spinal cord (lower motor neuron). In the UK the term motor neuron disease encompasses three main clinical presentations (amyotrophic lateral sclerosis/ALS, progressive muscular atrophy/PMA, and bulbar/pseudobulbar palsy) and a possible fourth (primary lateral sclerosis/PLS), which remains more controversial. Elsewhere "amyotrophic lateral sclerosis" is used synonymously with the term "motor neuron disease".

Clinical features

As it progresses, involvement of bulbar muscles makes aspiration pneumonia likely. Dysarthria makes the patient unintelligible. Patients often become wheelchair or bed-bound. Complications such as pressure sores are less common than in other neurologic conditions, as sensation remains intact. Cognitive function remains intact.

Respiratory muscles and the diaphragm are commonly affected.

Amyotrophic lateral sclerosis (ALS)

Upper and lower motor neuron signs within the same territory, e.g. marked wasting and fasciculations in one or more limbs (LMN) with spasticity and brisk reflexes (UMN). There may also be mixed bulbar features. (e.g. wasted, fasciculating tongue, spastic slow tongue movements, and brisk jaw jerk) with dysarthria. The features develop slowly over months (Fig. 9.8). As ALS progresses speaking aids, feeding tubes, and non-invasive respiratory support (NIPPV) may be needed earlier than with limb-onset patients. "Bulbar palsy" refers to involvement of the lower motor neuron (wasted, fasciculating tongue, floppy palate with nasal regurgitation) and "pseudobulbar palsy" to upper motor neuron. Most commonly occur.

Progressive bulbar and pseudobulbar palsy

Dysarthria and dysphagia develop over months. Initially there are few signs at other sites. Bulbar palsy means involvement of lower motor neurons of cranial nerves and pseudobulbar refers to disease of the upper motor neurons. Commonly there is a mixture of the two. Signs are stiff spastic tongue and palate, brisk jaw jerk or wasted, fasciculating tongue, floppy palate, and nasal regurgitation, or combinations of these. As the disease progresses, signs of ALS develop as well.

Progressive muscular atrophy (PMA)

Lower motor neuron syndrome, beginning asymmetrically in the small muscles of the hands or with foot drop and then spreads. Bulbar and upper motor neuron features may develop to produce a more typical ALS picture. Neurophysiology is needed to exclude a treatable condition, multifocal motor neuropathy with conduction block (MMN+CB), which can present in a similar fashion.

Primary lateral sclerosis (PLS)

A controversial subgroup of MND. It is a rare, pure upper motor neuron syndrome and is a diagnosis of exclusion.

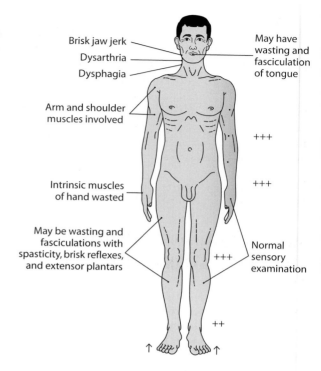

Fig. 9.8. Clinical findings in a patient with classical amyotrophic lateral sclerosis. There is a mixture of upper and lower motor neuron signs in the limbs and often a mixed bulbar and pseudobulbar picture (e.g. wasted fasciculating tongue, with a spastic palate). The latter may remain isolated or be the presenting feature of ALS.

Epidemiology

Prevalence 4 per 100 000 and annual incidence 1 per 100 000, increasing with age and peaking ages 55–75. Predominantly in men (2 : 1). It is a sporadic, acquired disease of uncertain etiology. In 5%–10% there is a genetic component. Over 100 mutations have been found on the Cu/Zn SOD-1 gene on chromosome 21.

Investigations

Neurophysiology. There should be near normal nerve conduction studies. EMG shows denervation in muscles supplied by more than one spinal level.

Management

There is no cure. Riluzole is a glutamate antagonist and increases survival by 3–6 months and seems more beneficial in bulbar-onset patients. It has no effect on disability.

Symptomatic treatment includes speech therapy and communication aids, modification of diet for safe swallowing. Patients may ultimately need a gastrostomy feeding tube and non-invasive positive pressure ventilation (NIPPV) for respiratory difficulties.

Physiotherapy, walking aids, orthoses (e.g. foot splints), wheelchairs are needed to aid mobility. Air bed mattresses to prevent pressure sores and house adaptations to allow patients to stay at home. Palliative care in terminal stages.

Outcome
MND is invariably fatal within 3–5 years of onset.

Myelopathy and cord compression (diseases affecting the spinal cord)

Knowledge of spinal anatomy is essential to understanding disorders affecting the spinal cord. It extends from the first cervical vertebra (C1) to the body of L1, where it is known as the conus medullaris. Below L1 the spinal canal is filled with nerve roots which have exited the cord at higher levels, the cauda equina.

Disease of the spinal cord above L1 produces upper motor neuron signs. Involvement below L1 affects nerve roots. Pain arises in cord disease only if there is involvement of nerve roots or bones.

The spinothalamic tracts carry pain and temperature sensation from the periphery and cross to the opposite side above the point of entry. Interruption of this pathway on one side results in loss of pain and temperature contralaterally.

The dorsal columns carry proprioception and vibration and remain on the same side of the spinal cord, posteriorly to the medulla where they cross. The corticospinal tracts descend from the cortex ipsilaterally crossing in the medulla at the "pyramidal decussation," and descend laterally. The tracts synapse segmentally in the anterior horn. All connections above the anterior horn cell are considered upper motor neuron, the anterior horn cell and nerve root, plexus and peripheral nerve the lower motor neuron.

Myelopathy
All types of myelopathy whether due to compression, inflammation, metabolic causes or a structural lesion produce similar symptoms and signs.

Clinical features
Epidemiology of spinal cord diseases (Table 9.6) In lesions extrinsic to the cord, motor features develop

Table 9.6. Epidemiology of spinal cord diseases

Cord Compression	Trauma	~3 per 100 000
	Disk prolapse (cervical and thoracic)	~1–2 per 100 000
	Extrinsic tumors (meningioma, Schwannoma, neurofibroma)	0.25–0.5 per 100 000
	Infective/ inflammatory lesions (abscess, TB, sarcoid)	~0.5 per 100 000
Intrinsic myelitis/ myelopathy	Multiple sclerosis	1.5 per 100 000
	Viral infection	0.1–0.4 per 100 000
	Connective tissue disease e.g. SLE	0.1 per 100 000
	Vitamin B12 deficiency (subacute combined degeneration of the cord)	0.1 per 100 000
	Vascular (anterior spinal artery infarction)	0.01 per 100 000 (higher during aortic surgery)
	Syringomyelia	1.5 per 100 000 (prevalence; incidence unknown)
	Neuro-syphilis	0.2 per 100 000 (higher in HIV + patients)
	HIV vacuolar myelopathy	10% adults with advanced disease

first and are more prominent. Sphincter dysfunction follows. Intrinsic diseases cause sphincter dysfunction earlier (sphincter pathways lie more centrally) and sensory features may be more apparent.

Paraparesis (spastic paraparesis or paraplegia) usually indicates a lesion of the spinal cord, whether extrinsic or intrinsic. Rarely, it may be due to a parasagittal lesion. Legs drag or feel heavy. There are upper motor neurone signs in both legs. Sphincter dysfunction may be present. It can be caused by a lesion in the thoracic or cervical region.

Tetraparesis (spastic tetraparesis; tetraplegia; quadraparesis; quadriplegia) indicates involvement in all four limbs. It is usually caused by a lesion in the cervical cord, or rarely the brainstem.

Brown-Séquard syndrome was initially described following experimental hemisection of the cord in animals. Pure Brown-Séquard syndrome is rare but partial forms are common:

- ipsilateral upper motor neuron signs – corticospinal tract
- ipsilateral loss of proprioception and vibration – dorsal columns
- contralateral loss of pain and temperature – spinothalamic tracts

Syringomyelia/syringobulbia

Syringomyelia is a fluid-filled cavity within the spinal cord and syringobulbia a similar cavity in the lower brainstem. The cervical cord is most commonly affected and may be associated with foramen magnum abnormalities such as Chiari malformation in which the cerebellar tonsils lie below the foramen.

The clinical picture evolves as the cavity expands affecting central structures first. There is preservation of pain and temperature in the sacral dermatomes because the ascending spinothalamic fibers from the sacrum lie peripherally. The clinical picture of *syringomyelia* includes the following: pain in the upper limbs exacerbated by coughing, sneezing or straining; dissociated sensory loss (loss of pain and temperature, preservation of touch, vibration, joint position sense) in a "cape-like" distribution over the arms and shoulders; when the cavity is small, it does not interrupt the ascending spinothalmic tracts nor the posterior dorsal columns; painless burns and cuts in the upper limbs due to dissociated sensory loss; wasting and weakness of the small muscles of the hand (involvement of the anterior horn cells); spastic paraparesis when the cavity has enlarged sufficiently to affect the descending laterally placed corticospinal tracts; unilateral or bilateral Horner's syndrome (involvement of ascending sympathetic fibers). Ultimately the dorsal columns may be affected.

Syringobulbia causes: bilateral wasting and weakness of the tongue, nystagmus, vertigo, facial sensory loss (over the nose and spreading outwards), palatal weakness and possible ataxia.

Slower onset neurological deficit – with lower motor neuron signs

Radiculopathy (Nerve root)

The spinal roots are named by the vertebral level from which they emerge from the cord. In the cervical region, the roots exit above each vertebral body (eight cervical roots although only seven cervical vertebrae). At other levels, they emerge below the vertebrae.

Clinical features

Regardless of etiology, the symptoms and signs of nerve root involvement are similar:

Pain severe, sharp, shooting, and/or burning radiating into the dermatome or muscle group supplied by the affected root, or numbness and/or weakness.

Signs – lower motor neuron in the affected myotome and sensory impairment in the affected dermatome with loss of relevant reflexes.

The most common patterns are:

(1) *Lateral cervical disk protrusion/prolapse*

The C6/C7 disk is most commonly affected causing pain (brachalgia) from shoulder to forearm and sensory disturbance, wasting and weakness of triceps, wrist and finger extensors, absent triceps reflex.

Without neurologic signs, most recover spontaneously. When delayed and when neurologic signs are present, surgical root decompression is required (see Chapter 11).

(2) *Lateral lumbar disk protrusion/prolapse*

The commonest involve compression of the L5 or S1 roots. Low back pain with radiation down the leg to the ankle. "Sciatica" is a misnomer. The sciatic nerve is not involved (see Chapter 11).

Most resolve with rest and analgesia.

Decompressive surgery may be required.

(3) *Central lumbar disk protrusion/prolapse*

If below L1 may result in compression of the cauda equina: back pain, radiation to relevant dermatomes, weakness and rarely retention of urine, bowel dysfunction, and impotence.

A picture identical to vascular intermittent claudication may occur if there is stenosis of the spinal canal, termed intermittent claudication of the spinal cord. Urinary retention in suspected central disk prolapse demands urgent MRI and decompression.

Plexopathy (Brachial and lumbosacral plexus)

Emerging spinal nerve roots join to form the brachial plexus and lumbo-sacral plexus.

Causes of plexopathy:

- Trauma (accidents/birth injuries esp brachial plexus)
- Inflammatory (neuralgic amyotrophy/brachial neuritis esp. brachial plexus)
- Metabolic (diabetic amyotrophy – lumbosacral plexus)
- Malignant infiltration (usually local spread)

- Compression (e.g. Pancoast tumor in the apex of the lung)
- Radiation damage (often delayed after treatment)
- Thoracic outlet syndrome (brachial plexus, e.g. cervical rib)
- Genetic (e.g. hereditary liability to pressure palsies)

Clinical features

Brachial plexus

(1) Upper plexus lesion (C5–6)

An upper plexus lesion may be caused by a traction injury on the arm at birth (Erb-Duchenne paralysis), falling on the shoulder, or other trauma. Signs: weakness, wasting deltoid, supraspinatus, biceps, brachioradialis, loss of biceps and brachioradialis jerks, sensory impairment C5, C6 dermatomes.

(2) Posterior cord lesion (C5–C8)

Signs: weakness, wasting deltoid, triceps, wrist extensors and extensor digitorum, loss of triceps jerk, sensory impairment in affected dermatomes.

(3) Lower plexus lesion (C8–T1)

May be caused by abduction of arm at birth (Klumpke's paralysis), trauma, cervical rib, Pancoast tumor. Signs: weakness, wasting hand, C8 and T1 sensory loss, Horner's syndrome if T1 involved.

Lumbosacral plexus

(1) Upper plexus lesion – weakness of hip flexion and adduction, anterior leg sensory loss
(2) Lower plexus lesion – weakness of hamstrings and foot muscles, with posterior leg sensory loss.

The most common patterns of brachial and lumbosacral plexopathy are:

- *Brachial amyotrophy* (neuralgic amyotrophy/brachial neuritis): unilateral inflammatory response after viral infection or vaccination, days of shoulder pain, followed by wasting and weakness of deltoid or other girdle or arm muscles. Recovery takes months.
- *Diabetic amyotrophy*: usually Type 2, older male diabetics during periods of poor control. Usually asymmetric, onset gradual or sudden with pain in back, hips, and thighs, unilateral wasting, weakness of proximal legs and hip girdle, knee jerk reduced or absent. Coexisting sensorimotor polyneuropathy is common.
- *Thoracic outlet syndrome/cervical rib*: a fibrous band or cervical rib from the transverse process of C7 to the first rib, stretches the lower part of the brachial plexus (C8, T1). There is pain along the ulnar border, sensory loss in T1 distribution, wasting of thenar muscles predominantly, possible Horner's syndrome. Treatment is surgical.
- *Pancoast tumor*: apical lung tumour can compress the lower part the lower part of the brachial plexus (C8, T1). Clinical features are as for cervical rib.

Peripheral neuropathy

Nerve fibers are myelinated or unmyelinated. Conduction is slower in unmyelinated nerves. Peripheral nerves contain three types of fiber.

The peripheral neuropathies may be hereditary, acquired, systemic, or restricted and may involve axonal degeneration, demyelination, or both.

If a single nerve is affected it is termed mononeuropathy, multiple single nerves mononeuritis multiplex. Polyneuropathy is diffuse, symmetric, usually distal, with proximal progression. Different presentations and results of nerve conduction studies allow a differential diagnosis.

Symptoms

Negative symptoms (loss of sensation):

Conditions affecting large myelinated fibers cause loss of touch and joint position sense (proprioception), leading to difficulty discriminating textures, feet and hands feeling like "cotton wool," unsteady gait especially at night when vision cannot compensate.

Small unmyelinated fiber involvement causes loss of pain and temperature appreciation, leading to painless burns or trauma and painless deformed joints (Charcot joints).

Positive symptoms (painful and unpleasant sensations):

Large myelinated fibre disease causes paresthesiae ("pins and needles") and other unpleasant sensations, and small unmyelinated fiber involvement painful positive symptoms of burning, tightness, feeling of walking on stones or glass, dysesthesia – pain on gentle touch, hyperalgesia – lowered threshold to pain, hyperpathia – pain threshold is elevated, but pain is felt in excess, lightning pains – sudden, very severe, shooting pains.

Motor symptoms – usually distal weakness and wasting, can be proximal especially where demyelination occurs.

Autonomic:

Postural hypotension with dizziness on standing
Urinary difficulties especially retention

Impotence

Diarrhea (occasionally constipation)

Diminished sweating

Signs

Sensory:

Functions of large myelinated fibers include:

– Vibration sense

– Joint position sense (proprioception)

– Two-point discrimination

Functions of small unmyelinated and thinly myelinated fibres include:

– Temperature perception

– Pain perception

Sensory loss classically in a "glove and stocking" distribution. Signs in the hands do not develop until sensory loss is up to at least mid-shin.

Loss "joint position sense causes of sensory ataxia" and positive Romberg's test.

Motor:

Depressed or absent reflexes, weakness, wasting

Fasciculations

Autonomic:

Postural hypotension. Other features of autonomic dysfunction can be confirmed in an autonomic laboratory

Epidemiology

Up to 8% of adults may have some form of neuropathy. Diabetes accounts for one-third. A further third are idiopathic. There are multiple disease associations and some are hereditary.

Pathology

Peripheral nerves can be disrupted by damage to the cell body (neuronopathy), the axon, the myelin sheath or the blood supply (e.g. vasculitis).

Neuropathies are classified according to the dominant pathologic process – axonal (Wallerian) degeneration or demyelination. If a nerve is severely demyelinated, secondary axonal degeneration may occur.

Axonal (Wallerian) degeneration:

When a nerve is injured the axon degenerates distally. Within 7–10 days this portion is inexcitable on nerve conduction studies.

Regeneration can occur, because the basement membrane of the Schwann cell survives along which the axon regrows 1 mm per day. In motor nerves affected by a chronic process remaining normal motor axons produce sprouts which reinnervate the denervated muscle fibers and are recorded as large polyphasic units on EMG.

In inherited demyelinating neuropathies the axons remain intact, but in some acquired demyelinating processes, secondary axonal loss occurs as in Guillain–Barré syndrome (GBS). Demyelination causes slowing of conduction and can be differentiated from axonal neuropathy on nerve conduction studies. Local demyelination occurs early in compression and entrapment neuropathies.

Polyneuropathies

The most common types of poly neuropathy, namely diabetes, alcohol, metabolic, and idiopathic, affect sensory nerves predominantly. Others cause a combination of sensory and motor symptoms. A few such as porphyria and lead poisoning affect only motor nerves.

Miscellaneous drugs, toxins and vitamin deficiencies can cause polyneuropathy. Drugs include amiodarone, antiretroviral agents (especially zalcitabine (ddc), stavudine (d4t) and didanosine (ddI)), chloroquine, cisplatin, dapsone, doxorubicin, ethambutol, isoniazid, paclitacel (Taxol), phenytoin, procainamide, pyridoxine excess (vitamin B6), suramin, tacrolimus, thalidomide, vincristine and vinblastine. Toxins include alcohol, arsenic, lead (usually purely motor), mercury, hexacarbons, organophosphates, thallium, and trichlorethylene. The relevant vitamin deficiencies are B1 (thiamine), B6 (pyridoxine), B12, and nicotinic acid.

Autonomic neuropathies are rarer and usually accompany mixed pictures such as in Guillain-Barré syndrome and hereditary sensory and autonomic neuropathy.

Other metabolic causes of polyneuropathy apart from diabetes are renal failure, hypothyroidism and porphyria. Rheumatological conditions include SLE, rheumatoid arthritis and vasculitic disorders. Cancer, especially of the lung and infections including HIV, leprosy, hepatitis C and Lyme disease add to the long list of causes and associations. Celiac disease and sarcoidosis are two inflammatory causes along with Guillain-Barré syndrome (GBS) discussed below.

Guillain-Barré Syndrome (GBS; acute inflammatory demyelinating polyradiculoneuropathy; AIDP)

This is a post-infective acute acquired inflammatory demyelinating process affecting peripheral nerves and nerve roots without involvement of the central nervous system. It can affect motor, sensory, and the autonomic nerves.

Clinical features

The classical presentation follows 1–3 weeks after an infective episode, usually an upper respiratory tract infection or diarrheal illness (often *Campylobacter jejuni*). It often starts with distal sensory symptoms (pins and needles and/or numbness). This usually ascends over days or weeks with progressive weakness, often worse proximally and involving facial and bulbar muscles in 50%. There is reduction or loss of the reflexes. In 25%, involvement of respiratory muscles requires ventilation.

Autonomic involvement (arrhythmias, sudden hyper- or hypotension, etc.) is rarer but indicates a severe course and increased mortality.

Symptoms may continue to progress for 6 weeks but recovery can occur over days to weeks, whereas severely affected patients may plateau over several months and be left with disability.

Other variants of GBS exist. In acute motor axonal neuropathy (AMAN) and acute motor and sensory axonal neuropathy (AMSAN), there is additional axonal loss, the course is often more severe, and recovery is protracted or incomplete. A further variant in 5% is Miller-Fisher syndrome with ophthalmoplegia, ataxia and lost reflexes without weakness.

Epidemiology

Incidence is 1.5 per 100 000. All age groups can be affected but men are more frequently affected.

Pathology

The pathogenic mechanisms have not been fully established but humoral and cell-mediated immune factors contribute. Antibodies cross-react with gangliosides in the nerve.

The dysimmune process lasts 4–6 weeks but the damage created often takes a long time to recover. If there is only demyelination, recovery is faster.

Investigations

Diagnosis is usually clinical and investigations often normal within the first week.

Lumbar puncture – the CSF protein is often markedly raised although may be normal early in the disease. Other CSF constituents are normal. A high CSF white cell count with a clinical picture of GBS is a common presentation at HIV seroconversion.

Neurophysiology (electromyogram; EMG) – classical features of demyelinating neuropathy may be absent early in the disease. Additional axonal loss may help to predict a poor recovery.

Management

Some are mildly affected and remain independent. More severely affected patients require monitoring, particularly while there is continued deterioration.

In paralyzed patients, attention must be given to the prevention of:

(1) pressure sores
(2) thrombosis and embolism
(3) aspiration

Monitoring vital capacity (VC) is essential. Weakening respiratory muscles risk respiratory arrest. VC below 1l indicates need for elective ventilation.

Immunomodulatory treatment involves modulation of the aberrant post-infectious autoimmune response with high-dose intravenous immunoglobulin (IVIg) or plasma exchange is effective. IVIg acts by complement inactivation, neutralization of idiotypic antibodies, cytokine inhibition, and saturation of Fc receptors on macrophages. Corticosteroids are of no value.

Outcome

Mortality is 10%. Death is more likely with severe disease, autonomic involvement, the elderly with co-morbidity. Within 1 year 80% recover fully but some have disability.

Charcot-Marie-Tooth disease (hereditary motor sensory neuropathy/CMT/HMSN)

The most common hereditary neurologic condition with incidence 10–20 per 100 000 worldwide. Classification of the hereditary motor sensory neuropathies by genetic profiling continues to undergo modification:

CMT-1 (A-D; A or B most common) – commonest form – autosomal dominant demyelinating neuropathy. Over 70% due to duplication of PMP-22 gene on chromosome 17.

CMT-2 (A-F) – autosomal dominant axonal.

CMT-X (1X-4X) – X-linked dominant associated with mutations of connexion-32 (CX-32).

CMT-4 (A-F and HMSN-R) – rare – autosomal recessive, hyertrophic, demyelinating.

Complex forms of CMT – associated with optic atrophy, retinitis pigmentosa, deafness and spastic paraparesis.

Features of Charcot-Marie-Tooth disease

Slowly progressive distal wasting of the lower limbs, and hands less often.

Foot deformities are invariable with pes cavus and clawing of the toes. These may be the only features in mild cases (Fig. 9.9). Clawing of the hands may also be seen.

Once wasting in the legs is severe, they resemble "inverted champagne bottles." Reduced or absent reflexes and variable loss of sensation. Sensory symptoms are rare.

(a)

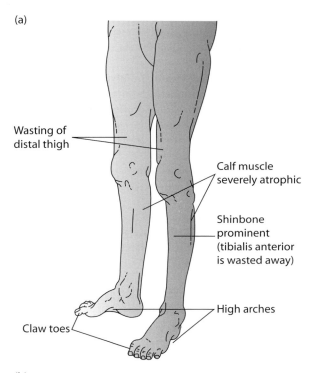

Wasting of distal thigh

Calf muscle severely atrophic

Shinbone prominent (tibialis anterior is wasted away)

High arches

Claw toes

(b)

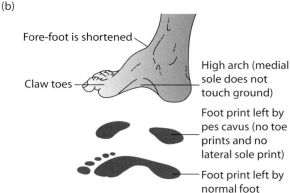

Fore-foot is shortened

Claw toes

High arch (medial sole does not touch ground)

Foot print left by pes cavus (no toe prints and no lateral sole print)

Foot print left by normal foot

Fig. 9.9. Pes cavus and leg appearance in hereditary motor sensory neuropathy.

Age of onset varies within families. Some only have foot deformities, others may be wheelchair-bound. Management is supportive.

Investigation

- Nerve conduction studies (NCS) – differentiate axonal degeneration from demyelination, characterize whether sensory and/or motor fibers are involved, and localize the sites of abnormality.
- Electromyography (EMG) – fine needle electrode into the muscle indicates if complete or partial denervation present (fibrillation potentials and positive sharp waves) and signs of reinnervation (large polyphasic units).
- Quantitative sensory testing (QST) – nerve conduction studies are only abnormal if larger myelinated fibers are affected. In pure small fiber neuropathy, QST includes assessing warm, cool, and pain thresholds.
- Nerve biopsy – when required, the sural nerve is the most accessible.
- Cerebrospinal fluid (CSF) examination – lumbar puncture is indicated if inflammatory demyelinating neuropathies are suspected.
- Blood tests – blood glucose or glucose tolerance test (diabetes), full blood count (hematological malignancy e.g. myeloma, leukemia, lymphoma or macrocytosis suggesting alcohol abuse), ESR (connective tissue diseases RA, SLE, vasculitis or a very high value suggesting myeloma), urea and electrolytes (renal failure), liver function tests (liver failure and alcohol abuse), vitamin B12 (deficiency), thyroid function tests (hypothyroidism), protein electrophoresis especially if ESR >50 mm/h (myeloma), rheumatoid factor (RF), antinuclear antibody (ANF) and anti neutrophil cytoplasmic antibodies (ANCA) for RA, SLE and vasculitis, antineuronal antibodies especially anti-Hu (paraneoplastic syndrome), antiganglioside antibodies (especially anti-GM1) for inflammatory demyelinating neuropathies.

Management

In idiopathic neuropathies and in many of the genetic neuropathies, treatment is supportive and symptomatic. When due to systemic disease, treatment is that of the underlying disorder.

Outcome

Dependent on the type and cause of the neuropathy. Guillain-Barré may be completely reversible. For many, particularly for those with idiopathic sensory neuropathies, there is often slow deterioration.

Mononeuropathies

Entrapment or compression is the most common cause, occurring when nerves pass through tight anatomic spaces. Localized demyelination, if prolonged may lead to distal axonal loss.

Carpal tunnel syndrome (median nerve compression at the wrist). Incidence is 125 per 100 000, caused by compression of the median nerve through the carpal tunnel at the wrist. It is usually idiopathic but can be associated with: pregnancy, arthritis of the wrist, diabetes mellitus, hypothyroidism, acromegaly.

Tingling, pain and numbness in the hand, especially at night and in the morning. Sensory loss may be found in the radial three and a half fingers, wasting and weakness of abductor pollicis brevis. Tapping over the carpal tunnel may reproduce tingling or pain (Tinel's sign).

Diagnosis can be confirmed by electrophysiology. Surgical decompression is the definitive procedure. Wrist splints and steroid injections may help temporarily.

- Ulnar nerve: this is less common. Entrapment usually occurs at the elbow leading to wasting and weakness of ulnar-innervated muscles and sensory loss in the ulnar one and a half fingers. It usually resolves or improves with conservative treatment and avoidance of pressure on the elbow. Surgical relocation of the nerve may help.
- Radial nerve: may be compressed against the humerus, e.g. when arm draped over the back of a chair ("Saturday night palsy") and results in wristdrop, weakness of finger extension and brachioradialis. Recovery is usually spontaneous.
- Common peroneal nerve: can become compressed as it crosses the fibular head due to prolonged squatting, a tight plaster cast, prolonged bed rest, or coma. It results in foot drop. Recovery is usual within months.
- Meralgia paraesthetica: caused by entrapment of the lateral cutaneous nerve of the thigh as it passes beneath the inguinal ligament, usually in overweight patients. Weight loss often helps.

Mononeuritis multiplex

Caused by
- Diabetes

- Vasculitis: polyarteritis nodosa, Wegener's granulomatosis, Churg-Strauss syndrome
- Connective tissue diseases: SLE, RA
- Sarcoidosis
- Malignancy/paraneoplastic disease
- HIV
- Leprosy
- Amyloidosis
- Neurofibromatosis
- several of these causes may also be associated with polyneuropathy
- Management and outcome depend on cause.

Myasthenia gravis

Acetylcholine is broken down by acetylcholinesterase bound to basal lamina in post-synaptic folds then stored in pre-synaptic vesicles until the next stimulus (Fig. 9.10). In myasthenia gravis antibodies reversibly block the post-synaptic acetylcholine receptors.

It is an antibody-mediated disease. There is thymic hyperplasia in 70% below age 40. In 10% a thymic tumor occurs, more often in older patients.

Clinical features

The classical symptom is fatiguable weakness, worsening after exercise and later in the day. It is often improved by rest, but this may take many hours. Some develop progression of weakness. Other features are ptosis (drooping of eyelid), difficulty closing eyes and mouth, diplopia, dysarthria, dysphagia, dysphonia, proximal limb weakness, weakness of the neck. There may be no signs at rest. Making a patient who has ptosis look up for 10–30 seconds may worsen the ptosis. Fatiguability at other sites can sometimes be demonstrated by exercising.

In generalized myasthenia when acute and severe, respiratory muscles may become affected and patients may require temporary ventilation. Some, especially older men, may have a pure ocular presentation with double vision and ptosis and never develop any generalized features.

Epidemiology

Prevalence is 1 per 10 000 with bimodal distribution between ages 15 and 30 and 60 and 75. Females predominate in the younger and males in the older. The former have an acute, fluctuating condition associated with HLA-B8 and HLA-DR3. Older patients tend to have a more ocular presentation, with little or no generalized involvement.

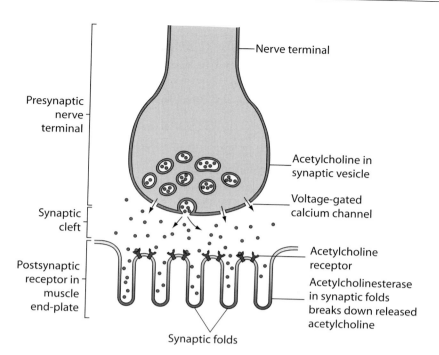

Nerve terminal

Presynaptic nerve terminal

Acetylcholine in synaptic vesicle

Voltage-gated calcium channel

Synaptic cleft

Postsynaptic receptor in muscle end-plate

Acetylcholine receptor

Acetylcholinesterase in synaptic folds breaks down released acetylcholine

Synaptic folds

Fig. 9.10. The normal neuromuscular junction.

Investigation

Serum acetylcholine receptor antibodies (AChRAbs) are diagnostic and, if present, no other diagnostic tests are required. These are present in 80% with generalized myasthenia and 20% with pure ocular myasthenia. Muscle-specific kinase antibodies (MuSK antibodies) should be requested if AChRAbs are absent.
Electromyography (EMG) may show decrement in amplitude of compound muscle action potential following repetitive stimulation and increased jitter using a single fiber needle electrode.
Tensilon (edrophonium) testing is rarely used because of the risks associated with it. Edrophonium is a fast acting, intravenous acetylcholinesterase inhibitor. Following an intravenous bolus, weakness is improved for a few minutes. It is most useful if there is measurable weakness, e.g. ptosis or ophthalmoplegia. Increasing acetylcholine levels can result in bradycardia and asytole so atropine is co-administered, with cardiac monitoring.
Thymus imaging by CT or MRI helps exclude thymic hyperplasia or thymoma.

Management

The aims are to improve symptoms and modulate the immune process.
Oral acetylcholinesterase inhibitors:
These provide symptomatic treatment and act by competitively antagonizing the acetylcholine receptor antibody. Neuromuscular blocking drugs during anesthesia are avoided.
Pyridostigmine is the drug of choice, with action lasting 3–6 hours. Side effects are salivation, abdominal pain, and possible worsening of weakness (cholinergic crisis).
Immunosuppression:
Corticosteroids produce improvement in 90% and remission in 80%. Temporary worsening of symptoms may occur after 7–10 days.
Other immunosuppressive drugs such as azathioprine may be necessary.
In rapidly progressive patients, intravenous immunoglobulin or plasma exchange are used.
Thymectomy improves prognosis in 70% in those with thymus hyperplasia. In older patients with a thymoma surgery is essential to remove a potentially malignant tumor, but rarely improves the myasthenia.

Outcome

Untreated there is 30% mortality within 3 years.
Many require indefinite corticosteroid treatment. Relapse and remission are common.

Other neuromuscular junction disorders

Lambert-Eaton Myasthenic syndrome (LEMS): in which antibodies are directed against pre-synaptic voltage-gated calcium channels. These result in failure of acetylcholine release. Variable muscle weakness

Table 9.7. Typical times of life when different myopathies become clinically evident

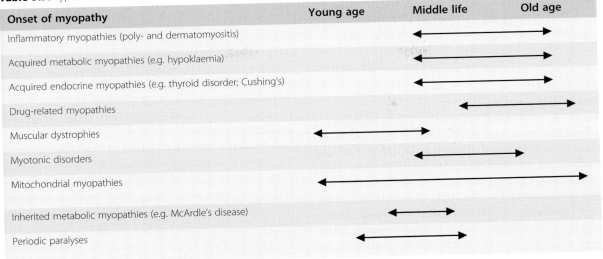

Onset of myopathy	Young age	Middle life	Old age
Inflammatory myopathies (poly- and dermatomyositis)		←	→
Acquired metabolic myopathies (e.g. hypoklaemia)		←	→
Acquired endocrine myopathies (e.g. thyroid disorder; Cushing's)		←	→
Drug-related myopathies		←	→
Muscular dystrophies	← →		
Myotonic disorders		← →	
Mitochondrial myopathies	←		→
Inherited metabolic myopathies (e.g. McArdle's disease)	← →		
Periodic paralyses	← →		

occurs often improving with exertion. It is rare. Three quarters are associated with occult neoplasia especially small cell carcinoma of the lung. Diagnosis is by demonstrating serum voltage-gated calcium channel antibodies and by EMG. Treatment is diaminopyridine, which blocks potassium channels and guanidine, which facilitates neuromuscular transmission.

Botulism: this follows a few days to weeks after ingesting food contaminated with *Clostridium botulinum* toxin or after wounds become infected with the bacterium. It is found in the soil. There is symmetric, descending flaccid paralysis and cranial nerve palsies, reduced weakness and respiratory weakness that may require ventilation. Consciousness is unaltered. Diagnosis is established by demonstrating toxin in feces, serum, or food. Treatment is supportive with intravenous anti-toxin. Mortality is 50%–70%. Inactivated botulinum toxin is used in medical practice and cosmetics. The effect lasts up to 3 months. Neurologic indications for therapeutic use of the toxin are cervical dystonia, blepharospasm, and spasticity.

Myopathy

A disturbance of the normal function of muscle produces a myopathy. There are many causes. In general, myopathies tend to cause proximal muscle weakness (Table 9.7).

Investigations should rule out reversible electrolyte or endocrine abnormalities, and include serum creatine kinase (CK), EMG for myopathic features or myotonia; and muscle biopsy and genetic testing where appropriate.

Hereditary myopathies
Muscular dystrophies

Duchenne's muscular dystrophy is an X-linked recessive condition (dystrophin gene) causing absence of dystrophin. The frequency is 20–30/100 000 liveborn males.

Patients are normal at birth and the disease is apparent by 4 years. Patients are wheelchair-bound by 10 years.

Often death occurs by 20 years due to respiratory failure or cardiomyopathy.

The signs are proximal weakness/pseudo-hypertrophy of the calves and "Gower's sign" – when rising to erect position, use of the hands to "climb" up legs. Often they develop cardiomyopathy. CK is grossly elevated (often >10 000 units per liter in boys; may be raised in female carriers)

EMG – myopathic
Muscle biopsy – absence of staining for dystrophin
Genetic test available
No cure – symptomatic treatment/genetic
    counseling.

Becker's muscular dystrophy: is also an X-linked recessive condition (dystrophin gene) in which dystrophin is altered rather than absent. The frequency is 15/100 000 liveborn males. It is similar to Duchenne's but much milder and has an onset in later childhood. Walking continues into teens and early adult life. Cramps are common with exercise. Cardiomyopathy may be worse than weakness. CK is elevated (may be lower levels than Duchenne's)

> EMG – myopathic
> Muscle biopsy – reduced levels of dystrophin
> Genetic test available
> No cure – treatment is symptomatic/genetic counseling.

Other muscular dystrophies

There is a growing recognition of a number of inherited dystrophies which affect different components of muscle. Their names indicate the pattern and distribution of weakness. Presentations vary from mild and slowly progressive to rapidly fatal with cardiac involvement. Facio-scapulo-humeral (FSH) muscular dystrophy is an autosomal dominant disease and is one example, another being limb-girdle muscular dystrophies which are of mixed inheritance.

Genetic tests exist for some, e.g. FSH.

There is no cure – symptomatic treatment/genetic counseling are all that can be offered.

Myotonic myopathies

Myotonic disorders include myotonic dystrophy (dystrophia myotonica) which is an autosomal dominant condition caused by expanded trinucleotide repeat (CTG) on chromosome 19 and showing 'anticipation' (successive generations more severely affected). Onset is between 20 and 50 years old and it progresses gradually.

It may range from extremely mild to a severe multisystem disease (with increasing number of expansions). The signs include myotonia – persistence of contraction, often for several seconds during attempted relaxation, worse in the cold. Other features may include distal muscle weakness which may progress proximally, wasting and weakness of the face and sternomastoid muscles, bilateral ptosis, frontal balding, cataracts, mild cognitive dysfunction, cardiomyopathy and cardiac conduction defects, gynecomastia, testicular atrophy, glucose intolerance, and bronchiectasis.

Investigation EMG may show myotonia and a genetic test is available.

Treatment is symptomatic.

Periodic paralysis

Hypokalemic periodic paralysis is an autosomal dominant condition in which there is an abnormal L-type calcium channel or sodium channel. The genetic fault is on chromosome 1 or 17. Onset is 10–20 years of age. It may remit after 35 years of age.

Weakness occurs after heavy carbohydrate meals or periods of rest following strenuous exertion. Attacks last 4–24 hours. During an attack, serum potassium falls to below 3.0 mmol/l. It is rarely fatal as diaphragm and respiratory muscles are spared. It is better to prevent than treat, with the carbonic anhydrase inhibitor acetazolamide. Replacement with potassium may be required.

Hyperkalemic periodic paralysis is an autosomal dominant condition involving abnormal voltage-gated sodium channels. The defect is on chromosome 17. Onset is in infancy or childhood and it may remit after 20 years of age. Weakness happens after exercising or during a fast, lasting from minutes to hours and shorter than hypokalemic periodic paralysis. Serum potassium rises above 5.0 mm/l. Attacks may be terminated by a carbohydrate load but glucose and insulin or calcium gluconate may be necessitated if severely raised potassium. Prophylaxis is acetazolamide or daily diuretic.

Metabolic inherited myopathies

Myophosphorylase deficiency (McArdle's disease) is an autosomal recessive condition. There is deficiency of myophosphorylase in skeletal muscle. Onset is in adolescence. Fatigue and muscle pain occur during exercise. Continued exertion causes 'true contractures' – fixed shortening of muscle. EMG is silent and there is absence of a normal rise in venous lactate during ischemic exercise (using blood pressure cuff). Diagnosis is by muscle biopsy or genetic testing. There is no cure.

Other metabolic myopathies are: phosphofructokinase deficiency, lactate dehydrogenase deficiency, and carnitine palmityl transferase deficiency. These are usually autosomal recessive. Thus young patients with a family history, muscle pain on exertion or fasting, and with myoglobinuria, should have investigation for one of the metabolic myopathies.

Diagnosis is by EMG, muscle biopsy, and genetic testing where available.

Mitochondrial myopathies

> Kearn-Sayres syndrome (KSS)
> Chronic progressive external ophthalmoplegia (CPEO)
> Myoclonic epilepsy and ragged red fibers (MERRF)

These are maternally inherited defects of mitochondrial DNA involving defects of the final oxidative pathway of the respiratory chain in mitochondria. They cause multiple different multisystem conditions particularly affecting muscle and the CNS. Patients are often, of short stature with a family history, diabetes, or deafness and myopathy.

There may be epilepsy, progressive ophthalmoplegia, GI disturbance, and cognitive dysfunction. Diagnosis is made by EMG, serum and CSF lactate: pyruvate ratio, muscle biopsy, and genetics on serum and muscle.

Acquired myopathies

Inflammatory myopathies (polymyositis, dermatomyositis, inclusion body myositis) affect a wide age range and are often associated with connective tissue diseases. These are discussed in Chapter 11.

Metabolic, endocrine, and drug related causes include Cushing's syndrome, thyroid disease, hypocalcemia, hypokalemia, steroid treatment, statins, and alcohol.

There is acquired metabolic disruption of muscle function causing proximal weakness with or without muscle pain. Most cases are reversible. Diagnosis is from drug history and appropriate endocrine tests. Management requires treatment of the underlying disorder, or withdrawal or reduction of the offending substance.

Movement disorders

These usually arise from lesions or diseases of the extrapyramidal system, which comprises the basal ganglia and their connections. They can be divided into two categories:

Akinetic-rigid syndromes – diminished movement and increased tone.

Dyskinesias – excessive movements outside voluntary control. These can be further subdivided depending on the type of movement. (1) Tremor – Tremor is common and a rhythmic oscillation of a body part. It can be a normal reaction to anxiety, due to medication or a pathologic condition. (2) Dystonia – A disorder dominated by sustained muscle contractions, which often cause twisting and repetitive movements or abnormal postures. Dystonic movements may be slow and writhing. When they are distal, they are termed athetosis. (3) Chorea – From the Greek word "a dance," consisting of irregular, unpredictable, brief, jerky movements. When movements are slow it is termed choreoathetosis. (4) Ballism – the least common from the Greek word "to throw," this involves wide-amplitude, violent, flailing movements. (5) Tics – repetitive, brief, isolated movements. (6) Myoclonus – sudden movement of one or more muscles.

Akinetic rigid syndromes

The most common is Parkinson's disease which is a specific pathologic entity. In practice there are several diseases with Parkinsonian clinical features.

All Parkinsonian conditions involve disruption of the extrapyramidal system, which includes the basal ganglia, the substantia nigra in the midbrain, and the connections between them and the cortex. The increased tone in these conditions causes rigidity.

Parkinson's disease (PD)
Clinical features

Patients complain of difficulty in initiating and alternating movements and of rigidity, predominantly of the limbs, and of difficulty with movements affecting limbs and face (facial hypomimia). The muscles of mastication, swallowing and speech, and the axial (trunk) muscles are also affected. Handwriting may be reduced in size (micrographia). Constipation and depression are common. Cognitive function is preserved until late disease. Examination often reveals a lack of facial expression. A hypophonic (soft) voice occurs, which is monotonous and accompanied by a slurring dysarthria and sometimes dribbling. In late disease dysphagia may be severe. Examination of the limbs reveals lead pipe rigidity in which tone is increased in all directions or cogwheeling where a superimposed tremor gives the movement a jerky sensation best demonstrated by slowly rotating the wrist. Power and reflexes are normal, there is slowing and paucity of all movements (bradykinesia and akinesia). There is often a stooped, shuffling, narrow-based gait with poor arm swing, difficulty initiating walking, turning, and stopping (festinant gait). In late features true Parkinson's there is a tendency to fall backward. Frequently these signs are accompanied by a coarse, resting, pill-rolling tremor (4–7 Hz) which is usually asymmetric and occurs at rest. Later in the disease postural instability and falls occur.

Epidemiology

It is the commonest of all movement disorders and is found worldwide increasing with age. Beyond age 50, approximately 1% are affected. There is moderate male preponderance and lifetime risk for a man is 2% and for women 1.3% with a prevalence of 1.6 per 100 population. Most have sporadic disease but there are kindreds with older onset disease due to

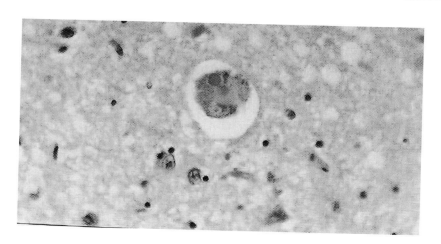

Fig. 9.11. Photomicrograph of a Lewy body (hematoxylin–eosin stain).

mutations of the alpha-synuclein gene and younger onset families with inherited recessive deletions of the *PARKIN* gene.

Pathology

There is progressive degeneration of cells within the pars compacta of the substantia nigra in the mid-brain. On macroscopic examination there is loss of black melanin-containing cells of the substantia nigra and microscopically reduced cell numbers and eosinophilic inclusion bodies, called "Lewy bodies" (Fig. 9.11).

Investigation

There are no diagnostic tests for any Parkinson disorders but a radionucleotide DAT-scan may reveal a suggestive pattern of dopamine loss.

Investigations may rule out the mimics which are hypothyroidism, small vessel cerebrovascular disease, or repeated head-injury as in boxers. A drug history will identify agents that disrupt dopaminergic transmission.

Management

The main aim is to restore dopamine : acetylcholine balance by replacing dopamine and occasionally reducing acetylcholine. The diagnosis should be reconsidered if early disease is unresponsive but later it can become resistant.

Levo-dopa (L-dopa) This is broken down to dopamine and has to be combined with a dopa-decarboxylase inhibitor to lessen risk of nausea, vomiting, and postural hypotension (Fig. 9.12).

Newer preparations contain a catechol-o-methyl transferase inhibitor to reduce peripheral side effects and lengthen duration of action.

With the advent of newer dopamine agonists use of L-dopa tends to be delayed because, with time, the duration of action reduces, the response becomes unpredictable, and patients experience marked "on–off" fluctuations comprising marked dyskinesias (excessive involuntary movements – chorea, dystonia) when "on" and immobility ("freezing") when off.

These abnormal responses to L-dopa take 5–10 years to develop and it remains the first-line drug in elderly patients and should not be delayed if younger patients are unresponsive or intolerant of dopamine agonists. Treatment is started gradually and increased slowly until an adequate response or side effects occur. L-dopa is best for treating rigidity and bradykinesia and has less effect on tremor.

Dopamine agonists Analogs of dopamine which directly stimulate different dopamine receptors, mimicking the action of dopamine. There are several:

(1) Bromocriptine: an ergot structure D2 agonist, D1 antagonist which can cause pulmonary, retroperitoneal, and pericardial fibrosis (2) Cabergoline: an ergot D2 agonist that may also produce pulmonary, retroperitoneal and pericardial fibrosis (3) Lisuride ergot D2 agonist, D1 antagonist capable of pulmonary, retroperitoneal, and pericardial fibrosis; caution in severe peripheral vascular disease and coronary disease (4) Pergolide: the ergot D1 and D2 agonist with fibrotic side effects of above drugs, caution with cardiac disease (5) Pramipexole: non-ergot D2 and D3 agonist can cause renal impairment (6) Ropinerole: non-ergot D2 agonist, caution in cardiac, renal, and hepatic impairment (7) Apomorphine: (subcutaneous), non-ergot D1 and D2 agonist.

All cause nausea, vomiting, and postural hypotension and pre-treatment with domperidone (a peripheral

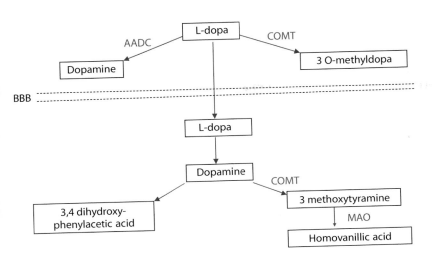

Fig. 9.12. The metabolism of L-dopa (BBB: blood–brain barrier; AADC: amino acid decarboxylase; COMT: catechol-o-methyltransferase; MAO: monoamine oxidase).

dopamine antagonist and anti-emetic) is helpful. Confusion and psychosis also occur. It is best to start treatment with an oral dopamine agonist used alone or in combination with other agents including L-dopa. As disease progresses, L-dopa is commonly added.

Anticholinergic drugs: some penetrate the blood-brain barrier (e.g. benzhexol) and can help tremor. They redress the imbalance of dopamine : acetylcholine. Dry mouth, constipation, urinary retention, visual blurring, hallucinations, and confusion limit their usefulness.

COMT inhibitors (catechol-o-methyl transferase): since dopamine is broken down peripherally by dopa-decarboxylase and COMT, an inhibitor of COMT, entacapone, was developed to reduce the peripheral breakdown of L-dopa. This increases the duration of action but not the quality of response.

MOAB inhibitors Selegiline inhibitors of monoamine oxidase B, blocking the and rasagaline central metabolism of dopamine.

Surgery
This may be considered in some severe but otherwise fit patients or in young patients who have failed medical treatments after initial response. The most common surgical procedure is insertion of subthalamic deep brain stimulators. Other techniques include pallidotomy, thalamotomy, and transplantation of fetal substantia nigra.

Outcome
Parkinson's disease invariably progresses with time. However, some remain mild or respond to increments of treatment.

Parkinsonian syndromes
The Parkinsonian plus syndromes:
Progressive supranuclear palsy (PSP). In this condition there is bradykinesia and rigidity which is mainly axial. No tremor is seen and there is a vertical supranuclear gaze palsy. Falls occur early in the disease process. Other features are pseudobulbar palsy with a "growling" dysarthria and a poor response to L-dopa. It is caused by deposition of "tau" protein in the nervous system. Median survival is 6 years.

Multisystem atrophy (MSA). There are three main variants. These are (1) Shy-Drager syndrome with predominant autonomic failure causing postural hypotension and urinary incontinence, axial rigidity, no tremor, and early falls (2) predominant cerebellar features with dysarthria and (3) predominant Parkinsonian features – similar to PD without tremor. MSA is associated with glial cytoplasmic inclusions in the brain. All of these have a poor or absent response to L-dopa.

Corticobasal degeneration (CBD). In this disorder there is marked asymmetric onset in one arm with apraxia ('alien limb') in the affected arm. There may also be stimulus-sensitive myoclonus, cortical sensory loss, slow initiation of eye movements, and akinesia with rigidity. Cognitive function is not affected until late in the course of the disease. Pick cells are found in the frontal region and brainstem. There is a poor L-dopa response.

Other Parkinsonian syndromes
Drug induced. All agents that antagonize dopamine can cause a syndrome with bradykinesia and rigidity

but usually less tremor. It can be difficult to distinguish from true PD but the age group affected is on average younger and orofacial dyskinesias are suggestive. Neuroleptic drugs (phenothiazines and atypical neuroleptics) are the most common causes. Others are antiemetics, especially metoclopramide and prochlorperazine.

Cerebrovascular disease

Small vessel cerebrovascular disease, particularly when involving deep gray matter and subcortical regions, can produce a Parkinsonian picture. There are often superimposed upper motor neuron features and a step-wise onset.

Wilson's Disease

An inherited autosomal recessive metabolic disease of copper which is deposited in brain, especially basal ganglia, cornea (Kayser-Fleischer rings), and liver. It is treated with D-penicillamine.

Dyskinesias

Tremor

Postural tremor is a tremor of the outstretched hands. It is usually bilateral and can be due to anxiety, secondary to beta agonists, antidepressants, alcohol, thyrotoxicosis, lithium, or withdrawl of benzodiazepines, alcohol, and opiates.

Rest tremor is due either to Parkinson's disease or a Parkinsonian syndrome.

Intention tremor is one which worsens or increases in amplitude as the hand approaches a target. This is indicative of a lesion of the cerebellum or cerebellar connections. It can be unilateral or bilateral depending on the cause.

Benign essential tremor is common and often inherited as an autosomal dominant trait, present on posture and action and not at rest and may be asymmetric. The head may also be tremulous (titubation). Often the tremor improves after alcohol. Beta-blockers may help.

Involuntary movements

Drug-induced

Acute dystonic reactions develop in 2%–5% of patients on neuroleptics such as phenothiazines and butyrophenones, or the antiemetics, metoclopramide and prochloperazine. These can occur after single or multiple doses.

The range of dystonias includes torticollis, oculogyric crisis, opithotonus, and trismus. Treatment is intravenous or oral anticholinergics.

Drug-induced Parkinsonism is discussed above.

Akathisia is a restlessness that occurs early in the use of neuroleptics. There is an irresistible need to move, which ceases with drug withdrawal.

Tardive dyskinesia develops after chronic exposure to neuroleptics and may be irreversible, even with drug withdrawal. There are rhythmic, involuntary movements of the tongue, face, and jaw.

Dystonia

This can be inherited or acquired, focal or generalized.

Primary torsion dystonia (DYT-1)

Inherited as an autosomal dominant trait (deletion on chromosome 9). It is particularly common in Ashkenazi Jews. It commences in the limbs during childhood and becomes widespread affecting all limbs and the torso over one to two decades. Treatment is often ineffective.

Dopa-responsive dystonia

An inherited dystonia (GTP-cyclohydrolase deficiency/ chromosome 14) that starts in the legs in early childhood. There is a permanent response to small doses of L-dopa.

Cervical dystonia ("torticollis")

A focal, acquired condition. It usually presents in the third to fifth decades with gradually progressing dystonic spasm in neck muscles. This causes the head to turn (torticollis) or be drawn backwards (retrocollis) or forwards (anterocollis). Botulinum toxin injections can provide relief.

Task-specific dystonia

An example of a task-specific dystonia is writer's cramp.

Chorea

The most clinically important is Huntington's disease. There are many secondary causes such as cerebrovascular disease, drugs, Sydenham's chorea, chorea gravidarum (during pregnancy).

Huntington's disease

A dominant inherited condition caused by an expanded trinucleotide repeat on chromosome 4. There is a relentless progression of dementia, chorea, and psychiatric manifestations developing in middle age. Death occurs within 12–15 years. Other movement disorders may co-exist. There is neuronal loss in the caudate and putamen and a reduction in GABA (gamma-aminobutyric acid) and acetylcholine levels. There is no effective treatment. Genetic testing is available

Tics

These are common and benign. They are repetitive abrupt, sudden, brief isolated movements which can sometimes be suppressed voluntarily.

Gilles de la Tourette syndrome is a rare autosomal dominant syndrome with incomplete penetrance. It begins in childhood or adolescence with multiple motor or vocal tics. The involuntary vocal utterances are often obscene words or phrases or sudden explosive grunts. There is an association with obsessive-compulsive tendencies, other psychiatric manifestations, and attention deficit disorder.

Myoclonus

Comprises sudden, brief, shock-like involuntary movement of single muscles or muscle groups, single or repetitive. These movements arise from the brain or spinal cord rather than the extrapyramidal system. They occur in a wide range of disorders and as a normal physiologic function before sleep (hypnogogic myoclonic jerk).

Post-anoxic myoclonus (Lance-Adams syndrome) follows severe cerebral anoxia, as after a cardiac arrest.

Myoclonic epilepsy may occur in different types of epilepsy.

Progressive myoclonic epilepsy may be combined with epilepsy, progressive cognitive decline, and several inherited metabolic diseases such as myoclonic epilepsy with ragged red fibers, sialidosis, and Lafora body disease.

Subacute sclerosing panencephalitis (SSPE) occurs up to 20 years after measles and is due to an immuno-logic response to the virus. It produces myoclonic jerking, dementia, spasticity, and rigidity. Death occurs within 2 years.

Creutzfeldt-Jakob disease (CJD) is a rare condition transmitted by prion protein. Increased public awareness is due to a new variant form that may have been transmitted from cattle affected by the equivalent disease, bovine spongiform encephalitis (BSE; "mad cow disease"). Sporadic CJD is found worldwide and its incidence has remained unchanged at 1 in a million. New variant CJD (vCJD) was not seen before 1994 and presents in the young. Clinical features include behavioral and psychiatric manifestations followed by myoclonus, ataxia, cognitive impairment, and prolonged illness (median 14 months). There were about 200 cases in the UK between 1995 and 2005. The predicted epidemic has not arisen.

Incoordination and unsteadiness

These can be due to abnormalities within the central or peripheral nervous system. Incoordination and unsteadiness are termed "ataxia" and classically associated with disorders of the cerebellum. However, loss of proprioception (joint position sense) in the periphery can cause similar unsteadiness and this is termed "sensory ataxia."

The main sensory input to the co-ordination system comes from muscle, tendon, and joint position sense receptors and ascends via the spinocerebellar tracts. Further input derives from the vestibular apparatus. Information from both sources passes through the cerebellar peduncles which acts as the integral center for postural control. Lesions of the brainstem and cerebellar connections can also cause an ataxic syndrome.

Cerebellar dysfunction

Caused by several pathologic processes, generalized or focal. Each cerebellar hemisphere controls the ipsilateral limb. There is no crossing of fibers so a lesion in the left cerebellar hemisphere causes left sided ataxia. By contrast, a generalized cerebellar syndrome causes bilateral abnormalities of eye movements, speech, co-ordination, and gait. If a lesion is confined to the vermis, unsteady gait may be the only feature.

Causes of generalized cerebellar syndromes are:

Alcohol – the most common cause which is usually reversible. Acute intoxication causes all the features of cerebellar dysfunction. After chronic overuse of alcohol, a persistent generalized cerebellar syndrome may develop often associated with cognitive impairment (Wernicke's Encephalopathy).

Drugs – particularly anti-epileptic drugs in the toxic range.

Inherited cerebellar ataxias – there are many but the best known is the autosomal recessive condition Friedreich's ataxia, caused by a trinucleotide repeat (pes cavus, pyramidal and dorsal column signs, cardiomyopathy, diabetes, optic atrophy). Others are mainly of dominant inheritance and known as the spino-cerebellar ataxias (SCA).

Developmental deformities – these may cause generalized or more focal cerebellar symptoms. Examples are Chiari malformations where the cerebellar tonsils lie below the foramen magnum, syringomyelia (50%), hydrocephalus (10%), and spina bifida (meningomyelocele). Dandy-Walker syndrome is characterized by an hypoplastic cerebellum, cystic dilatation of fourth ventricle, and hydrocephalus.

Focal cerebellar syndromes are:

Tumors – many can affect the cerebellum. In children, medulloblastomas and hemangioblastomas are most common. In adults, metastases are more frequent. Paraneoplastic cerebellar syndromes may also occur, associated with anti-Purkinje cell antibodies (anti-yo).

Vascular – hemorrhage is more common in the cerebellum than ischemic infarcts.

Inflammatory – multiple sclerosis is a common cause in young adults. Features may be focal or generalized. The demyelinating lesions are often in the brainstem, affecting the cerebellar pathways.

Infections – less common than other causes but include abscesses, bacterial and tuberculous, viral, PML (progressive multifocal leukoencephaloplathy) associated with JC virus (the initials of the first patient), HIV.

Clinical features

Abnormal eye movements are not always present and are unilateral in single hemisphere lesions. They may be (1) jerky pursuits – pursuit movements are slow, with jerky, catch-up saccadic movements on attempts to maintain fixation on a moving target (2) dysmetria of saccades – on attempting to move the eyes quickly to fixate on a target the eyes overshoot and oscillate several times before fixation is achieved. (3) nystagmus – this oscillation of the eyes is maximal on deviation of the eyes towards the side of the lesion. Nystagmus results from damage to the vestibular connections of the cerebellum.

Speech is slow and slurred and often said to be scanning, in which loss of intonation is accompanied by the breaking of words into syllables.

Impairment of movement control, includes difficulty initiating and terminating actions causing intention tremor – on placing the index finger on his/her nose and then the examiner's finger, the tremor increases as the finger approaches the target. Impaired movement is also demonstrable by dysdiadochokinesis – inability to carry out rapid alternating movements smoothly. Dysmetria is an inability to perform accurate targeted movements, which are jerky with overshooting of the target as in finger–nose and heel–shin tests, and rebound if outstretched arms are pushed down briefly.

Ataxic gait, which is wide-based and staggering. When mild, unsteadiness may be apparent only when walking heel-to-toe (tandem walking). Truncal ataxia causes difficulty sitting or standing without support.

Titubation is an anterior–posterior, nodding tremor of the head.

Hypotonia is a minor feature of cerebellar diseases producing "pendular" reflexes (the limb swings back and forth) but no functional sequelae.

Sensory ataxia

Describes unsteadiness of gait due to proprioception loss within the peripheral nerve or dorsal root ganglion (sensory neuronopathy). It may be the only feature or be part of generalized radiculo-neuropathy.

Clinical features

It can be differentiated from cerebellar ataxia because eye movements and speech are normal and incoordination occurs only when eyes are closed (Romberg test).

The most common causes of sensory ataxia are:

Acute inflammatory sensory neuropathy (Guillain-Barré variant) – a rare variant of Guillain-Barré syndrome can present with a subacute sensory ataxia with or without generalized demyelinating inflammatory polyradiculoneuropathy.

Paraneoplastic syndrome – can be part of a paraneoplastic syndrome due particularly to small cell carcinoma of the lung with anti-Hu antibodies.

Pyridoxine (vitamin B6) – excess ingestion of vitamin B6 can cause a sensory ataxic syndrome.

Primary Sjögren's syndrome – the main features are dry eyes and mouth but can very rarely cause a pure sensory ganglionitis.

Neurologic emergencies
Meningitis

Inflammation of the meninges. It can occur with infections, malignant infiltration, drugs, contrast media, blood following subarachnoid hemorrhage, systemic lupus erythematosus (SLE) and sarcoidosis.

Bacterial meningitis, especially *Neisseria meningitides* (meningococcal meningitis), is a medical emergency.

Epidemiology

The incidence of bacterial meningitis in the UK is 3–5 per 100 000. Viral meningitis incidence is 5–10 per 100 000.

Clinical features

- Meningism – there is a classical clinical triad that comprises meningism:
  - Headache – often severe
  - Neck stiffness – flexion of the neck is resisted by boardlike stiffness
  - Fever – may be high, with or without rigors. In non-bacterial meningitis fever may be absent or low
- Rash – most common with meningococcal meningitis and is purpuric and does not blanch on pressure
- Kernig's sign – with the patient supine the leg is bent at the hip and knee, lifted off the bed, and the knee straightened and ankle dorsiflexed. A positive test causes pain in the back
- Impaired consciousness – indicates cerebral swelling and possible impending herniation
- Focal neurologic signs – hemiparesis, dysphasia, hemianopia
- Partial or generalized seizures
- Cranial nerve signs
- Sensorineural deafness

Bacterial meningitis

A medical emergency, particularly when due to meningococcus. It can progress rapidly and has a high mortality rate especially in children.

Viral meningitis

Viral meningitis is rarely an emergency. It may present acutely or subacutely. It is usually self-limiting and lasts 4–10 days. Headaches may persist for weeks but sequelae are rare.

Tuberculous meningitis (TBM)

Typically causes a chronic meningitis but may present acutely and as an emergency with hydrocephalus because it can coat the basal meninges and block the flow of CSF. Meningitic signs take weeks or months to develop, following non-specific headache, confusion, malaise, anorexia, and fever. TBM can also cause cranial nerve palsies or radiculopathies. Tuberculomas sometimes act as space-occupying lesions.

Fungal meningitis

Cryptococcal meningitis is the most common and is associated with immunosuppression, particularly HIV. Presentation is similar to TBM. Raised intracranial pressure in the absence of blockage to CSF flow is common.

Investigation

Clinical features supported by lumbar puncture. Treatment should not be delayed until investigations are performed. Lumbar puncture should not be undertaken if there are signs of raised intracranial pressure because fatal "coning" may result. Papilledema may take days to develop and imaging of the brain is desirable before lumbar puncture. This will exclude raised intracranial pressure in most but not all cases.

Other investigations include the following:

CSF pressure

The pressure is characteristically elevated in all types of meningitis ($>200 \, mmH_2O$).

Staining of CSF

- Gram stain– Gram-positive diplococci – pneumococcus and Gram-negative intracellular diplococci – meningococcus.
- Ziehl–Neelsen stain – for acid-fast bacilli (AFB) – visualized in 20%.
- India ink stain – for fungi.

Culture

Blood and CSF for bacterial, fungal, and tuberculous meningitis but take, time – up to 6 weeks in tuberculosis.

Staining and culture of skin scrapings over petechial hemorrhages may help.

Serology and polymerase chain reaction (PCR)

Serology is carried out for viral and fungal meningitides. PCR is available for all forms of meningitis.

Investigation for distant source of infection

Imaging for sinusitis, chest infection, or skull fracture.

Management

Bacterial meningitis is a medical emergency. Delay in treatment increases the likelihood of death or permanent neurologic deficit. If bacterial meningitis is suspected, nothing must delay blind therapy with IV/IM penicillin, ceftriaxone or cefotaxime.

Viral meningitis is usually benign and self limiting. Treatment is symptomatic.

Tuberculous and fungal meningitis are most commonly associated with HIV immunosuppression. Tuberculous meningitis requires at least 9 months treatment with a combination of three or four agents: isoniazid (with pyridoxine cover), rifampicin, pyrazinamide and ethambutol. Cryptococcal meningitis is treated with amphotericin with or without flucytosine or fluconazole.

Contacts of patients with bacterial meningitis, including family, school, and work contacts, may require prophylaxis with oral rifampicin or ciprofloxacin.

Outcome

Depends on causative organism and severity of infection.

Bacterial meningitis has the highest mortality if untreated which overall is 15% with sequelae in 15% of survivors.

The majority with viral meningitis recover within 1–2 weeks. About 5% have residual deficits: malaise, fatigue, and headache.

In TBM, outcome depends on duration and severity. Full recovery occurs in 30%. In cryptococcal meningitis, confounding factors also include HIV/AIDS.

Encephalitis

Inflammation of the brain parenchyma, usually caused by viruses, but occasionally by bacteria, mycoplasma, histoplasma, or rickettsia. Incidence in the UK is 4 per 100 000.

There are two types:

Acute viral encephalitis – in which the virus attacks the brain directly.

Post-infectious encephalitis (also called acute disseminated encephalomyelitis or ADEM) – in which an infection outside the brain triggers an immune attack of the brain.

Causative organisms are usually common viruses, but may not be identified. In the UK the most common causes of adult encephalitis are:

Herpes simplex virus (30%) – most severe, highest
  mortality and morbidity
Echo virus
Coxsackie virus
Mumps virus

In the Far East, the most common cause is Japanese B encephalitis, caused by an arbovirus which causes epidemic encephalitis with a high mortality rate.

Clinical features

Encephalitis may be mild with headache and drowsiness. Some present as severe illness with depressed consciousness level, focal neurologic signs, or seizures.

Herpes simplex type 1 accounts for most of the severe cases in the UK.

Patients often have a prodromal illness with headache, malaise, myalgia, and pyrexia. Neck stiffness and photophobia occur if there is meningeal involvement. Virus-specific features may be seen such as parotid swelling in mumps or exanthemata in contagious viral disease.

Location and extent of parenchymal involvement determine the level of consciousness, confusion, limb weakness, dysarthria, dysphasia, seizures, ataxia, and brainstem signs.

Investigations

Definitive diagnosis is difficult. In half a causative organism is not identified. The following investigations are usually performed.

Lumbar puncture – to exclude bacterial meningitis and perform PCR for the herpes simplex virus and other common viruses. There is often a lymphocyte pleocytosis in encephalitis.

Brain scans (CT or MRI) – to exclude structural causes and to show the extent of any inflammation. Herpes simplex has a predilection for the temporal lobes and the imaging abnormalities are relatively specific for the diagnosis.

EEG – may show non-specific slow wave change or evidence of seizure activity. Abnormalities restricted to bilateral temporal lobes suggest Herpes simplex.

Serum biochemistry and thyroid antibodies to exclude metabolic and Hashimoto's encephalopathies.

The diagnosis is often based on clinical findings as investigations may be normal.

Management

Any suspected case of encephalitis should be treated immediately with intravenous acyclovir for potential herpes simplex infection. If the herpes simplex and varicella zoster CSF PCR are negative, aciclovir can be discontinued.

Supportive treatment includes care of the comatose patient, anticonvulsants for seizures, and control of cerebral edema.

Corticosteroids are used for ADEM but are controversial for direct viral infection.

Outcome

The prognosis is variable and depends on the causative organism and the extent of involvement.

In the UK, herpes simplex has an 80% mortality untreated, falling to 30% with treatment. In contrast, the mortality for mumps encephalitis is 2% even without specific treatment.

Neurologic morbidity is also variable. Memory disturbances and cognitive dysfunction are common sequelae to herpes simplex because of its predilection for the temporal lobes.

Status epilepticus

Status epilepticus is a state of continued or recurrent seizures, with failure to regain consciousness between seizures. Regardless of cause, it is treated similarly and rapidly. It is a medical emergency with 10–15% mortality.

The National Institute for Clinical Excellence (NICE) management guidelines are:

Early status/first stage (0–10 minutes)
- Secure airway and resuscitate
- Assess cardiorespiratory function
- Administer oxygen
- Establish intravenous access

Second stage (0–30 minutes)
- Institute regular monitoring
- Consider the possibility of non-epileptic status
- Emergency antiepileptic therapy
- Emergency investigations
- Administer glucose (50 ml of 50% solution) and/or intravenous thiamine (250 mg) as high potency intravenous Pabrinex, if any suggestion of alcohol abuse or impaired nutrition
- Treat acidosis if severe

Established status/third stage (0–60 minutes)
- Establish etiology
- Alert anesthetist and ITU
- Identify and treat medical complications
- Pressor therapy when appropriate

Refractory/fourth stage (30–90 minutes)
- Transfer to ITU
- Establish intensive care and, if available, EEG monitoring
- Initiate intracranial pressure monitoring where appropriate
- Initiate long-term, maintenance antiepileptic therapy
- Emergency antiepileptic drug therapy

Premonitory stage (pre-hospital):
- Diazepam 10–20 mg given rectally (repeated once 15 minutes later if status continues to threaten)
- OR

- Midazolam 10 mg given buccally
- If seizures continue, treat as below

Early status (0–30 minutes):
- Lorazepam IV (usually 4 mg bolus, repeated once after 10–20 minutes; rate not critical)
- Give usual antiepileptic medication if already on treatment
- For sustained control or if seizures continue, treat as below

Established status (0–60 minutes):
- Phenytoin infusion (between 15 and 18 mg/kg at a rate of 50 mg/minute) OR fosphenytoin infusion at a dose of 15–20 mg phenytoin equivalents (PE)/kg at a rate of 50–100 mg PE/minute
- AND/OR
- Phenobarbitone bolus of 10–15 mg/kg at a rate of 100 mg/minute

Refractory status (30–90 minutes)
- General anesthesia with one of:
- Propofol (1–2 mg/kg bolus, then infusion) titrated to effect
- Midazolam (0.1–0.2 mg bolus then infusion) titrated to effect
- Thiopentone (3–5 mg/kg bolus then infusion) titrated to effect; after 2–3 days infusion rate needs reduction as fat stores are saturated
- Anesthetic continued for 12–24 hours after the last clinical or electrographic seizure, then dose tapered

Emergency investigations:
- Blood gases
- Glucose
- Biochemistry screen (renal and liver function, calcium, magnesium)
- Full blood count and clotting
- Antiepileptic drug levels
- Toxicology – serum and urine
- CXR – for possible aspiration
- Other investigations – brain imaging and lumbar puncture if no raised intracranial pressure

Monitoring:
- Regular neurologic observations
- Pulse, blood pressure, and temperature
- ECG
- EEG – if available
- Blood gases, biochemistry, clotting, blood count, drug levels

Table 9.8. Distinguishing features, site of pathology and urgent investigations of severe neuromuscular weakness

Condition	Associated features	Site	Investigations
Guillain-Barré syndrome	Post-infectious motor weakness, areflexia	Nerve	Clinical, nerve conduction/EMG, lumbar puncture, *Campylobacter* serology
Myasthenia gravis	Ptosis, ophthalmoplegia, dysarthria, dysphagia, reflexes and sensation normal	Neuromuscular junction	Acetylcholine receptor antibodies, nerve conduction/EMG
Botulism	Areflexia, pupil dilatation, cranial palsies, paralytic ileus, urinary retention, sensory symptoms but no signs	Neuromuscular junction	Botulinum toxin in feces, serum, or suspect food
Myopathy/myositis	Normal reflexes and sensation	Muscle	EMG, CK, inflammatory markers, serum lactate and pyruvate (metabolic/mitochondrial myopathy), muscle biopsy

Severe neuromuscular weakness

Some neuromuscular conditions can deteriorate rapidly and lead to respiratory depression requiring ventilatory support. The most common are Guillain-Barré syndrome and myasthenia gravis. Others are botulism, polymyositis and metabolic myopathies. This section outlines their differentiation (Table 9.8)

Any emergency presentation with neuromuscular weakness requires repeated measurement of forced vital capacity (FVC). The results should be graphically documented, so that any downward trend in respiratory capacity can be acted on. If FVC falls below 1 litre, transfer to ITU should be arranged and ventilatory support provided if necessary.

Further reading

Crash Course: Neurology. 2nd edn. Christopher Turner, Anish Bahra and Katia Cikurel. Mosby, 2008.

Morrow J, Russell A, Guthrie E, *et al.* Malformation risks of antiepileptic drugs in pregnancy: a prospective study from the UK Epilepsy and Pregnancy Register. *J. Neurol Neurosurg Psychiatry* 2006; 77, 193–198.

Neurology and Neurosurgery Illustrated. 4th edn. K Lindsay and I Bone. Churchill Livingstone, 2004.

Neurological Differential Diagnosis. 2nd edn. John Patten. Springer, 1996.

Newer drugs for epilepsy www.nice.org.uk/TA076

Website for the Merck Manual – Neurology section – http://www.merck.com/mmpe/sec16.html

Contents

Eye problems are encountered across the field of medicine and surgery. A provisional diagnosis may be necessary before an expert opinion becomes available. Common presenting symptoms are red eye, loss of vision, or double vision. Examination (Tables 10.1 and 10.2) of the eye, even when asymptomatic, may provide supporting evidence for a systemic disease. There are also some eye conditions which should be considered in the management of the unconscious patient.

Red eye

Red eyes are the manifestation of infective, inflammatory, or congestive conditions in the eye and orbit. They are usually the sign of a local condition but sometimes may be the diagnosing factor in a systemic disease, most commonly sarcoidosis, tuberculosis, systemic lupus erythematosis (SLE), or Wegener's granumolatosis. The condition is not obvious to sufferers unless they are otherwise unwell.

Subconjunctival hemorrhage

Epidemiology

This appears suddenly as a bright red patch of blood under the conjunctiva and is usually symptomless but may cause a mild aching. It is rarely associated with hypertension or bleeding diatheses.

Management

In recurrent cases check medications for aspirin or warfarin, measure blood pressure and blood count. Reassure patient that it will resolve.

Conjunctivitis

Epidemiology

Bacteria, viruses, allergy, or chemical irritants may inflame the conjunctiva. Ophthalmia neonatorum is defined as a conjunctivitis in the first month of life and occurs from infection introduced during birth.

Pathology

Bacterial infections are most commonly caused by *Staphylococcus* spp., followed by *Streptococcus pneumoniae* and *Haemophilus* spp. Viral conjunctivitis is mostly due to adenovirus although in children molluscum contagiosum and herpes simplex may be the cause. Adult inclusion conjunctivitis is due to *Chlamydia trachomatis*. *Chlamydia* is also probably the commonest cause of ophthalmia neonatorum in Europe, other serious causative organisms are gonococcus and herpes virus. Allergic conjunctivitis may be of four types. An acute type 1 reaction, a seasonal reaction associated with asthma and eczema, a chronic response with follicles and papillae to an allergen or irritant, or finally vernal keratoconjunctivitis with giant cobblestone papillae on the conjunctival surface of the upper lid. Vernal means occurring in spring, when there is a high level of pollen in the air.

Clinical features

The visual acuity is not affected, except by discharge or excessive watering which can be wiped away, or by corneal infiltrates in adenoviral infection. The redness may be intense with swelling of the lids in bacterial infection but the eye movements are full with no double vision. The redness is most intense in the conjunctiva lining the lids. Eversion of the upper lid helps in diagnosis as white follicles just visible to the naked eye are the hallmark of viral and chlamydial

Table 10.1. Helpful markers in making a diagnosis

History	Examination
Onset and length of symptoms	Visual acuity
Effect on vision	Discharge
Nature of pain	Distribution of redness
Photophobia	Pupil reactions
Previous similar episodes	Corneal reflex Eye movements

Table 10.2. Signs and symptoms

	Visual acuity	Redness	Other
Subconjunctival hemorrhage	6/6	most intense	
Conjunctivitis	6/6	mild to moderate	discharge
Episcleritis	6/6	patchy superficial	
Anterior scleritis	6/6–6/12	moderate deep	
Uveitis	6/6-HM	around cornea	photophobia
Acute glaucoma	6/36-CF	generalized	nausea and vomiting

infection, small tufts of blood vessels called papillae are found in bacterial and mild allergic conditions, whilst giant papillae are found in vernal conjunctivitis. Viral conjunctivitis is bilateral in two-thirds of cases and may follow a fever and sore throat and is highly contagious. Chlamydial conjunctivitis is usually bilateral and protracted. Allergic conjunctivitis is itchy. Figure 10.1 shows types of conjunctivitis.

Investigations

Conjunctival swabs may be taken for identification of bacteria, viruses, and chlamydia but are not required in most cases of conjunctivitis. The exceptions are ophthalmia neonatorum, severe or persistent and unexplained conjunctivitis and if chlamydial infection is suspected. Infants with blocked tear ducts and sticky eyes do not require repeated bacteria swabs.

Management

In cases of ophthalmia neonatorum the child is referred to a pediatrician if systemically unwell as herpes viremia may be fatal and systemic involvement may also occur with *Pseudomonas*, *Neisseria gonorrhea*, and *Chlamydia trachomatis*.

Adult conjunctivitis is treated according to the expected cause. Topical antibiotics, commonly chloramphenicol, are used for suspected bacterial conjunctivitis. Topical steroid treatment of adenoviral infection is reserved for cases of severe inflammation or if the vision is affected by keratitis, as withdrawal of the steroid can cause an exacerbation of symptoms. Any with proven chlamydial infection should be referred for genital swabs before treatment of themselves and partner with azithromycin or an equivalent antibiotic. Allergic or toxic conjunctivitis may require preservative-free drops or steroid drops.

Outcome

Conjunctivitis does not affect the vision unless the cornea is involved, causing a keratitis. This occurs mildly in adenoviral keratitis, more severely in vernal

Fig. 10.1. Types of conjunctivitis.

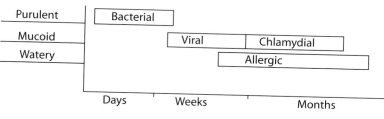

keratoconjunctivitis, and most severely in those areas where trachoma is prevalent.

Episcleritis and anterior scleritis

Epidemiology
Episcleritis typically affects young adults, is rarely associated with a systemic condition, but tends to recur. Anterior scleritis is more common in an older age group and is associated with rheumatoid arthritis, SLE, polyarteritis nodosa, Wegener's granulomatosis, sarcoidosis, and tuberculosis.

Pathology
Episcleritis is a dilatation of vessels in the tissue layer, which lies between the conjunctiva and the sclera. No structural damage is caused to the sclera. The vessels blanch with the application of guttae phenylephrine 2.5%. Anterior scleritis is usually diffuse but may be necrotizing or non-necrotizing. The necrotizing type, which is strongly associated with systemic vasculitis, shows areas of non-perfused thin sclera, which may perforate. The brawny redness of the sclera does not blanch with guttae phenylephrine.

Clinical features
Episcleritis causes a mild, gritty, aching pain with segmental redness and normal vision. Scleritis often causes a severe pain which interrupts sleep. Visual acuity is reduced if there is corneal thinning or an associated uveitis or posterior scleritis (Fig. 10.2).

Investigations
No investigations are required for episcleritis. In cases of scleritis an underlying vasculitis may exist. FBC, ESR, CRP, U&E, LFT, antinuclear antibodies, and anti-neutrophil antibodies may be helpful in exploring this possibility.

Management
The only treatment of proven efficacy in episcleritis is a non steroidal anti inflammatory agent (NSAID), which is used for moderate discomfort. Mild cases may benefit from ocular lubricants. Non-necrotizing scleritis usually responds to NSAIDs, but severe necrotizing disease has a poor untreated visual prognosis and requires admission for high dose steroids.

Outcome
Intermittent relapses are usual in episcleritis and nodular scleritis. Permanent visual loss may occur in necrotizing scleritis.

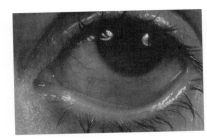
Fig. 10.2. Episcleritis (courtesy of Mr. P. Hamilton).

Uveitis

Epidemiology
Most cases are idiopathic but many systemic associations exist. Anterior uveitis, also called iritis, occurs in herpes simplex and zoster infections, sarcoidosis and tuberculosis, inflammatory bowel disease, ankylosing spondylitis and syphilis and is associated with rheumatoid arthritis, SLE Wegener's granulomatosis, sarcoidosis, and tuberculosis.

Pathology
There is inflammation of the anterior uvea with cells and fibrin in the aqueous. The cells form clumps, keratic precipitates, on the lower corneal endothelium and the iris sticks to the anterior capsule of the lens (Fig. 10.3). A posterior subcapsular cataract may form.

Clinical features
The main symptom is photophobia with a dull aching pain. The redness is mainly circumcorneal, known as a ciliary flush. Visual acuity is usually mildly reduced but may be down to hand movements if there is an excessive reaction with anterior chamber cells settling to form a hypopyon (Fig. 10.4). The latter occurs typically in ankylosing spondylitis. The pupil may be small and irregular if there are iris adhesions to the lens and the cornea hazy if there is an acute rise in intraocular pressure.

Investigations
The first attack of iritis requires a dilated examination of the posterior segment of the eye looking for vitritis, chorioretinitis, or retinal detachment. Repeated attacks may be associated with tuberculosis or sarcoidosis, in which a chest X-ray will be abnormal in 90% of cases. Other useful investigations are serum ACE, syphilis serology, FBC, ESR, and CRP.

Management
The pain of iritis is caused by spasm of the iris and is relieved by short acting cyclopentolate or long acting

301

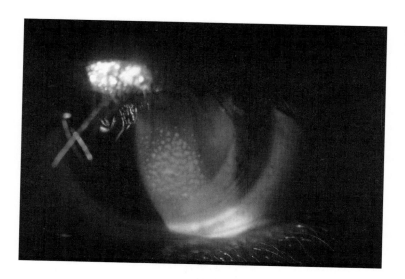

Fig. 10.3. Keratic precipitates (courtesy of Professor M. Stanford).

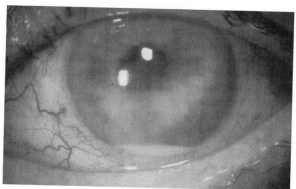

Fig. 10.4. Hypopyon (courtesy of Mr. P. Hamilton).

atropine. The inflammation is reduced by topical steroids of varying strength.

Outcome
Repeated attacks may cause reduction in visual acuity due to pupil adhesions to the lens and cataract formation.

Acute glaucoma
Epidemiology
The condition is more common in long-sighted (hypermetropic) elderly women.

Pathology
Aqueous humor drains out of the eye through the trabecular meshwork, which is in the angle between the cornea and the iris. The hypermetropic eye has a narrower than average drainage angle, which is further narrowed in old age by the swelling of the lens as it becomes cataractous. The drainage angle may close abruptly when the iris is bunched up by dilatation, either in low light conditions or by mydriatics. The acute rise in pressure from the normal (10–21 mmHg) to >60 mmHg causes pain and ischemia of the cornea and iris.

Clinical features
The main symptoms are nausea and vomiting caused by the sudden increase in intraocular pressure and these may mask the ocular pain, which is nonetheless severe. The visual acuity is reduced and the cornea cloudy to the naked eye with a mid-dilated and non-reactive pupil. The redness may be generalized or circumcorneal. The main attack may have been preceded by night-time haloes as the intraocular pressure increased transiently.

Investigations
Not required.

Management
Intravenous acetazolamide 500 mg and seek specialist help.

Outcome
Permanent severe visual loss due to retinal ischemia or a central retinal vein occlusion may occur if treatment is delayed.

A painful white eye
The most common cause is a reduced tear film and this may give the sensation of an aching pain behind the eye. Pathology outside the orbit can cause ocular pain as with the severe ocular pain of cluster headaches, trigeminal neuralgia and migraine.

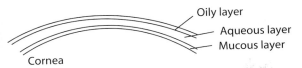

Fig. 10.5. Composition of the tear film.

Pain on eye movement is the first sign of optic neuritis.

Dry eyes
Epidemiology
The condition increases with age and is associated with blepharitis as well as the systemic conditions rheumatoid arthritis, Sjogren's syndrome, thyroid eye disease, graft vs host disease, and sarcoidosis.

Pathology
The tear film is composed of an inner mucous layer, an intermediate aqueous layer, and an outer oily layer, whose surface tension holds the watery layer in apposition (Fig. 10.5).

Clinical features
The main complaint is of gritty, burning, and tired eyes and even of watering, although the tears never overflow onto the cheek. The watering is an aqueous response to a lack of mucous layer. The thickness of the tear film above the lower lid is best seen with a slit lamp, surrogate measures using Schirmer's test are less informative. Staining of dry spots on the cornea and conjunctiva with fluorescein or the painful Rose Bengal stain show the extent of the drying.

Management
This is a chronic condition which is ameliorated but not cured by tear substitutes. There are various lubricating agents and it is difficult to predict which will help each individual. The preservative in most preparations may aggravate the symptoms, in which case refrigerated preservative-free drops are used. Mucous strands are treated with topical acetyl cysteine. In severe cases the lacrimal puncta can be stenosed with cautery or plastic plugs.

Outcome
A troublesome and persistent condition.

Blepharitis
Epidemiology
The condition occurs throughout life but is rare in young children. It is associated with dry eyes, acne rosacea, and atopic eczema.

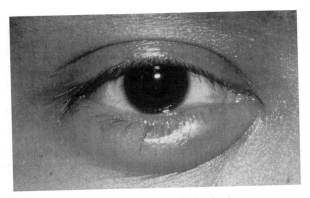

Fig. 10.6. Chalazion (Courtesy of Mr. P. Hamilton).

Pathology
There is a combination of staphylococcal infection, malproduction of lipids in the Meibomian glands, and tear film instability.

Clinical features
The eyes feel sore and gritty and the eyelids are red rimmed with various degrees of crusting. Chalazia, which are infected Meibomian glands, are common. The lid margins become notched and the eyelashes misdirected, and they may rub against the eye (Fig. 10.6).

Management
Cleaning of the lid margin is recommended with cotton wool buds and either baby shampoo or dilute sodium bicarbonate solution. Antibiotic ointment helps if there is an infected stye or chalazion. Chronic chalazia are treated with incision and curettage. Tear substitutes may ease the gritty sensation. In severe persistent exacerbations, a 3-month course of oral doxycycline reduces the inflammation.

Outcome
When persistent it can cause permanent structural changes to the lid margins.

Sudden loss of vision (Figs. 10.7, 10.8 and Table 10.3)
Central retinal artery occlusion (CRAO)
Epidemiology
This occurs most commonly in the seventh decade.

Pathology
The causes include giant cell arteritis, emboli from the heart or carotid arteries, and locally formed thrombus in hyperviscosity syndromes.

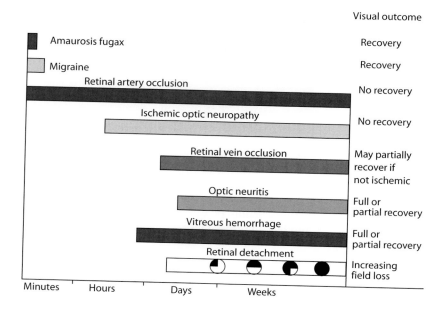

Fig. 10.7. Sudden visual loss: cause, duration, and outcome.

Sudden visual loss

Visual outcome

Cause	Visual outcome
Amaurosis fugax	Recovery
Migraine	Recovery
Retinal artery occlusion	No recovery
Ischemic optic neuropathy	No recovery
Retinal vein occlusion	May partially recover if not ischemic
Optic neuritis	Full or partial recovery
Vitreous hemorrhage	Full or partial recovery
Retinal detachment	Increasing field loss

Minutes Hours Days Weeks

Clinical features

There is a sudden profound loss of vision to counting fingers or less, a relative afferent pupillary defect, and a pale fundus caused by infarction of the retina (Fig. 10.9).

Management

Urgent ESR and CRP to exclude giant cell arteritis. FBC, glucose, lipids, vasculitis screen, carotid ultrasound, and echocardiography. There is no proven effective treatment.

Outcome

Recovery of vision is rare.

Central or branch retinal vein occlusion (CRVO or BRVO)

Epidemiology

This occurs most commonly over the age of 50 years.

Pathology

In 70% of cases the blockage is partial and the retina does not become ischemic. There are extensive hemorrhages throughout the retina but no cotton wool spots and only mild disk swelling. In 30% of CRVOs there is ischemia and visual loss is more profound. Poor prognostic signs are a relative afferent papillary defect, cotton wool spots, and marked disk swelling. It is very rare for the retina to become ischemic and the disk swollen after a branch vein occlusion.

Clinical features

The visual loss is often noticed on waking up or after a period of dehydration, and visual loss varies from mild to severe and may be progressive. Primary open angle glaucoma is an associated cause (Fig. 10.10).

Management

Exclude hypertension, diabetes, hyperviscosity syndromes, hyperlipidemia, clotting abnormalities in the under 50s and refer to an ophthalmologist for a fluorescein angiogram to determine which cases are ischemic and need pan-retinal photocoagulation.

Outcome

Untreated ischemic CRVOs develop painful neovascular glaucoma with profound visual loss. Non-ischemic CRVOs and branch vein occlusions may regain some vision.

Anterior ischemic optic neuropathy (AION)

Epidemiology

The majority of cases are hypertensive, non-arteritic with peak incidence in the 60–70-year age group but

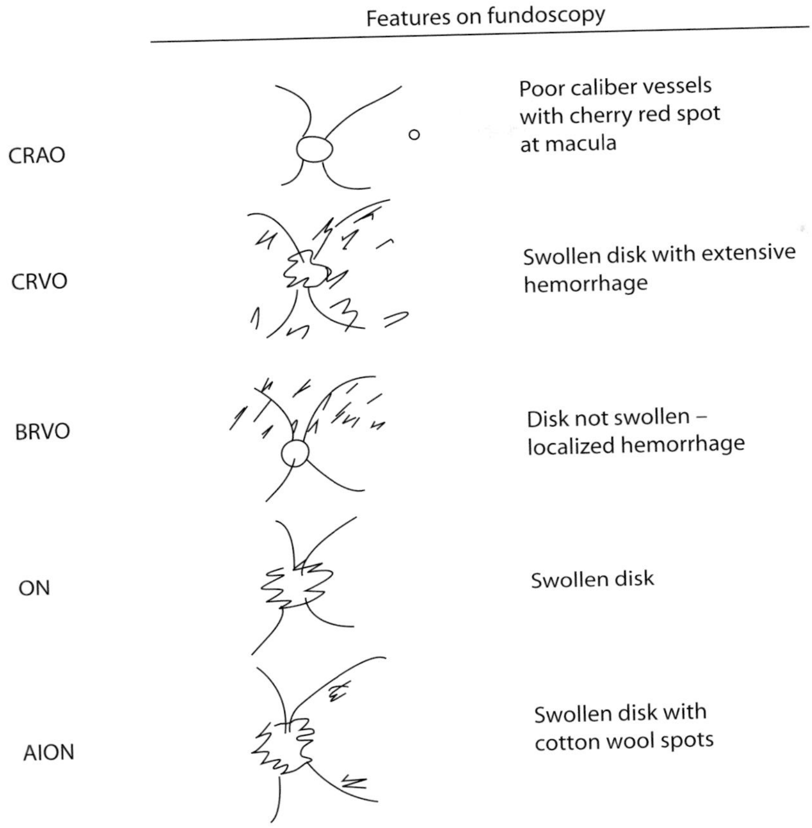

Features on fundoscopy

Fig. 10.8. Sudden visual loss: features on fundoscopy. (Abbreviations as in Table 10.2.)

CRAO — Poor caliber vessels with cherry red spot at macula

CRVO — Swollen disk with extensive hemorrhage

BRVO — Disk not swollen – localized hemorrhage

ON — Swollen disk

AION — Swollen disk with cotton wool spots

it may occur in younger age groups, particularly if there is a sudden drop in blood pressure. If the cause is giant cell arteritis, those over 70 are most frequently affected.

Pathology
There is occlusion of the posterior ciliary arteries serving the optic nerve head.

Clinical features
Loss of vision is sudden, may be noticed on waking and is more profound when the cause is arteritis. There is swelling of the optic disk, with localized hemorrhages and cotton wool spots. Visual field testing with a red pin shows an altitudinal loss and there is a relative afferent papillary defect (Fig. 10.11).

Management
If in any doubt that the cause is giant cell arteritis give 200 mg of IV hydrocortisone and admit for high-dose steroids. Treatment should not be undertaken as an outpatient as the elderly may suffer psychiatric and metabolic side effects. A temporal artery biopsy should be performed even after the start of treatment. Non-arteritic cases are screened for hypertension and diabetes and treated with low-dose aspirin.

Outcome
There is unlikely to be any improvement in the affected eye, the aim of treatment is to protect the contralateral eye.

Amaurosis fugax
There are multiple vascular, hematologic, neurologic, and ocular causes, many of which are treatable and are covered in other sections.
- Carotid artery disease causing slow flow in retinal artery
- Cardiac abnormalities with source of microemboli
- Vasculitis, either giant cell arteritis (GCA) or SLE
- Papilledema
- Hyperviscosity syndromes, coagulopathies, or anemia

305

Table 10.3 Signs in acute visual loss

Sign	Relative afferent pupillary defect	Unilateral swollen disk	Extensive retinal hemorrhages	Cotton-wool spots	Retinal exudates	Reduced color vision
Test	Swinging light		Fundoscopy			Ishihara color plates
CRAO	++	−	−	−	−	vision too poor to test
BRAO	+	−	−	−	−	+
CRVO	+ if ischemic	+	++	+ if ischemic	+	−
BRVO	−	−	+	+/−	−	+
AION	+	+	−	+	−	+
ON	+	+/−	−	+	−	+
Vit. heme	−			no view of fundus		−
RD	−	−	−	−	−	−

Notes:
CRAO: central retinal artery occlusion.
BRAO: branch retinal artery occlusion.
CRVO: central retinal vein occlusion.
BRVO: branch retinal vein occlusion.
AION: anterior ischemic optic neuropathy.
ON: optic neuritis.
Vit. heme: vitreous hemorrhage.
RD: retinal detachment.

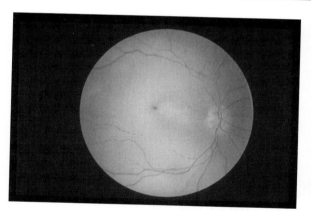

Fig. 10.9. Central retinal artery occlusion (courtesy of Mr. P. Hamilton).

Fig. 10.10. Branch retinal artery occlusion with cotton wool spots (courtesy of Mr. P. Hamilton).

Optic neuritis

Epidemiology

Optic neuritis is an inflammation of the optic nerve, which is likely to recover. The condition is usually monocular and is most common in adults between the ages of 20 and 40 years.

Pathology

Demyelinating optic neuritis is often associated with multiple sclerosis and there may be other neurologic dysfunctions. Viral infections, granulomatous inflammation (sarcoidosis, tuberculosis and syphilis), and adjacent sinusitis can cause an optic neuritis.

Clinical features

Subacute, sometimes severe visual loss which is associated with pain on eye movements. There is reduced color perception, particularly to red, a visual field loss with generalized constriction or a central scotoma.

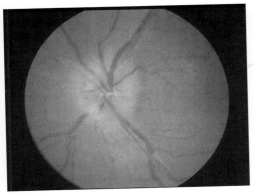

Fig. 10.11. Swollen optic disk (courtesy of Mr. P. Hamilton).

Table 10.4. Loss of vision

Type of visual loss	Condition	Common causes
Distance vision + glare	Cataract	Age-related, diabetes, steroids
Reading vision + recognizing faces	Macular degeneration	Age-related, smoking
General blurring	Diabetic retinopathy	Poor diabetic control
Loss of color vision	Optic neuropathy	Nutritional, toxic

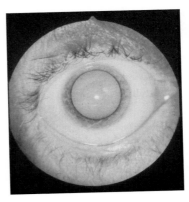

Fig. 10.12. Cataract (courtesy of Mr. P. Hamilton).

The swinging light test reveals a relative afferent pupillary defect (RAPD).

Management
Any case which has not resolved in 4 weeks requires investigation as for optic neuropathy.

Outcome
Most cases of optic neuritis resolve fully. With multiple sclerosis there may be permanent visual loss.

Retinal detachment
A condition requiring an urgent ophthalmologic review, in which visual loss is preceded by floaters and flashing lights and is more common in myopic individuals.

Gradual loss of vision (Table 10.4)
Cataract
Epidemiology
Cataract is the most common non-refractive cause of visual impairment worldwide.

Pathology
Any opacification of the crystalline lens is known as a cataract. There is a progressive yellowing and hardening of the lens with increasing age and the point at which this aging process is called a cataract is arbitrary. There are various scales for measuring the yellowing and focal opacification of the lens but they are mainly research tools. Therefore the popular understanding of cataract is of any opacification of the lens sufficient to cause visual symptoms. Factors associated with earlier onset are a family history, diabetes, and trauma.

Clinical features
Misting or blurring of vision of a gradual onset. Glare, particularly of car headlights, caused by scattering of light. An increasing myopia and difficulty with distance vision, which is not matched by difficulty with reading vision, which may remain good without glasses (Fig. 10.12).

Management
Cataract surgery is the fourth commonest procedure performed in the UK. It is a highly successful, usually day-case operation requiring a local anesthetic. There is a 0.3% risk of sight-threatening complications. The most serious complications are intraocular infection (endophthalmitis), choroidal hemorrhage, and retinal detachment.

Outcome
The cataract surgery rate in the UK is 4100/million population/year and post-operatively most people require glasses only for reading.

Age-related macular degeneration
Epidemiology
In the UK age-related macular degeneration (AMD) is the most common cause of visual loss in the over 75s and affects 20% of the elderly population.

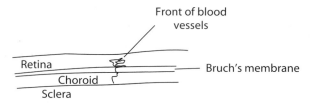

Fig. 10.13. Wet form of AMD.

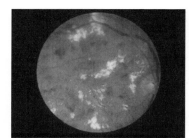

Fig. 10.14. Diabetic retinopathy with hemorrhages and exudates (courtesy of Mr. P. Hamilton).

Pathology

The macula is the area of the retina and choroid concerned with central vision. There are two main types of macular degeneration, exudative (wet) and non-exudative (dry) and both involve the retina, pigment epithelium, Bruch's membrane, and choriocapillaris. The majority (85%) of cases are of the dry type, with gradual loss of photoreceptors and pigment epithelium giving a patchy hyper- and hypopigmented atrophy. In the less common wet form, new blood vessels grow through defects in Bruch's membrane to form a subretinal neovascular membrane, which may hemorrhage or cause a localized exudative retinal detachment. Subsequent fibrosis causes a diskiform scar (Fig. 10.13).

Clinical features

There is a gradual loss of central vision, the main complaints being of progressive inability to read and recognize faces. In the wet form there may be a sudden marked deterioration with distortion or a dark area in the center of the visual field. The causes are a localized central retinal elevation or retinal hemorrhage.

Management

The only treatable AMD is the early wet type, when the visual acuity has not dropped below 6/60. Rapid referral to an ophthalmologist is required for anyone noticing new symptoms of distortion or central loss. Photodynamic therapy, a non-thermal laser, or various thermal lasers may achieve closure of the new vessels and prevent further progression in some cases.

Outcome

Registration as partially sighted or blind is required in only 15% of cases of AMD. Referral to low vision aids clinics should be considered early for advice on lighting, print types, and a variety of support societies.

Diabetes

Epidemiology

Diabetic retinopathy is the most common cause of blind registration for people between the ages of 25 and 65 years. Vision is impaired by maculopathy, which is more common in type 2 diabetes, or by vitreous hemorrhage and retinal traction, which are more common in type 1 disease.

Pathology

The microvascular abnormalities of diabetes result in capillary closure and abnormal permeability. Microaneurysms are seen as dot hemorrhages and, when they rupture, as flame-shaped hemorrhages. Capillary leakage leads to macular edema and lipid deposition, seen as exudates. Capillary closure is not visible clinically, except in a fluorescein angiogram. It may lead to small areas of retinal infarction, which are seen as cotton wool spots. Other signs of ischemia, which carry a poor prognosis, are venous loops and deep dark hemorrhages, which together form pre-proliferative retinopathy. Proliferative retinopathy is defined by fragile new vessels on the optic disk and on major vessels. Bleeding from these vessels into the vitreous causes fibrovascular proliferation resulting in a traction retinal detachment.

Clinical features

Gradual reduction in vision remains a frequent presentation of diabetes in the elderly population and is likely to be due to maculopathy. Retinal vein occlusions, for which diabetes is a risk factor, may have a subacute presentation with worsening vision over several weeks to months. Acute loss of vision is usually caused by a vitreous hemorrhage (Fig. 10.14).

Management

Control of blood sugar and blood pressure levels is the major factor in controlling all types of retinopathy. Untreated, maculopathy will cause visual loss. The aim of focal laser treatment is to seal leaking

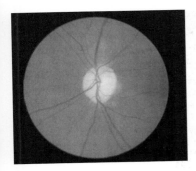

Fig. 10.15. Optic atrophy (courtesy of Mr. P. Hamilton).

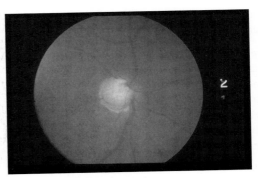

Fig. 10.16. Cupped optic disk (courtesy of Mr. P. Hamilton).

microaneurysms before edema and exudates become established. Macular ischemia is not amenable to treatment. In proliferative disease pan-retinal photo-coagulation is used to ablate the peripheral retina with the aim of reducing vaso-proliferative factors and causing regression of new vessels. Cataract surgery is commonly undertaken in diabetics and close monitoring should occur in the months following surgery as maculopathy can accelerate.

Outcome
The major risk factors for sight-threatening disease are duration and control of diabetes. Early detection and treatment of maculopathy may halt progression. Vitreo-retinal surgery for vitreous hemorrhage and retinal detachment is associated with multiple risks.

Optic neuropathy
Epidemiology
Optic neuropathy is a gradual and usually irreversible loss of optic nerve function. It occurs characteristically in middle age.

Pathology
Optic neuropathy has multiple causes including compression, infiltration, toxic, inherited, nutritional, and radiation induced. Common nutritional deficiencies are associated with excess intake of alcohol and tobacco. Compression may occur subacutely in thyroid eye disease.

Clinical features
Subacute or gradual, moderate to severe visual loss, which is associated with pain if there is an optic neuritis. There is reduced color perception, particularly of red, a visual field loss with generalized constriction or a central scotoma, and the swinging of a bright light from eye to eye reveals a relative afferent papillary defect (RAPD). The optic nerve initially appears normal but becomes pale over months (Fig. 10.15).

Management
Tobacco/alcohol neuropathy may improve with cessation of abuse and improved diet. Other causes which should be sought are syphilis, B12 and folate deficiency, sarcoidosis, and a compressive lesion.

Outcome
Most cases of optic neuritis resolve with variable amounts of visual loss. Optic neuropathy is less likely to show improvement.

Primary open angle glaucoma
A painless, progressive, and irreversible loss of peripheral and finally central field of vision. Seen on fundoscopy as a cupped optic disk (Fig. 10.16).

Double vision: binocular
Binocular double vision is only present with both eyes open.

Cranial nerve palsies
Epidemiology
The sixth nerve is the most susceptible due to its long course at the base of the brain. The third and fourth nerve palsies occur less frequently.

Pathology
Microvascular occlusions occur in diabetes and hypertension but recovery is expected. Compressive and infiltrative lesions persist.

Clinical features
There is double vision, which is not present when either eye is covered. The double vision is worse in looking in the direction of the weak muscle. Sudden onset of a painful third nerve palsy with pupil dilation is suggestive of a posterior communicating aneurysm. Papilledema suggests raised intracranial

pressure of any cause and may not be associated with a reduction in vision.

Management

In the case of a painful third nerve palsy there should be immediate referral to a neurosurgical centre. Temporal arteritis should be excluded in the over 60 year olds, diabetes, and hypertension in all cases. The optic disks should be examined to see if they are swollen. If there has been no recovery by 3 months, further investigation is warranted.

Outcome

The prognosis is good for microvascular causes and in cases where the intracranial pressure can be lowered.

Thyroid eye disease

Epidemiology

Eighty percent of people with thyroid eye disease, also known as Graves' ophthalmopathy, have signs of hyperthyroidism, 10% have Hashimoto's thyroiditis, and 10% have no detectable signs of abnormal thyroid function.

Pathology

There is characteristic infiltration and thickening of the extraocular muscles, which causes crowding in the orbit. The globe may protrude forward (proptosis) or there may be compression of the optic nerve at the orbital apex, causing reduction in vision.

Clinical features

The proptosis is often unilateral or asymmetric. Restriction of the extraocular muscles causes progressive diplopia with characteristic tethering of the inferior rectus. In active disease there may be compression of the optic nerve with reduction in color vision and visual field.

Management

Visual acuity and color vision should be examined regularly in each eye during active disease. Urgent referral for surgical decompression of the orbit or systemic steroid treatment is required if visual acuity or color vision deteriorate.

Outcome

Surgery on the extraocular muscles and eyelids is sometimes required when the disease has become inactive.

Central nervous system diseases

Lesions affecting central processing of extraocular muscle balance are uncommon and cause types of double vision that cannot be explained by weakness or restriction in individual muscles.

Double vision: monocular

This persists on covering one eye.

Monocular diplopia

Double vision sometimes persists even if one eye is covered. In this case the light is being split as it passes through the eye to form more than one image on the retina. The causes could be refractive errors, corneal irregularities, or opacities in the lens.

Ptosis
Disinsertion of the levator muscle

Epidemiology

The commonest cause of ptosis in the elderly population.

Pathology

The attachment of the levator palpebrae superioris muscle to the tarsal plate becomes thinned.

Clinical features

There is slowly progressive ptosis, the skin crease is raised or absent, and levator function is normal.

Management

Various surgical options are available to restore lid height.

Outcome

This is a surgically treatable condition.

Horner's syndrome

Epidemiology

A rare but significant cause of ptosis.

Pathology

There is disruption in the sympathetic pathways serving the dilator muscles of the pupil, eyelid elevators, and sweat glands of the forehead. The commonest site of a lesion is the level of the first rib but it can be at any level from the hypothalamus to the eye.

Clinical features

The pupil is mildly constricted and there is 1–2 mm of ptosis.

Management

The only condition that may need emergency treatment is a dissection of the carotid artery. A history of a recent whiplash injury to the neck should be sought and if positive low dose aspirin should be commenced before scanning of the carotid arteries. Chest X-ray is performed to exclude lesions of the lung apex.

Outcome

A cerebrovascular accident may follow a carotid dissection.

Myasthenia gravis

Epidemiology

The prevalence in Europe is 1 in 25 000 and women are affected more than men.

Pathology

It is an autoimmune disease whose target is the post-synaptic acetylcholine receptor of the motor end plate.

Clinical features

Variable ptosis and diplopia, worse at the end of the day. It is occasionally associated with rapidly progressive disease requiring ventilation. Weakness of other muscles should be sought as part of the examination. Relevant blood tests include acetlycholine receptor antibodies.

Management

Awareness of the possibility of acute deterioration and referral for a neurological opinion and muscle biopsy.

Outcome

Long-term medication may be required.

Other conditions

Conditions in which an ophthalmological opinion may be of use in confirmation of a diagnosis:

Granulomatous disorders

Tuberculosis, sarcoid, syphilis, toxoplasmosis, and brucellosis may cause an anterior or posterior uveitis.

Metabolic diseases

Hypercalcemia and Wilson's disease can cause corneal deposits. Hyperthyroidism causes superior limbic keratitis, proptosis, and restriction of eye movements and, in acute cases, optic nerve compression.

Vasculitis

Severe SLE is associated with retinal cotton wool spots and hemorrhages, Wegener's granulomatosis and rheumatoid arthritis cause scleritis and corneal melts, Behçet's can cause retinal vascular occlusions.

Hematological disorders

Retinal hemorrhages are found in conditions with low platelet counts and in hyperviscosity disorders when associated with venous occlusions. Roth's spots are found in cases of endocarditis.

HIV and AIDS

Asymptomatic cotton wool spots may indicate HIV retinopathy as do multiple molluscum contagiosum of the lids. Cytomegalovirus (CMV) and other viral causes of retinitis are usually symptomatic.

Swollen optic disks

Papilledema is a swelling of both optic disks due to raised intracranial pressure and is commonly asymptomatic, although transient obscurations in vision may occur. There may be an associated sixth nerve palsy.

The unconscious patient

There are two main ophthalmological considerations in an unconscious patient, one much more obvious than the other. Is the cornea protected and lubricated and is there a silent intraocular infection (endophthalmitis)?

Corneal protection

If the eyes are not completely closed, the conjunctiva and cornea dry and ulcerate. In the case of the cornea this presents a threat to vision. Ocular ointments, taping of the lids, and jelly preparations are of use in protection.

Endophthalmitis

Any unconscious patient with a bacterial, viral, or fungal septicemia requires a regular examination of the eye with dilated pupils to exclude intraocular seeding of the infection. The eye may be white with no suspicion of infection until the retina is inspected. If there is no red reflex, then it is highly likely that there is extensive vitreous activity. It is an occasional tragedy that patients regain consciousness to discover that they are blind.

Rheumatic

Terence Gibson

Contents

Table 11.1. What to look for when a patient complains of musculoskeletal pain

History	Examination
Onset: sudden or gradual	Distribution of symptoms
Age, gender	Deformity
Duration: continuous or intermittent	Swelling, effusion, redness
Peripheral joints, spine, or both	Muscle wasting or weakness
One, few, or multiple sites	Tenderness, range of movement
Stiffness, swelling	
Worse after rest/activity	Skin
Eye inflammation, rash	Nails
Diarrhea	Eyes
Disability, work, domestic circumstances	

A history of pain at one or more musculoskeletal sites may indicate a primary rheumatic diagnosis or it be a manifestation of a condition that mainly involves other parts of the body. In establishing the cause of the pain there are history and examination features which should be sought and documented (Table 11.1).

The duration of pain onset, the age of the patient and the distribution of symptoms may narrow the list of likely diagnoses. There are exceptions but the guide of Table 11.2 illustrates a general rule based on duration of pain onset.

Peripheral joint pain: sudden onset

Most of the causes of sudden onset (acute) arthritis affect one or a few joints simultaneously. The age of the patient and the sites of involvement can be indicative of the causes as shown in Fig. 11.1.

The investigation of sudden onset peripheral arthritis is urgent when a joint is red, hot, and contains an effusion. Fever, leukocytosis, and an acute phase response (high ESR or CRP) are common features. The key investigation is examination of synovial fluid if it can be aspirated

Joint pain

Pain is the principal symptom of all rheumatic disorders. It may affect the periphery, the spine, or both, and it may derive from the joints themselves, the bones, muscles, or the ligaments.

Table 11.2. Likely diagnosis based on mode of presentation

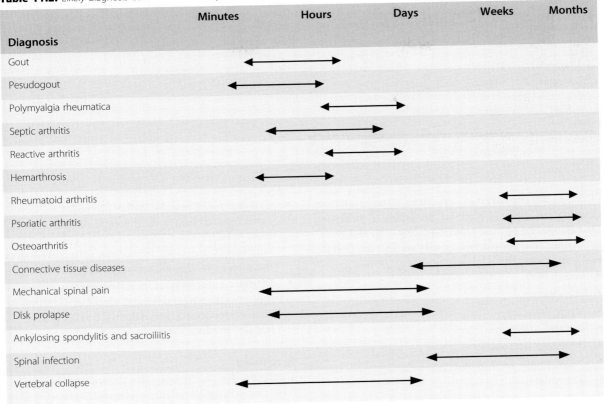

Diagnosis	Minutes	Hours	Days	Weeks	Months
Gout		←——————→			
Pesudogout	←————————→				
Polymyalgia rheumatica		←——————→			
Septic arthritis		←—————————→			
Reactive arthritis		←————→			
Hemarthrosis	←————→				
Rheumatoid arthritis				←————→	
Psoriatic arthritis				←————→	
Osteoarthritis				←————→	
Connective tissue diseases				←—————————→	
Mechanical spinal pain	←——————————→				
Disk prolapse	←——————————→				
Ankylosing spondylitis and sacroiliitis				←————→	
Spinal infection				←—————————→	
Vertebral collapse	←——————————→				

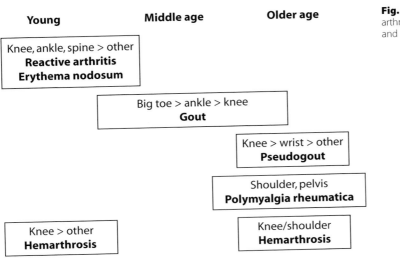

Fig. 11.1. Sudden onset peripheral arthritis – causes according to site of pain and age.

Table 11.3. Diagnostic investigations of sudden onset peripheral arthritis

	Synovial fluid				X-ray	Blood culture
	Appearance	WCC	Culture	Crystals		
Gout	Turbid/ purulent	++/ +++	Neg	Long needle shaped	Soft tissue swelling/ erosion	Neg
Pseudogout	Turbid/ purulent	++/ +++	Neg	Small rhomboid shaped	Chondro calcinosis/ OA	Neg
Reactive arthritis	Turbid	++	Neg	Nil	Normal	Neg
Septic arthritis	Turbid/ purulent	+++ +	Pos	Nil	Normal	Pos
Hemarthrosis	Blood	+		Nil	Normal or/OA	Neg

(Table 11.3). The naked eye appearance and immediate examination under a plain or preferably a polarizing microscope can provide rapid diagnosis (Fig. 11.2).

Conditions considered in this section on peripheral joint pain are:

- gout
- pseudogout
- septic arthritis
- reactive arthritis
- erythema nodosum
- polymyalgia rheumatica
- hemarthrosis

Gout

Gout presents as sudden painful swelling of the big toe, ankle, or other lower limb joint. It is caused by shedding of monosodium urate crystals into the joint cavity from microtophi on the joint lining. These accumulate when there is sustained hyperuricemia. When untreated, multiple joints may be affected causing deformities.

Clinical features

- Usually in middle life, male, obese, and often drinks alcohol to excess. Hypertension and alcoholic liver disease may be associated.
- The initial episode mainly affects the first metatarso-phalangeal joint (podagra). Subsequently, other joints of the foot, then the ankle and the knee may be involved.
- Acute gout is associated with one or more red, hot, swollen joints. The pain is extreme, fever is common.
- The upper limb joints are eventually affected. Deformities follow cumulative attacks. The condition may then become chronic with recurrent acute episodes.

- External tophi may be visible as chalky subcutaneous lumps on the ears, elbows, fingers, toes, or other sites. These commonly accompany long standing disease. Joint deformities give rise to the picture of chronic tophaceous gout.
- Diuretic induced gout in the elderly may cause tophi on the fingers, toes, or elsewhere with no or little evidence of acute arthritis. In this group, females predominate.

Epidemiology

Common but prevalence rates difficult to determine. The risk within populations correlates directly with the level of blood uric acid. It occurs more often in men because blood uric acid levels are higher in males until menopause when the levels become similar. The annual incidence for men is 1–3 and women 0.2 per 1000. There is a correlation of serum urate with body weight and affluence. It is rare in poor societies and in cultures which abstain from alcohol. People of Polynesian extraction and especially the Maoris of New Zealand are susceptible.

Pathology

Sustained hyperuricemia results in monosodium urate crystal deposition in collagen rich tissue, especially cartilage and synovium. Local trauma, infection, surgery, and reduction of blood uric acid cause fragmentation of deposits and liberation of crystals. These induce pronounced local inflammation. Crystal activation of synovial macrophages induces interleukin 8 (Il-8) and other chemoattractants resulting in neutrophil leukocytes entering the joints and ingesting the crystals.

Hyperuricemia is associated with inherent, relative impairment of uric acid clearance by the kidneys in 95% of gout. Increased hepatic purine synthesis induced by alcohol is contributory. Blood uric acid

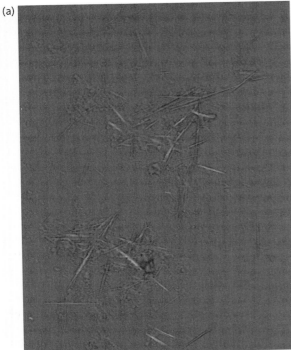

Fig. 11.2. Examples of synovial fluid crystals under polarizing microscopy. Sample from a tophus. The crystals lie within leukocytes aspirated from a swollen joint.
(a) monosodium urate in gout
(b) calcium pyrophosphate in pseudogout.

levels rise with obesity. All thiazide and loop diuretics elevate uric acid levels by reducing renal urate clearance. Rarely, an X-linked deficiency of a purine salvage enzyme, hypoxanthine guanine phosphoribosyltransferase (HPRT), will cause hyperuricemia and gout in childhood or adolescence (Fig. 11.3). Degrees of enzyme deficiency produce a spectrum of associated neurologic abnormalities. The Lesch–Nyhan syndrome is due to complete deficiency and comprises mental retardation, gout, and renal failure. Overactivity of the enzyme 5-phosphoribosyl-1-pyrophosphate is another X-linked trait that may cause gout in young males. Both are exceptionally rare.

Recurrent episodes of gouty arthritis may produce cartilage loss and permanent joint damage. Accumulations of urate (tophi) cause erosions of joint cartilage and bone with subsequent deformity.

Mild renal impairment is common due to associated hypertension, renal vascular disease, and less commonly, fibrosis due to urate crystals in kidney interstitial tissue.

Investigation

The clinical picture of acute gout affecting the big toe is distinctive, but confirmation can only be by demonstrating urate crystals within synovial fluid cells.

- The synovial fluid is turbid due to large numbers of white cells. Uric acid crystals may also be demonstrated in scrapings of tophi. A polarizing microscope with colored filters makes crystal identification easier but is not essential. Urate crystals tend to be slender, pointed, and are bright under a polarizing light microscope. They are "negatively birefringent" that is, in a color-compensated system they are yellow when aligned in one direction and blue when at 90°.

- Blood uric acid levels may be normal at the time of an attack. Conversely, not every patient with arthritis and hyperuricemia has gout. Withdrawal of alcohol, diuretic, or weight reduction may precipitate an attack by causing the blood and synovial fluid uric acid levels to fall.

- There may be peripheral neutrophilia, a very high CRP, or ESR.

- X-rays may show loss of joint space or erosions in chronic or recurrent tophaceous gout.

- Other biochemical features of gout may include hypertriglyceridemia and liver dysfunction.

- Mild renal impairment may be demonstrated by GFR estimation, but kidney failure is a rare consequence of primary gout.

315

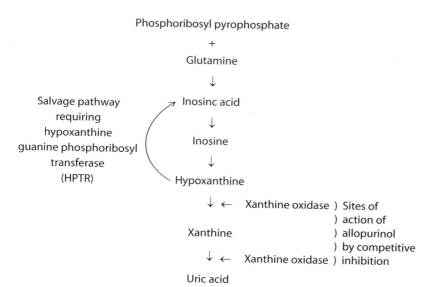

Phosphoribosyl pyrophosphate

\+

Glutamine

↓

Salvage pathway requiring hypoxanthine guanine phosphoribosyl transferase (HPTR)

Inosinc acid

↓

Inosine

↓

Hypoxanthine

↓ ← Xanthine oxidase) Sites of
) action of
Xanthine) allopurinol
) by competitive
↓ ← Xanthine oxidase) inhibition

Uric acid

Fig. 11.3. The *de novo* production of purines, their disposal as uric acid, and the sites of allopurinol action (XO – xanthine oxidase).

Management

There are two phases of management.

(1) Acute arthritis responds to joint aspiration, intra-articular corticosteroid and non steroidal anti inflammatory drugs (NSAIDs). Colchicine taken hourly is effective but not recommended. It invariably causes nausea, diarrhea or abdominal pain. When NSAIDs are contraindicated, a course (up to 2 weeks) of prednisolone is warranted. A single attack in a normouricemic individual does not warrant further measures if the blood uric acid level remains normal.

(2) Those with more than two annual episodes, visible tophi, deformed joints, or renal impairment should receive a blood uric acid lowering agent if there is persistent high serum uric acid level. Hyperuricemia associated with obesity and alcohol excess should be treated with dietary advice. Hypouricemic drug treatment should be indefinite. Allopurinol is the best hypouricemic drug. This inhibits uric acid production by competitive inhibition of xanthine oxidase (Fig. 11.3). Febuxostat is a new xanthine oxidase inhibitor, which may be useful when toxicity to allopurinol arises. This is more likely when there is renal impairment. Probenecid and sulfinpyrazone are alternative preparations, which increase uric acid excretion in the urine by blocking tubular reabsorption. These are less effective in renal impairment. Benzbromarone is an effective uricosuric agent in renal impairment and where there are huge tophi and renal

impairment IV uricase (Rasburicase) is justifiable. Reduction of blood uric acid increases the risk of further acute gout but this is lessened by concurrent colchicine in small dose. Concomitant hypertension and other associates of obesity should be sought and treated. The need for diuretic use should be reconsidered. Spironolactone may lessen the requirement for thiazide and loop diuretics.

Outcome

Acute gout is self-limiting but even with treatment may require several days or weeks to resolve. Recurrent episodes may continue for years despite successful reduction of blood uric acid. Tophi may require several years of treatment before disappearing.

Pseudogout

This is the second most common form of crystal synovitis. It occurs in older people. Crystals of calcium pyrophosphate dehydrate (CPPD) are shed from the joint cartilage and excite an inflammatory response analogous to that of gout. The knee is the most commonly affected. Calcification of joint cartilage (chondrocalcinosis) is usually seen but is not diagnostic.

Clinical features

A hot, swollen knee in an elderly person is most likely pseudogout. Usually only one joint is involved. As with gout, fever may be prominent. The wrist is the second most common joint to be affected. Involvement of other sites is uncommon.

Epidemiology

Women are affected slightly more often than men. It is mainly confined to those aged more than 60. It has a worldwide distribution.

Pathology

Calcification of cartilage (chondrocalcinosis) is an aging phenomenon. It is often associated with osteoarthritis (OA). One-third of those over age 80 have chondrocalcinosis of meniscal and joint lining cartilage. In order of frequency, knees, wrists, hips, symphysis pubis, shoulders, and finger joints may be involved. Calcification at these sites is due to deposition of crystalline calcium pyrophosphate dehydrate (CPPD). Shedding of crystals into the joint evokes acute inflammation as intense as that of gout. This phenomenon may be precipitated by trauma or an incidental febrile illness.

Widespread chondrocalcinosis in young or middle-aged patients with or without acute arthritis may denote evidence of hyperparathyroidism, hemochromatosis, or familial predisposition. The deposition of CPPD may be protective or cause OA. There are opposing views.

Investigation

The diagnosis can only be confirmed by examination of synovial fluid. This is sometimes so densely turbid as to suggest sepsis. CPPD crystals are more difficult to identify than sodium monourate. They may be few, small and rhomboid or oblong with blunt ends. They are "positively birefringent" and their color under a compensated polarizing microscope is the opposite of monosodium urate. ESR or CRP may be very high and neutrophilia is common. X-rays show chondrocalcinosis and OA of involved sites but are insufficient for diagnosis. In young or middle-aged patients estimation of serum calcium, phosphate, parathormone, ferritin levels, and thyroid function tests are necessary to exclude hyperparathyroidism, hemochromatosis, and hypothyroidism.

Management

Joint aspiration and intra-articular injection of corticosteroid are followed by rapid improvement. Most patients are elderly and NSAIDs may be used but with caution. Co-prescription of a proton pump inhibitor reduces gastric side effects. A short course of oral prednisolone is an alternative.

Unlike gout, there is no correctible metabolic derangement in most patients.

Outcome

Severe acute attacks improve within days but low grade inflammation may persist. The majority do not have recurrence.

Septic arthritis

Joint infection is often thought to be the cause of an acute swollen joint with fever but it is much less common than crystal synovitis. A primary focus of infection, bacteremia, and pre-existing joint disease are susceptibility factors.

Clinical features

- Evidence of pre-existing infection such as septicemia, skin ulcers, or pneumonia should raise suspicion.
- Usually only one joint is affected but two or multiple sites may be involved including non-synovial joints.
- The knee is the most common site but any joint may be affected.
- Acute arthritis of an upper limb joint other than the wrist is suspicious.
- A hot, swollen, single joint in otherwise quiescent chronic joint disease should raise the possibility of septic arthritis.
- Rigors, fever, and severe pain are common.
- A pustular or purpuric rash with or without a history of genital infection especially in the young raises the possibility of gonococcal infection. In this condition, polyarthralgia and a migratory arthritis may precede painful swelling of one or a few large or small joints.

Epidemiology

Joint sepsis accounts for less than 10% of acute arthritis. Patients with pre-existing or current infections, rheumatoid arthritis, and intravenous drug users are especially susceptible. No gender or age group is more likely to be affected except that gonococcal arthritis is confined to the sexually active.

Pathology

The most common organism is *Staphylococcus aureus* but *Streptococcus pneumoniae*, *Neisseria gonorrhea*, *Haemophilus influenzae*, and other microorganisms can all be implicated. It is not known why bacteremia may occasionally result in a septic arthritis, but previously damaged joints are receptive to infection. Failure to recognize joint sepsis results in progressive loss

(a)

(b)

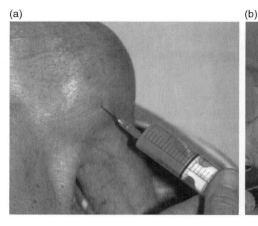

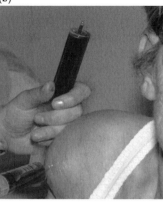

Fig. 11.4. Shoulder aspiration
(a) purulent synovial fluid in septic arthritis
(b) blood in hemarthrosis.

of cartilage, infection of underlying bone, and permanent joint damage.

Investigation

Suspicion of septic arthritis must always be confirmed by joint aspiration. Turbid or purulent synovial fluid is not sufficient evidence of infection (Fig. 11.4).

- The first step involves exclusion of crystals on microscopy.
- In a purulent sample, the diagnosis of sepsis must be presumed if crystals are absent.
- A Gram stain may confirm the presence of bacteria.
- Synovial fluid culture may yield evidence of infection even when organisms are not seen initially.
- Suspicion of gonococcal arthritis may require special culture media. Swabs of genital organs, mouth, and anus should also be obtained in this context.
- Blood cultures may provide evidence of bacteremia and should always be performed at the time of joint aspiration.
- Radiology of affected sites for narrowing of the joint space will indicate whether cartilage has been destroyed.

Management

Densely turbid or purulent synovial fluid in the absence of crystals should prompt immediate treatment with intravenous flucloxacillin and oral fucidic acid, even when bacterial identification has not yet been achieved. This choice of antibiotics reflects the likelihood of staphylococcal infection. The antibiotic regimen should be amended in the light of cultures and sensitivities. Intravenous treatment should continue for 7–14 days with regular joint aspiration, daily if necessary. Oral antibiotics should be substituted at the end of this period and continued for another 3–4 weeks, dependent on response. Surgical drainage and joint lavage should be arranged if aspiration fails or if the joint is inaccessible, e.g. the hip.

Outcome

Failure to recognize septic arthritis results in joint destruction, osteomyelitis, and secondary osteoarthritis. An unidentified focus of infection in a joint may lead to septicemia and death.

Reactive arthritis

The term reactive arthritis (Reiter's syndrome) indicates joint inflammation caused by an infection which has resolved and in which the relevant organism is not found within the joint itself. The arthritis associated with erythema nodosum has a similar distribution of joint involvement.

Clinical features

- A history of gastroenteritis or less commonly of urethritis may precede the sudden onset of painful swelling of joints (Table 11.4). Sometimes, no history of overt infection is present.
- The knees are the most commonly affected joints followed by the ankles then fingers and toes. Involvement is often asymmetric and may be accompanied by low back pain due to acute sacroiliitis.
- Plantar fasciitis and Achilles tendonitis occur in a minority and may be persistent.
- Gritty, red eyes with discharge due to conjunctivitis may coincide with the arthritis. When the illness

Table 11.4. Infectious organisms which have been associated with reactive arthritis

Salmonella species
Shigella dysenteriae
Campylobacter
Chlamydia trachomatis
Chlamydia pneumoniae
Clostridium perfringens

Table 11.5. Frequency of disease associations with Class 1 major histocompatibility gene HLA B27

Idiopathic ankylosing spondylitis	95%
Reactive arthritis	75%
Psoriatic spondylarthritis	50%
Inflammatory bowel disease spondarthritis	50%
Idiopathic anterior uveitis	50%

persists, anterior uveitis may occur as well as recurrent conjunctivitis.

- In sexually acquired reactive arthritis, there may be persisting evidence of a urethritis or in men, a balanitis.
- When the disease becomes chronic or recurrent, distal interphalangeal joint swelling or diffuse swelling of fingers and toes (dactylitis or sausage digits) often occur.
- A similar appearance of digits may be seen in the arthritis of psoriasis, inflammatory bowel disease, chronic sarcoidosis, and tuberculous joint infection.
- Sacroiliitis develops in 10% of chronic reactive arthritis, and ankylosing spondylitis may follow with stiffening of the spine.
- A rash identical to pustular psoriasis may occur on the soles of the feet (keratodermia blenorrhagica). Excess keratin may develop beneath the toe nails and sometimes the finger nails (onycholysis).
- The rash and nail changes, the interphalangeal joint involvement, the asymmetry of the arthritis, plantar fasciitis, tendonitis, and sacroiliitis are features which may also occur in psoriatic arthritis. There is also a clinical similarity to the arthritis of inflammatory bowel disease.
- The phenotypical overlap is, in part, reflected by the common association of these disorders with the gene for HLA B27 (Table 11.5).

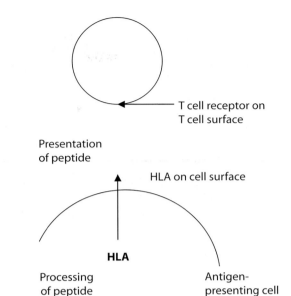

Fig. 11.5. The function of HLA class 1 and 2 molecules. HLA B27 is a class 1 gene and strongly associated with ankylosing spondylitis and related diseases. HLA DR4 is a class 2 gene and is linked with rheumatoid arthritis although the association is not as strong as that of HLA B27 with other rheumatic diseases. Both genes are involved in the presentation of peptides by macrophages or other cells. Class 1 genes present to CD8 and class 2 genes to CD4 T lymphocytes.

- The human leukocyte antigen (HLA) genes are within the major histocompatibility complex (MHC) on chromosome 6. *HLA B27* lies within the Class 1 region. Another HLA gene important for arthritis is *HLA DR4* and this is a Class 2 gene (Fig. 11.5).

Epidemiology

Men and women, usually young, are equally susceptible. The frequency is greater among populations where prevalence of *HLA B27* is relatively high, namely in the Northern Hemisphere. In areas of the developing world where infections are common, reactive arthritis is seen less often, probably because of the lower prevalence of *HLA B27*.

Pathology

Inflammation of involved joints is associated with CD4 T lymphocyte infiltration and increased vascularity of the synovium. Viable organisms are not found in the synovial fluid or synovium, but DNA and RNA traces of relevant bacteria have been identified in both. It is presumed that bacteria in the gut or urethra initiate an immune event involving macrophages or lymphocytes which migrate to the

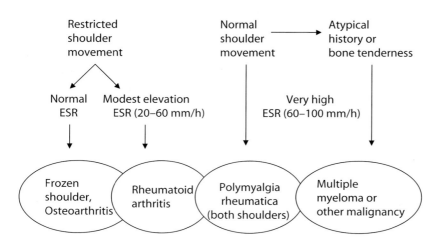

Fig. 11.6. Pain and stiffness of shoulders in subjects aged more than 60.

synovium. Approximately 75% carry the gene *HLA B27*, which is involved in the presentation of bacterial antigen by macrophages to CD8 positive T lymphocytes (Fig. 11.5). How this translates to a disease in which CD4 positive cells predominate in the synovium is unclear.

Investigation
There are no diagnostic investigations. Elevation of ESR and CRP corroborates the presence of inflammation. Aspirated synovial fluid is turbid and contains neutrophils but no organisms. The presence of *HLA B27* may enhance the diagnostic suspicion but it is not diagnostic. In chronic disease, radiologic bone erosions similar to those of rheumatoid arthritis may arise, and views of the pelvis and spine may show sacroiliitis and less commonly, progression of this to ankylosing spondylitis.

Management
The acute illness responds to simple analgesics, non-steroidal anti-inflammatory drugs, joint aspiration and intra-articular injection of corticosteroids. The chronic peripheral joint disease may respond to sulfasalazine, methotrexate, and probably to anti-TNFα preparations. Spinal involvement is helped by analgesics and non-steroidal anti-inflammatory agents but not by other agents.

Outcome
Eighty percent have an acute illness that resolves completely within a few weeks or months. For 15% it becomes a troublesome chronic arthritis with fluctuations in disease activity, toe, and finger joint swelling, and recurrent eye inflammation. In 5%, pain and

stiffness of the spine develop with all the features of idiopathic ankylosing spondylitis.

Polymyalgia rheumatica (PMR)
It is debatable whether polymyalgia rheumatica is an arthritis. Joint redness, swelling, warmth, and restricted joint movement are conspicuous by their absence. There is a frequent tendency to over-diagnose it amongst cases of frozen shoulder and rheumatoid arthritis. It is one of the few causes of a very high ESR. In a minority there is a clinical or histopathologic link with giant cell arteritis (GCA).

Clinical features
- The abrupt onset pain and stiffness of the shoulder or the pelvic girdle or both in a person older than 60 years is highly suggestive.
- Symptoms are worse after inactivity and there may be fatigue.
- There is a characteristic lack of clinical signs. Restricted movement of one or both shoulders suggests the alternative possibilities of frozen shoulder, osteoarthritis, or rheumatoid arthritis. The diagnosis of rheumatoid arthritis may become apparent only with time (Fig. 11.6).
- Pain and stiffness appear to derive from muscles but weakness and tenderness are absent. If either is present, polymyositis should be considered instead of PMR.
- The symptoms may be the prelude to giant cell arteritis. A history of headache, temporal artery, or scalp tenderness should always be sought. Sudden blindness or blurring of vision is a rare

event in the absence of scalp tenderness but it does occur and biopsy evidence of GCA exists in 10% of PMR patients who have exhibited no head pain or tenderness.

Epidemiology

The disorder is seen mainly in people of European extraction with a prevalence of less than 1% but with an increasing prevalence with each decade beyond 60. It is twice as common in women than men.

Pathology

No abnormality of muscles has been demonstrated and there is disputed evidence that the symptoms are due to inflammation of axial joints such as the sterno- and acromioclavicular joints. Mild inflammatory infiltrates have been found at these sites similar to rheumatoid arthritis. The intensity of the acute phase response is associated with a polyclonal increase of immunoglobulins. Rheumatoid factors are not found. The association of some cases of polymyalgia with giant cell arteritis has prompted the idea that the illness is a form of vasculitis, but beyond the occasional presence of inflammation of temporal arteries there are no histopathologic data to support this.

PMR shares immunogenetic susceptibility with rheumatoid arthritis, namely an association with *HLA DR4* which is found twice as often as in healthy controls.

Investigations

A very high ESR and/or CRP characterize the illness. The constellation of polymyalgic symptoms and a high ESR (usually 60–100 mm in the first hour) in a person over age 60 is highly suggestive. Another cause of a very high ESR, which may cause skeletal pain, is multiple myeloma (see Chapter 17). Other malignancies affecting the skeleton such as metastatic solid tumors may produce a similar picture.

A mild normocytic anemia, which may be normo- or hypochromic, increase of platelets, and mild liver dysfunction are regular findings.

Muscle enzymes, electromyography, muscle biopsy, and radiology of the skeleton are normal in PMR but are justifiable investigations if polymyositis, rheumatoid arthritis, multiple myeloma, or other neoplastic involvement of the skeleton are suspected.

Management

PMR symptoms resolve with 48 hours of prednisolone treatment. A dose of 40 mg daily is adequate. The ESR declines in parallel. If there is no response to treatment, the diagnosis is wrong and requires revision. The dose of prednisolone can be reduced quickly to the lowest necessary to keep the patient symptom free. It is better to monitor symptoms rather than ESR. The addition of azathioprine or methotrexate may allow reduction of prednisolone but is rarely necessary. Long-term steroid use, especially in the age group affected by PMR, requires the addition of a bisphosphonate to protect the skeleton against osteoporosis.

Outcome

A gratifying response to prednisolone and long-term low dose prednisolone (5–10 mg daily) maintenance is the rule. It is unwise to stop treatment within 1 year. Weaning off prednisolone may be attempted thereafter, but 60% will relapse and may require treatment for periods of 2–5 years. An unfortunate 10% of patients will require life-long prednisolone.

Erythema nodosum

Clinical features

- Arthritis with redness and edema around knees and ankles and less commonly around upper limb joints sometimes with low backache.
- Red nodules on shins or elsewhere on limbs.
- Fever.

Epidemiology

Prevalence is uncertain. It is three times more common in women and occurs in adolescents and middle life. It is rare in the elderly.

Pathology

The most common cause is acute sarcoidosis associated with bilateral hilar lymphadenopathy. Other causes or associations are streptococcal sore throat, TB, inflammatory bowel disease, Behçet's syndrome, enteric infections, or miscellaneous drugs. The skin lesions are those of a panniculitis with inflammation of fatty tissue. Hemorrhage accounts for the livid skin lesions and their subsequent similarity to bruises.

Investigation

The diagnosis is clinical. An acute phase response is usual. A chest X-ray and further investigation of likely causes such as throat swab or colonoscopy depends on associated symptoms.

Management

Analgesics and NSAIDs in most cases. Prednisolone in modest dose is occasionally required.

Outcome

Improvement can be anticipated. It is a self-limiting condition.

Hemarthrosis

This is a neglected and poorly recognized cause of acute joint pain in the elderly. Among younger people, it is the consequence of trauma, pigmented villonodular synovitis, hemophilia, or some other bleeding disorder.

Clinical features

- Pain and swelling affecting a knee or shoulder, occurring spontaneously in an older person.
- In young people, a history of trauma is often obtained. When caused by hemophilia, the diagnosis is usually well established. When hemarthrosis is recurrent, pigmented villonodular synovitis is possible. The knee is the joint most commonly affected by this rare condition.
- Warmth, swelling, tenderness, restricted movement, and presence of a joint effusion are the cardinal signs.

Epidemiology

There is no information about the frequency of hemarthrosis except that it occurs at both ends of the adult age spectrum.

Pathology

Concomitant osteoarthritis of the knee or shoulder is usual in the elderly. The latter is associated with loss of rotator cuff muscle and tendon tissues. The increased fragility of blood vessels associated with aging accounts for the bleeding.

In young patients with pigmented villonodular synovitis the synovium is hypertrophied and pigmented by deposits of hemosiderin.

Investigation

The diagnosis can only be achieved by joint aspiration. Radiographs in older patients will show osteoarthritis of the knee or shoulder. Radiographs of the latter may reveal upward migration of the humeral head and calcified fragments within and around the joint. This is sometimes referred to as Milwaukee shoulder. Villonodular synovitis in young people may cause radiologic erosion of bone. Other investigations are normal.

The definitive diagnosis of pigmented villonodular synovitis is obtained by direct vision arthroscopy and/or synovial biopsy.

Clotting factors and a platelet count should always be determined in both young and old.

Management

Aspiration of blood relieves pressure and reduces pain. In older persons recurrence is occasional but in pigmented villonodular synovitis it is the rule. In the latter, treatment is surgical synovectomy.

Outcome

In older patients, pain and disability due to underlying degeneration persist and may require joint replacement. In pigmented villonodular synovitis, recurrence after surgery may be treated with intra-articular radioisotope injections.

Peripheral joint pain: gradual onset

Painful joints which are gradual in onset may affect one, few, multiple, or cumulative sites. The age of the patient, the distribution of involvement, and the presence or absence of stiffness after inactivity and of swelling will indicate the probability of either an inflammatory joint disorder or osteoarthritis (Fig. 11.7). In general, a story of arthritis affecting multiple sites usually denotes one of the diseases caused by inflammation of the synovium. In these conditions, inflammatory markers such as ESR and C-reactive protein (CRP) are elevated and synovial fluid when aspirated is turbid due to the presence of many neutrophil leukocytes.

Rheumatoid arthritis (RA)

This is the most common form of polyarticular joint inflammation. It is the archetypical form of arthritis, causing synovial thickening, joint effusion, destruction, deformities, and disability.

Clinical features

- Pain, stiffness and swelling of small joints of the fingers and larger joints.
- Swelling and tenderness characteristically affect the second and third metacarpophalangeal joints.
- Nodules over the ulnar border of the forearms may be visible but need to be sought by palpation. They occur in 20% and are also found on Achilles tendons, finger pulps (especially in methotrexate-treated patients), and pressure areas. Nodules are found only in those who are rheumatoid factor positive.
- In chronic disease, deformity of finger joints with ulnar deviation and flexion or hyperextension occur due to subluxation of joints and misalignment of tendons. The metatarsals become

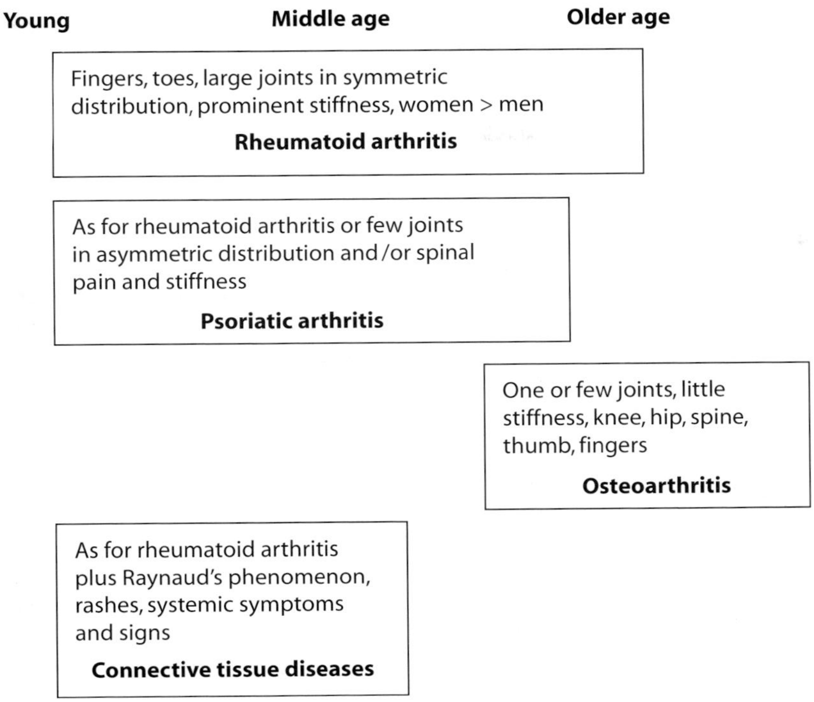

Young   Middle age   Older age

Fingers, toes, large joints in symmetric distribution, prominent stiffness, women > men **Rheumatoid arthritis**

As for rheumatoid arthritis or few joints in asymmetric distribution and /or spinal pain and stiffness **Psoriatic arthritis**

One or few joints, little stiffness, knee, hip, spine, thumb, fingers **Osteoarthritis**

As for rheumatoid arthritis plus Raynaud's phenomenon, rashes, systemic symptoms and signs **Connective tissue diseases**

Fig. 11.7. Peripheral joint pain of gradual onset.

prominent and painful with overlying callus. Joints such as wrists, elbows, shoulders, ankles, and other foot joints may become restricted. Leakage of synovial fluid from the knee causes lower limb edema simulating a deep vein thrombosis. The axial skeleton is not involved apart from the cervical spine.

- Extra-articular disease is more likely in sero-positive patients. Small pleural effusions, interstitial lung disease, asymptomatic pericarditis, eye redness and pain due to scleritis or corneal ulceration secondary to dry eyes (Sjogren's Syndrome), nail fold infarcts (Fig. 11.8), and leg ulcers due to cutaneous vasculitis. Vasculitis may be accompanied by mononeuritis or glove and stocking peripheral neuropathy (see Chapter 9). The central nervous system is not involved except by cervical cord compression due to subluxation of vertebrae secondary to local joint involvement. Subluxation may follow a fall or other trauma (Fig. 11.9).

- Felty's syndrome represents rheumatoid disease, splenomegaly, lymphadenopathy, leg ulcers, neutropenia, sometimes with thrombocytopenia. It is now rare.

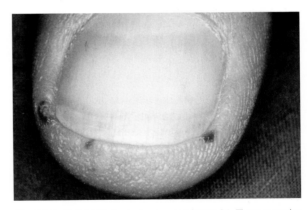

Fig. 11.8. Nail fold infarcts due to vasculitis in RA. These may also be seen in connective tissue diseases such as SLE.

- In Western countries rheumatoid arthritis remains the commonest cause of amyloidosis but like Felty's syndrome is now uncommon probably because of better disease control. Amyloid is an insoluble protein that is deposited in multiple organs such as the kidney causing nephrotic syndrome and renal failure. It is caused by high levels of serum amyloid, a protein which behaves as an acute reactant (AA disease). There are other

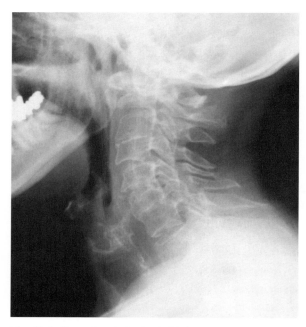

Fig. 11.9. X-ray of cervical spine in RA showing anterior subluxation of second and fifth vertebrae.

causes of amyloid and clinical associations of amyloidosis including more widespread additional organ involvement such as tongue, skin, and heart (AL disease). This occurs in association with multiple myeloma and monoclonal immunoglobulin synthesis.

Epidemiology

RA is a worldwide disease with an incidence of 1%. Young adults, those in middle life, and older people can be affected but the peak incidence is between ages 30 and 50. Women are affected twice as often as men. Extra-articular complications are less common in patients of Asian and African extraction. There is a small heritable predisposition, which may account for sporadic family clustering.

Pathology

Inflammation of synovium is the principal feature with increased vascularity, thickening of the synovial lining, and infiltration of the sub-synovium with lymphocytes, macrophages, and plasma cells. These changes are common to all chronic inflammatory joint diseases and can also be seen in chronic gout and osteoarthritis. T lymphocytes comprise a third of the cells and are mainly CD4 positive (helper) cells. Perivascular aggregations of cells resemble lymph node follicles.

Plasma cells may excrete rheumatoid factors. These are immunoglobulins (IgM, IgA, IgG) which react with the Fc region of the IgG globulin. The rheumatoid factor most easily measured is IgM and is found in the serum of 70%. These anti-IgG immunoglobulins are not specific and help to clear immune complexes containing microbial antigens, but no causative infection has been identified in RA. There is a strong association of rheumatoid arthritis with HLA DR4 and other MHC class 2 molecules with similar amino acid sequences (the shared epitope hypothesis). The MHC proteins of which the HLA system is part are important in the presentation of antigen to T cells, and both CD4 and CD8 lymphocytes need to be bound to HLA before they recognize antigens (see Fig. 11.5).

Inflamed hypertrophied synovium (pannus) encroaches on the cartilage surface. At the margins, the cartilage is thin and becomes denuded and the underlying bone is eroded by the pressure of tissue and the excretion of proteolytic enzymes.

The process of antigen internalization by macrophages or other cells and the processing into polypeptides and their representation on the cell surface involve many cytokines. Interleukin-1 (Il-1) generated by antigen-presenting cells stimulates T cells. Other pro-inflammatory cytokines which facilitate recruitment and activation of macrophages and both T and B lymphocytes are TNF-α, Il-2, Il-4, IFN (interferon), Il-6, and Il-2. There are many others, but pivotal to this cascade is TNF-α. Some cytokines such as Il-10 have an anti-inflammatory role. In common with other inflammatory diseases, multiple chemoattractants and adhesion molecules play a role in directing the accumulation of inflammatory cells.

Investigations

Mild normo- or hypochromic anemia, elevated ESR and C-reactive protein are to be expected in chronic inflammatory joint diseases. The presence of IgM rheumatoid factor (RF) in high titer is very suggestive of RA. A positive test in low titer may be found in health and connective tissue diseases. Anti-cyclic citrullated protein (CCP) has higher specificity than RF and will be deployed increasingly as a routine test. X-rays should be taken of hands and feet in suspected cases. Typical erosions of the fingers, especially the metacarpophalangeal joints, will consolidate the diagnosis. Erosive damage is often first detectable on the fifth metatarsal even when there is no foot pain and

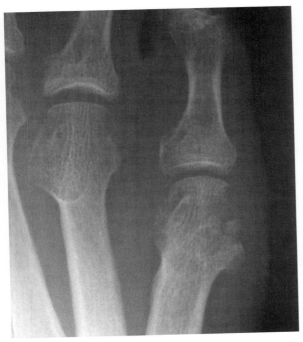

Fig. 11.10. X-ray of fifth metatarsal in RA showing typical erosions.

Table 11.6 Disease modifying anti-rheumatoid drugs (DMARDs)

Name	Major side effects
Methotrexate	Liver dysfunction, bone marrow suppression, gastro-intestinal, lung fibrosis
Sulfasalazine	Gastrointestinal, rashes, liver dysfunction
Azathioprine	As above
Leflunomide	As above but especially liver toxicity
D-Penicillamine	Proteinuria, neutropenia, thrombocytopenia
Sodium aurothiomalate	Rashes, proteinuria, bone marrow suppression
Hydroxychloroquine	Rashes, rarely visual impairment. Not so effective as other DMARDs
Anti-TNF-α preparations:	
Infliximab	Risk of opportunistic infection especially TB
Etanercept	
Adalimumab	
Anti CD20: Rituximab	

this is the reason why foot X-rays should always be requested (Fig. 11.10).

Management

Simple analgesics and non-steroidal anti-inflammatory drugs (NSAIDs) are used for pain control but, once the diagnosis is established, disease modifying anti-rheumatoid drugs (DMARDs) are required (Table 11.6). NSAID use is limited because of damage to the gastric and small bowel mucosa and the kidneys. The DMARD of first choice is methotrexate, which is given weekly with folic acid supplements on another day. It is recommended that methotrexate is given in combination with other DMARDs. The most popular combination is methotrexate, sulfasalazine and hydroxychloroquine with or without a small dose of prednisolone. Sodium aurothiomalate and penicillamine are now rarely prescribed. Nausea or other gastro-intestinal problems may occur, but monitoring every 8 weeks is essential to exclude bone marrow suppression and liver dysfunction. Unlike analgesics and NSAIDs, these have the ability to reduce inflammation and the acute phase response. They may also retard the destruction of cartilage and bone. It may be several weeks before benefits are apparent. Failure of DMARDS is an indication for an anti-TNF-α agent. There are three preparations: infliximab, which is given by intravenous infusion, etanercept and adalimumab, both of which are self-administered subcutaneously. Anti-TNF drugs are the most effective of all agents at slowing and stopping X-ray damage. Side effects include anaphylaxis, local rashes, and increased susceptibility to tuberculosis and other infections. Failure of anti-TNF is an indication for rituximab. This depletes circulating B cells and increases the risk of infection but not TB.

Many orthopedic procedures are available to alleviate pain and maintain mobility. The most successful of these are hip and knee joint replacements.

Systemic complications of the disease such as fibrosing alveolitis may require corticosteroid treatment and other immunosuppressive drugs such as cyclophosphamide. Intra-articular and intramuscular steroids are commonly used.

Outcome

Complete remission rarely occurs spontaneously but may be induced by DMARDs and more often by anti-TNF-α agents. Many patients have slow progression of disease despite symptomatic control. There is a spectrum of severity but disability may impair independence especially with advancing age and co-morbidity.

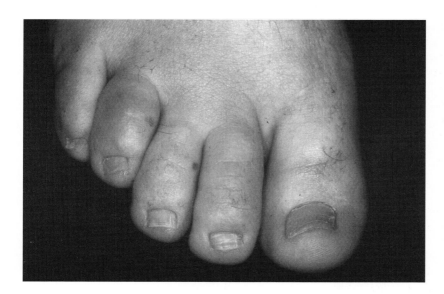

Fig. 11.11. Dactylitis (sausage) fourth toe in psoriatic arthritis.

Psoriatic arthritis

This condition causes much confusion and is often missed because of the heterogeneity of clinical manifestations and the absence of any relationship with the duration and severity of the psoriasis rash. It shares similarities with rheumatoid arthritis, reactive arthritis, and ankylosing spondylitis.

Clinical features

There are three main clinical patterns of disease.

- RA-like but with more frequent distal interphalangeal joint swelling and stiffness and an occasional severe picture called arthritis mutilans in which resorption of terminal digits and juxta-articular bone causes shortening of fingers and toes.
- Oligoarticular disease in which a few large or small joints may be affected in asymmetric fashion. Diffuse swelling of digits (dactylitis) may be a feature of this pattern, making the arthritis very similar to chronic reactive arthritis (Reiter's syndrome) (Fig. 11.11). Unlike reactive arthritis, there is no antecedant infection nor recurrent conjunctivits, balanitis, or mouth ulcers. This pattern and that which resembles RA occur with similar frequency.
- Sacroiliitis and ankylosing spondylitis with sternoclavicular, sternocostal and spinal pain and stiffness which are worse at night and after inactivity. In keeping with other causes of

spondarthritis, Achilles tendonitis and plantar fasciitis may occur. These cause pain which is worse after rest and there may be swelling of the Achilles tendon.

These three patterns are not mutually exclusive. For example, spinal pain and stiffness with restriction of spinal movement may be accompanied by a peripheral arthritis like that of RA.

The peripheral joint signs are of inflammation with warmth, swelling due to synovial thickening or joint effusions, tenderness, and restricted active and passive movement.

In any patient presenting with both peripheral and spinal symptoms, psoriasis offers the most likely explanation for this concurrence. The search should begin with the finger and toe nails where pitting or onycholysis (sheets of keratin beneath the nails) may be seen. Nail pitting is more likely when arthritis occurs especially affecting distal interphalangeal joints. Evidence of a typical scaly rash may be obvious, but there may only be a small patch in the scalp, around the hairline, the umbilicus, anal cleft, or the extensor surface of the elbows or knees. There is no relationship of the severity and activity of the rash with the extent or pattern of the arthritis. Arthritis may occur with any of the several patterns of psoriasis. Pustular psoriasis of the palms and soles is reminiscent of the rash of reactive arthritis and is further evidence of the relationship between these two disorders.

Epidemiology

Psoriasis is common and more prevalent amongst Europeans than amongst other races. Joint involvement occurs in 10%. The RA- like disease is seen more often in women and spondarthritis more often in men. There are immunogenetic links of the peripheral pattern of disease with HLA DR4 and of the spinal pattern with HLA B27. The rash precedes joint symptoms in 75%. There is association between both psoriasis and psoriatic arthritis and HIV infection.

Pathology

Psoriasis is an immunologic disorder in which increased cutaneous vascularity is followed by infiltration with lymphocytes which are mainly CD4 T cells. A similar sequence is thought to take place in the peripheral joints. The cellular pattern of chronic synovial inflammation is similar to RA. Cytokines in the skin and joints play a similar role to that described for RA.

Investigation

There is no specific diagnostic test. Mild anemia, raised inflammatory markers, and radiologic evidence of peripheral joint erosion and sacroliitis or ankylosing spondylitis should be sought. IgM rheumatoid factor is absent. Radiologic evidence of distal interphalangeal involvement or digital juxta-articular bone resorption (pencil in cup deformity of arthritis mutilans) may occur.

The intervertebral syndesmophytes of the spinal disease tend to be thicker than those seen in idiopathic ankylosing spondylitis. They may resemble the asymptomatic, thick, bridging osteophytes seen in aging spines or in diabetes mellitus and acromegaly, a radiologic phenomenon called diffuse intervertebral skeletal hyperostosis (DISH).

Management

Simple analgesics and non-steroidal anti-inflammatory drugs may be adequate for oligoarticular and spinal patterns of disease.

For the symmetric RA-like pattern the choice of disease modifying drugs (DMARDs) listed for RA should be considered. Methotrexate is the most attractive option and has the merit of improving the skin. Azathioprine, sulfasalazine, and cyclosporin may also benefit skin and joints. Hydroxychloroquine, and leflunomide may improve the peripheral joints. Anti-TNF-α drugs can improve the skin, the peripheral arthritis, and the spinal disease as well.

Outcome

The peripheral arthritis pattern resembling RA follows a similar course to RA, whereas the spondylitic disease resembles ankylosisng spondylitis in outcome. Oligoarticular disease follows a benign course and rarely changes its pattern. Patients with a mixed clinical picture are more likely to experience major disability.

Osteoarthritis (OA)

Unlike inflammatory conditions, the fundamental defect in osteoarthritis (OA) is cartilage failure. Radiologic evidence of OA affecting the spine is universal beyond the age of 60 but is not necessarily a cause of pain. Involvement of weight-bearing joints causes most disability. It is the commonest form of arthritis.

Clinical features

- When OA is symptomatic, pain, stiffness, and swelling develop gradually over months and years.
- Unlike inflammatory disease, pain is more likely to worsen after activity and less likely to increase after inactivity. Stiffness after rest is less severe than in joint inflammation.
- Hand swelling of the distal interphalangeal joints (Heberden nodes) is evidence of nodular generalized OA and patients with this are likely to have OA of the carpometacarpal joints of the thumbs and are susceptible to OA of the spine, knees, hips and other joints (Fig. 11.12).
- Deformity such as genu varus of the knees, muscle wasting, crepitus, restricted movement, and tenderness are common.
- Warmth and swelling due to joint effusions are indicative of secondary synovial inflammation. Swelling sometimes feels hard due to bony outgrowth from the joint margins (osteophytes), as in Heberden nodes.

Epidemiology

OA is associated with aging and previous joint injury. It is universal throughout the animal kingdom. Apart from hip involvement, women are more likely to be affected. Nodular generalized OA is seen more frequently amongst people of European extraction and in women especially. A family history of Heberden nodes is common, suggesting a strong genetic component. Involvement of the hip is less frequent amongst Asian and Black people. By contrast, OA of

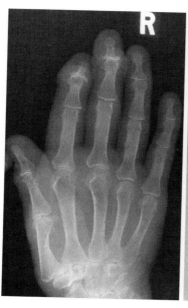
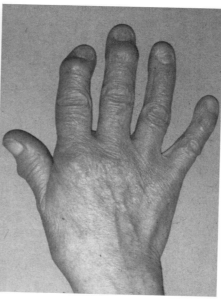

Fig. 11.12. Heberden nodes in nodular generalized OA (NGOA).

the knees is seen in all racial groups and there is a strong association with body weight and obesity. The relationship with obesity does not apply to other weight-bearing joints. Previous inflammation of a joint may cause secondary OA. Other predisposing factors are trauma, meniscectomy of the knee, acromegaly, hemochromatosis, and the rare condition ochronosis (alkaptonuria) in which homogentisic acid derived black pigment is deposited in the cartilage.

Pathology

The precise sequence of biochemical events preceding cartilage disintegration is not known. Cartilage comprises bundles of collagen between which are distributed aggrecan (large proteoglycans) molecules. The latter are made of core proteins to which are attached the glycosaminoglycan chains, keratan sulphate, and chondroitin sulphate. The core is attached to hyaluronic acid (Fig. 11.13).

Degenerating cartilage is characterized at an early stage by loss of glycosaminoglycans. Chondrocytes increase production of cartilage components and tend to clump together but eventually become less numerous. The proteoglycans become fragmented, splits appear from the surface of the cartilage to the underlying bone, and cartilage flakes off the surface. The bone attempts its own reparative process by becoming denser in the subchondral region and extending its surface area by generating new bone at the articular margins (osteophytes). The fissures in the cartilage

may extend into the bone where they expand giving rise to cysts. The synovium becomes inflamed in response to cartilage fragments in the joint cavity. Collections of lymphocytes and increased vascularity can make it indistinguishable from RA.

Investigations

There is no acute phase response and no reliable serologic marker for OA.

The diagnosis rests on clinical findings and the presence of characteristic radiological features, namely narrowing of joint space due to cartilage loss, osteophytes, sclerosis (hardening) of subchondral bone, and cysts. Not all radiologic OA is associated with pain, and interpretation of radiographs has to be circumspect. In general, the more severe the radiology the more likely it is to be clinically relevant.

MRI scans may reveal early OA, but radiographs remain the principal mode of imaging.

Management

Pain relief is the priority by use of NSAIDs or simple analgesia or both in combination. Education about the symptomatic benefits of weight reduction in OA of weight-bearing joints especially the knee should be stressed. Specific exercises to maintain muscle bulk are recommended. These may be taught by physiotherapists.

Intra-articular corticosteroids provide benefit that lasts for several weeks, but can only be justified in the presence of worsening pain and

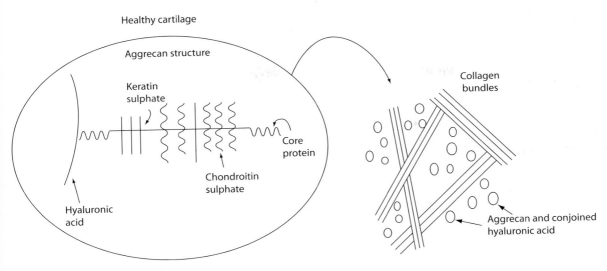

Fig. 11.13. The structure of cartilage.

evidence of synovial inflammation such as warmth or an effusion.

The use of intra-articular hyaluronate and oral glucosamine and chondroitin sulphate is controversial and poorly supported by controlled studies.

Joint replacements of hips, knees, shoulders, elbows, and other joints have transformed the lives of patients with OA, especially those with OA of hips or knees. Nocturnal pain is a strong indication for surgery.

Wheelchairs, domestic support, provision of extra steps, stair rails, stair lifts, and walking aids are supplementary measures, especially helpful to those who are too frail to undergo surgery.

Outcome
The usual course is of slow progression, but pain due to OA of the fingers may remit with time. Symptoms may fluctuate and patients do learn to avoid those activities which are associated with pain.

Connective tissue diseases
A number of multi-system disorders with overlapping clinical, serological, and pathologic features are categorized as connective tissue diseases. This is an unsatisfactory term for a group of conditions in which joint pain alone or an arthritis which resembles RA is common. The arthritis is distinguished from RA by a lack of permanent deformities and absence of radiologic bone erosions.

Systemic lupus erythematosus (SLE)
This is the archetypal connective tissue disease and is the most common apart from secondary Sjøgren's syndrome. It is most often seen in young women.

Clinical features
- The illness may evolve sporadically but arthritis occurs at some time in more than 90% and is the most common presenting problem. The fingers, wrists, elbows, and knees are most often affected with swelling, warmth, tenderness, and effusions. Unlike RA, the arthritis is not persistent and may resolve as other manifestations assume prominence.
- Skin rashes are the next most common problem. The most well known is the red, butterfly rash over the nose and face but diskoid lupus (a raised rash on face, scalp, or limbs that leaves scarring but may exist as an entity outside SLE), bullous eruptions, ischemic ulceration of digits and lower legs, livedo reticularis (Fig. 11.14), panniculitis (rare subcutaneous lumps), and patchy alopecia are together more common than the butterfly rash. Raynaud's phenomenon occurs in 50%.
- Photosensitivity is characteristic and both rashes and systemic disease may be precipitated by ultraviolet light.
- Ulcers of the mouth and nose.

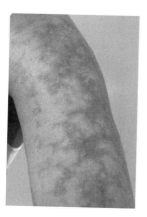

Fig. 11.14. Severe blotchiness of the skin (livedo reticularis) in a patient with SLE.

- Chest pain due to pleurisy or pericarditis. Clinical evidence of a unilateral pleural effusion is more common than a pericardial rub. Rarely, interstitial lung disease causing pneumonitis or lower lobe fibrosis (shrinking lung disease) or pulmonary hypertension.
- Myositis causing weakness, muscle pain, and tenderness.
- Renal involvement with nephritis, hypertension, and chronic renal failure.
- Nervous system features take many forms including epilepsy, psychosis, strokes, ataxia, headache, peripheral neurophathy, and retinal hemorrhage or exudates.
- Fatigue is usual and fever is common.
- The liver is one of the few organs not affected. Abdominal pain may be caused by vasculitis affecting mesenteric vessels.

Epidemiology

In North America the incidence is 30/100 000, whereas in Europe it is less. It is rare in parts of Africa and more common in Asia but in N. America and Europe, Black people are three times more susceptible than Whites. Women account for 90% of cases. Onset occurs nearly always during the reproductive years. A range of drugs including hydralazine and minocycline may cause an SLE-like illness.

Pathology

- Autoantibody production and infiltration of involved sites by lymphocytes are usual. Whether the antibodies drive the disease is uncertain.
- Deposition of immunoglobulins, principally IgG and immune complexes, at involved sites including blood vessel walls may initiate the inflammatory process.
- Cutaneous and internal organ vasculitis causes ischemic damage and there is a range of renal histopathology (World Health Organization Classification grades 1–5).
- Absence of any diagnostic central nervous system histopathology is characteristic. Thrombotic lesions of small veins and venules have been described in the brain, but not vasculitis.

Investigations

A positive antinuclear factor (ANF) screening test is followed by measurement of antibodies against double-stranded DNA (ds DNA), which are found in 90% of SLE. A positive ANF may also be due to anti-Ro (SSA), -La (SSB), -U1RNP and -histones. Although these are found in 10%–60% of SLE patients, they have stronger associations with other connective tissue diseases. Anti-histones are associated with drug-induced SLE. Anti-Sm occurs in about 20% and is more specific for SLE. The Ro, La, and Sm antibodies are named after the first patients in whom they were discovered. High titers of IgG, IgM, or IgA antiphospholipid antibodies and the lupus anticoagulant define a syndrome of recurrent venous and arterial thrombosis and recurrent spontaneous abortion. The IgG antibody seems to be the most relevant. This may occur in SLE or as an independent condition. Other features of this syndrome may include livedo reticularis, heart valve vegetations, stroke syndromes, and multi-organ failure.

- Reduced serum complement (C3, C4, and total complement) is common in active disease. Subjects with hereditary low serum complement components are prone to SLE.
- Anemia, low platelet and neutrophil counts, high serum creatinine and urea, renal and skin biopsy evidence of immune complex deposition and inflammatory cell infiltration, estimation of GFR, proteinuria, and celluria, elevated CSF protein and cells, abnormal electroencephalogram (EEG), CT, or MRI of brain. The MRI may reveal small areas of abnormality similar to those of multiple sclerosis. Abnormal chest radiograph (pleurisy), ECG (pericarditis), or echocardiogram (pericardial effusion, valve vegetations, or so-called Libman Sachs endocarditis), elevated creatine kinase (CK), abnormal electromyogram (EMG) or muscle biopsy in myositis are amongst

the investigations helpful in confirming the diagnosis and specific organ involvement.

Management

No treatment may be required in mild or quiescent illness. Prednisolone in the lowest dose compatible with well-being is required by most at some time.

Hydroxychloroquine helps rash and arthritis, azathioprine reduces the prednisolone requirement, intravenous cyclophosphamide and mycophenalate contribute to containment of renal disease, and cyclophosphamide may also help nervous system manifestations. Intravenous immunoglobulins, anti-TNFα, and retuximab may benefit some patients.

For patients with symptomatic antiphospholipid syndrome, long-term anticoagulation is indicated.

Chronic renal failure may require dialysis and renal transplantation.

Outcome

Serious morbidity and premature death may be due to central nervous system or kidney involvement. Infection remains the most common cause of premature death. With increased survival, a high frequency of ischemic heart disease has been noted.

Scleroderma

The outward features are of skin tightening and Raynaud's phenomenon but major organs can be affected. It is an uncommon disease.

Clinical features

- Raynaud's phenomenon is present in all cases.
- Arthralgia, mild polyarthritis, stiffness, and swelling of the hands or feet are often early features.
- Weakness, pain, and stiffness may indicate associated polymyositis.
- There may be a prodromal phase when the above features unfold over months and the diagnosis is obscure.
- Tightening of the skin of the fingers (sclerodactyly) and the face may develop insidiously or with devastating speed. There may be telangiectasia on the face, limbs or trunk. Digital pulp atrophy or infarction occur if the Raynaud's phenomenon is severe. In the chronic disease, subcutaneous calcification may be visible on the hands, arms, or elsewhere.
- The extent of the skin disease gives an indication of whether internal organ involvement is likely. Skin tightening of the face and arms alone is called limited scleroderma. Apart from the esophagus,

which is always involved, the intestine, lungs, heart, or kidneys are unlikely to be affected. By contrast, skin involvement of the trunk indicates the more severe illness of diffuse scleroderma in which the lungs and small intestine are likely to be affected. Use of the term CREST syndrome (Calcinosis, Sclerodactyly, Esophagus, Telangiectasia) to denote milder disease has been superseded by the concept of limited and diffuse scleroderma.

- Indigestion may indicate esophageal reflux. Dysphagia is an uncommon complaint, even though esophageal motility is abnormal in most cases.
- Dyspnea is usually caused by lung fibrosis, but heart failure due to cardiomyopathy occasionally occurs. The lung involvement is characterized by fine crackles at the lung bases. Dyspnea in the absence of respiratory findings may be caused by pulmonary hypertension, which occurs more often in limited scleroderma. Pulmonary hypertension may also arise secondary to lung fibrosis.
- Abdominal distension, steatorrhea, and weight loss indicate small bowel involvement, which is due to bacterial overgrowth. Colonic disease is relatively uncommon but causes constipation.
- Renal failure associated with hypertension may develop rapidly. So-called renal crises usually occur in early disease when skin change is also progressing rapidly. They are more likely when steroids have been prescribed.
- Chest pain may be caused by pleurisy or pericarditis. Pleural and pericardial rubs may be audible or signs of pleural effusion may occur.
- Features of Sjøgren's syndrome are common, but facial pain or numbness due to fifth cranial nerve entrapment occurs uncommonly.
- There are occasional associations with primary biliary cirrhosis and cancer.

Epidemiology

Women are affected four times as often as men. All races are susceptible and there is no geographic clustering. The prevalence is 10 per 1 000 000 of the population.

Pathology

Inflammation of involved tissues is followed by fibrosis. Blood vessels of all sizes may be narrowed by intimal thickening and vasospasm resulting in ischemic injury. The cause is unknown.

Investigation

- Elevated ESR, CRP, and immunoglobulins reflect the degree of inflammation.
- Antinuclear antibodies are found in 95%, often with a speckled pattern. The presence of anticentromere antibody is characteristic of limited scleroderma.
- Chest X-ray, respiratory function tests, and echocardiogram should be performed in all cases to determine the presence or severity of lung or heart disease especially of asymptomatic pulmonary hypertension.
- CT scan of chest, esophageal manometry, barium studies, bile acid breath tests for malabsorption, serum creatine kinase, electromyogram, muscle biopsy for confirmation of myositis as indicated.

Management

Raynaud's phenomenon should be treated by cold avoidance, calcium channel antagonists, or intravenous prostacyclin. Antacids, proton pump inhibitors help esophagitis, NSAIDs, prednisolone, and immunosuppressive agents for pleurisy, pericarditis and myositis; high dose prednisolone and pulses of intravenous cychophosphamide may retard lung fibrosis; calcium channel blockade, bosentan, and intravenous or inhaled prostacyclin and sildanefil or other phosphodiesterase inhibitors may improve pulmonary hypertension; bosentan and sildanefil can also improve severe Raynauds and digital ischemia; ACE inhibitors are life saving in renal crisis but renal dialysis may be required sometimes indefinitely.

The fibrosis of the skin is resistant to treatment but claims have been made for many drugs, especially D-penicillamine.

Outcome

The outlook of limited scleroderma is better than the diffuse disease because, although the skin may worsen slowly and pulmonary fibrosis may develop in late disease, death due to major organ dysfunction is uncommon. The exception to this favorable prognosis is development of pulmonary hypertension. In diffuse scleroderma, spontaneous improvement of the skin often occurs. Involvement of internal organs may not progress but regression is unusual. Deaths due to scleroderma are most commonly due to pulmonary fibrosis and the sequelae of renal crises.

Myositis

Muscle inflammation may be a manifestation of SLE, scleroderma, mixed connective tissue disease, or it may be unassociated, when it is known as polymyositis. An entity of myositis with a distinct rash is known as dermatomyositis. Inclusion body myositis (ICM) is another variant. These are all uncommon.

Clinical features

- Weakness of proximal muscles with associated stiffness. Pain may also occur and be difficult to separate from arthritis which is common. Muscle tenderness is mild. Polymyalgia rheumatica does not cause weakness and is easily distinguished from polymyositis.
- Function is often impaired, so that climbing stairs, bathing, and dressing are difficult.
- Dysphagia, a nasal voice, or nasal regurgitation of food indicate striated palatal muscle or esophageal smooth muscle involvement.
- Dyspnea is a serious symptom but not usually evident at onset. It may be due to inhalation of food and subsequent pneumonia, weakness of respiratory muscles, or associated interstitial lung disease.
- In dermatomyositis a red rash occurs over the extensor surface of the fingers and forearms and sometimes on the neck, shoulders, and face. The upper eyelids may be red or mauve in color. On the fingers there may be skin cracks (mechanic's hands), nail fold infarcts due to vasculitis (see Fig. 11.8), and raised nodules over the knuckles called Gottron's papules.
- Swelling of finger joints resembling RA.
- The presence of fine crackles at the lung bases indicates fibrosing alveolitis or heart failure due to myocardial involvement.
- In chronic cases there may be palpable subcutaneous calcification. There is a rare childhood entity of dermatomyositis which is different from the illness of adults and in which extensive subcutaneous calcification is common.
- In 10% of dermatomyositis patients there is an obvious or hidden malignant disease.

Epidemiology

In European populations the incidence is 2 per million per year. It is more common amongst Black people and twice as frequent in women, with peak onset in middle life.

Pathology

Chronic inflammatory infiltrates with B and T cells and decaying or dead muscle fibers are found patchily and in varying degrees of severity. Dermatomyositis is pathologically distinct from polymyositis, and inclusion body myopathy (IBM). In the former B cells predominate in a perivascular arrangement whereas in polymyositis and IBM there is predominance of CD8 T cells distributed mainly in the muscle itself.

Investigation

- Elevated serum creatine kinase (CK) is usual. Alanine transaminase is also raised. The CK can increase 200- and 100-fold above the upper limit.
- Electromyography (EMG) usually reveals abnormal motor unit potentials (MUP) which are scattered and reduced in amplitude and duration. These are not diagnostic.
- Muscle biopsy of tender or weak muscles reveals pathology in 90% of cases.
- MRI scanning may reveal abnormal muscle and may help selection of biopsy sites. The choice of site must avoid previous EMG needle insertion.
- CK estimation, EMG, and biopsy should all be performed because one or more of these may be normal.
- All should undergo chest radiograph to exclude cancer, interstitial lung disease, or inhalation pneumonia. Heart failure is rare. Depending on the clinical picture, high resolution CT of chest, respiratory function tests (RFT), ECG, and echocardiogram may be warranted. Cardiac conduction defects occur.
- Serology is of limited value. Positive ANF and anti-ENA antibodies are common as in other connective tissue diseases. Anti-Jo-1 is an antibody linked to lung involvement. This or another anti-aminoacyl-tRNA synthetase antibody can be associated with interstitial lung disease in any connective tissue disease, and is known as the antisynthetase syndrome.
- Muscle weakness due to metabolic or endocrine causes may be difficult to distinguish from myositis clinically. Inclusion body myopathy has similar features but has a slower onset, normal CK, and distinct muscle histology.

Management

Modest dose prednisolone 20–60 mg with methotrexate, azathioprine, or ciclosporin usually evoke a response. Intravenous immunoglobulin may help and be life saving. Rehabilitation exercises help to restore strength.

Outcome

A minority require critical care management including respiratory and inotropic support, especially when sepsis intervenes. Patience and continued anti-inflammatory treatment are required. Improvement may be slow. The CK level is not by itself a reliable index of disease activity. In the majority, mild relapses or low grade disease persistence occur over a prolonged period of years.

Sjøgren's syndrome

Dryness of the eyes, mouth and other mucosal surfaces is called keratoconjunctivitis sicca (KCS). This may occur with aging, but when associated with inflammation and fibrosis of the lacrimal and salivary glands it is called Sjøgren's syndrome. It is considered primary when it exists in isolation and secondary when it occurs with RA or a connective tissue disease.

Clinical features

- Dryness and grittiness of eyes.
- Dry mouth, gingivitis, caries, and premature loss of teeth.
- Parotid swelling
- Arthritis or arthralgia
- In primary Sjøgren's there may be a purpuric rash on the lower part of the legs and ankles due to leukocytoclastic vasculitis.
- Peripheral neuropathy or rarely interstitial lung disease may also be features.
- Renal tubular acidosis is a complication that is usually asymptomatic.

Epidemiology

Taking primary and secondary disease together, Sjøgren's syndrome may affect as many as 0.5% of the population, involving women several times more often than men.

Pathology

The lacrimal and salivary glands including those of the lips become infiltrated with mainly CD4 positive T-cell lymphocytes. B cells are also present and these produce large amounts of immunoglobulins including polyclonal and monoclonal IgM with rheumatoid factor activity (capable of binding to the Fc fragment of IgG). These may form cryoglobulins, i.e. immune complexes that precipitate on cooling. The presence of cryoglobulins correlates with the presence of cutaneous leukocytoclastic vasculitis.

Investigation

- Screening for dry eyes entails the Schirmer test in which a strip of filter paper placed in the middle of the lower lid allows a measure of eye moisture. In secondary Sjøgren's syndrome this test when positive may suffice.
- Ophthalmologic examination with a slit lamp and Rose Bengal staining may corroborate dryness and surface damage to the cornea.
- Investigation of salivary dysfunction can be undertaken with saliva flow rates.
- Sialographic imaging may reveal anatomic derangement of major glands.
- The diagnosis of Sjøgren's syndrome can be corroborated by lip biopsy which demonstrates minor salivary gland chronic inflammation.
- Anti-Ro (anti-SS A where SS stands for Sjøgren's syndrome) and anti-La (SS B), are found in 50% of cases. These antibodies are also found in SLE, scleroderma and mixed connective tissue disease. The antigens for these closely related antibodies are ribonucleoprotein particles. In primary disease, positive tests for RF and ANF occur in 70% and 90%, respectively.

Management

Treatment is symptomatic with artificial tears, artificial saliva, and pilocarpine. Oral hygiene and regular mouth moistening may reduce dental caries. Corticosteroids and immunosuppressive agents are effective for the extra-glandular features of primary Sjøgren's syndrome.

Outcome

There is no cure for either primary or secondary Sjøgren's syndrome. The principal risk of the primary disease is the development of B-cell lymphoma. This occurs in 10%. Progressive enlargement of a parotid gland or cervical lymphadenopathy justify biopsy to exclude this possibility.

Mixed connective tissue disease (MCTD)

This is a disputed entity since it describes a group of patients with features of SLE and scleroderma, often with polymyositis. Individual cases may evolve into one or other of the two major connective tissue diseases. Historically, the concept of MCTD has been associated with the presence of an antibody, anti-U1-RNP.

Clinical features

None of the findings outlined below is specific.

• Polyarthritis	>90%
• Raynaud's phenomenon	80%
• Swollen fingers	70%
• Sclerodactyly	50%
• Polymyositis	70%
• Interstitial lung disease	60%

Renal and neurologic involvement are uncommon.

Epidemiology

Since the illness is often seen as a convenient label for a clinical constellation of an evolving connective tissue disease, the frequency is hard to determine but is less than 10 per 1 000 000 adults. It is ten times more frequent in women and has no racial predilection.

Pathology

There is no specific histopathology. In some diagnostic criteria, the presence of high titer antibody against a uridine rich ribonucleoprotein (U1RNP) is mandatory. The antigen is similar to that of anti-Sm, both being ribonucleoproteins involved in the splicing of messenger RNA.

Investigation

Appropriate investigations are driven by the pattern of clinical disease and may involve those described for myositis, scleroderma, and SLE.

Management

Initial descriptions emphasized the responsiveness of MCTD to corticosteroids. The indications for prednisolone and immunosuppressive use are those described for the individual connective tissue diseases.

Outcome

The initial descriptions of MCTD emphasized an excellent prognosis with a high percentage of remission. Even when evolution to recognizable SLE or

Table 11.7. Vasculitis disorders

	Main clinical features	Size of vessel and ANCA status
Giant cell arteritis (GCA, temporal arteritis, cranial arteritis)	Polymyalgia rheumatica headache, loss of vision	Large artery ANCA negative
Henoch Schonlein Purpura (HSP)	Purpura, arthritis, abdominal pain, nephritis	Small artery ANCA negative
Cutaneous leukocytoclastic vasculitis	Purpura	Small artery ANCA negative
Wegener's granulomatosis	Arthritis, respiratory symptoms, eye inflammation, nephritis, eosinophilia	Small artery PR2 ANCA positive
Churg-Strauss syndrome	Asthma, arthritis, neuropathy, pulmonary infiltrates, eosinophilia	Small artery MPO ANCA positive
Microscopic polyangiitis	Nephritis, neuropathy, lung involvement	Small artery MPO ANCA positive
Polyarteritis nodosa	Livedo reticularis, orchitis, neuropathy	Small artery ANCA negative
Behçet's syndrome	Arthritis, mouth and genital ulcers	Large and small arteries, veins ANCA negative
Takayasus arteritis	Ischemic events	Aorta and large arteries ANCA negative

scleroderma does not occur, persistent symptoms are the rule, sometimes with glomerulonephritis.

Vasculitis

The connective tissue diseases and RA may all be associated with vascular inflammation and in RA and SLE this may be clinically important. In addition, there are several, mostly uncommon, diseases in which vasculitis is the principal aspect of the pathology. All are associated with joint or muscle pain or arthritis. They are categorized on the basis of the size of vessels affected and the presence or absence of antibodies against neutrophil cytoplasmic antigens (ANCA).

In general, the vasculitis associated with RA and connective tissue diseases affects small arteries, arterioles, and venules. In RA this causes skin ulceration, peripheral neuropathy, or mononeuritis and, rarely, digital gangrene. In connective tissue diseases such as SLE, a vasculitis may also affect the kidneys. The following account discusses the primary vasculitic diseases in order of their frequency. The clinical manifestations are disparate (Table 11.7).

Giant cell arteritis (GCA)

The vasculitis overlaps with polymyalgia rheumatica (PMR) and is considered to be a manifestation of the same disease complex.

Clinical features
- Headache, especially but not exclusively in the temporal region in an elderly person.
- Scalp or temporal artery tenderness with thickening of the artery.
- Muscle pain and stiffness before, during, or following a headache in 10%.
- Pain in the jaw and face when eating.
- Visual impairment or blindness in one eye in fewer than 10%.

Epidemiology
Almost exclusively in White people, women more than men, mainly over age 60, prevalence less than 1%.

Pathology
There is thickening of the temporal arterial intima often with luminal thrombosis. All layers of the artery are infiltrated with T-cell lymphocytes, plasma cells, and giant cells.

Investigations
As with PMR, a very high ESR is usual and, when this is found in an older person with headache, the diagnosis is likely. When suspected, a temporal artery biopsy should be performed before or within 48 hours of starting treatment.

Management

Prednisolone 40 mg is usually adequate and should begin as soon as the diagnosis is suspected. The dose should be reduced to the lowest that maintains control of symptoms and ESR. Bone protection with a bisphosphonate drug should not be overlooked.

Outcome

Treatment is required for at least 2 years. A small number of patients may develop upper limb ischemia due to brachial artery involvement. Rarely, aortic dissection due to aortitis may occur. Ultrasonography has shown a high percentage of asymptomatic neck vessel involvement.

Cutaneous vasculitis

Lower limb purpura, which may coalesce to form ecchymoses, can be due to vasculitis of small vessels. All may be associated with joint pain especially of knees and ankles. The most distinctive of these is Henoch Schonlein purpura (HSP) which occurs mostly in children but also in adults. Leukocytoclastis vasculitis is a pathologic description that is often used to describe a clinical entity.

Henoch Schonlein Purpura

Clinical features

- Purpura lower aspect legs, buttocks
- Abdominal pain
- Joint pain
- Nephritis

Epidemiology

More common in men and children.

Pathology

Deposition of IgA-containing immune complexes in blood vessels and kidneys. It appears to be precipitated by preceding upper respiratory tract infection with a range of organisms.

Investigation

There is no specific diagnostic test. The presence of protein and blood in the urine indicates renal involvement. Persistence of these findings warrants monitoring of renal function and biopsy.

Management

Symptomatic treatment is all that is required. A minority may need corticosteroids for control of joint pain. Evidence of progressive renal involvement warrants high dose steroids and immunosuppressive treatment.

Outcome

The majority resolve spontaneously within days or a few weeks. Renal involvement in adults is more likely to be progressive than in children.

Leukocytoclastic vasculitis

The pathologic appearance is of fibrinoid necrosis of the vessel walls with infiltration by polymorph leukocytes.

Clinical features

- Palpable purpura of the legs similar to HSP.
- Arthritis knees, ankles, and occasionally other joints.
- Occasional peripheral neuropathy or mononeuritis.
- Associated diseases may include Sjøgren's syndrome, SLE, or other connective tissue disease, hepatitis C, HIV, SBE, underlying malignant disease.

Epidemiology

More often in women with a prevalence of fewer than one per 100 000 adults.

Pathology

The appearance of the vessels described above is due to immune complex deposition.

Investigation

Serologic markers for connective tissue disease, HIV, hepatitis C. Serum complement levels may be low. Cryoglobulins are difficult to detect but should be requested and may be present especially in hepatitis C infection.

Wegener's granulomatosis

This is another rare vasculitis. It may be localized to the upper respiratory tract, but is more often a systemic, multi-organ disease.

Clinical features

- Epistaxis, sinusitis, deafness, nasal depression
- Eye inflammation – scleritis or uveitis
- Fever
- Arthritis
- Cough, hemoptysis, dyspnea, stridor
- Glomerulonephritis
- Mononeuritis multiplex

The differential diagnosis is wide and the diagnosis often delayed or difficult to confirm. Collapse of the nose is also seen in the even rarer disorder of relapsing polychondritis, which has other overlapping features including eye inflammation, sinusitis, glomerulonephritis, and stridor due to tracheal stenosis. Painful, red, swollen ears and aortic regurgitation, however, are two distinguishing features of relapsing polychondritis.

Epidemiology

It arises mainly in White people, men as often as women, and usually in middle life.

Pathology

Vasculitis at involved sites affects mainly small arteries. Granulomas in the upper respiratory tract and the lung comprise accumulations of multiple cell types including giant cells.

Investigation

When the diagnosis is suspected on clinical grounds, the most helpful serologic test is the anti neutrophil cytoplasmic antibody (ANCA). There are two relevant ANCA antibodies, one against proteinase-3 (PR3-ANCA or C ANCA) and the other against myeloperoxidase (MPO-ANCA or P ANCA). Previous terminology emphasized the neutrophil staining pattern and the prefix "C" indicated cytoplasmic and "P" perinuclear. It is the PR3-ANCA (C ANCA) which is typical of Wegener's granulomatosis. The MPO ANCA lacks the same specificity and is found in Microscopic Polyangiitis and Churg-Strauss syndrome but not predictably. MPO ANCA has also been described in other diseases (see Table 11.7).

Radiographs or CT scans of the chest may reveal opacities sometimes with cavitation. When respiratory symptoms are the presenting problem, the radiologic appearance may initially be interpreted as pneumonia or cancer. Radiographs, CT, or MRI scans of the sinuses may demonstrate mucosal thickening and bone erosion.

Biopsy of involved sinuses may be diagnostic.

Management

Weekly intravenous pulses or daily oral cyclophosphamide provide the most successful treatment. Supplementary corticosteroids are also used. Once activity is controlled, long-term azathioprine is substituted for cyclophosphamide.

Outcome

Remission is usual but relapse is common. Superimposed infection, renal and respiratory failure cause long term morbidity. Ten-year survival is 80%.

Churg-Strauss syndrome

This is another small vessel vasculitis which shares some features of Wegener's. It is characterized by antecedent asthma, sinusitis, and nasal polyposis sometimes for a decade or more. Mononeuritis multiplex, glomerulonephritis, purpuric rash, and arthritis are the main features. Eosinophilia is usual and chest radiography may reveal pulmonary infiltrates in 50% of cases. The MPO-ANCA test is positive in a high percentage of cases. Corticosteroids and sometimes cyclophosphamide are used to control the disease.

Microscopic polyangiitis

In this disorder, glomerulonephritis tends to predominate but mononeuritis multiplex, pulmonary infiltrates, joint and muscle pain may also occur. MPO-ANCA is found in high frequency. Prednisolone, cyclophosphamide, azathioprine, mycophenolate are used in treatment.

Polyarteritis nodosa

This is the vasculitis that is best known yet it is now rarely seen or described. It may be associated with hepatitis B infection. Joint and muscle pain, livedo reticularis of the skin (see Fig. 11.4), mononeuritis multiplex, nephritis, and abdominal pain are regular features. Arteriography may reveal small aneurysms at involved sites and these are almost diagnostic. Management is dictated by severity and site. The cascade of prednisolone, cyclophosphamide, azathioprine, and other immunosuppressants is the usual therapeutic approach.

Behçet's syndrome

This is an uncommon disease occurring in men and women equally, usually before age 40. Clustering occurs in the East and in Mediterranean countries but elsewhere it is rare. Clinical features in order of frequency are arthritis, mainly of large joints, mouth and genital ulcers, iritis, thrombophlebitis, erythema nodosum, colitis, aneurysm of the abdominal aorta, arterial and venous occlusion, and stroke syndromes. There are no serologic or histologic diagnostic findings. The pathergy reaction involves the development of a skin pustule at the site of a sterile needle prick. It is not a reliable test in Europe but is said to be helpful in establishing the diagnosis in Turkey. It is characterized by periods of remission and relapse. Treatment with prednisolone, azathioprine, cyclophosphamide, colchicine, ciclosporin, and anti TNF agents thalidomide have yielded variable success. In

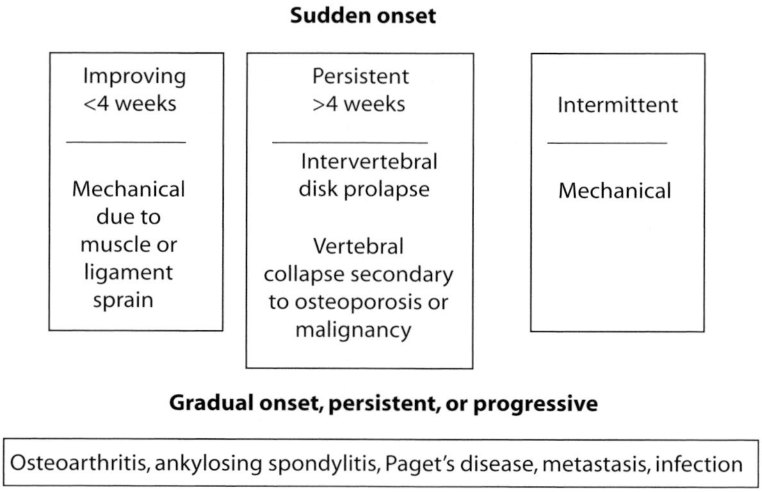

Sudden onset

| Improving <4 weeks ——— Mechanical due to muscle or ligament sprain | Persistent >4 weeks ——— Intervertebral disk prolapse — Vertebral collapse secondary to osteoporosis or malignancy | Intermittent ——— Mechanical |

Gradual onset, persistent, or progressive

Osteoarthritis, ankylosing spondylitis, Paget's disease, metastasis, infection

Fig. 11.15. The probable cause of lumbar pain according to mode of onset.

Japan it is a relatively common cause of blindness. The mortality rate is low.

Takayasu's arteritis (pulseless disease)

This is found almost exclusively in the East. It affects women in adolescence or early 20s and only rarely affects men. Joint pain, fever, and ischemic events such as exercise induced arm pain, TIA, or stroke are the usual presenting symptoms. Signs include absence of peripheral pulses and bruits over carotid, subclavian, and abdominal vessels in young women with an elevated ESR or CRP. The diagnosis is confirmed by arch aortogram or periperhal arteriography. These demonstrate typical narrowing and occlusion of vessels. Treatment with prednisolone may be supplemented with immunosuppressive drugs, such as azathioprine, if improvement is slow. The prognosis is good but relapse common.

Spinal pain

Low back and neck pain are part of the human condition and are experienced by all adults at some time. The need for medical consultation is sometimes driven by depression, anxiety, or intolerable domestic or work environments. In at least 10% of patients with chronic pain no cause is established.

The mode of onset, age of the patient and distribution of symptoms are important clues to diagnosis (Fig. 11.15). The vast majority of episodes are mechanical, benign, and self limiting. However, spinal pain may be caused by serious disease and there is need for vigilance and an awareness of the features that should raise suspicion.

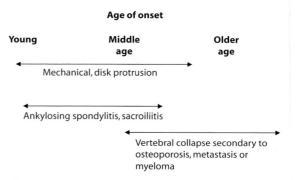

Fig. 11.16. Causes of spinal pain related to age of onset.

The history

Young, middle aged and thus those most physically active are the patients whose neck and low back pain is most likely to be due to mechanical factors or intervertebral disk protrusion (Fig. 11.16). From middle age onward, both sudden and gradual onset spinal pain are more likely caused by osteoporosis, malignancy, or infection. A history of cancer, weight loss, fever, rigors, immunosuppression, diabetes, alcoholism are amongst the features which should raise suspicion of serious pathology. A history of peripheral joint pain or swelling, eye inflammation, Crohn's disease, ulcerative colitis or psoriasis should suggest associated sacroiliitis or ankylosing spondylitis (AS). Spinal stiffness is a variable accompanying feature of spinal pain but when severe and worse in the morning or after inactivity, especially in a young male, AS or sacroiliitis should be suspected. Nocturnal pain in a young person is also suspicious of AS but in a middle-aged or older person, malignant disease should be excluded.

Referral of pain into the arm or leg does not necessarily denote nerve root or spinal cord involvement. Such referral is common and from the neck, pain may extend to the occiput, the scapula, and the forehead. Pain derived from the shoulder may be difficult to distinguish, especially since it is often experienced in the upper arm. Pain from the lumbar spine may be referred to one or both buttocks. Pain referred below the elbow or knee, pain accentuated by coughing, sneezing, or straining or associated tingling or numbness in hand, arm, foot or leg suggest neurologic involvement. Pain or paresthesiae in the legs made worse by walking suggests "intermittent claudication of the cauda equina" due to spinal stenosis.

The examination

Observation rarely yields a diagnosis. In the dorsal region, a kyphosis may be indicative of vertebral collapse, osteoarthritis, or ankylosing spondylitis.

In the dorsi-lumbar region, a scoliosis may be congenital and associated with rotation of the vertebrae (congenital kyphoscoliosis). It may also represent an unconscious response to pain, the patient leaning to the side of the pathology to reduce muscle, ligamentous, or nerve root tension.

Rarely, swelling over paravertebral or sacroiliac areas denotes the presence of an abscess or malignancy.

Any painful spinal problem causes protective muscle spasm and restriction of movement. Forward and lateral flexion, extension and rotation should be examined and the movement causing most pain documented. Local tenderness of the spine, paravertebral, and sacroiliac areas will often be found but this has poor localizing value.

Estimation of straight leg raising is of some value in low back conditions with referred leg pain. If reduced to less than 90° on one side or if the maneuver induces paresthesiae it suggests nerve root irritation.

Evidence of muscle wasting, weakness, and diminished or absent reflexes imply nerve root or cord impingement. The most common cause of wasting of the hand muscles (T1 root) is cervical spondylosis (OA of the spine). The most common cause of thenar wasting is OA of the first carpo-metacarpal joint but carpal tunnel syndrome due to median nerve compression may also be a cause. Weakness of toe dorsiflexion (L5 root) and an absent ankle jerk (S1 root) are common. Disturbance of bladder function, weakness with increased tone, accentuated reflexes and/or extensor plantar responses are indicative of cord

compression. Usually this is due to trauma, cancer, or abscess formation and is a medical emergency.

Sensory impairment in cervical spine OA or disk protrusion usually affects the hand, with numbness of first and second fingers (C6), middle finger (C7), or the ring and little finger (C8). Distinction from median nerve (carpal tunnel syndrome) and ulnar nerve lesions (most often at the elbow due to trauma) can be distinguished by history and careful examination (Chapter 9). Investigation of spinal pain is simple.

1. Spinal X-rays of the relevant section with a view of the pelvis if sacroiliitis or AS is suspected and a chest X-ray in smokers or where there is any suspicion of serious disease.
2. Hematology, CRP, ESR, bone biochemistry, vitamin D, and parathormone where metabolic bone disease is suspected.
3. MRI scan of spine if neurological symptoms or signs are a feature. CT scan is less helpful.
4. Radionucleotide bone or PET or MRI scan if X-rays are non-diagnostic and disseminated malignancy or a focus of infection is suspected.
5. Nerve conduction studies to help distinguish peripheral nerve from spinal cord or nerve root pathology.

Spinal pain: sudden onset

The likely causes of pain beginning suddenly are outlined in Fig. 11.15.

Mechanical neck and lumbar spinal pain

Clinical features

- Abrupt onset, sometimes after identifiable physical activity or trauma. Referral into surrounding anatomic areas such as shoulder, upper arm, buttock.
- Local tenderness, restricted movement, normal neurologic examination.

Epidemiology

All men and women at some time especially in the time of most physical activity and during the working life.

Pathology

Strain or rupture of ligament, muscle, or joint capsule fibers. Sustained postures that impose a stretch on soft tissues of neck or lumbar region are often occupational such as desk work or driving.

Investigations

Exclusion of alternative disorders as above where clinical suspicion or persistent pain indicate. Imaging may reveal intervertebral disk space narrowing with osteophytes in subjects of middle age and older. Such changes are often asymptomatic and therefore irrelevant.

Management

Simple advice about posture, weight reduction, avoidance of bending, lifting heavy shopping or luggage, attention to occupational factors, such as raising a desk or altering position of a keyboard. Exercise is often advocated. A variety of physical treatments including heat, massage, manipulation, acupuncture, collars, corsets may have transient benefits. Bed rest is not advised.

Outcome

Resolution of pain within weeks or a few months and a trend toward improvement within 4 weeks can be anticipated in 90%. Persistence of pain demands sequential investigation to exclude alternative pathology. Recurrence is common throughout life giving intermittent pain.

Disk prolapse

Clinical features

- Sudden pain in the neck referred to arm or hand or pain in the lower back referred down the length of the leg (sciatica). Antecedent history of neck or back pain or identifiable strenuous activity.
- Paresthesiae of hand, leg, or foot.
- Symptoms persist for weeks.
- Restriction head or lumbar movement, reduced unilateral straight leg raising, neurologic deficit.

Epidemiology

There are no data that distinguish the frequency of spinal pain due to disk prolapse. The age distribution is the same as for mechanical back and neck ache.

Pathology

The structure of intervertebral disks includes a gelatinous central nucleus pulposus surrounded by fibrous tissue, the annulus fibrosus. The weakest area of the annulus is at the posterolateral margin. It is at this site that the nucleus may bulge and cause local and neurologic symptoms and signs by impinging on emerging nerve roots. Less commonly, there may be posterior protrusion of lumbar disks contributing to spinal stenosis and "intermittent claudication of the cauda equina." Even more rarely a posterior cervical disk protrusion compresses the cord with resultant paresis.

Investigations

Hematology, biochemistry, plain chest, spine, and pelvis radiographs help to exclude serious disease. An MRI scan of the relevant part of the spine is the best means of confirming an intervertebral disk protrusion.

Management

The approach is identical to that of mechanical spinal pain. Epidural and local injections of anaesthetic and corticosteroids may alleviate pain of cervical and lumbar lesions. Lumbosacral disk protrusions can be excised surgically if pain persists for many weeks or months. Surgical treatment of cervical disk lesions is less popular.

Outcome

Symptoms due to root impingement resolve with conservative management in 90%. Signs such as loss of ankle or biceps reflexes may persist indefinitely.

Vertebral crush fracture

Clinical features

- Pain is most often experienced by osteoporotic women in middle to late life. It is sudden and severe.
- The dorsal spine is the most commonly affected site.
- Kyphosis (gibbus) of the spine, local tenderness.
- Weight loss, known cancer, smoking, middle age, male gender, absence of osteoporosis risk factors should raise possibility of neoplastic disease.

Epidemiology

Women of European or Asian extraction, early menopause, thin body habitus are features that increase susceptibility to osteoporosis, which is defined as a bone mineral density (BMD) of less than 2.5 standard deviations below the mean of a young normal adult. Osteopenia is defined as a BMD 1–2.5 SD below the mean. Black people have a relatively high bone density and both vertebral deformity and hip fracture are rare in people of African descent.

Radiologic evidence of vertebral crush fracture is much more common than clinically reported. In White women it increases from 7% in middle life to 60% in those aged more than 90. Post-menopausal

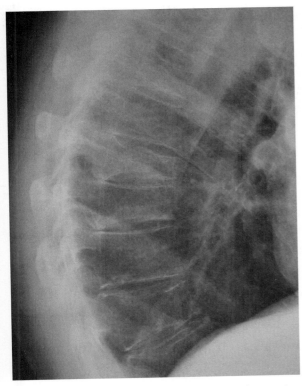

Fig. 11.17. X-ray of a spine showing vertebral crush fractures in osteoporosis.

women are particularly susceptible to rapid bone loss during corticosteroid treatment. In men the prevalence is half that for women.

Pathology

Isolated crush fracture of a vertebra may be due to metastatic malignant deposits of tumor displacing bone, plasma cell expansion eroding cancellous bone in myeloma, and most commonly osteoporosis. This represents the progressive loss of bone with age from a peak level in youth. Bone turnover is complex and influenced by many factors such as exercise, body weight, dietary calcium, vitamin D, co-morbidity, corticosteroid drugs, hormones especially estrogen, and genes. Both mineral and collagen are lost with age and bone resorption by osteoclasts is accelerated with loss of estrogen at menopause.

Investigation

Plain radiographs can contribute to confirmation of vertebral collapse and its cause (Fig. 11.17). Sclerosis of the bone is suggestive of malignant metastasis from prostate, breast, other organs, or lymphoma. Paget's disease needs to be considered when bone is sclerotic

and, although a cause of pain, it does not usually cause vertebral collapse. Paget's disease may affect any part of the skeleton and is a common radiologic incidental finding. It is caused by osteoclast dysfunction. Single or multiple sites may be affected. The pain of Paget's disease responds to bisphosphanate treatment. These are drugs which reduce osteoclast activity and bone resorption.

Bone biochemistry, hematology, ESR, vitamin D, parathormone (PTH), and technetium bone scan are further investigations driven by the clinical indications.

Hypercalcemia and raised alkaline phosphatase may suggest malignancy, as does a high ESR. A very high ESR (>80) is consistent with myeloma and serum protein electrophoresis and urine examination for Bence-Jones protein should then be done. If metastasis from a solid tumor is suspected, prostate specific antigen (PSA) should be requested, mammogram in a woman. A technetium radioisotope bone scan will allow detection of secondaries at other skeletal sites. Bone scans tend to be normal in myeloma. If the vertebral collapse is recent, a bone scan will reveal increased isotope uptake at that site, whatever the etiology.

A low vitamin D level with raised PTH may contribute to osteoporosis and is seen in older, institutionalized, or home-bound subjects. It is also a feature of osteomalacia as discussed below. Hyperparathyroidism may cause bone pain, but not acute vertebral collapse. MRI or CT scan are imperative if there are neurologic signs especially affecting the pyramidal tract or if there is a sensory level. These imply cord compression and are found in malignancy and infection with abscess formation but not osteoporosis.

Bone mass density (BMD) of the spine and femoral neck is usually obtained by dual photon absorptiometry (DEXA scan). Comparison of values with the mean of young adults provides the t-score on which the diagnosis of osteoporosis depends. The z-score is a comparison of BMD with an age-matched population.

Management

Exclusion of malignant disease is necessary in a minority since the age, gender, and radiologic vertebral deformities are sufficiently characteristic to ascribe the problem to osteoporosis in most cases.

Pain control can be difficult. Escalating use of analgesics including opiates is used. Subcutaneous calcitonin may also reduce pain.

Bone density can be improved by several agents. There are limited data on whether these reduce the risk of further vertebral crush or other fractures. Calcium and vitamin D supplementation alone may improve bone density but have a limited impact on fracture rates. They may lessen the frequency of falls by improving muscle power. When given with a bisphosphanate such as oral etidronate, alendronate, risedonrate, ibandronic acid, pamidronate, or annual IV zolendronic acid bone density improves or stabilises. These are antiresorptive agents by virtue of their suppression of osteoclasts. Their prevention of further fracture is real but modest. For patients aged less than 65, who are intolerant of bisphosphanates, raloxifene is another option. This is a selective estrogen receptor modulator (SERM) with a range of effects on several organs and which is antiresorptive of bone. It can reduce vertebral fracture rates. For patients aged over 65 with multiple fractures despite the above treatment, the anabolic agent teriparatide may be considered. This is a recombinant preparation of human PTH. Another anabolic agent is strontium ranelate. This, like teriparatide is recommended only when biphosphonates have been ineffective or poorly tolerated.

Metastatic malignant causes may be treated with radiotherapy or chemotherapy and surgical decompression if the spinal cord is compromised. Associated hypercalcemia requires i.v. pamidronate and fluids.

Outcome

In osteoporotic crush fracture pain improves over days. Mobility can be quickly restored. Bone density may increase over months but does not guarantee protection from recurrence. Spinal deformity may become pronounced. Osteoporosis is not painful unless associated with fracture.

Vertebral metastatic malignancy has a poor prognosis, but is dependent on the underlying nature of the tumor and its treatment.

Spinal pain: gradual onset, persistent, or progressive

Osteoarthritis (cervical and lumbar spondylosis)

Osteoarthritis may affect the facetal and intervertebral joints.

Clinical features
- Pain and stiffness, intermittent and often worse after exertion.
- Restricted movement and local tenderness.
- Signs of OA elsewhere especially Heberden nodes.
- Neurologic symptoms and signs indistinguishable from those described for spinal disk protrusion.
- Cervical myelopathy especially when osteophytes cause thickening of ligamentum flavum or subluxation of vertebrae.
- Spinal stenosis with leg pain on walking.

Epidemiology

Spinal OA is ubiquitous and some radiologic evidence of intervertebral OA is universal in those aged >75. In the majority there are no symptoms. An occupation entailing bending, lifting, or carrying heavy loads is a predisposing factor.

Pathology

The changes are identical to those of peripheral joints.

Management

As for mechanical spinal pain. Surgical decompression of the cervical spine or cauda equina may be necessary in myelopathy or lumbar stenosis. Surgical fusion of vertebrae is a disappointing procedure. Prosthetic intervertebral disks are available for insertion, the results uncertain.

Outcome

Pain that is present for more than a year tends to persist indefinitely.

Ankylosing spondylitis

This is a relatively common cause of spinal pain in young men.

Clinical features
- Low back, dorsal, or neck pain worse at night and in the morning.
- Stiffness worse after inactivity.
- Reduced spinal movement, lumbosacral spine mainly but all areas affected.
- History of peripheral arthritis affecting knees, ankles, or other joints.
- Painful heels (plantar fasciitis), Achilles tendonitis, other joints.
- Previous reactive arthritis, known psoriasis, ulcerative colitis, Crohn's disease.
- History of iritis.

(a)

(b)

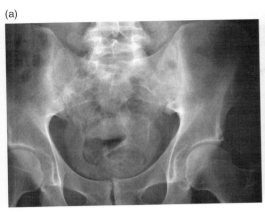
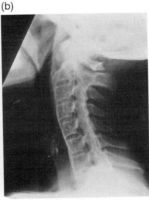

Fig. 11.18. X-ray of (a) pelvis showing bilateral sacroiliitis. (b) ankylosis of cervical spine.

Epidemiology

Prevalence is about 1%, five times more frequent in men, more common in those of European and Asian extraction, relatively uncommon amongst Black people. Presentation occurs before age 40.

Pathology

There is a 95% association with the histocompatability antigen HLA B27 (see Table 11.5). This relationship is weaker in non-White populations. The associations with bowel disease, infection, and psoriasis are of interest.

Synovial inflammation of peripheral joints is similar to that of RA. Inflammation of the sacroiliac, facetal, and intervertebral joints is followed by ossification of spinal ligaments and disks. Stiffening occurs before ossification is visible on X-ray.

Inflammation of ligament or muscle attachments (enthesitis) is thought by some to be the basic pathologic process. Bone outgrowths on the margins of the vertebrae extend vertically and unite.

Investigations

X-rays of pelvis or lumbar spine to confirm bilateral sacroiliitis. CT or MRI scans of sacroiliac joints may confirm the diagnosis if X-rays are equivocal (Fig. 11.18). X-ray of the spine may be normal or show syndesmophytes and ossification of disks and spinal ligaments to form a "bamboo spine." This may be confused with the thick, asymptomatic bridging osteophytes of diffuse intervertebral skeletal hyperostosis (DISH) a radiologic phenomenon seen mainly in older people and diabetics.

Hematology, ESR, or CRP may provide evidence of anemia and inflammation. Some rely upon detecting the presence of HLA B27, but this occurs in about 10% of the healthy European population and is therefore of limited value as a discriminator.

Management

The tenets of treatment are simple:

1. A well-tolerated NSAID
2. Regular mobilizing exercises.

Occasionally, corticosteroids are required. For patients who cannot tolerate NSAIDs or who have severe progressive disease, anti-TNFα agents are warranted. They are effective in a higher proportion and side-effects are fewer than in RA. Sulfasalazine may improve the peripheral arthritis but not the spine.

Outcome

A majority have mild disease that does not disrupt daily activities. Some with more severe disease develop hip involvement requiring joint replacement. Rarely, aortitis leads to aortic regurgitation.

Paget's disease

Clinical features

This is a bone disorder of osteoclasts in older people. It is usually asymptomatic but can cause pain especially in the spine and long bones. The skull may be affected and become visibly enlarged. Deafness may be a complication. Bowing of long bones and osteoarthritis of adjacent joints may occur due to softening and deformity of the bone. It may feel warm compared with unaffected areas.

Epidemiology

The prevalence is 5%. It is more common in men and increases in frequency with age. It is rare below age 50.

Pathology

There is increased activity of osteoclasts and disorganised bone as osteoblasts respond. It may be caused by a slow virus but none has been confidently implicated.

Investigation

The X-ray appearance of sclerotic areas of bone with coarse trabeculation and increased bone size are characteristic. The increase of dimension helps distinguish it from metastatic cancer. The serum alkaline phosphatase may be elevated depending on extent of skeletal involvement. A bone scan shows increased uptake of isotope treatment. The potent biphosphanates such as zolendronic acid are very effective but other biphosphanates can be of benefit. Pain is the only indication for treatment.

Outcome

Most respond to treatment. There is a rare association with osteosarcoma.

Malignancy

This is a rare cause of spinal pain.

Clinical features

- Persistent pain, often at night
- Known pre-existing cancer or a story of weight loss, anemia, pronounced acute phase response.

Epidemiology

Some solid tumors are likely to metastasize to bone, namely prostate, breast, lung, kidney, thyroid, colon, and bladder. Primary tumors are rare. Lymphoma may be confined to the spine.

About 70% of tumors are ultimately associated with spinal metastases.

Pathology

Seeding of cancer cells by the circulation occurs. Lymphoma develops *in situ*. Myelomatosis may cause slow onset of spinal pain.

Investigations

Clinical suspicion, abnormal bone biochemistry, raised acute response. Radiographs may show sclerotic lesions with prostate, breast, colon, lymphoma, and sometimes lung tumors. Thyroid, bladder, and myeloma cause osteolytic areas. Radionuclear and MRI scanning are both performed to help confirm and establish extent of disease.

Management and outcome

As for a malignant disease causing sudden onset pain.

Infection

Persistent pain with fever in a susceptible person may be due to local infection.

Epidemiology

The frequency of spinal infection increases with age. It is more common amongst diabetics and whenever there has been bacteremia. In Western communities *Staphylococcus aureus* is the commonest microorganism, but in the developing world it is tuberculosis. Other organisms include *E.coli, Streptococcus, Salmonella, Brucella.*

Clinical features

- Chronic spinal pain.
- Fever, weight loss, rigors.
- Root or cord symptoms and signs if abscess develops or if vertebral destruction results in subluxation.
- Psoas abscess presenting in groin if infection spreads along psoas sheath from vertebrae.

Pathology

The organism is usually blood borne and infects the intervertebral disk before invading adjacent bone.

Investigation

X-rays may show characteristic loss of disk space and erosion or partial destruction of adjacent vertebrae. X-ray evidence of unilateral sacroiliitis should raise suspicion of infection. MRI or CT imaging will define the extent of damage and soft tissue swelling as well as abscess formation. A collection of pus in the epidural space can cause pressure on the spinal cord with subsequent paresis. Blood culture may isolate a pyogenic organism. Needle aspiration or biopsy will identify the infecting organism or, in the case of mycobacterial infection, reveal a granuloma with or without caseation.

Management

Surgical drainage of any pyogenic collection and appropriate antibiotics for a period of 6 weeks or, in the case of TB of the spine, for 9 months. Stabilization of relevant vertebrae may be necessary using bone grafting.

Shoulder pain

Pain confined to one or both shoulders is common and is most often due to abnormalities of the periarticular structures.

How to distinguish the likely cause

Whether or not pain is confined to one or both shoulders, the rapidity of onset, age of patients and

Table 11.8. Characteristics of different causes of shoulder pain

	Onset	Bilateral/ unilateral	Age	Painful restriction	Elevated ESR/CRP	X-ray
Frozen shoulder (adhesive capsulitis)	Slow	Unilateral	Middle life	Concentric	No	Normal
Supraspinatus tendonitis	Slow	Unilateral	Middle life	Abduction	No	Normal
Calcific supraspinatus	Sudden	Unilateral	Middle life	Abduction	Yes	Calcification of tendon
Bicipital tendonitis	Slow	Unilateral	Middle life	Flexion	No	Normal
Hemarthrosis	Sudden	Unilateral	Older	Concentric	No	Upward migration
Milwaukee shoulder	Slow	Unilateral	Older	Concentric	No	Peri-articular calcification
Rotator cuff degeneration	Slow	Bilateral	Older	Concentric	No	Upward migration humerus
PMR	Sudden	Bilateral	Older	None	Yes	Normal
RA	Slow	Bilateral	Middle life	Concentric	Yes	Normal
OA	Slow	Unilateral	Older	Concentric	No	Loss of joint space

whether there is restriction of movement in one or more directions can help establish a diagnosis. (Fig. 11.6 and Table 11.8).

Frozen shoulder
This is common but can be surprisingly disabling.

Clinical features
- Usually unilateral
- Sometimes after trivial trauma or strain.
- Progressive pain and immobility of shoulder, nocturnal discomfort, and difficulty with dressing.
- Impaired, painful active, and passive movement in all directions.
- When associated with diabetes, diabetic retinopathy and renal disease or neuropathy are more likely.

Epidemiology
There is a strong association with diabetes mellitus. In the non-diabetic population the prevalence is 1%–2%. Onset before age 40 is uncommon.

Pathology
The joint capsule becomes adherent to the overlying rotator cuff muscles for unknown reasons.

Management
An intra-articular injection of a long acting cortico-steroid helps the pain. Regular mobilizing exercises may help restore movement.

Outcome
Improvement invariably occurs and full recovery is the rule, but it may take up to 2 years. Involvement of the contralateral shoulder may arise at some future date.

Tendonitis
One or more of the rotator cuff muscle tendons may become inflamed, especially in those of working age either as a result of repetitive or unaccustomed use of the arm.

Clinical features
- Pain in a shoulder, worse on active abduction, flexion or rotation, usually of insidious onset may be due to inflammation of the supraspinatus tendon.
- A painful arc on active abduction and against resistance.
- Tenderness over the insertion of the supraspinatus tendon.
- Calcific supraspinatus tendonitis is recognized by its sudden onset and exceptionally severe pain.

345

- Bicipital tendonitis causes pain that is worse on active flexion, especially against resistance. The long head of the biceps is tender to palpation on its course anterior to the shoulder.

Epidemiology

The frequency of shoulder tendonitis is unknown except that it commonly occurs amongst sports people and those engaged in physical work. Calcific supraspinatus on the other hand has no known predisposing characteristics.

Calcific tendonitis is due to deposition and leakage of calcium hydroxyapatite into the surrounding soft tissues or subacromial bursa. The reason for calcium deposition is unknown.

Investigation

X-ray of the shoulder may reveal calcification of the supraspinatus tendon but it requires ultrasound or MRI scanning to demonstrate edema, swelling, or tears of the tendons. In calcific tendonitis there may be elevation of ESR, CRP, and neutrophilia.

Management

Local corticosteroids into or around the tendon, NSAIDs, physical treatments, and surgery to relieve impingement summarize the therapeutic approaches available depending on response to initial conservative management.

Outcome

If there is no impingement and no major tear, the response to corticosterid injections is good. Surgical decompression also has an excellent outcome when it becomes necessary.

Rotator cuff degeneration

A majority of people aged >80 have limitation of shoulder movements.

Clinical features

- Restricted movement in all directions.
- Difficulty dressing and bathing.
- Variable pain but often insufficient to make patient complain.
- Graduation of severity with hemarthrosis and chronic effusion at severe end of spectrum.

Epidemiology

A majority of subjects experience tears and attenuation of rotator cuff muscles with advancing age.

Pathology

As the muscles become thin, the humeral head moves upward and may impinge on and erode the acromion. These changes may be associated with fragments of cartilage and calcium hydroxyapatite from the skeleton in synovial fluid. Occasionally, acute hemarthrosis complicates the picture. The constellation of rotator cuff degeneration and liberation of calcium into the joint is sometimes referred to as Milwaukee shoulder.

Management

Local corticosteroid injections may help for a period of days or weeks. There is no certain remedy.

Outcome

It is surprising that patients do not complain more. Progression is common to the extent that assistance is required for dressing and toileting.

Other regional pain syndromes

Non-articular pain other than that of the shoulder is common and affects all age groups. To the uninitiated, the symptoms may be confused with arthritis affecting the joints.

Elbow – pain and tenderness over the lateral aspect of the elbow, sometimes over the lateral epicondyle, is called tennis elbow or lateral epicondylitis. It is due to a small tear and inflammation of the attachment of wrist dorsiflexor muscles. Pain is accentuated by resisted dorsiflexion of the wrist. It can be treated by identifying and avoiding the physical activity that caused the problem, a local injection of corticosteroid, and a range of physical treatments. It improves within 6–12 months with and without treatment. Medial epicondylitis (or golfers' elbow) has an identical pathology affecting the insertion of the wrist flexor muscles. Management is the same.

Wrist – carpal tunnel syndrome due to median nerve compression at the wrist, OA of the first carpometacarpal joint, and De Quervain's tenosynovitis are sometimes difficult to distinguish. All may cause pain at the wrist and the forearm. The first two are associated with wasting of the thenar eminence. Carpal tunnel is characteristically worse at night or on awakening and may be associated with paraesthesiae of the fingers, sensory impairment in a median nerve distribution, pain or tingling when the front of the wrist is tapped (Tinel's sign). Any condition that causes narrowing of the carpal tunnel may be causative including wrist arthritis, fluid retention of pregnancy, hypothyroidism. It is more common amongst diabetics (Chapter 9).

The thumb base is a common site of involvement, especially in nodular generalized OA. Inability to grip, open jars, and use the hand in other tasks are regular complaints amongst women in middle or older age groups. Immobilization in a splint, local steroid injection, analgesics are the treatments but none is wholly effective.

De Quervain's tenosynovitis also causes pain on using the hand. There is pain, tenderness, and sometimes swelling and crepitus over the abductor and extensor pollicis tendons with pain on resisted thumb abduction. It is frequently seen in office workers who use keyboards, but other occupational activities involving hand use may also cause the tendon inflammation. Management is best achieved by local steroid injection and avoidance of relevant activities.

Pain in the hand or arm caused by work practices is often claimed to be due to a syndrome called repetitive strain injury (RSI). It is doubtful that this represents an entity and is more likely attributable to one or more of the better recognized disorders described above.

Fingers – work related inflammation of one or more of the flexor tendons may cause pain, tenderness, swelling, and restricted flexion and extension. One effect of this is triggering. An affected digit cannot be extended without assistance because a nodule on the tendon prevents movement within the tendon sheath. The condition may arise *de novo* amongst diabetics adding to the panoply of upper limb conditions to which diabetics are susceptible. The thickened fingers in this context are referred to as diabetic cheiroarthropathy. Sometimes flexion deformities develop and these are difficult to distinguish from Dupuytren's contracture in which thickening and contraction of the palmar fascia causes permanent finger flexion. The management of flexor tendon inflammation includes infiltration of the tendon sheaths with steroids. Triggering or flexion deformity may require surgical release procedures.

Chest wall – Pain and tenderness of the chest wall most often presents to emergency departments as possible ischemic heart disease. Tenderness of the sternocostal or costochondral junctions is the only finding and investigations are normal. This is sometimes called costochontritis. Psoriatic arthritis and anklyosing spondylitis may also cause pain and tenderness of the sternocostal and sternoclavicular joints occasionally with swelling.

Hip – any pain in the pelvic girdle is described by patients as hip pain. Uusally, examination of the hip is normal. Pain in the buttock most often derives from the spine or sacroiliac joints. Pain over the greater trochanter is almost exclusive to women and disturbs sleep. There is associated tenderness and the phenomenon is called trochanteric bursitis. It can be distinguished from a tear of hip abductor muscles by inability to stand on the affected limb without pain. Injection of steroid into the tender area is usually effective but recurrence is usual.

Ankle and foot

Achilles tendonitis – This can be associated with ankylosing spondylitis, reactive arthritis, or psoriatic arthritis but most often there is no obvious explanation. The tendon is often thickened, and tender. It can be treated by avoidance of shoes without heels, a paratendon injection of hydrocortisone, and physical treatments such as ultrasonography. A complication is tendon rupture, a problem made more likely by corticosteroid injection.

Tendonitis of tibialis anterior or peroneal muscles is frequently confused with ankle arthritis. It may be caused by pes planus and valgus deformity of the ankles (flat feet). Insertion of medial arch supports, foot exercises, and local steroid injections have a modest chance of succeeding. It tends to be a recurring problem.

Plantar fasciitis – Like Achilles tendonitis, pain in the heel may be associated with ankylosing spondylitis, reactive arthritis, or psoriatic arthritis. Similarly, it occurs more often in the absence of these disorders. It may be due to increasing body weight or excessive walking and standing. Weight reduction, shoes with heels, heel pads, and local injections of steroid will improve matters in most patients. It tends to improve over several months, whatever treatment is pursued.

Diffuse pain

Skeletal pain which is widespread and not derived from peripheral or axial joints demands careful consideration. In middle and late life, serious pathology needs exclusion especially on a background of weight loss, anemia or known cancer. This may include hematology for anemia, neutropenia or thrombocytopenia as evidence of marrow infiltration; liver biochemistry; thyroid function; Vitamin D3 level; ESR and CRP and protein electrophoresis to explore for systemic disease or evidence of myeloma, X-rays of the chest and skeleton, bone scan, CT or MRI of

Table 11.9. Biochemistry of bone disease

	Alkaline phosphatase	Serum calcium	Serum phosphate	Vitamin D3	PTH
Osteoporosis	N	N	N	N	N
Osteomalacia	↑	↓ or N	N	↓	↑
Paget's disease	N or ↑ dependent on extent	N	N	N	N
Hyperparathyroidism	N or ↑	↑	↓	N	↑ or high N

Note:
N = Normal.

relevant areas of the skeleton, abdomen, or chest (Table 11.9).

Diffuse pain with an elevated serum calcium should be pursued with a PTH assay. A high or high normal level indicates hyperparathyroidism. The serum phosphate may be low. A chest X-ray to rule out lung cancer as a source of bone metastases or the site of PTH related polypeptide giving rise to the picture of hyperparathyroidism. Bone scan may identify sites of secondary spread of solid tumor in the skeleton but is normal in myeloma. The further investigation and management of hyperparathyroidism is found (see Chapter 11).

A low or normal serum calcium may also be associated with an elevated serum PTH when the cause of diffuse pain is osteomalacia. A low vitamin D level can then be anticipated. There may also be elevation of serum alkaline phosphatase derived from bone. When the serum vitamin D is low in the absence of elevated PTH, it is unlikely to have pathologic relevance. Osteomalacia is seen most commonly in South Asian women living in non-tropical countries. It occurs both in Muslims, who may cover most exposed areas, and in Hindus, who do not. Relative lack of sunlight and loss of cutaneous vitamin D synthesis accounts for the disease. It is rarely found in women from the south and west of Africa. Occasionally, the problem is due to malabsorption. This occurs in all races. Diffuse pain, proximal muscle weakness, and sometimes a waddling gait are the main clinical features. An X-ray of the pelvis or of long bones may show isolated lines of demineralization called Looser zones or Milkman pseudofractures. Treatment is successfully achieved by oral calcium and vitamin D supplements or in the presence of malabsorption by injections of vitamin D.

Hypothyroidism is another well-recognized cause of diffuse pain. Elevated TSH, low T4, macrocysosis, and raised serum CK may each be of diagnostic value.

When pain is associated with tenderness at multiple sites including the shoulders, occiputs, trapezius, lateral aspect elbows, sacroiliac joints, greater trochanters, and the medial aspect of the knees, fibromyalgia is a diagnosis that may be usefully invoked. The syndrome affects about 2% of the population and women three times more often than men. It is associated with fatigue, altered sleep patterns, depression, and irritable bowel syndrome in 50%. No pathology has been defined, but an explanation could rest with the hypothesis of pain amplification. It is an attractive proposition for an illness that attracts skepticism. The concept rests on demonstrable increase of muscle and skin pain perception and other evidence such as increased substance P in CSF. Management entails education, analgesia, antidepressants, and structured exercise programs. Symptoms can be modified by treatment but tend to persist indefinitely.

References

NICE guidance: Secondary prevention of osteoporotic fragility fractures in postmenopausal women Jan 2005 and Alendronate, etidronate, risedronate, raloxifene and strontium ranelate for the primary prevention of osteoporotic fragility fractures in post menopausal women Oct 2008: www.nice.org.uk.

NICE guidance: Rheumatoid arthritis. The management of rheumatoid arthritis in adults Feb 2009: www.nice.org.uk.

Rheumatology, edited Hochberg, Silman, Smolen, Weinblatt, Weisman, conrech, 2008 Elsevier

Contents

Nutritional

Weight gain

Excessive weight gain is an increasingly frequent phenomenon. Most patients with weight gain have simple obesity and will not require further investigation.

Accumulation of fluid due to cardiac, renal, or hepatic failure may also cause weight gain. These conditions are usually be pre-existing and it is unusual for weight gain alone to be a presenting feature.

Drugs, particularly glucocorticoids, estrogens, and progestogens, can also cause weight gain but should be suspected from the history.

Hypothyroidism and Cushing's syndrome are two endocrine disorders that can present with weight gain and patients should be screened for these where there has been a recent increase in weight unexplained by alterations in lifestyle or life events or if there are clinical features to suggest an underlying endocrine disturbance (Fig. 12.1 and Table 12.1).

Simple obesity

Introduction

Obesity has increased rapidly in prevalence and is now a major public health problem in developed and developing countries.

It increases morbidity and mortality through the risk of developing type 2 diabetes mellitus, hypertension, heart, gall bladder, musculoskeletal diseases, and some forms of cancer. Obesity also carries social stigma and causes psychologic morbidity.

Epidemiology

In the UK more than one in five adults is clinically obese. The rate of obesity increases with age, but younger people with obesity are also increasing dramatically. The percentage of adults classified as obese has doubled since the mid 1980s.

Clinical features

Obesity is measured using body mass index (BMI) calculated by dividing body weight in kilograms by height in meters squared. Weight is classified according to BMI (Table 12.2).

Pathology

Obesity is a disease and not a self-inflicted condition. There is widespread stigmatization and negative attitudes towards obese patients who report disrespect from health professionals towards their problems.

The cause of obesity is not well delineated. Body weight appears to be largely predetermined. There is a genetic component which determines the controlling physiological and biochemical mechanisms. No specific gene defect has yet been found, but obesity does tend to run in families. This is partly genetic but families do share cultural, socio-economic, and psychological factors which are important.

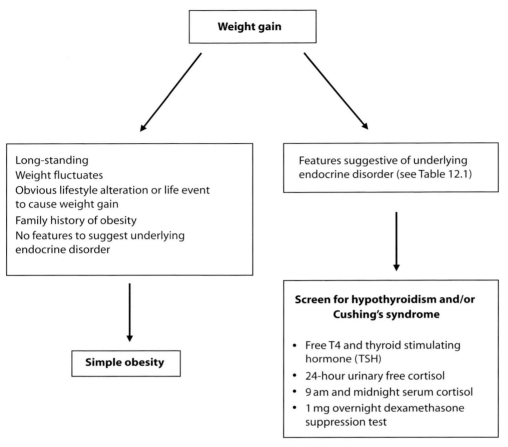

Fig. 12.1. How to distinguish simple obesity from endocrine causes of weight gain.

Table 12.1. Clinical features which suggest an underlying endocrine cause of weight gain

Hypothyroidism	Cushing's syndrome
Tiredness, lethargy	Central distribution of body fat
Coarse dry skin	Moon face
Non-pitting edema	Thin skin and easy bruising
Cold intolerance	Tiredness
Constipation	Proximal muscle weakness
Hoarse voice	Hypertension
Menorrhagia	Hirsutes and menstrual disturbance
Carpal tunnel syndrome	Highly colored striae (see Fig. 12.3)
Depression	Mental disturbance
Goiter	Glucose intolerance
Slow relaxing reflexes	Osteoporosis

Table 12.2. Categories of BMI

BMI kg/m^2	Weight category
<18.5	Underweight
18.5–24.9	Normal weight
25–29.9	Overweight
30–39.9	Obese
>40	Morbidly obese

Investigation

Clinical assessment should indicate whether the weight gain is related to simple obesity and recent environmental triggering factors should be sought. Most will not require investigation. Patients should also be assessed for features of underlying endocrine disturbance (Table 12.1). If there is any suspicion then screening investigations should be initiated (Fig. 12.1).

Management

One must bear in mind the health risks, social stigmatization, and the realities of treating the condition. The patient must be motivated to lose weight or treatment will fail. It is best to devise realistic management regimens and goals with the aim of improving lifestyle. Measures such as diet and exercise must be maintained long term. Short-term dramatic alterations in diet and exercise regimens are usually followed by relapse.

Motivation to improve lifestyle measures and behavior modification can be gained through self-help groups, dietetic services, and psychologic counseling.

Anti-obesity drugs can assist in clinically obese patients but must be used in conjunction with other lifestyle measures. Orlistat inhibits pancreatic lipase and reduces absorption of dietary fat. Its use is limited by gastro-intestinal side effects, mainly oily stools, fecal urgency, and flatulence due to undigested fat. Sibutramine is a centrally acting appetite suppressant thought to act by inhibiting uptake of norepinephrine and serotonin. It may cause increased heart rate and hypertension.

These measures are frequently disappointing in maintaining weight loss and in improving morbidity. Some patients, particularly the morbidly obese (BMI $>40\,kg/m^2$) benefit from gastric reduction surgery (bariatric surgery). This usually involves gastric banding or gastric bypass, restricting the quantities of food that can be eaten.

Hypothyroidism

Introduction

Hypothyroidism is the clinical picture resulting from insufficient circulating free thyroid hormones. This can be due to insufficiency of the thyroid gland itself (primary hypothyroidism) or lesions of the pituitary or hypothalamus (secondary hypothyroidism). The causes are listed in Table 12.3.

The commonest cause of hypothyroidism is an organ-specific autoimmune destructive process within the thyroid gland (Hashimoto's thyroiditis).

Myxedema is sometimes used synonymously with hypothyroidism but is more correctly used to describe the thickened "doughy" consistency of the skin, which occurs in advanced stages of hypothyroidism.

Clinical features

- The clinical features are described in Table 12.1.
- Development of hypothyroidism is often insidious with gradual progression of non-specific

Table 12.3. Causes of hypothyroidism

Common
Autoimmune hypothyroidism (Hashimoto's disease)
Idiopathic primary (atrophic) hypothyroidism
Post-radioiodine, radiotherapy, or surgery
Uncommon
Thyroiditis
Drug-induced (lithium, iodides, amiodarone)
Congenital defect in hormone synthesis
Iodine deficiency
Hypothalamic or pituitary defect

symptoms such as tiredness, which are easy to overlook. They may be erroneously attributed to aging and diagnosis requires a high index of suspicion.
- Weight gain is a feature but is usually modest.
- Mild degrees of hypothyroidism are often identified on routine blood tests.
- With progression, features become more pronounced and patients progressively unwell.
- Patients with Hashimoto's disease will usually have a small diffusely enlarged painless thyroid (goiter).
- Slow relaxation of tendon reflexes is characteristic but only seen with advanced hypothyroidism. It is best demonstrated at the ankle.
- Undiagnosed hypothyroidism can lead to altered consciousness, confusion, dementia, and coma sometimes precipitated by intercurrent illness.
- Severe disease can lead to pleural and pericardial effusions and ascites.

Epidemiology

Autoimmune destruction of the thyroid (Hashimoto's disease) is the commonest cause in parts of the world where iodine intake is sufficient. It occurs at any age but peaks in middle age and is much commoner in women (ratio 5:1). It can be associated with other organ-specific autoimmune conditions such as type 1 diabetes, Addison's disease, and pernicious anemia. There is often a family history of thyroid disease indicating a genetic predisposition.

Chronic iodine deficiency, which is endemic in some parts of the world, can cause a goiter and hypothyroidism (Table 12.3). Iodine deficiency is rare in the UK where salt is iodized.

Pathology

Hashimoto's disease involves infiltration of the thyroid by lymphocytes causing autoimmune type destruction. This progresses over months or years with a gradual loss of thyroid function and a slow fall in production and release of free thyroid hormones. There may be an early transient phase of thyrotoxicosis due to a severe inflammatory response causing thyroid follicular disruption and release of excessive thyroid hormones.

Patients with Hashimoto's disease often exhibit circulating antibodies against thyroid antigens (thyroid autoantibodies). These are thought to be involved in pathogenesis, although their importance and role are not delineated.

Transient thyroiditis may occur in other situations typically in association with a viral infection. This type of thyroiditis usually causes an acute painful thyroid accompanied by other features of systemic infection. It will usually settle spontaneously or on treatment of the infection, but there may be a transient episode of thyrotoxicosis followed by hypothyroidism and then restoration of the euthyroid status. Some suffer permanent damage and hypothyroidism. Painless forms of thyroiditis can also occur, namely Riedel's thyroiditis, which is characterized by fibrous change within the thyroid, and lymphocytic thyroiditis, which often occurs in the post-partum period.

Hypothyroidism commonly follows treatment of thyrotoxicosis with drugs such as carbimazole. This is usually transient and responds to reductions of dose. The administration of radioactive iodine or subtotal thyroidectomy for thyrotoxicosis often causes permanent hypothyroidism. Hypothyroidism may also occur after radiotherapy given to the neck for other reasons, e.g. lymphoma, when it may occur soon or many years later. These patients require long-term follow-up.

Lesions of the pituitary and hypothalamus are unusual causes. The commonest is an anterior pituitary adenoma or its treatment by surgery and radiotherapy, damaging thyrotrophs and reducing thyroid stimulating hormone (TSH) secretion. Radiotherapy for any tumor within the head can cause hypopituitarism if the pituitary is in the radiation field and this may occur many years later.

Amiodarone and lithium can both cause hypothyroidism and patients treated with these drugs should have thyroid function tests beforehand. Amiodarone can also cause thyrotoxicosis.

One in 5000 babies is born with a hereditary defect of thyroid hormone synthesis. Undetected neonatal hypothyroidism leads to severe developmental abnormalities (cretinism) but should be detected by neonatal screening.

Investigations

Once the clinical suspicion has been aroused, the diagnosis is usually straightforward.

Measurement of blood levels of the free (non-protein bound) thyroid hormones; free T3 (fT3), and free T4 (fT4) are low whatever the cause of hypothyroidism.

The TSH level is raised and often very high in any cause of *primary* hypothyroidism. The pituitary and hypothalamus sense the low free thyroid hormone levels and further stimulate the failing thyroid gland by secreting more TSH.

In pituitary or hypothalamic disease the free thyroid hormone levels are low but the TSH level is not raised (usually low or in the lower part of the quoted normal range). If TSH is the only test done, this diagnosis may be missed.

Measurement of thyroid autoantibodies helps to identify Hashimoto's disease as the cause of thyroid failure.

Patients with Hashimoto's disease may go through a phase of so-called subclinical or compensated hypothyroidism where TSH is slightly raised but where the thyroid is able to continue producing sufficient free thyroid hormones to maintain these within the low normal range. This can continue for many years. Some patients have symptoms due to a subtle lack of thyroid hormones.

Hypercholesterolemia and a macrocytic anemia may also be seen.

Management

Treatment of hypothyroidism, whatever the cause, is easy. Standard treatment is synthetic thyroid hormone tablets (levothyroxine) once daily. This is commenced in a small dose of 25–50 μg once daily and increased by 25–50 μg increments. It is important to correct hypothyroidism slowly, particularly in the elderly and in those at risk of heart disease, since rapid correction can precipitate angina or myocardial infarction. Patients with very severe hypothyroidism or so-called myxedema coma may require more rapid correction in the initial period.

The object of treatment is to restore euthyroidism. The best way of determining optimal treatment in primary disease is to measure serum TSH and aim for a low normal level (usually 1–2 mU/l), which is thought to be the most physiological.

TSH measurements and increments in dosage should be performed every 2 months since it takes

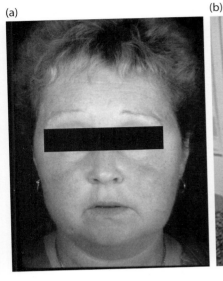
(a)

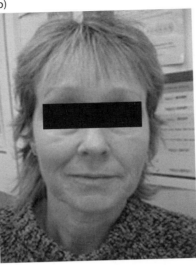
(b)

Fig. 12.2. (a) *Shows a patient with the moon face, facial plethora and, hirsutes as characteristic of Cushing's syndrome.* (b) *Shows the same patient 2 years after removal of an ACTH-secreting pituitary adenoma.*

this long for TSH levels to achieve a new steady state. TSH cannot be used to guide treatment of secondary hypothyroidism.

In Hashimoto's disease the requirement for thyroxine gradually increases as the disease process continues.

It is important that patients with hypothalamic or pituitary hypothyroidism do not receive thyroid replacement until other deficiencies of the pituitary–adrenal axis have been corrected, since thyroxine therapy alone may precipitate acute adrenocortical insufficiency.

Outcome

Depends on the underlying cause; for most the outlook is good. Patients with Hashimoto's disease who are stabilized on optimal replacement therapy with thyroxine should expect a normal quality of life and life expectancy.

Cushing's syndrome
Introduction

This is caused by the effects of excessive circulating glucocorticoids. The commonest cause of a Cushingoid appearance is the chronic administration of glucocorticoids as treatment of asthma, inflammatory bowel disease or connective tissue diseases. The decision to treat with long term steroids must consider the balance between benefits and side-effects. The endogenous causes of Cushing's syndrome are 1. Pituitary adenoma 2. Adrenal adenoma, carcinoma or nodular hyperplasia 3. Ectopic ACTH from a tumor elsewhere, usually a small cell carcinoma of the lung or carcinoid tumor.

Clinical features
- The main clinical features are listed in Table 12.1 p. 352.
- Disfigurement (Fig. 12.2) may cause psychologic and physical distress.
- Weight gain is central and progressive and may be considerable but Cushing's seldom causes extreme obesity.
- The striae are different from those which occur in obesity and pregnancy. They are larger, more highly colored, and out of keeping with the degree of obesity (Fig. 12.3).
- Psychologic features, mainly lethargy, mood swings, depression, and anxiety are invariably present and are frequently underestimated.

Epidemiology

Cushing's disease due to administration of glucocorticoids is common. The endogenous causes are rare. Pituitary adenomas account for 60% of all cases of endogenous Cushing's syndrome and this etiology is usually termed Cushing's *disease*. It affects women more often than men (approximately 4 : 1) with peak incidence in the third and fourth decades.

Adrenal adenomas, or more rarely nodular hyperplasia or carcinomas, account for 30%, the remainder being ectopic ACTH-producing tumors.

Pathology

Pituitary-dependent Cushing's syndrome (Cushing's disease) is caused by excessive ACTH production

(a)

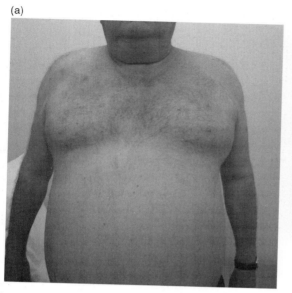

(b)

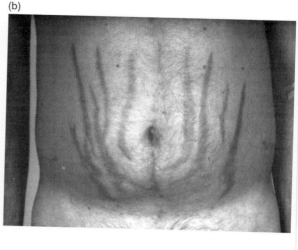

Fig. 12.3. (a) Central obesity, proximal muscle wasting, (b) Characteristic highly colored striae of Cushing's syndrome.

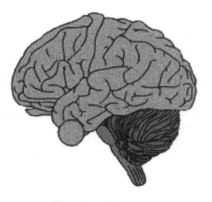

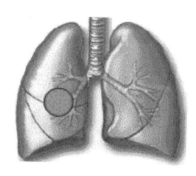

Fig. 12.4. Diagrammatic representation of the causes of endogenous Cushing's syndrome.

Pituitary adenoma. ACTH secreting. 60% of cases.

Small cell carcinoma of the lung or carciniod. ACTH secreting. 10% of cases.

Adrenal adenoma, nodular hyperplasia or carcinoma. Cortisol secreting. 30% of cases.

from a, usually small, pituitary adenoma (Fig. 12.4). These rarely cause any mass effect. Some appear to have hyperplasia of the ACTH-producing cells (corticotrophs) without any discrete adenoma. The primary defect may reside in the hypothalamus with over-stimulation of corticotrophs. Regardless of the cause, the excessive ACTH cause adrenocortical hyperplasia and hypercortisolism.

Adrenal adenomas function autonomously and produce excessive quantities of cortisol. This results in feedback suppression of ACTH secretion from the normal pituitary gland. The cortex of the unaffected adrenal gland atrophies as a result. Adrenal nodular hyperplasia also results in excessive cortisol production by both adrenals with similar suppression of ACTH. Adrenal carcinomas tend to be larger than adenomas at the time of diagnosis and produce larger quantities of cortisol.

Ectopic ACTH is exceedingly rare. The usual source is a small cell carcinoma or carcinoid tumor of the lung. The onset may be rapid and the classical phenotype of Cushing's syndrome may be minimal or absent. Patients may have hypokalemic alkalosis due to the mineralocorticoid effect of the high cortisol levels.

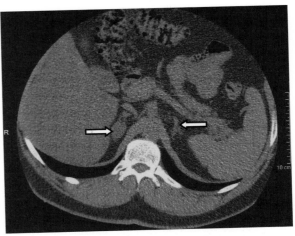

Fig. 12.5. CT scan showing cortisol secreting adenoma in right adrenal gland (left arrow). Left adrenal is normal (right arrow).

Investigations

Iatrogenic Cushing's syndrome caused by the administration of exogenous steroids must first be excluded. This is usually easy from the history, but the use of topical and inhaled steroid preparations can rarely cause a Cushingoid appearance and may be overlooked.

The diagnosis of an endogenous cause is a two-step process. The first step is demonstration of excessive glucocorticoid production. Once this is established, investigation centers around determining the etiology.

The diagnosis can be complex due to lack of specificity of many of the tests and confounding factors including the potential for cyclical disease. For these reasons, particularly in difficult cases, the diagnosis is made using a combination of tests.

Depression, obesity, excessive alcohol, and drugs such as estrogens and carbamazepine can all result in false-positive testing and should be excluded before proceeding.

The best screening tests are:

(1) Demonstration of excessive total urinary cortisol excretion over a 24-hour period.
(2) Loss of normal diurnal variation of cortisol levels.
(3) Lack of suppression of cortisol in response to the administration of dexamethasone.

Cortisol levels are highest on waking in the morning and fall to a nadir during the first hour or two of sleep. One of the earliest demonstrable abnormalities in Cushing's syndrome is the lack of a fall in cortisol levels in the evening. This is best detected by measuring midnight cortisol values with the patient asleep: easiest to perform as an in-patient!

A failure of suppression of a 9 am cortisol level after administration of 1 mg of dexamethasone at 11 pm (overnight dexamethasone suppression test) is also indicative of Cushing's syndrome and can be performed as an outpatient. A more prolonged form of this test, the low dose dexamethasone suppression test (0.5 mg 6-hourly for 48 hours), uses similar principles.

Once the diagnosis of Cushing's syndrome has been established, the source must be found. A high dose dexamethasone suppression test (2 mg 6-hourly over 48 hours) will often show suppression of hypercortisolemia of pituitary origin but not when the source is adrenal or ectopic.

Serum ACTH measurement is useful because it is suppressed by hypercortisolemia of an adrenal source but often high in the presence of a pituitary adenoma. Ectopic sources will often produce very high ACTH levels.

Imaging is an essential part of localizing the abnormality. MRI is best for imaging the pituitary although, even with modern scanners, the abnormality may not be seen in a proportion of cases. A CT will demonstrate an adrenal lesion (Fig. 12.5) and a chest radiograph often reveals an ectopic source. Small carcinoid tumors can be difficult to localize.

Management

Patients with severe Cushing's need to be treated urgently since there is considerable morbidity and much psychologic and physical distress.

Treatment depends on the underlying etiology.

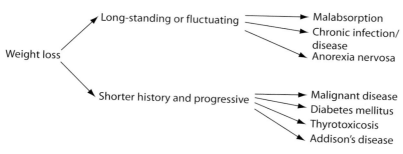

Fig. 12.6. Weight loss.

Pituitary tumors are best treated surgically usually via a transphenoidal route. This should be done by specialized pituitary surgeons. Patients who are not cured by surgery or who develop recurrent disease may undergo further surgery or radiotherapy to the pituitary gland.

Solitary adrenal adenomas can usually be cured by unilateral adrenalectomy leaving a contra-lateral adrenal gland. However, patients *must* be treated with glucocorticoid and mineralocorticoid replacement both during and after operation since the corticotrophs and remaining adrenal cortex are suppressed and atrophied by the prior hypercortisolemia. This treatment must continue until there is evidence that the pituitary–adrenal axis has recovered. Without such replacement therapy, acute adrenocortical insufficiency can occur.

Adrenal carcinomas are often difficult to excise or have metastasized by the time of diagnosis. They carry a poor prognosis.

Medical treatment of Cushing's syndrome is less effective but may be indicated while patients are being prepared for surgery or if other treatments have failed or are not possible. Ketoconazole, metyrapone, aminoglutethimide, and mitotane all block steroid synthesis. Mitotane is also cytotoxic and so is used in adrenal carcinomas. The response to these agents is poor.

Treatment of ectopic tumors depends on the histologic type and stage of the underlying tumor.

Outcome

Depends on the etiology, severity and the duration of disease.

The majority of adrenal adenomas can be surgically resected and patients cured. The features of Cushing's syndrome gradually resolve, although this can take a notoriously long time. Patients with a pituitary source have a 60% chance of cure in the best centers with most of the remainder responding to radiotherapy. A significant proportion suffer recurrence at some stage and there is morbidity from hypopituitarism as a result of treatment.

There is a growing realization that patients with treated Cushing's syndrome have ongoing physical and psychologic problems as a result of their condition.

Adrenal carcinomas and ectopic tumors carry a poor prognosis, but small carcinoid tumors can be resected and the patient cured.

Weight loss (Fig. 12.6)

Weight loss may occur for innocuous reasons such as dieting or stressful life events or changes in activity levels. Weight loss without such simple explanation or in the presence of other symptoms may be indication of underlying pathology. A careful history and examination are required in the assessment of weight loss (Fig. 12.7).

Appetite is a useful discriminatory symptom, characteristically reduced in malignant disease but relatively preserved in other conditions and increased in hyperthyroidism.

Thyrotoxicosis (hyperthyroidism)

Introduction

Describes the tissue response to excessive levels of circulating free thyroid hormones: free T4 (fT_4) and free T3 (fT_3). The elevated levels of free thyroid hormones induce a hypermetabolic state and overactivity of the sympathetic nervous system causing the features listed below. Like hypothyroidism, this clinical picture can have several causes (Table 12.4). Graves' disease is by far the commonest cause of thyrotoxicosis.

Clinical features

- Weight loss with increased appetite
- Tremor of hands
- Sweating and heat intolerance
- Anxiety, irritability, easy fatigue, poor concentration. Often noticed by family members
- Diarrhea

Teenager　　　Young adult　　　Middle age　　　Older age　　**Fig. 12.7.** Assessment of weight loss.

| Anorexia nervosa |
| Type 1 diabetes |

| Malabsorption |
| Thyrotoxicosis/Addison's |

| Malignant disease |
| Type 2 diabetes |

| Chronic infection/disease |

Table 12.4. Causes of thyrotoxicosis

Common

　　　Graves' disease

　　　Toxic multinodular goiter

　　　Toxic adenoma

Uncommon

　　　Drug induced (amiodarone)

　　　Other causes of thyroiditis

　　　Iodide induced

　　　Thyrotoxicosis factitia

Very uncommon

　　　Functioning follicular carcinoma

　　　TSH-secreting pituitary tumor

　　　Struma ovarii

　　　Choriocarcinoma or hydatidiform mole

　　　Pituitary resistance to thyroid hormones

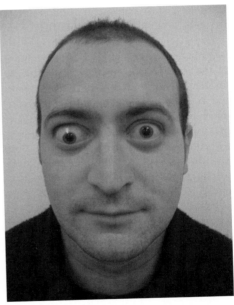

Fig. 12.8. Ophthalmopathy of Graves' disease showing lid retraction (sclera visible above the iris) and exophthalmos (sclera visible below the iris) in the left eye with difficulty in elevating the eye on the right due to tethering of the extraocular muscles. The patient was asked to look straight at the camera.

- Palpitations and tachycardia often most prominent when resting in bed. Cardiac dysrhythmias, particularly atrial fibrillation. Cardiac failure may occur in the elderly
- Eye signs (Fig. 12.8): irritation, corneal injection and chemosis, periorbital oedema, lid lag, lid retraction, exophthalmos, and diplopia. Apart from lid lag and retraction, which occur in any form of thyrotoxicosis, eye changes are peculiar to Graves' disease
- Thyroid enlargement (goiter) which is typically smooth, firm, and symmetric with a bruit due to hypervascularity in Graves' disease or nodular

in the case of a toxic adenoma or toxic multinodular goiter.

- Proximal myopathy
- Pre-tibial myxedema involves raised, thickened, reddened, and well-demarcated lesions in the dermis usually occurring over the anterior tibial area. There is thickening of the dermis with a lymphocytic infiltration, increased hyaluronic acid and edema. It is confined to Graves' disease

and can occur in other areas, taking on a variety of appearances.

Epidemiology

Graves' disease is relatively common: one or two cases per 1000 individuals per year in the UK. It occurs at any age, peaking in the third and fourth decades. It is more common in women (F : M, 7 : 1). There is often a family history and there is linkage to HLA haplotypes.

Etiology and pathology

Graves' disease is also called Basedow's disease and accounts for 85% of thyrotoxicosis in the UK. Thyroid-stimulating IgG immunoglobulins (TSIs) are present in the circulation. These stimulate the TSH receptors in thyroid tissue causing increased production and release of free thyroid hormones as well as stimulating growth and increased vascularity of the gland.

Graves' disease is curiously and classically associated with eye changes (ophthalmopathy) possibly due to shared antigen between thyroid and retro-orbital tissues. There is expansion of retro-orbital tissues with increase in connective tissue and in the size of extra ocular muscles with lymphocytic infiltration and edema. Only 50% develop clinical signs of eye disease and it does not necessarily follow the course of the thyrotoxic illness. The increased volume of the retro-orbital tissues may push the globe forward (exophthalmos) causing the characteristic staring appearance (Fig. 12.8). There may be tethering of extraocular muscles causing abnormal eye movements and diplopia. More extreme forms of exophthalmos may result in failure of apposition of the eyelids, leading to irritation, infection, or even ulceration of the cornea. The increased retro-orbital pressure can cause pressure on the optic nerve and threaten vision.

Lid retraction and lid lag are due to sympathetic over-stimulation of levator palpebrae superioris.

Approximately 5% of patients with Graves' disease develop an infiltrative dermopathy (pre-tibial myxedema, see above).

In a multinodular goiter one or more nodules may start to function autonomously and secrete excessive quantities of free thyroid hormones. Thyroid adenomas can also behave in such a fashion.

Thyroiditis, caused typically by viral illnesses, amiodarone, or following pregnancy, results in damage to follicular cells, which release excessive amounts of stored thyroid hormones. This can also occur in Hashimoto's thyroiditis, although the thyrotoxicosis is often transient and may be followed by hypothyroidism or return to the euthyroid state.

Investigations

Patients with Graves' disease can often be distinguished clinically, particularly if there is ophthalmopathy. Careful assessment of the thyroid gland may help in the differential diagnosis. Diffuse thyroid enlargement and a thyroid bruit are also suggestive of Graves' disease. Palpation may identify a toxic adenoma, toxic multinodular goiter, or the tenderness of thyroiditis.

The diagnosis is confirmed by laboratory finding of high serum fT_3 and fT_4 levels and a suppressed TSH due to feedback inhibition of the elevated thyroid hormones on the pituitary and hypothalamus.

Occasionally, the fT_4 levels are normal but the fT_3 levels are elevated (so-called T_3 toxicosis).

The finding of elevated or even normal TSH levels in the presence of elevated free thyroid hormones should raise the possibility of the very unusual conditions: a TSH-producing pituitary tumor, a choriocarcinoma or hydatidiform mole, or pituitary resistance to thyroid hormones.

If there is any doubt about the cause of thyrotoxicosis, then other tests should be considered. The presence of thyroid autoantibodies helps to confirm Graves' disease. Thyroid isotope uptake scanning will show diffuse increased uptake of tracer in Graves' disease but reduced or absent uptake in a destructive thyroiditis. Toxic nodules will show increased uptake in the nodule but suppression of the rest of the gland, and a toxic multinodular goiter will show similar focal uptake of iodine in the autonomously functioning nodules.

Management

The treatment options for Graves' disease are thionamide antithyroid drugs (carbimazole, methimazole, and propylthiouracil), radioiodine, or surgery.

In the UK carbimazole is the usual treatment for an initial episode of thyrotoxicosis due to Graves' disease. The initial dose is 20–60 mg daily, adjusted at frequent intervals in order to render the patient biochemically and clinically euthyroid. Carbimazole inhibits production of thyroid hormones within the thyroid and perhaps has an effect to modulate and improve the underlying autoimmune process. Once the patient is euthyroid, a maintenance dose is continued for 6–18 months and then withdrawn in the hope of sustained remission. Antithyroid drugs can cause hypothyroidism, which responds to dose reduction. Patients receiving carbimazole are warned about potential side effects, which include skin rash and, rarely, agranulocytosis. The latter may manifest as fevers, sore throats, or mouth ulcers. Patients who develop any of these features should immediately stop the drug and undergo a white blood cell count. Failure to recognize agranulocytosis may have fatal consequences.

60% relapse after treatment with antithyroid drugs. These should then be treated with a therapeutic dose of oral radioactive iodine which is safe and will prevent further relapses in the majority. The main drawback of radioiodine which, is taken up by and then destroys thyroid cells is that it often causes hypothyroidism, usually a few months to several years after treatment. Hypothyroidism is easily treated and is preferable to relapsing thyrotoxicosis.

Radioiodine is the treatment of choice for toxic nodules and toxic multinodular goiters since it is preferentially taken up by the hyper-functioning nodules with relative sparing of the rest of the gland. This results in high cure rates at low risk of hypothyroidism.

Thyroidectomy is reserved for large goiters causing pressure symptoms, cosmetic reasons, or where other treatments have failed.

Patients suffering from thyroiditis may require temporary treatment until the underlying disease process has resolved. Amiodarone-induced thyrotoxicosis is becoming increasingly common, is often refractory to treatment with antithyroid drugs, but may respond to glucocorticoid therapy.

Outcome

Most patients can eventually be cured using one or more of the treatment regimens and will go on to lead normal lives in both duration and quality.

Addison's disease

Introduction

This is a failure of the adrenal cortex and the hormones it secretes. It is named after Thomas Addison, a nineteenth-century physician, who first described the condition in a classic monograph while working at Guy's Hospital in London. In Addison's day the commonest cause of adrenal failure was tuberculous destruction. The most common cause is now organ-specific autoimmune disease. Although an uncommon condition, its diagnosis is of the utmost importance since patients will die without treatment whereas replacement therapy restores normal life expectancy.

Clinical features

- Weight loss and anorexia
- Tiredness/lethargy/weakness
- Usually insidious in onset but may present with an acute Addisonian crisis (hypotension and acute circulatory failure) precipitated by intercurrent illness or surgical procedure
- Skin pigmentation may be generalized but in some patients is patchy and appears on pressure areas like elbow and belt areas or in palmar creases, scars, and buccal mucosa (Fig. 12.9)
- Dizziness and postural hypotension due to salt and water depletion and loss of intravascular volume
- Abdominal pain and vomiting
- Oligomenorrhea

Epidemiology

Addison's disease is rare with an incidence of 0.8 cases per 100 000 population. Most occur sporadically but an autoimmune etiology can be linked to other organ-specific autoimmune conditions such as hypothyroidism, type 1 diabetes, hypoparathyroidism, pernicious anemia, and patchy depigmentation of the skin (vitiligo) (Fig. 12.10).

Pathology

Autoimmune destruction of the adrenal cortex accounts for 70% (Table 12.5); the adrenal medulla is spared. The destruction advances insidiously over months or years before symptoms arise. The failure of glucocorticoid and mineralocorticoid secretion leads to progressive renal sodium loss, potassium retention, dehydration, and hypotension. Patients are unable to mount a glucocorticoid stress response during intercurrent illness, surgery, or injury. If it has progressed to an advanced stage, then an incidental illness can precipitate cardiovascular collapse (Addisonian crisis), which can be fatal. Some patients still die from undiagnosed Addison's disease.

It can also be caused by bilateral tuberculous destruction affecting the whole gland including the medulla.

In malignant disease, metastases to the adrenals are relatively common but seldom cause adrenal insufficiency. Necrosis or hemorrhage may occur during other severe illnesses particularly septicemia.

(a)   (b)

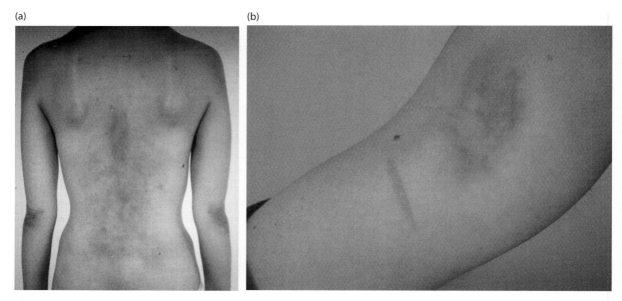

Fig. 12.9. (a) Patchy pigmentation in a patient with newly diagnosed Addison's disease. This patient had lost 20 kg in weight, had severe postural hypotension, a serum sodium of 122 and potassium of 7.8 mmol/l. Note the pigmentation over the pressure points on the elbows. (b) Pigmentation in a scar of a patient with Addison's disease.

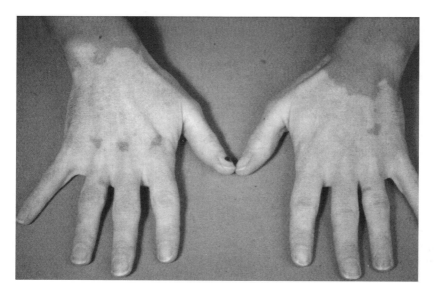

Fig. 12.10. Vitiligo of the hands in a patient with Addison's disease.

Hemorrhage into the adrenal glands during meningococcal septicemia is known as the Waterhouse–Friedrichsen syndrome.

Pituitary or hypothalamic disease leading to reduced ACTH secretion and long-term corticosteroid administration causing suppression of the pituitary–adrenal axis can also cause hypoadrenalism. Adrenal function may need to be checked when withdrawing such steroid treatment. These so-called secondary causes of hypoadrenalism are not associated with skin pigmentation and this can be a useful distinguishing feature.

Investigations
Blood tests characteristically show hyponatremia and hyperkalemia. Plasma urea levels are often raised as a result of plasma volume contraction and blood glucose may be low. Random blood cortisol levels may be

Table 12.5. Causes of adrenocortical insufficiency

Usual

    Autoimmune (sporadic or in association with other autoimmune conditions)

Less common causes (both glands need to be affected)

    Tuberculosis

    Metastases

    Adrenal hemorrhage

    HIV

    Adrenal vein thrombosis

Secondary causes

    Suppression by exogenous glucocorticoid administration

    Pituitary/hypothalamic disease

difficult to interpret due to the normal diurnal variation and the retention of some secretory capacity. When stressed or stimulated, the cortisol levels may still rise to the normal range. Normal levels of cortisol *do not* exclude Addison's disease particularly in a patient who is unwell. Acutely unwell patients with normally functioning adrenal glands should have relatively high levels of cortisol and normal levels may be inappropriately low.

ACTH levels are often high or very high in primary adrenal disease indicating reduced feedback of cortisol at the level of the pituitary and hypothalamus. ACTH levels are low or normal in secondary causes of hypoadrenalism.

Patients with primary adrenocortical insufficiency disease also have aldosterone deficiency and plasma renin activity is elevated.

The gold standard test of adrenal reserve is the short synacthen test, maximally stimulating the adrenal cortex by injecting 250 µg of synthetic ACTH (synacthen). Plasma cortisol levels are measured before the injection and at 30 and 60 minutes post-injection. A normal response is a rise to a peak cortisol value of at least 550 nmol/l.

Management

An Addisonian crisis is a medical emergency. Patients require urgent hospital admission and intensive treatment and monitoring. Intravascular volume and sodium depletion should be treated with intravenous normal saline. Hydrocortisone, initially 100 mg qds, is administered intravenously, reducing with improvement.

Intravenous dextrose may also be required if there is hypoglycemia.

Mineralocorticoid replacement is not required immediately, since intravenous saline will correct the metabolic defect of aldosterone deficiency and large doses of glucocorticoids also have some mineralocorticoid effect.

After recovery, patients are placed on standard adrenocortical replacement therapy with fludrocortisone 50–200 µg daily and hydrocortisone 15–25 mg daily in divided doses, the largest being given after awakening to mimic the normal diurnal variation of cortisol. Doses of both are tailored to individuals.

Patient education is important: medication is for life and cessation can be life threatening. Intercurrent illness, injury, surgery, or emotional stress increase requirements for glucocorticoids. Patients should increase the dose of medication during such events and seek help if unable to take medication for any reason. Parenteral steroids may need to be administered temporarily.

Outcome

Provided patients are appropriately advised and managed and able to comply with medication, life expectancy and quality are normal.

Swelling in the neck (Fig. 12.11)

A lump in the neck is often discovered or noticed incidentally by the patient or sometimes by a doctor carrying out a routine examination. In most cases the origin of the lesion will be suggested by the anatomical situation or other clinical characteristics. Sebaceous cysts and lipomas will be in the skin and may occur anywhere. Lymph nodes will follow their anatomical distribution and are often multiple. Salivary gland swellings will be in the parotid, submandibular or submental salivary glands. Thyroid enlargement (goiter) is over the anterior portion of the neck, usually over the cricoid cartilage and just below the larynx. Generalized thyroid swelling will usually retain the anatomy of the thyroid with a lobe palpable on either side of the trachea connected by an isthmus. A characteristic feature of the thyroid is that the gland moves upwards on swallowing. Thyroglossal cysts are typically in the midline and move upwards on protrusion of the tongue. Lesions related to the carotid artery may be pulsatile, although it is important to distinguish transmitted pulsation from a lesion adjacent to the carotid. Branchial cleft cysts are congenital cysts in the lateral part of the neck and occur anywhere from the parotid area to the mediastinum. Cystic hygromas are congenital

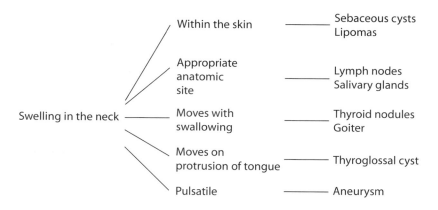

Fig. 12.11. Swelling in the neck.

Table 12.6. Causes of thyroid nodules

Colloid nodules

Thyroid cyst

Thyroid adenoma

Part of a multinodular goiter

Thyroid cancer

Metastatic lesion

lymphangiomas. A laryngocele is herniation of the laryngeal mucosa through the thyrohyoid membrane, resulting in a reducible, tense mass in the neck. The mass recurs on sneezing or blowing of the nose.

Ultrasound or CT scanning of the neck can be used to confirm the origin of the lesion and gain further information about its characteristics. A fine needle aspirate or a biopsy of solid lesions may be necessary to make a diagnosis, particularly if malignancy is suspected.

Thyroid nodules

Introduction

Thyroid nodules are very common and the vast majority are benign. Small nodules can be detected on high-resolution ultrasound scanning in around 20% of an unselected adult population. Most of these nodules will be undetectable by clinical examination. The most important aspect of thyroid nodules is to differentiate benign from malignant lesions.

Clinical features

Many thyroid nodules are noticed incidentally. Most are asymptomatic, but hemorrhage into a cyst may cause discomfort and tenderness.

Most patients with thyroid nodules will have normal thyroid function. Adenomas can produce excessive quantities of thyroid hormones (toxic adenoma). Extensive infiltration of the thyroid by malignant lesions may cause hypothyroidism.

Tethering of the mass or thyroid to other structures in the neck is suggestive of malignancy as is associated lymphadenopathy.

Epidemiology

Thyroid nodules are more common in women, but the likelihood of malignancy is higher in men. Approximately 5% of thyroid nodules are cancerous.

Pathology and etiology

Table 12.6 shows a list of the causes of thyroid nodules.

Colloid nodules, cysts and multinodular goiters are very common. Hemorrhage may occur into cysts causing acute enlargement.

There are five main categories of thyroid cancer:

- *Papillary*: the commonest form of thyroid cancer is more common in middle-aged women. It spreads to local lymph nodes but seldom to distant sites. The prognosis is generally good.
- *Follicular*: also more common in middle-aged women, spreads by means of distant metastases.
- *Medullary cell carcinoma*: tumor of the C-cells of the thyroid that secrete calcitonin. Twenty per cent are familial and genetic screening is required.
- *Thyroid lymphoma*: the risk of this is increased in Hashimoto's disease.
- *Anaplastic*: occurs in an older population. It infiltrates locally and tends to be aggressive with a very poor prognosis.

Table 12.7. Causes of a goiter

Simple goiter
Iodine deficiency
Multinodular goiter
Autoimmune thyroid disease
Thyroiditis
Drugs such as lithium
Thyroid cancer

Investigations

The first investigation is usually an ultrasound scan to determine size, extent, and consistency of the nodule and whether it is cystic or associated with any other thyroid nodules.

A nuclear medicine isotope uptake scan may also be useful. Solid nodules, which are less avid for iodine than the surrounding thyroid (cold nodules), are more likely to be malignant.

All palpable nodules should undergo fine needle aspiration (FNA) to determine their histologic nature. If this is indeterminate, then surgical removal may need to be considered. FNA of difficult or small nodules can be carried out under ultrasound guidance.

Thyroid function tests should be carried out.

Management

Nodules that are benign on FNA can be followed with serial clinical assessment and ultrasound scanning.

The management of thyroid cancer is highly specialized and should be carried out by an appropriate multidisciplinary team. Treatment typically involves surgery to remove the thyroid and any associated disease in the neck. Surgery may be followed by high dose radioiodine therapy in papillary or follicular cancer to ablate residual disease.

Outcome

The prognosis of thyroid cancer depends on the histologic type and degree of spread at the time of diagnosis. Papillary cell carcinoma has the best prognosis with a 5-year survival of 90%. Patients with anaplastic disease fare worst with a 5-year survival of <1%.

Goiter

Introduction

A goiter is the name for any enlargement of the thyroid gland.

Clinical features

A goiter (Table 12.7) is also often noticed incidentally by the patient, another person, or a doctor whom the patient consults for another reason.

Smooth, diffuse enlargement suggests a simple goiter, iodine deficiency, autoimmune disease, or thyroiditis. A nodular feel or asymmetry makes the most likely cause a multinodular goiter or, rarely, thyroid malignancy. Malignancy is further suggested by tethering of the thyroid to underlying structures, lymphadenopathy, or hoarseness of the voice from recurrent laryngeal nerve damage. Tenderness occurs with thyroiditis. A bruit in the thyroid occurs with Graves' disease.

These conditions can lead to hypo- or hyperthyroidism.

Large goiters can cause compression of the trachea or esophagus leading to symptoms of breathlessness or choking particularly on lying down, stridor, or difficulty swallowing.

Epidemiology

Iodine deficiency is the most common cause of a goiter worldwide.

Pathology and etiology

A goiter is referred to as a simple goiter when there is generalized smooth homogeneous enlargement with normal function and no obvious underlying cause.

Iodine deficiency occurs in inland or mountainous areas such as the Himalayas, the Andes, central Africa, and Eastern Europe. Iodine deficiency is rare in countries such as the UK where salt is iodized.

A multinodular goiter, as its name implies, is caused by multiple benign nodules within the thyroid substance. These are of varying size and can sometimes result in massive enlargement of the thyroid. The goiter may be asymmetric and can cause compression in the neck or extend down behind the sternum into the mediastinum.

Autoimmune thyroid disease and any cause of thyroiditis can cause diffuse thyroid enlargement. It is typical for the gland to be slightly enlarged in Hashimoto's disease. The size of the goiter in Graves' disease is highly variable.

Thyroid cancer may present as a thyroid nodule or mass but may cause more diffuse thyroid enlargement. There may be infiltration of local structures, spread to regional lymph nodes or more distant metastases.

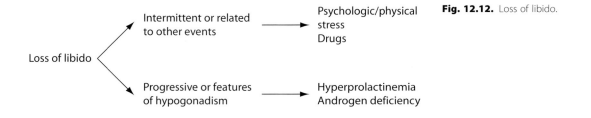

Fig. 12.12. Loss of libido.

Investigations

Consider the following investigations:

- Thyroid function tests
- Thyroid autoantibodies
- Thyroid ultrasound scan
- CT scan
- Fine needle aspiration

The clinical features, thyroid function tests and thyroid autoantibodies are usually all that is required to diagnose thyroid autoimmune disease and thyroiditis. An ultrasound scan will clarify whether or not the gland is homogeneous or contains a mass or multiple nodules. A mass will require fine needle aspiration (FNA) or biopsy. It is standard practice to carry out an FNA on the dominant nodule in a multinodular goiter.

A CT scan may be required to delineate the extent of a large multinodular goiter, particularly its degree of retrosternal extension and encroachment on other structures such as the trachea.

Management

For autoimmune disease and thyroiditis, see p. 354 and p. 360. For thyroid cancer, see under thyroid nodules (p. 364). A simple goiter needs no treatment. Iodine deficiency needs supplementation. A multinodular goiter needs no specific therapy provided thyroid function is normal and an FNA has shown benign results, but a large or enlarging multinodular goiter causing compressive problems should be removed.

Outcome

Non-malignant causes of a goiter have an excellent prognosis. Even patients requiring thyroidectomy for a large multinodular goiter should have a normal life expectancy.

Loss of libido (Fig. 12.12)

Many day-to-day factors influence the libido of an individual. Events causing emotional, psychologic, or physical upset are a common cause of loss of

Table 12.8. Important aspects of history taking and examination in a patient with loss of libido

History	Examination
Gender, age	Height and arm span
Onset sudden/gradual/relates to other events	Degree of body hair
Severity, progression, duration	Muscular development
Frequency of shaving	Visual field testing (pituitary tumor)
Pubertal development	Gynecomastia
Fertility	Testicular examination
Previous testicular problems	
Symptoms of a pituitary tumor	
Alcohol/cannabis abuse	
Drug history	

libido. Most men and women will suffer from a degree of lack of libido intermittently during their lives and recognize the cause. This usually improves or resolves when the precipitating factor is no longer present.

Loss of libido or sex drive can be a problem in both men and women but is more often a presenting feature of underlying endocrine dysfunction in men. This is due to the fact that men are largely dependent on circulating androgen levels for the maintenance of libido, whereas in women the situation is more complex. Certain well-recognized conditions cause low testosterone levels in men. Women with ovarian, pituitary, or hypothalamic dysfunction present with amenorrhea or infertility rather than loss of libido.

Loss of libido in men has to be distinguished from erectile dysfunction, where the list of etiologies is quite different; for example, the autonomic neuropathy of diabetes frequently causes erectile dysfunction while libido is relatively maintained. Loss of libido will, however, often also lead to erectile dysfunction.

The history and examination are very important in determining the cause of loss of libido (Table 12.8).

Table 12.9. Causes of hyperprolactinemia

Common

    Pregnancy and breast feeding

    Prolactinoma

    Drugs

    Stress

    Renal failure

    Macroprolactinemia

Uncommon

    Head injury

    Pituitary stalk compression

    Hypothyroidism

There may be an obvious temporal relation to stressful life events, starting medication, or the development of some other intercurrent illness. Temporary or intermittent loss of libido is less likely to indicate underlying endocrine dysfunction.

The presence of features suggesting androgen deficiency (pp. 368–9) indicates the need for further investigation. Enquiries as to development of secondary sexual characteristics during puberty should also be made.

Libido tends to reduce with age, although there is considerable inter-individual variation. It is likely that many other environmental factors come into play.

Many drugs have been implicated in both loss of libido and erectile dysfunction. It is, however, sometimes difficult to know how much the symptomatology is due to the drug and how much is due to the underlying condition that the medication is being used to treat. Drugs that have been particularly implicated are beta-blockers and antidepressants. Any antiandrogenic drugs will obviously lower libido.

Hyperprolactinemia

Introduction

Release of prolactin by the lactotrophs of the anterior pituitary gland is controlled mainly by an inhibitory factor (dopamine) secreted by the hypothalamus.

There are several causes of hyperprolactinemia (Table 12.9).

Clinical features

Hyperprolactinemia causes galactorrhea, menstrual irregularities (oligomenorrhea or amenorrhea), and infertility in women. Men can also develop galactorrhea, infertility, and hypogonadism.

The mechanism of hypogonadism in hyperprolactinemia is complex and not well understood. It probably includes an effect to inhibit gonadotrophin secretion from the pituitary and perhaps an inhibitory effect on the action of gonadotrophins at the level of the gonad.

Men with prolactinomas tend to present later than women. This is because men are less likely to develop galactorrhea and less likely to complain of loss of libido than women presenting with menstrual disturbance and infertility. Men consequently tend to have much larger tumors at the time of diagnosis. Larger tumors can compress and impair the function of the anterior pituitary and enlarge superiorly into the suprasellar space where they characteristically exert pressure on the optic chiasm causing a bitemporal visual field defect. Patients with large tumors may also present with headaches or even ophthalmoplegia due to pressure on the third, fourth, and sixth cranial nerves.

Epidemiology

Hyperprolactinemia and prolactinomas are much commoner in women. Part of the explanation may relate to the earlier presentation detailed above. Microprolactinomas are increasing in incidence, perhaps due to earlier diagnosis and the development of high-resolution MRI scanning enabling detection of tiny tumors within the anterior pituitary.

Pathology and etiology

Prolactin levels are elevated and can become very high during pregnancy and breast feeding. Physical and mental stress can cause a mild elevation of prolactin. The stress of a venepuncture is sometimes enough to stimulate prolactin release in a patient who is anxious about this procedure.

Prolactinomas are the commonest cause of a moderate to high prolactin level. They are the commonest type of anterior pituitary adenoma. Ninety-nine percent of prolactinomas are benign and typically enlarge only very slowly over many years. In women, most are now diagnosed at a very early stage and at a time when they are less than 1 cm in diameter (microprolactinoma) (Fig. 12.13(a)). They can, however, grow to an enormous size and cause pressure effects (Fig. 12.13(b)).

Antipsychotic agents such as chlorpromazine, haloperidol, risperidone, and amisulpride and the antiemetic agents metoclopramide and domperidone can all inhibit the effects of dopamine on lactotrophs and result in hyperprolactinemia.

Damage or compression of the pituitary stalk can inhibit the passage of dopamine in the portal system

(a)

(b)

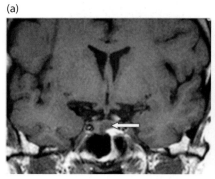
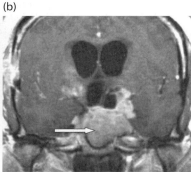

Fig. 12.13. (a) A typical non-enhancing microprolactinoma in the anterior pituitary (arrowed). (b) A massive contrast-enhancing prolactinoma (arrowed) extending superiorly into the suprasellar space and brain causing hydrocephalus with dilated ventricles.

from the hypothalamus to the anterior pituitary. This results in the lactotrophs escaping from dopamine inhibition and resultant hyperprolactinemia. Typical causes are head injuries sectioning the stalk or non-prolactin secreting pituitary tumors causing stalk compression.

Hypothyroidism can cause a mild degree of hyper-prolactinemia due to increased TRH (thyrotrophin releasing hormone) which stimulates prolactin secretion by lactotrophs. Of patients with renal failure 25%–70% have mildly raised prolactin levels thought to be due to reduced renal clearance.

Macroprolactin is a term given to high molecular weight forms of prolactin found in some patients with hyperprolactinemia. The commonest cause is an IgG, which binds prolactin in the circulation, reducing its clearance and causing artificially high levels. Macroprolactinemia is though to be benign and explains at least some of the hyperprolactinemia that was previously labeled as idiopathic.

Investigations

Consideration should be given to performing the following:

* Repeat prolactin and measurement of macroprolactin
* Pregnancy test
* Thyroid function tests
* Serum creatinine
* MRI scan of the pituitary

Management

The treatment of hyperprolactinemia will depend on the underlying cause. In those who require prolactin lowering therapy, dopamine agonist agents are the treatment of choice, simulating the effect of dopamine on the lactotrophs in the anterior pituitary.

Prolactinomas, in contrast to other pituitary tumors which usually require surgical removal, are most effectively treated with dopamine agonists. These are is cabergoline, bromocriptine, and quinagolide. Cabergoline is usually used as first choice, due to its efficacy and tolerability. These agents are highly effective in reducing prolactin levels to normal, restoring gonadal function, and reducing the size of the tumor. Even patients with massive prolactinomas should have a trial of dopamine agonist therapy, unless there are clinical indications which necessitate urgent surgical debulking (Fig. 12.14). Dopamine agonists can cause nausea, vomiting, abdominal discomfort, and dizziness. Fibrotic conditions such as retroperitoneal and heart valve fibrosis have been reported but are very rare. Cabergoline appears to be best tolerated and is used as the treatment of choice in the UK.

Outcome

The outcome of hyperprolactinemia depends on the underlying cause. Microprolactinomas have a very favorable outcome. Ninety-five percent are easily controlled on dopamine agonist therapy, which may have to be continued indefinitely but results in tumor shrinkage, and restoration of gonadal function and fertility.

Androgen deficiency

The main circulating androgen in adult men is testosterone. Testosterone is produced in Leydig cells in the testes under the control of luteinizing hormone produced by the anterior pituitary. There is a circadian rhythm of testosterone with levels higher in the morning than in the late afternoon and evening. There is also a steady decline in testosterone levels once past middle age. The main causes of testosterone deficiency are listed in Table 12.10.

(a) (b)

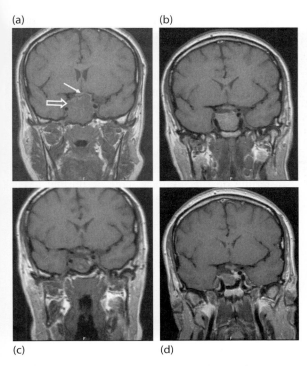

(c) (d)

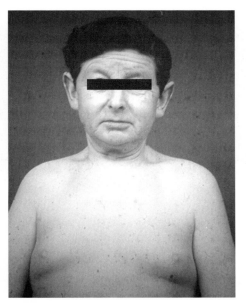

Fig. 12.15. Patient with testosterone deficiency due to a pituitary tumor. Note the poor facial hair growth, lack of body hair, and poor muscular development.

Fig. 12.14. (a) Coronal MRI scan showing a large prolactinoma (open arrow) extending into the suprasellar space and displacing the optic chiasm (solid arrow); (b), (c) and (d) show the tumor 1, 4, and 8 months respectively after continuous cabergoline therapy.

Table 12.10. Causes of low total testosterone

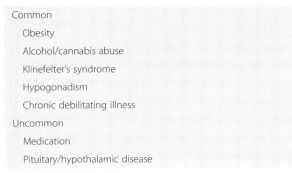

Common
Obesity
Alcohol/cannabis abuse
Klinefelter's syndrome
Hypogonadism
Chronic debilitating illness
Uncommon
Medication
Pituitary/hypothalamic disease

Clinical features

Patients with severe androgen deficiency have a very characteristic youthful, prepubertal facial appearance caused by lack of facial hair (Fig. 12.15). Patients with minor degrees of androgen deficiency may not show any significant physical signs. Other characteristic features are:

- Loss of libido
- Reduced facial, body, and pubic hair (ask about frequency of shaving)
- Poor muscular development
- If testicular deficiency occurs prior to puberty, then patients may be tall with increased limb length relative to height due to late fusion of epiphyses (eunuchoid body proportions) and have a higher pitched voice
- Gynecomastia
- Small testes in primary or secondary hypogonadism and Klinefelter's syndrome (see below)
- Osteoporosis

Epidemiology

Klinefelter's syndrome is the commonest cause of male hypogonadism and has an incidence of 2 per 1000 live births. Many individuals with Klinefelter's syndrome remain undiagnosed throughout life.

Pathology and etiology

Of circulating testosterone 98%–99% is bound to carrier proteins, mainly sex-hormone binding globulin (SHBG). The small unbound fraction is the active component, since it binds to the androgen receptor on target tissues. Most laboratories measure total testosterone (bound plus free). It is notoriously difficult to interpret total testosterone levels as there are many factors which may influence the levels of total testosterone and SHBG including the following:

Table 12.11. Causes of primary and secondary hypogonadism

Primary hypogonadism

    Consequences of treatment of testicular tumors or testicular torsion

    Klinefelter's syndrome

    Trauma

    Bilateral orchitis (usually mumps)

    Congenital anorchia

Secondary hypogonadism

    Pituitary tumors or their treatment

    Hemochromatosis, sarcoidosis, tuberculosis, histiocytosis X, Kallman's syndrome

- Timing of the sample. There is a circadian rhythm of testosterone. Levels may be 50% lower in the late afternoon and evening than at 9 am.
- Age. Levels of testosterone decline with age, this is likely to be physiologic.
- Obesity and glucocorticoids reduce SHBG and, therefore, levels of total testosterone.
- Alcohol has a direct toxic effect on Leydig cells.
- Cannabis and anabolic steroid abuse inhibit LH secretion by the anterior pituitary thereby reducing testosterone production.

Causes of hypogonadism are shown in Table 12.11. Damage to the testes can cause primary hypogonadism. Both testes must be damaged to cause androgen deficiency. The commonest causes are trauma, consequences of treatment for testicular tumors, or testicular torsion. Mumps and other infections can cause bilateral orchitis, damaging the testes. The testes may be congenitally absent (congenital anorchia). Klinefelter's syndrome is a developmental defect caused by an extra X chromosome. The karyotype is usually 47 XXY. The condition is very heterogeneous with some patients being well virilized and others having a very eunuchoid appearance with gynecomastia and very small testes. Patients with Klinefelter's syndrome are usually infertile.

Any pituitary or hypothalamic disease affecting gonadotrophin-releasing hormone (GnRH) or gonadotrophin secretion can cause *secondary* hypogonadism and low testosterone levels. The commonest causes are pituitary tumors or their treatment by surgery or radiotherapy. Hemochromatosis, sarcoidosis, tuberculosis, and histiocytosis X can also cause pituitary and hypothalamic damage but are rare. Kallman's syndrome is a rare developmental defect

resulting in isolated GnRH deficiency and associated with anosmia (lack of a sense of smell).

Investigations

Measurement of total testosterone should be standardized at 9 am, measurement of SHBG can help to evaluate low levels. Interpreting testosterone levels must be done with caution and in the context of the clinical situation.

Elevated levels of LH and FSH confirm primary hypogonadism due to lack of negative feedback of testosterone on the pituitary. Low or normal levels of gonadotrophins in the presence of significantly low testosterone levels should raise the possibility of pituitary or hypothalamic disease and consideration of an MRI scan of this area. Patients with suspected Klinefelter's syndrome require karyotyping.

Management

Not all patients with low testosterone will require treatment. Treatment of physiologic decline in testosterone levels with age is not currently recommended. Treatment may need to be directed at the underlying cause.

Patients with significant biochemical and clinical androgen deficiency require replacement therapy to restore libido and sexual function, restore normal secondary sexual characteristics (testicular size does not improve), and prevent or treat osteopenia.

Oral testosterone is ineffective due to a large hepatic extraction. Treatment options include depot intramuscular injections daily transdermal gel or patch applications, daily buccal or sublingual medication, or 6-monthly implants.

Outcome

The prognosis is generally good depending on the underlying problem. Patients with primary hypogonadism on long-term testosterone treatment should have a normal life expectancy.

Asymptomatic findings

Hyperglycemia

A raised blood glucose (hyperglycemia) is often found on routine screening in patients who have no relevant symptoms. Hyperglycemia usually indicates the presence of diabetes mellitus but temporary hyperglycemia can be caused by stress during infections or trauma and precipitated by drugs, particularly corticosteroids. Patients should be retested for diabetes once the precipitating factor is removed.

Diabetes mellitus

Introduction

Diabetes mellitus is a metabolic disorder characterized by chronic high blood glucose levels. It is the commonest endocrine abnormality and its incidence is increasing dramatically around the world, mainly due to a rise in the prevalence of type 2 diabetes. It causes a huge health and economic burden mainly due to its chronic complications. There are two main forms: types 1 and 2, which, although both result in hyperglycemia, have distinct pathophysiologic mechanisms.

Clinical features

- Hyperglycemia leads to an osmotic diuresis and the classic symptoms of thirst and polyuria.
- Type 2 is usually insidious in onset and may be diagnosed incidentally or on screening before the blood glucose has become high enough to induce symptoms.
- Patients may feel tired and unwell.
- Hyperglycemia leads to increased risk of infection particularly balanitis, vaginal candidiasis, and skin abscesses. These may be presenting features.
- The initial event may be acute metabolic decompensation (diabetic ketoacidosis), particularly in patients with type 1 diabetes.
- Patients with type 2 diabetes may present with the long-term complications because of its insidious onset.
- Type 2 diabetes becomes more prevalent with advancing age and is strongly associated with obesity.
- Type 1 has a peak incidence in early teenage years, but can occur at any age. Patients with type 1 are usually thin and have lost weight at the time of diagnosis.

Epidemiology

Approximately 3%–4% of the population of the UK have type 2 diabetes and this is increasing due to obesity. About 2.5 million people are known to have type 2 diabetes in the UK with approximately 1 million more undiagnosed. The prevalence of type 2 diabetes is much higher in certain ethnic groups. UK residents of Asian and Afro-Caribbean origin aged over 60 years have a prevalence approaching 25%. Type 2 diabetes, which used to be very uncommon in those aged less than 40, is increasing in this age group and even in children. Type 1 diabetes is less common, making up 10% of all cases.

Table 12.12. Classification of diabetes mellitus (Alberti & Zimmet, 1998)

Type 1
Immune mediated or idiopathic
Type 2
Predominantly insulin resistance or insulin secretory defect
Other specific types
Maturity onset diabetes in the young (MODY)
Genetic defects of beta cell function or insulin action
Diseases of the exocrine pancreas
Endocrinopathies: Cushing's syndrome, acromegaly
Drug or chemical-induced diabetes
Gestational diabetes mellitus

Pathology

The classification of diabetes (Alberti & Zimmet, 1998) is shown in Table 12.12. Type 1 and type 2 diabetes comprise the majority, but it can also be caused by pancreatic damage due to pancreatitis, carcinoma, or hemochromatosis. Cushing's syndrome (see p. 355) and acromegaly both cause glucose intolerance and diabetes.

Type 1 – caused by immune-mediated destruction of the insulin-producing beta cells within the islets of Langerhans in the pancreas. The exact etiology remains unknown. There is a genetic component and association with some HLA haplotypes and 50% concordance in monozygotic twins. There is also a likely environmental trigger. Once a critical mass of beta cells has been destroyed, circulating insulin levels fall and blood glucose rises. Insulin deficiency also causes production of ketone bodies by the liver leading to acidosis. Untreated, patients become progressively dehydrated and acidotic leading to coma, circulatory collapse, and death.

Type 2 – also has a genetic component with frequent history in family members. Some genetic defects have been discovered which explain the development of diabetes in isolated families, but these are not present in the majority with type 2 diabetes. Obesity, sedentary living, and poor diet high in refined carbohydrate are strongly associated with risk of type 2 diabetes.

The pathophysiology of type 2 is different from that of type 1 diabetes. There is both a resistance to the effects of insulin in peripheral tissues and an inability of the beta cell to produce sufficient insulin to maintain normal blood glucose levels. These defects become more severe with disease chronicity. In contrast to type 1, the beta cells produce insulin until relatively late in the disease process. This is the reason why they are less likely to develop the ketoacidosis associated with insulin deficiency. Type 2 diabetes usually develops over many years and patients are asymptomatic in the early stages. There is a 20% prevalence of complications by time of diagnosis.

Glucocorticoid therapy causes insulin resistance and may precipitate diabetes. Gestational diabetes occurs for the first time during pregnancy and usually resolves post-partum. Such patients are at risk of developing type 2 diabetes later in life.

Table 12.13. Clinical features of acromegaly

Enlarging hands and feet (ask about increased ring and shoe size)

Facial features: coarsening of features particularly nose, lips, tongue, and supraorbital ridges, expansion of the mandible (prognathism), wide spacing of teeth

Skin features: excessive sweating, greasiness of skin, skin tags, acne

Signs of mass lesion: headache, visual field defect, cranial nerve palsies

Carpal tunnel syndrome

Hypertension

Organomegaly: goiter, cardiomyopathy

Osteoarthritis

Glucose intolerance/diabetes mellitus

Acromegaly is a rare condition almost always caused by a growth hormone-secreting pituitary adenoma. It is usually insidious in onset and presents with features listed in Table 12.13 and shown in Fig. 12.16. Diagnosis is clinical and supported by lack of suppression of growth hormone levels during an oral glucose tolerance test and a pituitary tumor on MRI scanning. Treatment is primarily surgical removal of the adenoma. Second-line treatment is radiotherapy to the pituitary. Medical therapy is available in the form of long-acting somatostatin analogs or a growth hormone receptor antagonist, pegvisomant.

Complications of diabetes – The metabolic abnormalities of diabetes lead to an increased risk of damage to blood vessels. The complications (Table 12.14) are traditionally divided into consequences of atheroma (macrovascular disease) and damage to the capillaries (microvascular disease).

Patients with diabetes have a two- to four-fold increased risk of macrovascular disease. This results in morbidity and mortality due to myocardial infarction, cerebrovascular and peripheral vascular disease. Increased atheroma is due to a clustering of risk factors: hypertension, dyslipidemia, obesity, and hyperglycemia. The association of these risk factors is often termed the metabolic syndrome.

The microvascular complications are peculiar to diabetes and are manifest as damage to retinal capillaries (retinopathy), glomerulus (nephropathy), and peripheral sensory nerves of the legs (neuropathy).

(a) 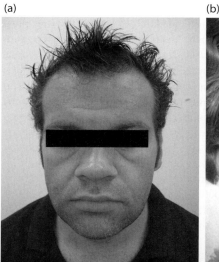   (b)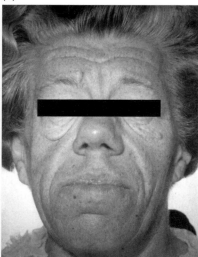

Fig. 12.16. (a), (b) Facial features of two patients with acromegaly showing generalized coarse features due to thickening of the soft tissues. There is particular enlargement of the nose, lips, and mandible (prognathism) in patient (b).

Table 12.14. Complications of diabetes mellitus

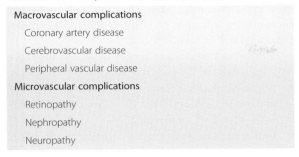

Macrovascular complications

    Coronary artery disease

    Cerebrovascular disease

    Peripheral vascular disease

Microvascular complications

    Retinopathy

    Nephropathy

    Neuropathy

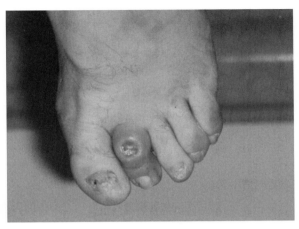

Fig. 12.18. Typical neuropathic ulcer in a patient with diabetes due to peripheral sensory neuropathy and deformity of the toe resulting in pressure on footwear and ulceration. There is swelling and redness of the toe indicating infection.

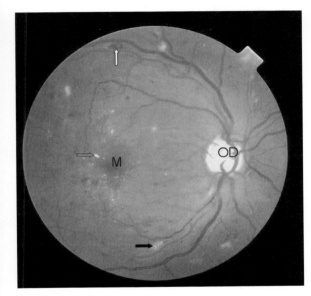

Fig. 12.17. Retinal photograph showing preproliferative retinopathy. OD = optic disk, M = macula, top arrow = intra-retinal hemorrhage, middle arrow = hard exudates, bottom arrow = cotton wool spot of retinal ischemia.

The risk and progression of these complications are related to poor glycemic control, but hypertension also has an influence.

Diabetic retinopathy is the commonest cause of blindness in the UK under age 50. Retinopathy (Fig. 12.17) first manifests itself as small microaneurysms on the retinal capillaries. These are seen as small red dots on retinal examination. As retinopathy progresses, small hemorrhages appear within the retina (often termed blot hemorrhages) as well as leakage of plasma (hard exudates). These are termed background retinopathy. As damage to the microvasculature progresses, areas become ischemic and sites of infarction develop. These are seen as white areas (termed soft exudates or cotton wool spots) now called preproliferative retinopathy. Ischemia eventually precipitates the formation of fragile new blood vessels, stimulated by the release of growth factors, termed proliferative retinopathy. This is a real and imminent threat to vision, since these vessels can rupture causing large pre-retinal hemorrhages leading to blindness. Retinopathy affecting the macula (maculopathy) can reduce visual acuity and warrants urgent attention.

Diabetic nephropathy is caused by very slowly progressive damage to the renal glomerulus. There is mesangial expansion and basement membrane thickening. Untreated, this leads to renal failure which is still a common cause of death in type 1 diabetes.

Diabetes can damage many nerves. The pathogenesis remains obscure but may include a metabolic insult to the nerve tissue itself as well as disruption of the microvasculature supplying the nerves (vasa nervorum). The commonest manifestation is bilateral distal sensory neuropathy causing numbness or tingling of toes spreading slowly proximally. Patients may be unaware of the neuropathy and there is risk of foot damage and ulceration (Fig. 12.18).

This is increased if peripheral vascular disease is also present. Poor healing and complicating infection can lead to cellulitis (Fig. 12.19), osteomyelitis, tissue necrosis, and gangrene, sometimes necessitating amputation. These are responsible for some of the morbidity and mortality associated with diabetes and anxiety to patients and their families. Diabetes can also cause motor neuropathy in the limbs and sometimes isolated mononeuropathies, particularly

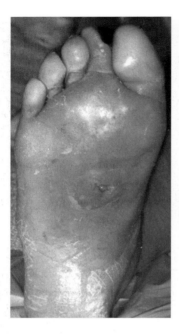

Fig. 12.19. Plantar ulcer with marked surrounding cellulitis in a patient with diabetes, neuropathy, and peripheral vascular disease.

third and sixth cranial nerve palsies. Autonomic neuropathy also occurs leading to erectile dysfunction and other unpleasant and intractable manifestations such as vomiting due to gastroparesis, constipation or diarrhea, postural hypotension, and difficulties with bladder emptying.

Investigations

The diagnosis of diabetes is easy when blood glucose is unequivocally raised in the presence of characteristic symptoms, particularly in type 1 diabetes.

If the patient is asymptomatic and blood glucose values equivocal, then care must be taken. The diagnosis must be secure, since there are medical and legal implications for the patient. Blood glucose cut-off levels have been set to assist discrimination between normal and diabetes (Alberti & Zimmet, 1998). The current diagnostic criteria are based on studies showing that the risk of retinopathy increases at a certain glycemic threshold.

The main diagnostic criteria :

- fasting venous plasma glucose >7 mmol/l (overnight fast 8–14 hours).
- random venous plasma glucose >11.1 mmol/l.
- an oral glucose tolerance test (OGTT) in patients where random or fasting values are close to the cut-off values. 75 g of oral glucose are administered after an overnight fast. A fasting venous plasma glucose of >7 mmol/l *or* a 2-hour post-load glucose of >11.1 mmol/l is diagnostic.

An abnormal value needs confirmation at least once if the patient is asymptomatic. Patients should be free from infection or trauma, which can cause a transitory rise in blood glucose.

Two other categories of abnormal glucose tolerance have been defined between normality and diabetes:

- impaired glucose tolerance where the fasting glucose is <7 mmol/l but the 2-hour OGTT value is >7.8 and <11.1 mmol/l.
- impaired fasting glycemia where fasting glucose is >6.1 and <7 mmol/l.

These two categories indicate an increased risk of progressing to overt diabetes and developing macrovascular disease.

Management

Modern treatment requires input from a multidisciplinary team including doctors, diabetes specialist nurses, dietitians, podiatrists, and psychotherapists. Patient education is important for developing an understanding of the disease and encouraging responsibility for self-management and lifestyle. Management also requires support and surveillance, and risk reduction for complications.

The better the long-term glycemic control, the less likely are long-term complications, particularly microvascular disease. Glycemic control is best assessed by measuring HbA1c or glycosylated hemoglobin, which reflects the degree of glycemic control over the previous 6–8 weeks. This should be checked every 2–6 months, aiming to maintain it between 6.5 and 7.5%.

Dietary advice takes into account vagaries such as eating habits, ethnicity, social circumstances, and other lifestyle factors. Appropriate weight-reducing calorie restricted diets can markedly improve insulin resistance and beta cell function. Dietary advice in type 1 diabetes focuses on teaching carbohydrate counting at each meal as part of a daily meal plan.

All patients with diabetes should be encouraged to take regular exercise. This improves insulin sensitivity and lowers blood glucose.

Oral hypoglycemic agents The introduction of healthy lifestyle measures will often allow patients with type 2 diabetes to achieve good glycemic control without medication. There is, however, an inexorable decline in glycemic control with time and most require oral hypoglycemic agents eventually. These should augment lifestyle measures and not replace them. The main oral hypoglycemic agents in current use are:

- **Biguanides**: Metformin is used first line in obese patients since it does not cause weight gain and may even assist weight loss. It does not cause hypoglycemia. The mechanism of action is controversial but may include reduced hepatic gluconeogenesis, increased peripheral glucose disposal, and appetite suppression. The main side effects are nausea, abdominal pain, and diarrhea. It should be stopped in patients with renal, hepatic, or cardiac failure where there is a small risk of lactic acidosis developing.

- **Sulphonylureas**: Gliclazide, glipizide, and glimepiride are now favored over the older and longer-acting glibenclamide and chlorpropamide, which are more likely to cause prolonged hypoglycemia particularly in the elderly. They are insulin secretagogs acting on beta cell receptors to stimulate insulin release. They tend to promote weight gain and are used in non-obese patients or in addition to metformin. They can cause hypoglycemia but are effective and well tolerated.

- **Meglitinides**: Repaglinide and nateglinide are newer insulin secretagoges, which have a more rapid onset but shorter duration of action than sulphonylureas.

- **Thiazolidinediones**: Rosiglitazone and pioglitazone act on peroxisome proliferator-activated receptor-gamma (PPARγ) nuclear receptors to improve insulin sensitivity. They cause fluid retention and should not be used in heart failure.

- **Dipeptidylpeptidase-4 inhibitors**: Sitagliptin and vildagliptin are inhibitors of dipeptidylpeptidase-4 (DPP-4) which degrades naturally occurring hormones called incretins. These drugs increase the effect of incretins, which allows a rise of insulin and lower glucagon levels.

  Rosiglitazone has fallen out of favor due to a possible association between its use and increased risk of myocardial ischemia. Both drugs have been associated with a risk of fractures, especially in women.

- **Acarbose**: Acarbose is an inhibitor of alpha glucosidase in the intestine. It delays digestion and absorption of sucrose and starch. Its use is limited by frequent flatulence and diarrhea.

Exenatide – This is an incretin mimetic which is administered by injection to lower blood glucose in patients with type 2 diabetes. Exenatide mimics the effect of a hormone called GLP-1. It stimulates

Table 12.15. Types of insulin

Insulin type	Kinetics	Trade name in UK
Rapid-acting analog	Onset: 10–15 min Peak: 60–90 min Duration: 4–5 h	Humalog (insulin lispro) NovoRapid (insulin aspart)
Fast-acting soluble insulin	Onset: 0.5–1 h Peak: 2–4 h Duration: 5–8 h	Humulin S Human Actrapid
Intermediate-acting isophane	Onset: 1–3 h Peak: 5–8 h Duration: up to 18 h	Humulin I Human Insulatard
Long-acting insulin analog	Onset: 90 min Duration: 24 h	Lantus (insulin glargine) Levemir (insulin detemir)
Premixed insulin containing variable ratio of rapid-acting analog or soluble to intermediate	Depends on type of insulins in mix and ratio	Humalog Mix25 Novomix 30 Humulin M3 Human Mixtard 30

pancreatic beta cells to secrete insulin in response to raised blood sugar. It also reduces the production of glucagon, slows gastric emptying and reduces appetite. Exenatide is an alternative to insulin in type 2 diabetes patients who cannot be treated adequately by dietary measures and oral medication. An advantage over insulin is that it induces weight reduction whereas insulin has the reverse effect. Exenatide can cause nausea, vomiting, abdominal pain, bloating, diarrhea and pancreatitis.

Insulin – Exogenous insulin is essential for the survival of patients with type 1 diabetes. Increasing numbers with type 2 diabetes also receive insulin as efforts to improve glycemic control are intensified amongst an ever-growing diabetic population.

There are many types of insulin and regimens (Table 12.15). The regimen and dose should be tailored to individuals.

Most patients with type 1 diabetes are now started on a basal bolus regime, which typically consists of a long-acting insulin analog administered before retiring to bed to provide some background insulin over a 24-hour period. Bolus doses of a rapid-acting insulin analog are then added immediately before meals to try to limit the hyperglycemia which follows carbohydrate ingestion.

Regimens for type 2 diabetes are more variable. Many require large doses to overcome insulin resistance. A common approach is to prescribe a long or intermediate insulin at night to control nocturnal and fasting glucose values with continued oral hypoglycemic agents during the day. The continuation of metformin when commencing insulin therapy may improve sensitivity to insulin and limit the weight gain associated with insulin initiation.

Most patients administer insulin subcutaneously, using portable pen devices, in the abdomen, outer thigh, or outer upper arm. Home blood glucose monitoring is performed using small portable glucose testing meters. Patients learn how to deal with the effects of alcohol and exercise on glucose levels and insulin requirements. They are also taught to avoid and deal with low blood glucose (hypoglycemia) and intercurrent illness which tends to increase blood glucose.

Acute metabolic complications

Hypoglycemia – Episodes of excessively low blood glucose are common when taking insulin particularly when striving for tight glycemic control in order to prevent microvascular complications. It can also occur with oral hypoglycemic agents especially sulphonylureas and meglitinides but is less common. The majority of hypoglycemic episodes are caused by delayed or inadequate meals. Other precipitating factors are unaccustomed exercise and alcohol ingestion. Hypoglycemia occurs when blood glucose falls to around <3 mmol/l. In the early stages, patients experience hunger, sweating, tremor of the hands, headache, tingling of the lips, dizziness, and weakness. Most episodes are mild and recognized and treated by patients with glucose sweets or a glucose-containing drink followed by longer-acting carbohydrate to prevent recurrence. If blood glucose falls further, then a change in behavior may occur with tiredness, confusion, drowsiness, disorientation, irritability, and aggression. Untreated hypoglycemia may progress to coma and epiletiform seizures. Even at this stage patients usually recover without permanent sequelae once treated, but permanent brain damage and death may occur if it is severe and prolonged. Severe episodes require intravenous glucose (100 ml of 20% dextrose as a bolus) or intramuscular glucagon (1 mg).

Ketoacidosis – those with type 1 diabetes are most at risk. Common precipitants are cessation of insulin and intercurrent illness or infection. Ketoacidosis may be the initial presenting feature of type 1, but can develop in those with type 2 diabetes particularly after progression to relative insulin deficiency. This leads to a catabolic state resulting in hyperglycemia, osmotic diuresis, dehydration, and ketone body (acetoacetate and β-hydroxybutyrate) formation by the liver leading to acidosis. Symptoms due to hyperglycemia are associated with anorexia, nausea, vomiting, and abdominal pain which can cause diagnostic difficulties. Untreated, drowsiness, coma, and eventually cardiovascular collapse and death follow. Signs of volume depletion, sighing respiration (Kussmaul respiration), and breath odor of acetone may occur. Evidence of precipitating illness or infection may be present. Urgent treatment is of the utmost importance, particularly correction of the often profound dehydration. Management includes:

- Check blood glucose, urea, and electrolytes, blood gases, full blood count, urine and blood cultures, ECG, and chest X-ray.

- Start intravenous 0.9% saline according to the degree of dehydration. Usually 1 liter in the first hour initially. The degree of volume depletion in young patients with ketoacidosis is often as much as 5 liters. Change fluids to dextrose saline when blood glucose falls below 15 mmol/l.

- Start an intravenous sliding scale of short-acting insulin (usually 50 units of actrapid in 50 ml 0.9% saline administered via a syringe driver). Infuse initially at 6 units/hour and adjust according to blood glucose response.

- Check serum potassium every hour. There is a real danger from hypokalemia as insulin drives glucose and potassium into cells. Potassium must be added to the infusion fluids in sufficient quantities to maintain the serum potassium within the normal range.

- If the patient is unconscious, then close monitoring and appropriate supportive measures such as a nasogastric tube to prevent aspiration, a urinary catheter to monitor fluid balance, and heparinization may be required. Further investigation and treatment of possible precipitating factors needs to be considered.

Hyperosmolar non-ketotic coma and lactic acidosis – These usually occur in elderly patients with type 2 diabetes. They are usually precipitated by an intercurrent illness supervening on a degree of chronic hyperglycemia. Patients are usually extremely hyperglycemic and hyperosmolar, but are not ketotic. Occasionally, such patients have raised lactate levels causing acidosis (lactic acidosis). Management is similar to that of ketoacidosis with some important differences. Correction of profound dehydration is again of the utmost importance but complicated by the fact that these patients are often elderly and less able to tolerate the administration of large quantities of intravenous fluids. This is particularly so if there is cardiac disease. There is a high risk of venous thromboembolism and anticoagulation should be instituted. This condition carries a high mortality.

Chronic complications

Macrovascular risk – the increased mortality in diabetes, particularly in those with type 2 diabetes, is due to macrovascular disease and especially myocardial infarction. An important aspect of management is therefore to review cardiovascular risk and not just glycemic control. Factors which need to be considered are age, ethnicity, family history of cardiovascular disease, smoking, abdominal adiposity, lipids, and blood pressure. The modifiable risk factors need to be aggressively managed including smoking cessation, use of lipid lowering agents, antihypertensives, and antiplatelet agents.

Retinopathy – good glycemic control, as with all microvascular complications, helps prevent retinopathy and reduces the risk of progression once this has occurred. Timely use of laser therapy reduces the risk of progression to visual impairment hence detection and monitoring of retinopathy is critically important. Patients should undergo an annual check of visual acuity and retinal examination preferably by digital retinal photography after mydriasis (pupillary dilatation) with tropicamide eye drops. Patients with new vessel formation or its consequences need to be referred for urgent ophthalmologic review and consideration of laser therapy. Rapidly worsening background retinopathy, retinopathy affecting the macular area of the retina, preproliferative retinopathy, or any unexplained deterioration in visual acuity also merit specialist assessment.

Nephropathy – annual screening for nephropathy is essential. Patients should undergo annual measurement of urinary albumin excretion. A rise in urinary albumin excretion occurs at a very early stage in the pathophysiology of diabetic nephropathy. This is often accompanied by a relative rise in blood pressure. Glycemic control should be optimized. Blood pressure needs to be treated aggressively with angiotensin converting enzyme (ACE) inhibitors or angiotensin II receptor blockers both of which have a favorable effect on renal hemodynamics and reduce the rate of progression of renal damage.

Diabetic foot disease – diabetic foot disease is notorious. It can lead to ulceration, infection, gangrene, and amputation. Patients who suffer such problems often spend long periods in hospital and consume a large proportion of healthcare resource. The most important aspect of these more severe manifestations is that they are largely preventable. Patients must be screened for the development of peripheral neuropathy and peripheral vascular disease on an annual basis. Patients who develop neuropathy or peripheral vascular disease need education in the principles of good foot care to try to prevent future damage and ulceration. There is, as yet, no specific treatment for peripheral neuropathy, although any unpleasant dysesthesia or pain can be treated with small doses of amitriptyline, gabapentin, or carbamazepine. Peripheral vascular disease requires attention to cardiovascular risk factors and consideration of revascularization procedures such as angioplasty or bypass grafting. Foot ulceration needs treatment in a specialist unit. The following measures are often required or should be considered:

- Relieve pressure on the ulcerated area to promote healing (bed rest, appropriate footware, or other pressure relieving devices).
- Regular debridement and dressings by appropriately experienced podiatrists.
- Deep swabs of the affected areas and appropriate antibiotics.
- X-ray or other imaging of the foot to look for underlying osteomyelitis.
- Assess vascular supply by Doppler or arteriography.
- Angioplasty or vascular surgery if non-healing ulcer, critical ischemia, or ischemic pain at rest.
- Surgical debridement or amputation if there is deep infection or osteomyelitis not responding to antibiotics, worsening infection threatening limb and life, intractable ischemic pain, critical ischemia, or gangrene (Fig. 12.20).

Outcome

Diabetes reduces life expectancy mainly due to the risk of chronic macro- and microvascular complications. The incidence and progression of chronic complications can be reduced by up-to-date management

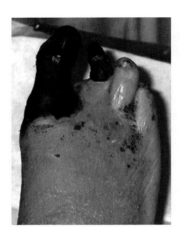

Fig. 12.20. Dry gangrene of the first and third toes in a patient with diabetes, peripheral neuropathy, and peripheral vascular disease.

aimed at optimizing glycemic control, and aggressively controlling modifiable cardiovascular risk factors. Regular screening for complications is essential.

Diabetes is a chronic disease and has the potential to interfere with day-to-day activities and quality of life. Treatment must therefore be holistic and aim to minimize such interference providing appropriate education, training, practical help, and psychologic input where this is required.

Optimal management requires the services of a skilled multidisciplinary team and improves the outlook in diabetes, although such resources are still not uniformly available. Screening for type 2 diabetes, particularly in high-risk groups, is urgently required since earlier intervention would reduce morbidity.

Attempts to cure diabetes, particularly type 1 diabetes, are ongoing. Whole pancreas transplants are being carried out with increasing frequency. The majority of these are carried out at the same time as renal transplantation for end-stage diabetic kidney disease when patients are already damaged by advanced complications and the prognosis is limited. Solitary pancreas transplants are seldom carried out due to the morbidity and mortality attached to the procedure and immunosuppressive drugs, which have to be given to prevent rejection. The most promising prospect of a cure is the development of islet cell transplants.

Hypercalcemia

Introduction

Hypercalcemia is now frequently detected as an asymptomatic finding during biochemical screening. Once detected and confirmed, investigation must be undertaken to determine a definitive diagnosis, since

the commonest causes of hypercalcemia are primary hyperparathyroidism and malignant disease.

Clinical features

Mild hypercalcemia is usually asymptomatic. The higher the calcium, the more likely patients are to experience clinical manifestations:

- Tiredness, weakness, general malaise, non-specific bony aches and pains.
- Polyuria and thirst.
- Weight loss, anorexia, nausea, vomiting, abdominal discomfort, and constipation.
- More severe hypercalcemia can cause drowsiness and confusion, dehydration, hypotension, and cardiac dysrhythmias.
- Long-standing hypercalcemia can lead to renal stones and nephrolithiasis causing renal colic and renal failure, and to erosion and thinning of the bones.
- Parathyroid adenomas are not usually palpable in the neck.

Epidemiology

Primary hyperparathyroidism and malignant disease account for around 90% of all cases of hypercalcemia. Primary hyperparathyroidism is common and its incidence has increased, probably due to the widespread introduction of multi-channel analyzers and increased biochemical screening detecting patients who would have previously remained undiagnosed. The prevalence of primary hyperparathyroidism is estimated at 2–10 per 10 000 of the population. Its peak incidence is age 40–60 and it is two to three times more common in women.

Etiology and pathology

Calcium circulates in the blood bound to carrier proteins (mostly albumin). A small ionised fraction circulating freely is the active moiety. Calcium is measured as the total amount of bound and ionized fractions. Alterations in the plasma albumin concentration can therefore alter the total calcium level, and the important calcium level is therefore one which has been corrected for albumin concentration.

The causes of hypercalcemia are listed in Table 12.16 and Fig. 12.21.

Thiazide diuretics cause only mild hypercalcemia by reducing renal calcium excretion. Primary hyperparathyroidism is usually due to a small adenoma in one of the four parathyroid glands, but can rarely be caused by multiple adenomas, four-gland hyperplasia or parathyroid carcinoma.

The adenoma secretes parathyroid hormone (PTH) autonomously resulting in high circulating PTH levels. PTH acts at a variety of sites but mainly on the kidney to increase renal tubular calcium absorption and increase phosphate excretion. PTH also stimulates bone turnover, particularly osteoclast activity, thereby mobilizing calcium into the circulation. This causes cortical bone loss, which may increase the risk of fracture. Cortical bony erosions, best seen in the hands, may occur and lead to cyst formation (osteitis fibrosa cystica). Severe bony changes are seldom seen nowadays due to earlier diagnosis. Urinary calcium excretion is high and there may be renal calcium deposition (nephrocalcinosis) or renal stone formation.

Patients with long-standing renal failure or who have received a renal transplant may develop so-called tertiary hyperparathyroidism where autonomous PTH secretion occurs due to long-standing stimulation of the parathyroids as a result of altered calcium homeostasis that occurs in this situation.

Hypercalcemia due to malignant disease is most often caused by carcinoma of the lung or breast.

Table 12.16. Causs of hypercalcemia

Common
Primary hyperparathyroidism
Malignant disease
Thiazide diuretics (mild hypercalcemia only)
Uncommon
Tertiary hyperparathyroidism (renal failure)
Thyrotoxicosis
Multiple myeloma
Sarcoidosis
Milk–alkali syndrome
Vitamin D excess
Familial hypocalciuric hypercalcemia

Fig. 12.21. Flow diagram for diagnosing the causes of hypercalcemia.

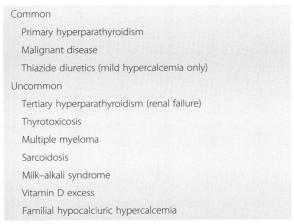

Hypercalcemia

Thiazide diuretic
Milk and antacids
Excessive vitamin D

Stop and recheck

Not on interfering agents

Persistent hypercalcemia → **Check parathyroid hormone**

Suppressed

Excludes hyperparathyroidism
Investigate for other causes

Raised or inappropriately normal

Hyperparathyroidism confirmed (exclude familial hypocalciuric hypercalcemia by measuring urine calcium excretion)

The mechanism is either widespread bony metastases stimulating calcium release or by humoral secretion by the tumor of a peptide similar to parathyroid hormone termed parathyroid hormone-related peptide (PTHrP). This peptide may be produced in huge quantities and can cause very severe hypercalcemia.

Other causes of hypercalcemia are much less common. Thyrotoxicosis can cause hypercalcemia thought to be due to increased bone turnover. Most patients with thyrotoxicosis do not develop hypercalcemia and, where this does occur, it is usually mild.

Sarcoidosis can cause hypercalcemia due to production of 1–25-dihydroxycholecalciferol by activated macrophages. Milk–alkali syndrome is unusual and, as it name suggests, is caused by the simultaneous consumption of large quantities of milk and alkaline antacids. The antacids promote the absorption of calcium and can cause quite marked hypercalcemia. This quickly settles once the causative agents are withdrawn.

Familial hypocalciuric hypercalcemia (FHH) is a rare but important cause of hypercalcemia since it is easily mistaken for primary hyperparathyroidism and many of these patients are subject to unnecessary surgery. FHH is an autosomal dominant condition caused by heterozygous inactivating mutations of the calcium sensing receptor. There is relative insensitivity of the parathyroid calcium receptor to calcium resulting in "resetting" of the serum calcium level, which then runs at a level above the normal range. The PTH levels are usually normal or slightly high. Urinary calcium excretion is not raised and this is helpful in distinguishing this condition from primary hyperparathyroidism. FHH is thought to be a benign condition.

Investigations

A diagnostic pathway for investigating hypercalcemia is shown in Fig. 12.21. Assessment of hypercalcemia should be based on repeated calcium levels, corrected for the prevailing albumin level, and obtained without undue venous stasis.

The history should exclude ingestion of thiazide diuretics, excessive milk and alkali, or vitamin D products. Hypercalcemia due to malignant disease will usually occur in patients who are already known to have malignancy. Although hypercalcemia is seldom the presenting feature of malignant disease, patients with hypercalcemia should have a thorough clinical examination, including examination of the breasts.

Measurement of PTH is the definitive investigation. Suppressed levels exclude hyperparathyroidism.

Raised levels are virtually diagnostic of hyperparathyroidism, although the rare FHH should be excluded by the measurement of urinary calcium to creatinine clearance ratio. A ratio of <0.01 in the absence of renal disease suggests FHH. Another potentially confusing factor is that PTH levels may be in the upper normal range, but this is still inappropriately high in the presence of hypercalcemia when PTH levels should be suppressed due to feedback inhibition of raised calcium on PTH secretion.

Patients with hyperparathyroidism may also have a low serum phosphate level and a metabolic acidosis. The increased bone turnover may also cause a raised alkaline phosphatase. A renal ultrasound scan to look for renal stones and a bone density scan are also helpful in assessment of the need for parathyroidectomy.

The diagnosis of hyperparathyroidism is essentially biochemical but high-resolution ultrasound scanning and sestamibi isotope scanning can help localize the adenoma which may assist surgery.

Investigations for other causes of hypercalcemia might include thyroid function tests, tumor markers, PTHrP, bone or CT scanning for malignant disease, and a CXR and serum angiotensin-converting enzyme level for sarcoidosis.

Management

Patients with primary hyperparathyroidism who are symptomatic from hypercalcemia or have evidence of end-organ damage such as osteoporosis, renal impairment, nephrocalcinosis, or renal stones should undergo parathyroid surgery, which is usually curative.

In asymptomatic patients the situation is more controversial since the long-term risks in this situation are not well documented. Current recommendations advocate surgery be performed in the following circumstances:

- Age under 50 years.
- Corrected serum calcium >0.25 mmol/l above the normal range.
- Renal calcium excretion >10 mmol/day.
- Creatinine clearance reduced $>30\%$ compared to age and sex-matched controls.
- Bone density more than 2.5 standard deviations below the peak bone mass (T score <-2.5) in any of the lumbar spine, hip, or distal radius.

The treatment of hypercalcemia due to causes other than hyperparathyroidism centers around removing or treating the cause.

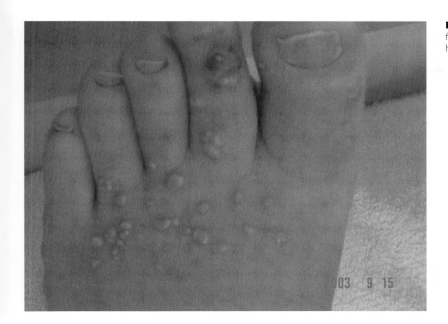

Fig. 12.22. Eruptive xanthomata on the foot of a patient with severe hypertriglyceridemia.

Severe hypercalcemia can be a medical emergency. Calcium levels in excess of 3 mmol/l usually result in patients being dehydrated. Severe hypercalcemia should be treated initially by rehydration with intravenous 0.9% saline. Saline alone can reduce serum calcium levels by the order of 1 mmol/l. Treatment with furosemide or other loop diuretics, once rehydration is complete, helps to increase urinary calcium excretion and lower blood levels. Bisphosphonates are also extremely useful agents in reducing high calcium levels by inhibiting bone turnover. An intravenous infusion of 15–60 mg of disodium pamidronate is the standard treatment. Corticosteroids are sometimes helpful, particularly if the hypercalcemia is due to myeloma, sarcoidosis, or vitamin D intoxication. Calcitonin can also be used but is less effective.

Outcome
The prognosis in hypercalcemia depends on the underlying cause. The outlook in primary hyperparathyroidism is good. Cure rates in those with solitary adenomas are 95%–98% when removed by experienced specialized endocrine surgeons.

Hypercholesterolemia (hyperlipidemia)
Introduction
Raised total and low density lipoprotein (LDL) cholesterol levels are independent risk factors for the development of atheroma and its consequences. Most members of the public are now aware of the significance of an elevated cholesterol. Screening tests for cholesterol are widely available and around 50% of the population have cholesterol levels above recommended targets.

Clinical features
Most patients with hypercholesterolemia are asymptomatic. Physical signs are usually absent, although some patients develop a premature arcus senilis or xanthelasmata on the eyelids. Tendon xanthomata may occur in those with familial hypercholesterolemia and eruptive xanthomata in those with hypertriglyceridemia (Fig. 12.22).

Epidemiology
The risk of coronary heart disease increases as cholesterol rises above 5.2 mmol/l. Around 25% of the middle-aged population of the UK have total cholesterol levels above 6.5 mmol/l, which significantly increases risk of coronary heart disease.

Pathology
Cholesterol and triglycerides circulate bound to proteins and these complexes are termed lipoproteins. Abnormalities of lipids and lipoproteins account for a large proportion of coronary heart disease. The most important lipoproteins are low-density lipoproteins (LDL), which are rich in cholesterol and correlate strongly with the risk of coronary artery disease. High-density lipoprotein (HDL) is mainly phospholipid and correlates *inversely* with the risk of coronary

Table 12.17. Secondary causes of hyperlipidemia

Diabetes mellitus

Hypothyroidism

Renal disease

Biliary obstruction

Alcohol

artery disease. Raised triglycerides also confer an increased risk of coronary artery disease.

Individual cholesterol and lipoprotein levels are largely genetically determined, although obesity, sedentary living, and a diet high in saturated fat intake have an adverse effect. In most patients the genetic defects are polygenic. The most common abnormalities are of a mild to moderate elevation of total and LDL cholesterol (total cholesterol typically between 6.5 and 9 mmol/l). Some patients have mixed hyperlipidemia with elevation of LDL cholesterol and triglycerides and reduced HDL. Polygenic origins combined with adverse lifestyle factors are often found in this situation.

There are some uncommon isolated gene defects, which lead to specific abnormal lipid and lipoprotein profiles and risk. Familial hypercholesterolemia is a dominantly inherited condition, which results in very high cholesterol (typically >9 mmol/l). These patients have a defect in the LDL receptor gene resulting in reduced catabolism of LDL cholesterol. There is risk of premature coronary artery disease with over half of men dying before the age of 60 years. Familial combined hyperlipidemia with elevation of cholesterol and triglycerides is autosomal dominant. Elevation of triglycerides alone can occur in familial hypertriglyceridemia, again autosomal dominant, and rarely familial lipoprotein lipase deficiency where there is massive elevation of triglycerides, eruptive xanthomata (Fig. 12.22), and a consequent increased risk of pancreatitis.

Hypercholesterolemia may occur secondary to other conditions (Table 12.17). Part of the metabolic derangement in type 2 diabetes includes a tendency towards increased total and LDL cholesterol, reduced HDL cholesterol, and raised triglycerides. In addition, the LDL in type 2 diabetes is smaller and more dense and thought to be more atherogenic. These abnormalities are at least part of the explanation for the increased cardiovascular morbidity and mortality.

Hypothyroidism is associated with raised levels of total and LDL cholesterol which improve on treatment with thyroxine. Patients with chronic renal disease show abnormalities of cholesterol and triglycerides, and nephrotic syndrome in particular is associated with elevations of cholesterol levels. Obstruction of the biliary tree by chronic conditions such as primary biliary cirrhosis can increase cholesterol. Alcohol excess causes mainly hypertriglyceridemia.

Investigations

Patients at high risk of cardiovascular disease should be screened for hypercholesterolemia. Total cholesterol and triglycerides are often the initial assessment, but measurements of HDL improve estimation of cardiovascular risk. Lipids should ideally be measured after an overnight fast. In practice, this makes little difference to cholesterol levels and decisions based on non-fasting cholesterol values are acceptable.

Grossly elevated levels require further investigation for types of specific dyslipidemia.

Management

The management of hypercholesterolemia is traditionally divided into primary prevention of atherosclerosis before this is clinically manifest or the secondary prevention of further damage once complications of this process have occurred. Reducing total and LDL cholesterol and raising HDL cholesterol have been shown to be effective in reducing the risk of developing coronary heart disease in those at high risk and in reducing the risk of further events once the clinical features of this condition are manifest.

Patients with coronary heart disease should all be treated with cholesterol-lowering agents. There is now a huge amount of evidence supporting the benefits of using lipid lowering statins which lower LDL cholesterol and reduce coronary heart disease.

For individuals who have not yet developed clinically overt complications of dyslipidemia, it is important that individual cholesterol levels are not treated in isolation but that a global assessment of future cardiovascular risk is obtained taking into account all known cardiovascular risk factors for an individual patient. These should include age, gender, ethnicity, smoking, diabetes, hypertension, HDL cholesterol, and family history of premature vascular disease. All treatable risk factors should be addressed and the use of aspirin considered.

The decision to treat cholesterol should be made according to risk prediction. Risk prediction charts (British National Formulary, 2009) can be used to aid decision-making processes in individuals, but these charts should not replace balanced clinical judgment for individual patients.

Patients who have a predicted cardiovascular risk of >20% (equivalent to a coronary heart disease risk of >15%) over the next 10 years should be considered for specific therapy to lower cholesterol regardless of the cholesterol level. Advice on diet, weight loss, and exercise should be given. These lifestyle measures may reduce cholesterol, but often have little significant impact. Rhabdomyolysis can rarely occur with statins and patients should be advised to report unexplained muscle pain, tenderness, or weakness.

Individuals with a coronary heart disease risk of <15%, but close to this level, should be given lifestyle advice and reassessed annually.

Other cholesterol modifying medications are available. Ezetimibe is an agent that inhibits intestinal absorption of cholesterol and can be used when a statin is insufficient to control cholesterol or cannot be used.

Fibrates such as bezafibrate, ciprofibrate, fenofibrate, and gemfibrozil are the treatment of choice in hypertriglyceridemia. Nicotinic acid can lower cholesterol and triglycerides and raise HDL cholesterol but often causes vasodilatation. Fish oil preparations can help lower triglycerides.

Outcome

There is now a wealth of evidence to show that lowering of cholesterol, particularly with the use of statins, reduces coronary heart disease in those at high risk. It does not, however, *prevent* the development of this condition. It remains to be seen whether or not earlier intervention or more aggressive cholesterol lowering, as well as treatment of other risk factors, can reduce the incidence still further.

Further reading

Alberti KGMM, Zimmet PZ. Definition, diagnosis and classification of diabetes mellitus and its complications. Part 1: Diagnosis and classification of diabetes mellitus. Provisional report of a WHO consultation. *Diabetic Med.* 1998, **15**:539–533.

Ajjan R. *Endocrinology and Diabetes*. John Wiley and Sons Ltd, Wiley-Blackwell, 2009.

Bilezikian JP, Potts JT, El-Hajj *et al*. Udelsman R and Wells SA. Summary statement from a workshop on asymptomatic primary hyperparathyroidism: a perspective for the 21st century. *J Clin Endocrinol Metab* 2002, **87**:5353–5361.

British National Formulary, No. 57, March 2009.

Wass J, Turner H. *Oxford Handbook of Endocrinology and Diabetes*. Oxford University Press, 2009.

Contents

Introduction

Poisoning is one of the commonest medical emergencies in the UK and accounts for 10%–20% of acute medical admissions. The most common causes of poisoning in the UK are outlined in Table 13.1. Assessing poisoned patients and managing them is an exciting challenge because they often have complex psychosocial issues, together with general medical problems, and have taken toxins in sizeable doses. They require the best of clinical skills to provide the best outcome. Sadly, poisoned patients do not always meet with the sympathies of admitting doctors because they may be perceived to have "self-inflicted illness." This is a morally unacceptable view. Self-poisoned patients are most likely to respond to a pragmatic, non-judgmental approach. Often an overdose is taken at a time of stress, e.g. due to exams or relationship difficulties. Patients often need a helpful ear, supportive medical care, and follow-up support. Some may need on-going psychiatric evaluation and support.

Some patients, such as those who have taken paracetamol, may need treatment with an antidote. However, in general, the antidotes in toxicology are few (Table 13.2) and the outcome depends on the ability of the clinician to deliver meticulous supportive care.

How to identify a poisoned patient

Clues that alert us to a toxic exposure having occurred include the following.

- Patient may admit to having taken an overdose.
- Patient may be distressed or tearful.
- Overdose is commoner in younger patients, slightly more common in women than men, but may be of more serious suicidal intent in the elderly.
- Past or current history of depression or other psychiatric diagnoses.
- Past history of overdose or self-harm.
- Past history of personal abuse e.g. victim of sexual abuse as a child.
- Underlying alcohol problem.
- Social problems, e.g. lack of housing, relationship difficulties, social isolation, etc.
- Overdose is more common in lower socioeconomic classes and where there is deprivation.
- Needle marks on arms (men), groins (often women) indicating an injection habit.
- Admission from the workplace (occupational exposure).
- The family or ambulance staff may have brought the patient in with empty packets of drugs.

Assessing a poisoned patient

Substances involved in poisoning vary widely between different countries. The important five for the UK are listed in Table 13.1. In assessing poisoned patients it is important to take a good history and perform a meticulous physical examination. Clinical features of poisoning that identify which toxin may have been taken in a

Table 13.1. The most common causes of poisoning in the UK

Analgesic drugs, including acetaminophen and non-steroidal anti-inflammatory drugs – these account for half of all poisoning cases

Cardiovascular toxic drugs, especially tricyclic antidepressants – approximately 10% of cases of poisoning

Drugs of misuse

Carbon monoxide – the commonest cause of death by poisoning

Alcohol – the co-ingestant in 50% of cases of self-poisoning

Table 13.2. Common antidotes available for treatment of poisoning

Poison	Antidote
Acetaminophen	N-acetylcysteine
Carbon monoxide	Oxygen, hyperbaric oxygen
Tricyclic antidepressants	Sodium bicarbonate
Cyanide	Nitrites, hydroxocobalamin, sodium thiosulphate
Opioids, e.g. heroin, morphine	Naloxone
Iron	Desferrioxamine, deferoxamine
Digoxin	Fab fragments (digibind®)

non-comatose patient are shown in Fig. 13.1. How to confirm this diagnosis is then shown in Table 13.3.

When patients are unconscious and no history is available, the diagnosis of the substance causing the poisoning depends on exclusion of other causes of coma and consideration of circumstantial evidence. Figure 13.2 shows how to look out for diagnostic clues. In assessing comatose patients it is vital to remember that other medical causes of coma need to be excluded (see Table 13.4).

General management of the poisoned patient

Most require little more than symptomatic and supportive care. First remember to assess:

- Airway
- Breathing
- Circulation

The principles of preventing absorption or enhancing elimination (Table 13.5) depend on to what the patient has been exposed, by what route and how long ago and whether that substance binds to charcoal or not (Table 13.6). Antidotes are few (Table 13.2) but

can be life saving. To assess the degree of suicidal intent, prior to formal psychiatric evaluation of the patient, the Beck's depression scale is commonly used (Table 13.7). If the score exceeds 4, the patient requires special nursing to protect against self-harm.

Indications for intubation and assisted ventilation are:

- Glasgow Coma Scale <8, or falling rapidly
- Post-cardio-respiratory arrest
- Recurrent seizures
- Hypoxia – not corrected with oxygen mask and high flow oxygen therapy
- Hypercarbia – p_{CO_2} >6.6 kPa or hypocarbia p_{CO_2} <2.5 kPa
- Inability to protect airway
- Shock, i.e. tachycardia, hypotension, metabolic acidosis.

Optimizing the cardiac output and blood pressure means maintenance of oxygen delivery as well as maintenance of adequate organ perfusion and blood pressure. Hypotension usually responds to filling with IV fluids, then treatment of any cardiac arrhythmia with an inotrope or vasoconstrictor if required. Epinephrine (adrenaline) increases the heart rate and stroke volume. At low doses, the primary effect is to increase cardiac output, while at higher doses there is additional potent vasoconstriction. If, despite adequate filling, the blood pressure remains low then vasoconstrictors should be used, e.g. norepinephrine. This has no effect on cardiac output, but is useful in generating perfusion of the brain, liver, and kidneys. However, it should be used at the lowest possible dose to achieve the desired effect as it reduces renal blood flow, splanchnic blood flow, and impairs peripheral perfusion.

Complications of poisoning and their management
Vomiting

If vomiting fails to respond to simple measures such as sucking ice cubes, metoclopramide 10 mg i.v. or ondansetron 8 mg i.v. by slow injection may be particularly effective, the latter especially in paracetamol or theophylline poisoning.

Agitation

Talk to the patient calmly, and before sedating a patient exclude possible causes of agitation such as hypoglycemia, full bladder, pain, hypoxia. Give diazepam (0.1–0.2 mg/kg) IV, repeated as necessary.

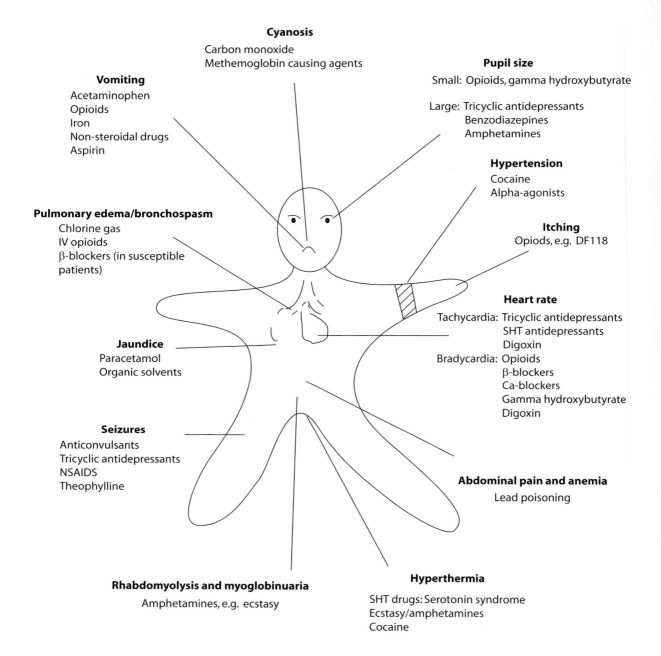

Cyanosis
Carbon monoxide
Methemoglobin causing agents

Pupil size
Small: Opioids, gamma hydroxybutyrate

Large: Tricyclic antidepressants
Benzodiazepines
Amphetamines

Vomiting
Acetaminophen
Opioids
Iron
Non-steroidal drugs
Aspirin

Hypertension
Cocaine
Alpha-agonists

Pulmonary edema/bronchospasm
Chlorine gas
IV opioids
β-blockers (in susceptible patients)

Itching
Opiods, e.g. DF118

Heart rate
Tachycardia: Tricyclic antidepressants
SHT antidepressants
Digoxin
Bradycardia: Opioids
β-blockers
Ca-blockers
Gamma hydroxybutyrate
Digoxin

Jaundice
Paracetamol
Organic solvents

Seizures
Anticonvulsants
Tricyclic antidepressants
NSAIDS
Theophylline

Abdominal pain and anemia
Lead poisoning

Rhabdomyolysis and myoglobinuaria
Amphetamines, e.g. ecstasy

Hyperthermia
SHT drugs: Serotonin syndrome
Ecstasy/amphetamines
Cocaine

Notes

(1) In mixed overdoses the diagnostic features may become blurred.
(2) In early Acetaminophen poisoning there may be no clinical
signs of poisoning.

Fig. 13.1. Diagnostic clues to the poison taken in patients who are not/not yet comatose.

Table 13.3. Diagnostic tests to confirm the toxin in Fig. 13.1

Possible toxin diagnosis from Fig. 13.1	Associated features	Confirmatory investigation
Acetaminophen	Right upper quadrant tenderness, vomiting, renal angle tenderness	Plasma acetaminophen concentration. If jaundice/history of ingestion more than 12 hours ago then also do LFTs and PTR or INR
Anticonvulsants	Ataxia, nystagmus, dysarthria, hyponatraemia, heart block	Plasma levels of drug e.g. carbamazepine used for confirmation but there is poor correlation between level and degree of toxicity
Agents causing methemoglobinemia	History of use of "poppers" (amyl nitrite), medication with dapsone	Blood methemoglobin concentration
Tricyclic antidepressants	Cardiac rhythm disturbance, hot dry skin, hypotension, urine retention	ECG shows tachycardia and may show QRS prolongation (>140 ms)
5HT antidepressants	Sometimes may be accompanied by serotonin syndrome characterized by rigidity, hyperthermia, and autonomic instability	ECG shows tachycardia, no QRS prolongation
Drugs of abuse	Agitation/sedation, conjunctival injection with cannabis, cardiac pain/vascular complications	Urine dip test qualitatively confirms presence of amphetamines, benzodiazepines, cannabis, cocaine, or opioids. For legal purposes confirmation by HPLC is needed
Aspirin (salicylate)	Tinnitus, sweating, purpura, respiratory alkalosis, metabolic acidosis	Plasma salicylate concentration
Opioids	Coma, respiratory depression, pin-point pupils	The best diagnostic test is administration of the antidote, naloxone
Lead	Blue line on gums, abdominal pain, anemia	Serum lead concentration, blood film may show basophilic stippling
Carbon monoxide	History of house fire, high serum lactate	COHb – this is good for confirmation but there is poor correlation between level and degree of toxicity
Iron	Metabolic acidosis, vomiting, hepatic injury, rusty colored urine	Serum concentration of iron, abdominal X-ray may reveal radio-opaque iron tablets
Digoxin	Heart block, malignant arrhythmias, reduced cardiac output	Serum digoxin concentration, ECG

Note:
There are no readiliy available diagnostic tests for NSAIDs, gammahydroxybutyrate, beta-blockers, or calcium channel blockers.

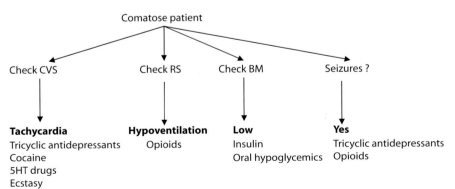

Fig. 13.2. Diagnostic clues to the poison taken in patients who present comatose.

Table 13.4. Differential diagnosis of common causes of coma

Likely diagnosis		Associated features	Investigations of choice to confirm
Drug overdose	(1) Tricyclic antidepressants	(1) tachycardia, fits, hypotension, warm dry skin, urine retention	(1) ECG – tachycardia and may show QRS prolongation (>140 ms)
	(2) 5HT drugs	(2) serotonergic features – rigidity, autonomic instability, hyperthermia	(2) ECG – tachycardia
	(3) Opioids	(3) pin-point pupils, respiratory depression, coma	(3) Response to naloxone
	(4) Toxic alcohols	(4) profound metabolic acidosis, anion/osmolar gaps	(4) Methanol/ethylene glycol blood concentration
	(5) Hypoglycemic agents and insulin	(5) history of diabetes	(5) Blood glucose
	(6) Benzodiazepines	(6) nil	(6) nil
	(7) Carbon monoxide	(7) evidence of exposure to CO/fire	(7) COHb level in blood
CNS causes	Cerebral contusion	Trauma history	CT head scan, preferably with contrast
	Extradural hematoma	May have focal neurologic signs, trauma history	CT head scan, preferably with contrast
	Subdural hematoma	May have focal neurologic signs	CT head scan, preferably with contrast
	Cerebral infarction or hemorrhage	May have focal neurologic signs	CT head scan, preferably with contrast
	Subarachnoid hemorrhage	May have focal neurologic signs, neck stiffness, photophobia, may have "hit on head with a hammer" history	CT head scan, preferably with contrast and lumbar puncture
	Brainstem infarction/hemorrhage	May have focal neurologic signs	MRI head scan
	Cerebral venous sinus thrombosis	May have focal neurologic signs	CT head scan, preferably with contrast
	Meningitis	Neck stiffness, photophobia, characteristic meningococcal rash	CT and lumbar puncture
	Encephalitis	History of "cold sores" or other viral illness	CT and lumbar puncture, and EEG
	Cerebral abscess	May have history of trauma to the skull, patient may have focal neurologic signs, neck stiffness, other stigmata of infection	CT head scan, preferably with contrast
	Brain tumor	May have history of severe headaches, worse in the morning, focal neurologic signs	CT head scan, preferably with contrast
	Epilepsy (especially post-ictal)	History of epilepsy	CT head scan and EEG

Diabetes	Diabetes mellitus	Hypoglycemia, ketoacidosis, hyperosmolar coma	Blood glucose concentration, arterial blood gases, urea and Electrolytes
Uremia		Often pre-existing history of renal disease or recent exposure to a nephrotoxic drug	Urea and electrolytes, ECG may show tall tented T waves of concurrent hyperkalemia
Hypothermia		Shivering, ECG change (J waves) – history suggestive of lying around for many hours or immersion in cold water etc.	Rectal temperature
Others	Hypothyroidism	May be concurrent goiter, a history of other autoimmune diseases, patient often >40 years of age	Thyroid function tests, thyroid autoantibody tests
	Hyponatremia	Often concurrent hypokalemia	Serum and urine osmolality, urea and electrolytes
	Hepatic failure due to viral agents	Jaundice, renal dysfunction, clotting abnormalities	Liver function tests, ABGs, PTR, hepatitis A,B,C serology, CMV, toxoplasma

Table 13.5. Principles of preventing absorption or enhancing elimination of toxins

Route of exposure	Preventing absorption	Enhanced elimination
Skin	Remove clothing, wash copiously with soap and water	–
Eye	Irrigate with saline for at least 20 minutes, examine under slit lamp for corneal injury	–
Ingestion	If a life-threatening amount of a toxin has been taken within the last hour, consider gastric lavage	If a toxin has a low volume of distribution and low protein binding, it may be effectively cleared by hemodialysis, e.g. salicylates
	If a significant overdose has been taken within the last hour and the substance binds to activated charcoal (AC), give 50 g AC orally. If carbamazepine, dapsone, phenobarbitone, quinine, or theophylline has been taken, give 50 g charcoal every 4 hours with sorbitol/lactulose, i.e. multiple dose activated charcoal	If a toxin binds avidly to charcoal, it may be removed by charcoal hemoperfusion, e.g. carbamazepine
	If a large ingestion of iron, lithium, packets of drugs, or SR preparations such as verapamil or theophylline have been taken, consider whole bowel irrigation with polyethylene glycol	If a toxin is highly protein bound, it may be cleared effectively by MARS (albumin dialysis system)
Inoculation	Local excision and debridement if high pressure injury in a digit	If the toxin is a weak acid, its renal elimination is enhanced by alkaline diuresis, e.g. salicylates
Inhalation	Oxygen – nebulized bronchodilators if wheeze	

Table 13.6. Substances not bound by activated charcoal

Acids
Alkalis
Metals and metallic salts, e.g. Hg and mercuric chloride, lithium
Toxic alcohols, e.g. methanol, ethylene glycol
Cyanide

Dystonias

These are common after overdoses with antipsychotic drugs and some anti-emetics. Oculogyric crises, torticollis (wry neck), trismus (jaw clenching) respond to procyclidine (5–10 mg IV) or benztropine (1–2 mg IV).

Seizures

These are common after poisoning with a wide variety of agents. A non-sustained fit does not require pharmacologic intervention. However, persistent (>5 min) and recurrent seizures require treatment. The drug of choice is diazepam (0.1–0.2 mg/kg) repeated as required. If seizures are persistent or recurrent despite adequate doses of benzodiazepines, IV phenytoin should be used (15 mg/kg). Status epilepticus requires paralysis and ventilation with EEG monitoring.

Rhabdomyolysis

Patients with rhabdomyolysis (muscle necrosis) as evidenced by a positive urine dipstick test for blood (cross-reacts with hemoglobin or myoglobin) and a raised serum creatine kinase, should be kept well hydrated with IV fluids to limit the risk of acute renal failure. For severe rhabdomyolysis (serum creatine kinase > several thousands), urinary alkalinization may be considered.

Serotonin syndrome

This is characterized by agitation, hyperreflexia, hypertonia, sweating, tachycardia, and hyperpyrexia. It should be treated by withdrawal of the offending drug, diazepam, application of cooling measures. Rarely, cyproheptadine may be required.

Specific toxins
Acetaminophen

Acetaminophen is frequently taken in overdose, often with another drug or alcohol. After a latent phase, clinical features of poisoning emerge unless the antidote N-acetylcysteine has been given within 12 hours of the overdose.

Clinical features

The clinical features include nausea, vomiting, and jaundice. There may be right upper quadrant tenderness from hepatic injury and hepatic failure may occur. More rarely, renal failure may occur.

Table 13.7. Beck's depression scale

Parameter	Scoring	Beck's score (add up all those relevant below)
0	Isolation	Someone present
1		Someone nearby or in vocal contact
2		No-one nearby in visual/vocal contact
0	Timing	Intervention probable
1		Intervention not likely
2		Intervention highly unlikely
0	Precautions against discovery	None
1		Passive precautions (avoiding others)
2		Active precautions, e.g. locking door
0	Acting to gain help after the attempt	Notified potential helper regarding the attempt
1		Contacted but did not specifically notify helper regarding the attempt
2		Did not contact or notify helper
0	Final acts in the anticipation of death	None
1		Thought about or made some arrangement
2		Definite plans made, e.g. changing will
0	Active preparation for attempt	None
1		Minimal
2		Extensive
0	Suicide note	None
1		None written, written but torn up or thought about
2		Note present
0	Overt communication of intent before attempt	None
1		Equivocal communication
2		Unequivocal communication

Note:
If the sum of all the scores for each parameter is greater than 4, it indicates significant suicidal intent.

Epidemiology

Acetaminophen poisoning is the commonest cause of poisoning in the UK, accounting for up to half of all overdoses. Between 100 and 150 patients die in the UK each year as a result of hepatic injury from acetaminophen.

Pathology

Acetaminophen is converted to the toxic metabolite N-acetyl-p-benzoquinoneimine (NAPQI), which causes hepatic injury (centrilobular necrosis) once protective intracellular glutathione is depleted. If the patient is taking enzyme-inducing agents, more NAPQI is produced, or if they are glutathione depleted (e.g. anorexia), they are at greater risk from acetaminophen. The toxic dose is 150 mg/kg body weight (75 mg/kg for "at-risk" groups).

Investigations

Patients presenting with acetaminophen overdose, or an overdose of white tablets, should have a acetaminophen blood concentration checked. Those presenting late (>15 hours since ingestion) need to have liver function tests, prothrombin time (PTR) or INR, urea and electrolytes, creatinine, and arterial blood gases checked.

Management

The management of a patient with acetaminophen overdose is summarized in Fig. 13.3. If a patient presents within 1 hour of the acetaminophen overdose, activated charcoal can be given in addition to the management shown in the figure. The antidote of choice, N-acetylcysteine, provides complete protection against toxicity if given within 10 hours of the overdose; its

Has an acetaminophen overdose been taken (>75 mg acetaminophen/kg body weight ?) within the last 8 hours?

→ NO
check for other overdoses/
clinical issues

Yes

Has the overdose been taken within the last 8 hours?

→ NO

Yes

telephone NPIS (UK) for advice

Check a plasma acetaminophen level against the time since overdose when the blood sample was taken on the nomogram below. Plot high-risk patients (enzyme induction, glutathione depletion) against the "high-risk" treatment line.

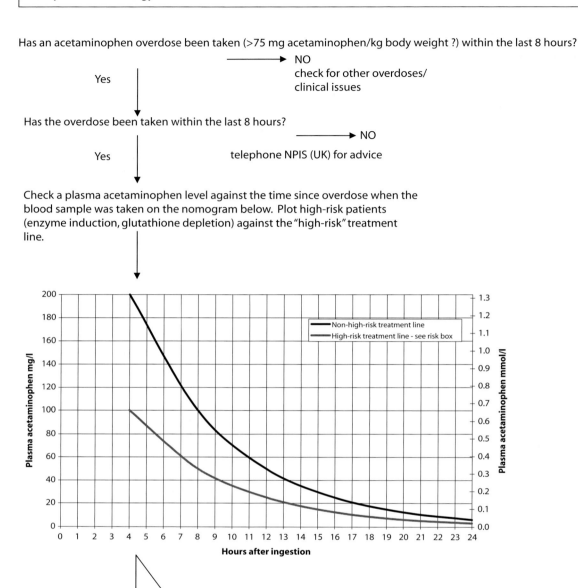

If the blood level is at/near the treatment line start treatment with the IV antidote N-acetylcysteine. Watch for anaphylactoid reactions (flushing, bronchospasm, hypotension).

If the blood level is well below the treatment line, then do not start the antidote.

Fig. 13.3. Algorithm for managing an acetaminophen overdose.

efficacy declines thereafter. If a patient presents more than 8 hours after ingestion, N-acetylcysteine administration should not be delayed to wait for the result of the acetaminophen blood concentration result but started immediately and the National Poisons Information Service phoned for advice (UK) (see references for the number). Liver transplantation should be considered in individuals who develop acute liver failure due to late acetaminophen poisoning.

If multiple ingestions of acetaminophen have taken place over several hours or days (i.e. a staggered overdose), there is no merit in measuring the plasma acetaminophen concentration as it will be uninterpretable. Such patients should be given *N*-acetylcysteine if the acetaminophen dose exceeds 150 mg/kg body weight in any one 24-hour period, or 75 mg/kg body weight in "high-risk groups."

Outcome

Patients presenting within 10 hours of the overdose who receive the full treatment with IV *N*-acetylcysteine over 20¼ hours have complete recovery and can be discharged at the end of the infusion, without further tests, provided any vomiting has settled and there is no abdominal/renal angle tenderness. Patients who present later than this have increasing risk of hepatic injury and developing fulminant hepatic failure. Some survive with ITU level care, but liver transplantation is the preferred option if a suitable donor organ is available.

Non-steroidal anti-inflammatory drugs (NSAIDs)

Mefenamic acid and ibuprofen overdose account for approximately 10% of all overdoses in the UK.

Clinical features

Most overdoses have little more than mild gastro-intestinal upset including mild abdominal pain. Vomiting and diarrhea may occur. Of patients taking a NSAID overdose (particularly mefenamic acid), 10%–20% may have fits, which are usually self-limiting. Renal failure can occur. Acidosis may occur with large ingestions. Drowsiness, lethargy, ataxia, nystagmus, blurred vision, and tachycardia may rarely occur. Serious features including coma, prolonged fits, apnea, and bradycardia are very rare. Deaths have occurred.

Epidemiology

Ingestion is particularly common among young women.

Pathology

Gastro-intestinal effects and renal effects are due to the inhibition of cyclo-oxygenase.

Investigations

Although NSAID concentrations in plasma can be measured, the half-life of the drugs in overdose is so short that it is of no clinical value to measure this. Liver and renal function tests and a full blood count should be checked in large ingestions (>10 tablets) or where there is any clinical concern.

Management

Give 50 g of activated charcoal if >100 mg/kg body weight of ibuprofen or more than 10 tablets of other NSAIDS have been taken in the last hour. Maintain the airway and assist ventilation if necessary. Treat non-self-limiting seizures with diazepam i.v. (0.1–0.2 mg/kg). Oral proton pump inhibitors such as omeprazole may ease symptoms of gastro-intestinal irritation.

Outcome

Most patients do very well and can be discharged within 12 hours. Those with complications need to be admitted for longer than this.

Tricyclic antidepressants

Tricyclic antidepressants such as amitriptyline, imipramine, and dothiepin are still commonly prescribed to depressed patients and are very toxic in overdose, deaths occurring from CVS and CNS features of the drug. Management of tricyclic antidepressant overdose is a good example of meticulous supportive care determining outcome.

Clinical features

Ingestion of more than 10 mg/kg body weight is likely to cause significant toxicity. Features include anticholinergic effects (warm, dry skin, tachycardia, blurred vision, dilated pupils, urine retention, and depressed respiration and level of consciousness), seizures, and arrhythmias. Features of severe poisoning include coma, cardiac arrhythmia, fits, and hypotension due to myocardial depression (Fig. 13.4). ECG abnormalities are common in moderate to severe poisoning, particularly prolongation of the QRS interval. Supra- and ventricular arrhythmias occur and may be the cause of sudden death. Death can occur within a few hours of admission and may result from ventricular fibrillation, intractable cardiogenic shock, or recurrent seizures.

Epidemiology

Tricyclic antidepressant overdose is the second most common overdose in the UK. It is the commonest cause of death in patients who have taken an overdose but reach hospital alive. Those most likely to present are those for whom the drug has been prescribed to treat depression.

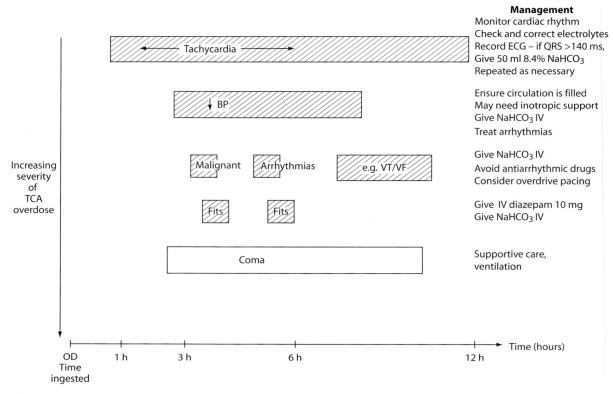

Fig. 13.4. Typical time course, severity, and management of tricyclic antidepressant overdosage.

Pathology

Toxicity is due to the anticholinergic features of the drug, together with alpha-adrenergic effects and direct myocardial depression.

Investigations

Measurement of the plasma level of a tricyclic antidepressant is not helpful in the management of an overdose. An ECG should be performed in all but the most trivial overdose. A QRS interval of >140 ms carries an increased risk of arrhythmias and fits. Arterial blood gas analysis should be performed in patients with marked symptoms and particularly in those with seizures, coma, or a widened QRS complex on ECG.

Management

Maintenance of the airway, breathing, and circulation is critical. Activated charcoal should be given if the patient has ingested more than 10 mg/kg within the last hour.

Cardiac monitoring is essential if significant ingestion (more than five tablets) has taken place and is seldom needed beyond 24 hours post-ingestion.

All anti-arrhythmic drugs are arrhythmogenic and should be avoided if possible because the patient already has potential cardiotoxicity from the tricyclic antidepressant.

Sodium bicarbonate (50 ml of 8.4% IV) should be given to all patients with QRS prolongation, arrhythmias, or hypotension (Fig. 13.4). Give repeated doses by bolus, aiming to keep the pH between 7.45 and 7.55. If multiple arrhythmias occur a transvenous pacing wire is required (Fig. 13.4). If ventricular tachycardia occurs and a pacing wire is not *in situ*, give 50–100 ml of 8.4% sodium bicarbonate IV and then lignocaine 100 mg IV.

Outcome

The elderly and those with pre-existing heart disease are at greater risk of toxicity.

5HT drugs or selective serotonin re-uptake inhibitors (SSRIs)

Antidepressant drugs such as fluoxetine, citalopram, and venlafaxine are commonly taken in overdose.

They do not have the anticholinergic actions of the tricyclic antidepressants and are thus much less cardiotoxic. In many countries, tricyclic antidepressants are being replaced with the less cardiotoxic selective serotonin re-uptake inhibitors (SSRIs). However, in large doses SSRIs can still cause toxicity.

Clinical features

Drowsiness and sinus tachycardia are the most common effects in overdose, but the extent is much less than in tricyclic antidepressant poisoning. Nausea and diarrhea are common. Seizures can occur, but are more common in venlafaxine overdose. Dizziness, tremor, agitation, bradycardia, and hypertension have been reported. The serotonin syndrome may be caused by the administration of two or more drugs that increase serotonin concentrations in the CNS or by overdose of any drug with serotonergic activity.

Epidemiology

Commonly taken in overdose, especially amongst those who have received prescriptions for the drugs.

Pathology

They act by increasing serotonin (5HT) within the CNS.

Investigations

None, unless level of consciousness is significantly impaired, e.g. Glasgow Coma Scale (GCS) <8.

Management

Supportive and symptomatic measures are required. Give 50 g activated charcoal if an adult has ingested more than 10 tablets within the last 1 hour. Observe for 6 hours. Rarely coma, hypotension, and fits will require treatment.

Outcome

5HT antidepressants cause fewer deaths in overdose than tricyclic antidepressants.

Drugs of abuse

Cannabis

The term "cannabis" refers to all psychoactive substances derived from the dried leaves and flowers of the plant *Cannabis sativa*. Marijuana refers to any part of the plant used to induce effects, and hashish is the dried resin from the flower tops.

Clinical features

When smoked, onset of relaxation and "well-being" occurs within 10–30 minutes; after ingestion the onset is 1–3 hours. The duration of effect is 4–8 hours. Low doses produce euphoria, perceptual alteration, and conjunctival injection, followed by relaxation and drowsiness, hypertension, tachycardia, slurred speech, and ataxia. High doses produce acute paranoid psychosis, anxiety, confusion, hallucinations, and distortion of time and space. Intravenous misuse of the crude extract of cannabis may cause nausea and vomiting, diarrhea, abdominal pain, fever, hypotension, pulmonary edema, acute renal failure, disseminated intravascular coagulation, and death. Psychologic dependence is common but tolerance and withdrawal symptoms are unusual.

Epidemiology

Cannabis is often smoked with tobacco and is very widely used.

Pathology

Cannabis has an active metabolite, delta-9 tetrahydrocannabinoid (Δ9THC), which is responsible for its CNS depressant effect.

Investigations

Most patients have only mild symptoms. Unless severe systemic effects are present, no investigations are needed. Cannabinoid metabolites may be detected in the urine for several days after acute exposure, but urine levels do not correlate with the degree of toxicity.

Management

For patients with drug-induced psychosis, reassurance is usually sufficient but diazepam may be used for sedation. Hypotension usually responds well to intravenous fluids. All patients who have injected cannabis should be admitted, and careful management of fluid and electrolyte balance is essential, owing to the risks of acute renal failure and pulmonary edema, which are managed conventionally.

Outcome

Serious poisoning resulting from ingestion or smoking of cannabis is extremely rare. A few deaths occur either in combination with other drugs or from IV preparations. Most patients with cannabis toxicity do not present to a medical service.

Benzodiazepines

Benzodiazepine (diazepam, clonazepam, temazepam) dependence tends to result from over-prescription. Polydrug abusers also commonly misuse these drugs.

Clinical features

Drowsiness and mid-position or dilated pupils are common and occur within 3 hours of ingestion. Ataxia, dysarthria, nystagmus, and confusion are also observed. Coma may follow, but in lone benzodiazepine overdose a GCS grade below 10 is very rare. Minor hypotension and respiratory depression may occur. Respiratory arrest is uncommon but can occur after shorter-acting agents such as midazolam.

Epidemiology

Benzodiazepines are taken alone or in combination with other agents in approximately 10% of overdose cases in the UK. Deaths occur only when they are taken with other drugs or alcohol, or if taken by a susceptible population such as the elderly or by patients with respiratory failure.

Pathology

Benzodiazepines bind at a site close to the GABA receptor in the CNS. The depressant effect on the CNS may impair respiration and induce coma.

Investigations

Benzodiazepines in the blood are hardly ever measured. There is a qualitative urine test, which tests for benzodiazepines, but again this is rarely used.

Management

Gastric lavage is not advised in pure benzodiazepine overdose. Activated charcoal, if required, can be given within 1 hour of the overdose, particularly in a mixed overdose. Impaired consciousness is treated conventionally, with particular attention to maintenance of the airway. Observation should be for at least 6 hours after ingestion of the drug, or for 24 hours in more serious cases. Oxygen saturation monitoring using a pulse oximeter is useful for ascertaining the adequacy of ventilation. Flumazenil is a specific benzodiazepine antagonist, but it is not used in the vast majority of cases of poisoning with benzodiazepines. Flumazenil must never be used in patients with a history of convulsions or toxin-induced cardiotoxicity, or in those who have co-ingested tricyclic antidepressants. In such circumstances, seizures and ventricular arrhythmias can be precipitated.

Outcome

In general, lone benzodiazepine overdoses are remarkably safe and near-full recovery takes place within 24 hours. Difficulties occur when other CNS depressants, such as tricyclic antidepressants, opioids, or alcohol, are taken in addition or when an overdose occurs in susceptible groups such as the elderly or those with chronic obstructive pulmonary disease.

Cocaine/crack cocaine

Cocaine (hydrochloride) is usually purchased as a white powder or as colorless crystals and may be sniffed or snorted using a tube into the nose, from which it is rapidly absorbed, or injected intravenously. "Crack" is cocaine that has been separated from its hydrochloride base (free-base), melted, and smoked in a pipe or mixed with tobacco in a cigarette to give a rapid onset of effect similar to intravenous use. Crack is usually sold in "rocks" containing 150 mg of cocaine or as a "line" of cocaine for snorting that contains 20–30 mg of the drug.

Clinical features

After intranasal use, the effects occur within minutes and last 20–90 minutes. Following intravenous use or oral use, the peak "high" occurs within 10 and 45–90 minutes, respectively, and after smoking crack, a peak "high" occurs within 10 minutes. In most cases the effects begin to resolve in about 20 minutes, except when taken intranasally. In fatal poisoning, the onset and progression of symptoms are accelerated and death may occur in minutes. Survival beyond 3 hours indicates that the patient is unlikely to die.

Mild to moderate intoxication with cocaine causes euphoria, agitation, aggression, cerebellar signs, dilated pupils, vomiting, pallor, headache, cold sweats, twitching, pyrexia, tachycardia, hallucinations, and hypertension. Features of severe intoxication are shown in Fig. 13.5. A toxic psychosis occurs with high levels of consumption, and tactile hallucinations (formication) may be prominent.

Epidemiology

One should consider cocaine toxicity in young healthy adults who present with symptoms of ischemic heart disease. It is no longer the pastime of the city rich but can occur in any rural or urban population.

Pathology

Cocaine has alpha activity, which causes profound hypertension. It causes vasospasm which may result in myocardial ischemia or infarction.

Investigations

Patients with features suggestive of cocaine intoxication must have their blood pressure measured early and frequently, and an ECG performed (Fig. 13.5). Those with chest pain should be investigated appropriately

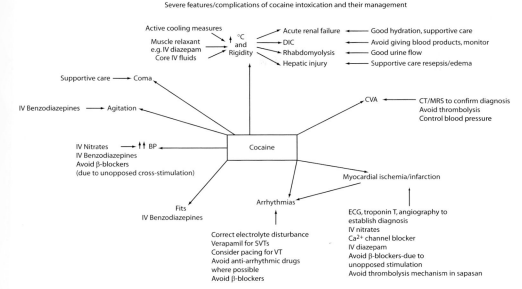

Severe features/complications of cocaine intoxication and their management

Fig. 13.5. Severe features/complications of cocaine intoxication and their management

(Fig. 13.5). Cocaine can be detected in the urine by simple drug abuse screening tests.

Management
50 g activated charcoal should be given orally to any patient presenting within 1 hour of oral ingestion, irrespective of the amount taken. All patients should be observed with ECG monitoring for a minimum of 2 hours. ECG changes can, however, be misleading in cocaine toxicity. Blood pressure, heart rate, and body temperature should also be monitored and the patient observed carefully for the development of specific complications, which should be managed as shown in Fig. 13.5.

Outcome
The toxic dose is variable and depends on individual tolerance, the presence of other drugs and the route of administration. Ingestion of any amount over 1 g is potentially fatal.

MDMA (ecstasy)
MDMA (3,4-methylenedioxymethamphetamine, ecstasy) is a "designer" amphetamine also known as E, Adam, white dove, white burger, or red and black. It is commonly taken at dance parties because it produces feelings of euphoria and emotional intimacy, together with distorted sensations. Amphetamines and the newer designer amphetamines are virtually indistinguishable in their clinical effects. There is no evidence that they are addictive.

Clinical features
Effects occur within 1 hour of ingestion and last 4–6 hours following doses of 75–150 mg but up to 48 hours after the ingestion of 100–300 mg. However, tolerance is common, and most regular users need to take considerably higher doses. Agitation or drowsiness is also common. The majority of patients who have taken ecstasy become profoundly dehydrated, but a small proportion develop hyponatremia, usually through drinking excessive amounts of water in the absence of sufficient exertion to sweat off the fluid. Antidiuretic hormone secretion may also contribute to the development of hyponatremia. Other features of intoxication with amphetamines or ecstasy include nausea, hyperreflexia, muscle pain, trismus (jaw-clenching), dilated pupils, blurred vision, sweating, dry mouth, agitation, visual hallucinations, paranoid psychosis, and anxiety. Severe intoxication is characterized by the same features as cocaine toxicity (Fig. 13.5) with perhaps less propensity for myocardial ischaemia. A serotonin-like syndrome can also be caused by ecstasy.

Epidemiology
Use of ecstasy and other amphetamines remains common in the UK. Only a small proportion of users develop problems with the drug, perhaps due to dehydration, hyperthermia, or some sort of genetic susceptibility such as a metabolic myopathy.

Pathology

Ecstasy and other amphetamines cause serotonergic neurons in the CNS to release 5HT.

Investigations

It is important to measure serum urea and electrolytes, creatine kinase, and blood glucose, a full blood count and liver function tests, and observe all symptomatic cases with ECG, blood pressure, and temperature monitoring for at least 6 hours post-exposure. A 12-lead ECG is required.

Management

The complications described above should be treated as for cocaine (see Fig. 13.5). Selective serotonergic antagonists (e.g. cyproheptadine/ketanserin) may be used to reduce temperature and rigidity by central mechanisms in those with a 5HT-like syndrome.

Outcome

Several tens of deaths have occurred from ecstasy in the UK between 2000 and 2005. Some have been due to hepatic injury, others to cerebral edema.

Opioids

These include heroin, morphine, methadone, codeine, pethidine, dihydrocodeine, and dextropropoxyphene. They give a rapid, intensely pleasurable experience, often accompanied by heightened sexual arousal. Physical dependence occurs within a few weeks of regular high-dose injection and, as a result, the dose is escalated and the addict's life becomes increasingly centered upon obtaining and taking the drug.

Clinical features of opioid overdose

Accidental overdose is common. The hallmarks of opioid analgesic poisoning are:

- depressed respiration
- pinpoint or small pupils
- depressed consciousness level
- signs of intravenous drug misuse (e.g. needle track marks)

Severe poisoning is indicated by respiratory depression, hypotension, non-cardiogenic pulmonary edema, and hypothermia. Death occurs by respiratory arrest or from aspiration of gastric contents. Poisoning with dextropropoxyphene (the opioid moiety of co-proxamol) may also result in cardiac conduction effects, particularly QRS prolongation, ventricular arrhythmias, and heart block. Symptoms of opioid poisoning can be prolonged for up to 48 hours, particularly after ingestion of methadone, which has a long half-life.

Epidemiology

Accidental overdose is common. Opioids are beginning to overtake carbon monoxide as the commonest cause of death by poisoning in the UK.

Pathology

Opioids bind to receptors in the CNS (μ and κ amongst others) and periphery, causing CNS depression, analgesia, and respiratory depression.

Investigations

Unconscious patients should always have their acetaminophen concentration checked because of the prevalence of combination opioid/acetaminophen drugs. Oxygen saturation and arterial blood gases demonstrate the adequacy of ventilation in those whose respiration has been compromised. Qualitative screening of the urine is an effective way to confirm recent use. Occasionally, measuring opioids and their metabolites in blood is required for medicolegal purposes, particularly when there is a fatality.

Management

Steps should be taken to ensure a clear airway and, if necessary, provide respiratory support. Supplementary high-flow oxygen should be administered. The need for endotracheal intubation can often be avoided by prompt administration of adequate doses of the opioid antagonist naloxone (see Fig. 13.6). Oxygen saturation monitoring and arterial blood gases demonstrate the adequacy of ventilation in those whose respiration has been compromised. The treatment of coma, fits, and hypotension is detailed elsewhere. Non-cardiogenic pulmonary edema in severe cases does not usually respond to diuretic therapy, and non-invasive ventilatory support with continuous positive airway pressure (CPAP) may be required.

Naloxone is a specific opioid antagonist that reverses the above features of opioid toxicity. Its use is shown in Fig. 13.6. Administration of too much naloxone should be avoided as it can precipitate a withdrawal reaction, characterized by gastro-intestinal effects, sweating, and fits. After the initial IV bolus, an infusion of naloxone may be needed because the half-life of the antidote is much shorter than the half-lives of most opioids. Naloxone has been reported to cause pulmonary edema and ventricular arrhythmias, but such events are infrequent and not enough to outweigh its use.

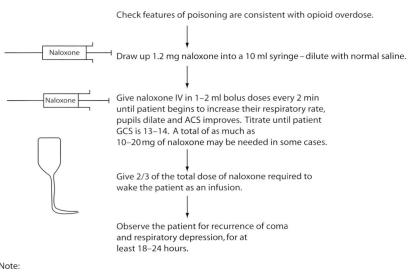

Check features of poisoning are consistent with opioid overdose.

Fig. 13.6. How to give naloxone in opioid poisoning

Draw up 1.2 mg naloxone into a 10 ml syringe – dilute with normal saline.

Give naloxone IV in 1–2 ml bolus doses every 2 min until patient begins to increase their respiratory rate, pupils dilate and ACS improves. Titrate until patient GCS is 13–14. A total of as much as 10–20 mg of naloxone may be needed in some cases.

Give 2/3 of the total dose of naloxone required to wake the patient as an infusion.

Observe the patient for recurrence of coma and respiratory depression, for at least 18–24 hours.

Note:
(1) IV is the prefered method for naloxone administration.
(2) It can be given undiluted down an endotracheal tube in emergencies.
(3) Administration of too much naloxone should be avoided because it can precipitate a withdrawal reaction, characterized by sweating and seizures.

Outcome

Most deaths occur in the community. Those reaching hospital alive usually survive.

Carbon monoxide and smoke

Carbon monoxide is a colorless, non-irritant, odorless gas; sources include smoke from fires, car exhausts, and the incomplete burning of gas fires or cookers.

Clinical features

Clinical effects from carbon monoxide exposure range from the more subtle cardiovascular and neurobehavioral effects at low ambient concentrations to unconsciousness and death after exposure to high concentrations. The early clinical features of acute carbon monoxide poisoning are headache, nausea, and vomiting (often mistaken for "gastric flu"), ataxia, and nystagmus. Later features are drowsiness, hyperventilation, hyper-reflexia, and shivering. Central and peripheral cyanosis occur. Some patients are disinhibited, agitated, or aggressive rather than drowsy. In severe cases (Fig. 13.7) convulsions, coma, hypotension, respiratory depression, ECG changes (ST segment depression, T-wave abnormalities, ventricular tachycardia, or ventricular fibrillation), and cardiovascular arrest may occur. Cerebral edema is common and focal neurologic signs can be present. Significant abnormalities on physical examination include impaired short-term memory and cerebellar signs (past-pointing and unsteadiness of gait, particularly heel–toe walking). Any one of these signs would classify the episode as severe. Rigidity, hyper-reflexia, and an extensor plantar response may occur in mild, moderate, or severe cases. Carbon monoxide poisoning in pregnancy is likely to cause miscarriage or premature labor due to fetal hypoxia. Patients recovering from carbon monoxide poisoning may suffer neurologic sequelae including tremor, personality changes, memory impairment, visual loss, inability to concentrate, and Parkinsonian features. Chronic ("low level") carbon monoxide poisoning causes symptoms which are difficult to distinguish from influenza, i.e. nausea, vomiting, headache, lethargy, and aches and pains. Angina may become more severe. Neurobehavioral effects may be seen, especially in the aged. Behavior that requires sustained attention or performance is most sensitive to disruption by carbon monoxide.

Epidemiology

The risk of carbon monoxide poisoning is greatest where surrounding air ventilation is poor, particularly in the home. As well as carbon monoxide, smoke produced in house fires contains a mixture of soot and organic particles, together with other gases such as hydrogen sulfide. Carbon monoxide is the most common cause of death by poisoning in the UK and many other countries.

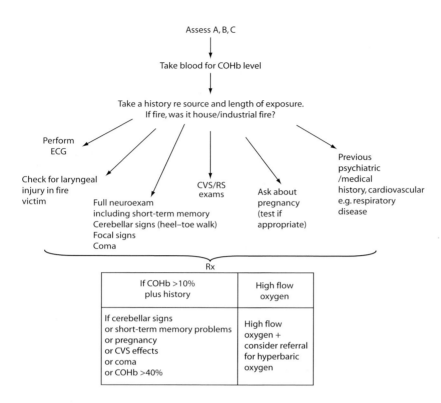

Assess A, B, C

↓

Take blood for COHb level

↓

Take a history re source and length of exposure.
If fire, was it house/industrial fire?

Perform
ECG

Check for laryngeal
injury in fire
victim

Full neuroexam
including short-term memory
Cerebellar signs (heel–toe walk)
Focal signs
Coma

CVS/RS
exams

Ask about
pregnancy
(test if
appropriate)

Previous
psychiatric
/medical
history, cardiovascular
e.g. respiratory
disease

Rx

If COHb >10% plus history	High flow oxygen
If cerebellar signs or short-term memory problems or pregnancy or CVS effects or coma or COHb >40%	High flow oxygen + consider referral for hyperbaric oxygen

Fig. 13.7. Assessing and managing a carbon monoxide poisoned patient.

Pathology

Carbon monoxide reduces the oxygen-carrying capacity of the blood by binding to hemoglobin to form carboxyhemoglobin (COHb), and impairs the function of cytochrome oxidases. This impairs oxygen delivery from blood to tissues and its utilization within tissues. It acts as a chemical asphyxiant.

Investigations

The carboxyhemoglobin (COHb) concentration is of value in confirming the diagnosis of acute carbon monoxide poisoning, although it may not be elevated sufficiently to be diagnostic in chronic cases. However, the degree of COHb elevation measured at hospital does not correlate well with the severity of poisoning, even acutely. This is because blood COHb concentrations fall rapidly on cessation of exposure and patients may also receive oxygen therapy in ambulances whilst being transferred to hospitals. Normal values are up to 3%–5% and can be as high as 6%–10% in smokers; COHb levels below 10% are not usually associated with symptoms. An ECG should be performed in anyone with acute poisoning, especially in patients with pre-existing heart disease. Serious poisoning also requires arterial blood gas

analysis. Oxygen saturation readings by pulse oximetry are misleading (see below).

Management

The most important first step in treating carbon monoxide poisoning is to move the patient away from the source of exposure. It is vital to ensure that the airway, breathing, and circulation are adequately maintained and give supplementary oxygen as soon as possible. The half-life of COHb whilst breathing air ranges from 4–6 hours. On 100% oxygen at ambient pressure, the half-life of COHb is reduced to approximately 40 min. Thus, oxygen should be given in high flow, e.g. 12 liters per minute, ideally through a tightly fitting facemask such as a CPAP mask. It should be continued until the COHb is less than 5% and for at least 6 hours after exposure. Sometimes 12–20 hours are required for this to take place. Unfortunately, pulse oximeters measure both carboxyhemoglobin and oxyhemoglobin and so a normal saturation value does not give grounds for reassurance. Care should be taken to avoid excessive intravenous fluid administration, particularly in the elderly, because of the risk of pulmonary edema. Most deaths occur in those who have arrested at the scene or who are unconscious on arrival at hospital. Blood pressure should be monitored and convulsions controlled with diazepam.

The use of hyperbaric oxygen is controversial; Figure 13.7 lists the current indications for considering such therapy. The theoretical value of hyperbaric oxygen is that at 2.5 atmospheres the half-life of COHb is reduced to 20 minutes and it also increases the amount of dissolved oxygen by about ten times. The logistic difficulties of transporting sick patients to hyperbaric chambers should not be under-estimated.

Outcome
Carbon monoxide remains the commonest cause of death by poisoning in the UK. Both acute and chronic exposure can result in serious neurologic sequelae.

Alcohol/ethanol
Ethanol is found not just in alcoholic drinks but in many household preparations, e.g. mouthwash and antiseptics.

Clinical features
The fatal dose of absolute ethanol is 6–10 ml/kg body weight. Ethanol is rapidly absorbed and generally absorption is 80%-90% complete in 1 hour. Mild effects (blood alcohol <1.5 g/l) include impaired co-ordination and reaction time. Moderate effects (blood alcohol 1.5–3 g/l) include dysarthria, ataxia, diplopia, flushing, sweating, and tachycardia. Severe effects (blood alcohol 3–5 g/l) include hypothermia, drowsiness progressing to coma and metabolic acidosis, and respiratory or circulatory arrest. Severe hypoglycemia may lead to convulsions.

Epidemiology
Ethanol is commonly taken with other drugs in overdose.

Pathology
Ethanol has a CNS depressant effect. Its effect is additive with other CNS depressant drugs.

Investigations
Blood or breath alcohol level should be determined if the patient is symptomatic. At blood alcohol levels of >1.5 g/l all patients should have urea and electrolytes, glucose, and ABGs performed.

Management
Gastric lavage is not useful as ethanol is rapidly absorbed and activated charcoal does not absorb alcohol. Observation is recommended for at least 4 hours post-ingestion, or until the patient is asymptomatic. Protect the airway to prevent aspiration. Intubation and ventilation may be required for respiratory depression. Ensure the patient is well hydrated. Acidosis will usually respond to correction of the hypoglycemia and hypovolemia but additional sodium bicarbonate may occasionally be required. Convulsions usually respond to the correction of hypoglycemia. Diazepam 10 mg IV may occasionally be necessary. Supportive care is usually enough and hemodialysis should be reserved for life-threatening cases. It should be considered if the blood ethanol level is >5 g/l or arterial pH <7.0.

Outcome
With supportive care, most ethanol poisoned patients recover within 12 hours.

Further reading
American Academy of Clinical Toxicology & European Association of Poisons Control Centres and Clinical Toxicologists. Position statement: Single-dose activated charcoal. *J Toxicol Clin Toxicol* 1997; **35**, 721–741.

American Academy of Clinical Toxicology; European Association of Poisons Centres and Clinical Toxicologists. Position statement and practice guidelines on the use of multi-dose activated charcoal in the treatment of acute poisoning. *J Toxicol Clin Toxicol* 1999; **37**(6), 731–751.

Flanagan RJ, Jones AL. *Antidotes*. London: Taylor-Francis 2001.

Jones A, Dargan P. *Churchill's Pocketbook of Toxicology*. Churchill Livingstone 2001.

Wallace CI, Dargan PI & Jones AL. Paracetamol overdose: an evidence based flowchart to guide management. *Emerg Med J* 2002; **19**, 202–205.

Wu AH, McKay C, Broussard LA *et al*. National Academy of Clinical Biochemistry Laboratory Medicine Practice Guidelines: recommendations for the use of laboratory tests to support poisoned patients who present to the emergency department. *Clin Chem* 2003; **49**(3), 357–379.

UK National Poisons Information Service 0870 600 6266; database TOXBASE®.

Sexually transmissible infections

Andrew de Burgh-Thomas and Jan Welch

Contents

Introduction

Sexually transmissible infections (STIs) are common and rates are increasing in the UK. The highest incidence occurs in inner city areas where socio-economic, educational, cultural, and ethnic factors contribute to frequent partner change.

Sexually transmissible infections involve at least three people, the individual with the infection, the person from whom they caught it, and that person's other partner or partners. As STIs are often asymptomatic, especially in women, partner notification is crucial to prevent both reinfection and the sequelae of ongoing infection. STIs are often multiple and finding one should prompt the search for others; they have also been shown to facilitate the transmission of HIV infection.

Common presentations of sexually transmitted infections are discharge, lumps, sores, rashes, or pain in the pelvis (women) or testes (men). Other conditions can present similarly, so a careful sexual history is an important factor in determining the most likely diagnosis.

The aims of management are to alleviate physical and emotional distress, to resolve or ameliorate infection, and to offer education and advice to protect both the patient and others from future harm. Any potential for embarrassment can be minimized by a competent and non-judgmental approach.

Discharge is a common presentation in both men and women, although the causes are very different. Men presenting with urethral discharge commonly have a sexually transmitted infection such as chlamydia, gonorrhea, or non-specific urethritis. Although vaginal discharge frequently has an infective cause, such infections are uncommonly sexually acquired causes of discharge:

Urethral (males):
Non-specific urethritis
Chlamydia
Gonorrhea
Vaginal (females):
Physiologic*
Bacterial vaginosis*
Candidiasis*
Trichomoniasis

Urethral discharge – men
What to look for when a man complains of discharge (Fig. 14.1)

Urethral discharge is a common presentation in men. Associated symptoms are **dysuria** (a stinging sensation on passing urine) and **urethral irritation** (itching or burning in the urethra). Common causes are

---

* *Not sexually acquired*

History	Examination
Age	Overt discharge, staining of underwear
Duration: days to weeks	Meatitis
Quantity: mild or profuse	Testicular tenderness/swelling
Colour: clear/white or yellow	
Itching or tingling	
Pain on passing urine	
Nocturia/urgency/hematuria	
Testicular pain	
Symptoms elsewhere, e.g. eyes, joints	
Recent unprotected sex, especially new partner	

chlamydia and gonorrhea, although some men have these infections without signs or symptoms. Other urinary symptoms such as frequency, urgency, and nocturia can suggest additional causes such as urinary tract infection and diabetes mellitus.

Gonorrhea

Gonorrhea causes urethritis and cervicitis, asymptomatic throat infections, and proctitis. It can be diagnosed immediately by microscopy in the majority of men but only 50% of women.

Clinical features

- Men with gonorrhea usually present with sudden onset profuse yellow/green urethral discharge (80%) and dysuria (50%) but may be asymptomatic (<10%).

- Women are commonly asymptomatic (up to 50%), so their infection is frequently diagnosed as the result of screening or partner notification. Women may complain of vaginal discharge, lower abdominal pain, or dysuria.

- Rectal infection (proctitis) may result from receptive anal intercourse in both men and women, or from self-inoculation from cervical and/or urethral infection, for example, via fingers or toilet paper. Proctitis may be asymptomatic or associated with rectal discharge, pain, or discomfort (proctalgia).

- Pharyngeal infections are usually asymptomatic (>90%).

- Eye infection can result from auto-inoculation, e.g. by fingers, and usually causes intense pain and redness together with a profuse purulent discharge. If not properly treated, ocular infection can perforate the globe.

- Complications in men include epididymo-orchitis (pain and swelling of the epididymis and testis)

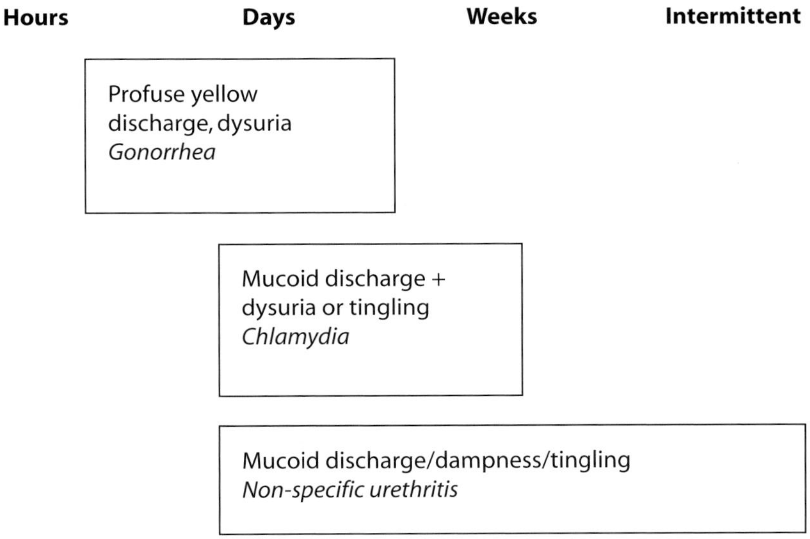

Hours	Days	Weeks	Intermittent

Profuse yellow discharge, dysuria
Gonorrhea

Mucoid discharge + dysuria or tingling
Chlamydia

Mucoid discharge/dampness/tingling
Non-specific urethritis

Fig. 14.1. Likely diagnosis of urethral discharge based on presentation.

401

Table 14.1. The management of gonorrhea (GC)

Infection	Screening	Treatment	Guide to partners within
Gonorrhea (GC)	Test for chlamydia and gonorrhea prior to treatment	400 mg cefixime stat	• 3 months if patient asymptomatic • 2 weeks from onset of symptoms

and infection of the glands within the frenulum (tysonitis).

- Complications in women include infection of the secretory glands of the labia majora (Bartholinitis), ascending infection of the Fallopian tubes (salpingitis), and pelvic inflammatory disease (PID).
- Systemic complications of gonorrhea, such as rash and arthritis, are uncommon.
- Mother to child transmission can result in neonatal ophthalmia presenting usually days after birth.
- Gonorrhea in an older child is strongly suggestive of child sexual abuse.

Epidemiology

Gonorrhea is associated with recent new sexual partners, lack of condom use, and total number of sexual partners. It is more common in young black men and women from socioeconomically disadvantaged areas and men who have sex with other men.

The incubation period is 2–10 days.

Pathology

Gonorrhea is caused by a Gram-negative intracellular bacterium, named *Neisseria gonorrhoeae*. It is a diplococcus more commonly known as the "gonococcus." It is a delicate organism, best grown at 35 °C on nutrient agar plates containing a selective growth medium incubated in an atmosphere enriched with 5% carbon dioxide. *N. gonorrhoeae* is distinguished from other *Neisseria* species such as *Neisseria meningitides* by tests of sugar utilisation.

The gonococcus infects susceptible mucous membranes lined by columnar or cubical epithelium such as the urethra, cervix, rectum, and pharynx, or immature epithelium. The stratified epithelium of the mature vulva and vagina is not susceptible, and so it does not cause vaginal infection in women. A high vaginal swab can miss an infection that a cervical sample would identify. In prepubertal girls the immature epithelium can be infected which results in symptomatic vulvo-vaginitis with discharge.

Investigations

Samples are usually taken from the urethra in men and the cervix and urethra of women; sampling of additional sites such as the rectum and pharynx will depend on the sexual history. Urethral specimens are taken with a smooth plastic loop or tiny swab inserted into the tip causing momentary discomfort. The sample is smeared onto a slide and spread onto a culture plate. The slide is examined by microscopy for the presence of the Gram-negative intracellular diplococci, together with pus cells, on which the preliminary diagnosis is made.

Culture confirms the diagnosis and permits antibiotic resistance to be identified. Nucleic acid amplification tests (NAATs) can identify both chlamydia and gonorrhea from a *"first pass"* urine sample in men or a cervical/vulvo-vaginal swab in women. The NAAT test does not provide information on antibiotic sensitivity.

Management

A single dose of cefixime is sufficient to cure urethral, cervical, or ano-rectal infection, although pharyngeal infection may require further treatment. It can be given in the clinic and be directly observed. The antibiotic used will depend on local current resistance patterns. Concurrent chlamydial infection occurs in 40% and is treated at the same time. Women should be advised that antibiotics may reduce the effectiveness of oral contraception.

Partner notification is vital to prevent reinfection and reduce the pool of infection in the community. Early detection and treatment of infection minimizes the potential for damage to the fertility of women. Patients should be advised to abstain from sex until they and their partners have completed treatment (Table 14.1).

Outcome

First-line treatment should cure at least 95% of genital gonorrhea. Persistent symptoms may be due to re-infection from an untreated partner, or due to resistant infection.

Table 14.2. The management of chlamydia infection

Infection	Screening	Treatment	Guide to partners within
Chlamydia	Test for chlamydia and gonorrhea prior to treatment	Azithromycin l g stat or doxycycline 100 mg 7/7	• 6 months if patient asymptomatic • 4 weeks from onset of symptoms

Chlamydia

Chlamydia trachomatis (CT) is a common genital infection, being found in 10%–15% of sexually active young women in the UK. It is a common cause of male urethritis, but most women and about half of men are asymptomatic.

Clinical features

- The classic presentation of chlamydial infection is a man with a mucoid urethral discharge and dysuria. Fifty percent of men are asymptomatic.
- Eighty percent of women are asymptomatic; symptoms may include post-coital/intermenstrual bleeding, lower abdominal pain, or purulent vaginal discharge.
- Adult eye infection can result from auto-inoculation, e.g. by fingers.
- Rectal infection is usually asymptomatic, but may cause pain or discomfort and anal discharge (proctitis).
- A complication in the male is epididymo-orchitis; in the female pelvic inflammatory disease and Fitz-Hugh-Curtis syndrome (perihepatitis).
- Reiter's syndrome (reactive artritis) is the triad of urethritis, conjunctivitis, and arthritis; additional features include penile rash (circinate balanitis) and keratotic rash on the feet (keratoderma blennorrhagica).
- Maternal carriage of CT can result in neonatal infection of the eye or lung (ophthalmitis or pneumonitis). Partner notification is therefore crucial.

Epidemiology

The prevalence is 15% in those under age 20. Risk factors are age <25, a new sexual partner. Condoms are protective. It is the largest preventable cause of subfertility and ectopic pregnancy. The damage can be silent and permanent damage increases exponentially with subsequent infection.

Pathology

Chlamydia trachomatis is a small obligate intracellular bacterium, which characteristically infects the urethra, cervix, rectum, or eye. It is not visible on conventional Gram staining. Chlamydia must be diagnosed either in cell culture, which is laborious and now rarely used, or by colorimetric enzyme immunoassays, or by using the newer nucleic acid amplification tests (NAATs).

Investigations

Samples depend on available tests; swabs and transport media vary. Ideal are those with high specificity and sensitivity such as NAAT. Specimen collection is non-intrusive *"first pass"* urine for men and self-collected vulvo-vaginal swabs from women. Cervical and urethral swabs require skill and time.

Management

Uncomplicated infection – single dose azithromycin. Seven-day course doxycycline is cheaper but adherence reduced. Alcohol may worsen urethral symptoms.

A longer course of treatment is used for complicated infection such as epididymo-orchitis or pelvic inflammatory disease. Women should be advised that the antibiotics used reduce the effectiveness of combined oral contraception.

Patients should be provided with information about the importance of sexual contacts being treated. Partner notification is vital. Patients should be advised to abstain from sex until they and their partners have completed treatment (Table 14.2).

Outcome

Short-term is excellent, although improvement may be slow in men. Reassurance that slow resolution of symptoms do not mean persistent infection minimizes frequent attendances. Repeat chlamydia infection months later may identify reinfection, from an untreated partner.

Non-specific urethritis

Non-gonococcal specific urethritis (NSU) is a diagnosis only made in men, as white cells are often present in the female urethra. Characteristically, a man presents with discharge and/or dysuria, and on

microscopy an excess of polymorphonuclear leukocytes (PMN) is found in the urethra, but no Gram-
negative diplococci.

Clinical features

- Urethral discharge is usually less profuse than
  in gonorrhea, and mucoid rather than purulent
- Dysuria or urethral irritation is commonly present

Epidemiology and pathology

The underlying cause varies with the population and
whether a first or recurrent presentation. *Chlamydia
trachomatis* can be found in 50% of first episodes, *Urea-
plasma urealyticum* and *Mycoplasma genitalium* in
10%–20%, respectively, and *Trichomonas vaginalis*. In
1%–17%. Less common causes include herpes simplex,
candida, urinary tract infection, and non-infective
causes: urethral stricture, foreign body, or psychosexual
problems. No infection is identified in 20%–30%.

Investigations

In men a sample from the anterior urethra is examined as for gonorrhea. Diagnosis is made when at least
five PMN are found on high-power microscopy without gonococci; the test is less sensitive if urine has
been passed within the previous 4 hours.

Samples should also be sent for chlamydia and
gonorrhea culture.

Management

As for chlamydia. Information about NSU should be
provided, with advice about partner notification and
abstinence from intercourse until treatment of partner.

Outcome

About 20% of men with NSU develop persistent or
recurrent symptoms; chlamydia is rarely found. Urea-
plasmas and *M. genitalium* may be responsible, so
symptomatic patients are treated with erythromycin
or a longer course of azithromycin and metronidazole
for *Trichomonas vaginalis*. Further treatment is usually unnecessary provided that re-infection has been
excluded; men should be reassured and discouraged
from urethral massage or use of disinfectants as these
can perpetuate symptoms.

Vaginal discharge

What to consider when a woman complains of vaginal discharge

Some vaginal discharge is normal (physiological discharge). It varies throughout the menstrual cycle.

Vaginal discharge is likely to be caused by infection
if it is itchy, sore, smelly, or profuse. It may be precipitated by alterations in normal vaginal flora caused
by antibiotics.

Discharge is often associated with dysuria.
Women can distinguish between **internal dysuria**,
affecting the urethra, for example from chlamydia,
and **external dysuria due to vulval** stinging from
candida (Fig. 14.2).

Management of vaginal discharge is described in
Table 14.3.

History	Examination
New/recurrent	Vulval redness/edema
Relationship to menstrual cycle	Splits in skin
Itching	Characteristics of discharge, e.g. profuse, odor, homogeneous, frothy
Smell: fishy/yeasty	
Quantity: mild/profuse	
Soreness/dysuria	
Method of contraception	
Sexual history	
Recent antibiotics	

Bacterial vaginosis

Bacterial vaginosis (BV) or *Gardnerella vaginalis*, is
the commonest cause of vaginal discharge in women
of child-bearing age. Men are not affected.

Clinical features

Women with BV complain of a discharge and an
unpleasant fishy odor usually worsened by sexual
intercourse, but usually no soreness. Half have no
symptoms. On examination there is no inflammation,
but a grayish-white discharge. The characteristic
aroma is caused by anaerobes.

Epidemiology

BV is not sexually transmitted but is more common
in the sexually active, especially if other STIs are
present. Risk factors for BV include younger age,
black ethnicity, douching, multiple male partners, or
at least one female partner in the past year, a past
pregnancy, and smoking. Hormonal contraception
that reduces menstrual loss and condoms reduce
the risk.

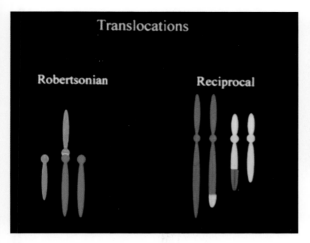

Fig. 1.2. Figurative examples of Robertsonian and reciprocal translocations.

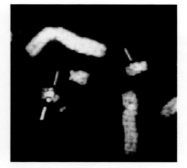

Fig. 1.3. In the FISH study, probes for specific DNA sequences on the chromosome of interest are labeled with a fluorescent dye. The probe is hybridized with the DNA sequences on a slide and analyzed under the fluorescent microscope. In a normal cell, two signals should be detected. If only one signal is present, it denotes missing information or deletion. This can be used to detect deletions at the ends of the chromosomes (telomeres) or within the chromosome (interstitial).

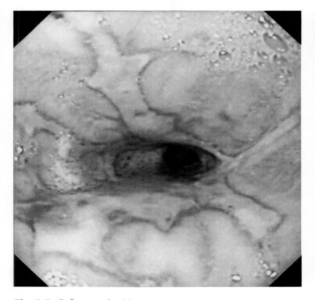

Fig. 3.7. Reflux esophagitis.

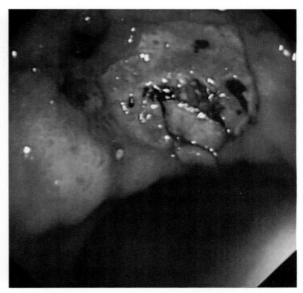

Fig. 3.10. Endoscopic appearance of gastric cancer.

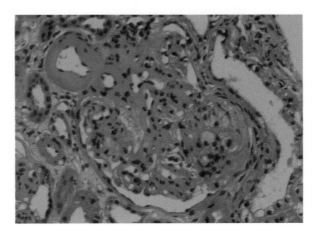

Fig. 4.3. Glomerulus from a patient with diabetic nephropathy showing hyalinosis of the afferent and efferent arterioles (top left), diffuse mesangial expansion, and a secondary sclerosing lesion (bottom right) (H and E ×200).

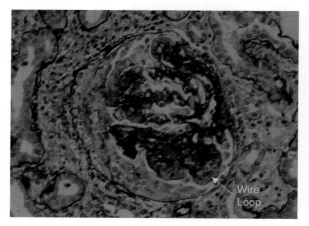

Fig. 4.4. Glomerulus showing a diffuse proliferative lupus nephritis with a wire loop in the capillary wall (arrow), and a crescent (PAS ×200).

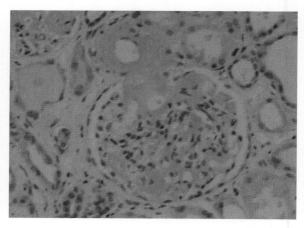

Fig. 4.6. Congo red stain of a glomerulus in a case of amyloidosis demonstrating amyloid deposition in the arteriole and mesangium (Congo red ×200).

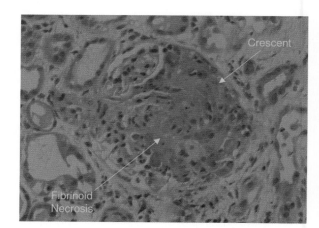

Fig. 4.10. Glomerulus in a case of systemic vasculitis showing fibrinoid necrosis (long arrow) and a crescent (short arrow) (H and E ×200).

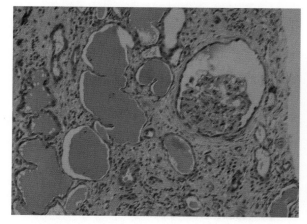

Fig. 4.5. Renal biopsy of a case of HIV-associated nephropathy (HIVAN). The glomerulus is collapsed leaving a large acellular Bowman's space. The tubules show gross microcystic dilatation and contain pink amorphous casts. There is marked tubulointerstitial fibrosis (H and E ×100).

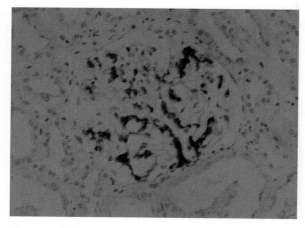

Fig. 4.15. IgA mesangial deposits (immunoperoxidase ×200).

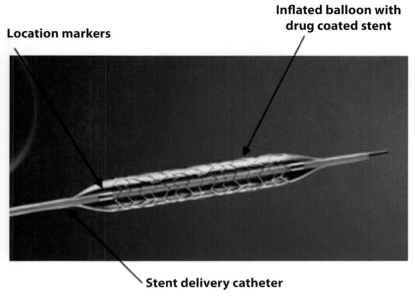

Location markers

Inflated balloon with drug coated stent

Stent delivery catheter

Fig. 5.9. Close-up view of a coronary artery stent.

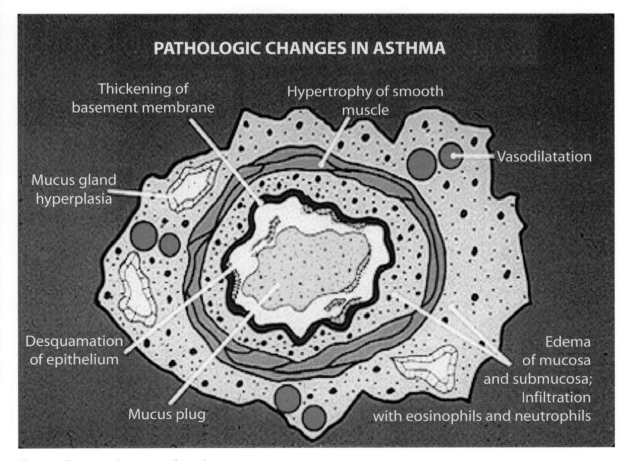

PATHOLOGIC CHANGES IN ASTHMA

Thickening of basement membrane

Hypertrophy of smooth muscle

Vasodilatation

Mucus gland hyperplasia

Desquamation of epithelium

Mucus plug

Edema of mucosa and submucosa; Infiltration with eosinophils and neutrophils

Fig. 6.2. Changes in the airway wall in asthma.

Fig. 7.2. Operative view of the middle ear demonstrating cholesteatoma (arrowed) with its characteristic skin-like appearance.

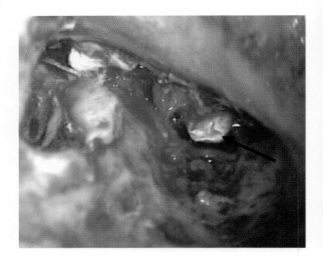

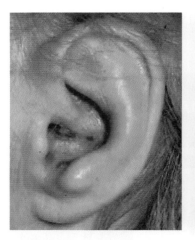

Fig. 7.4. Vesicles of the pinna characteristic of Ramsey–Hunt syndrome.

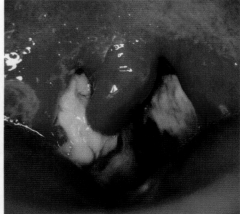

Fig. 7.6. Infected tonsils covered in slough – characteristic of glandular fever.

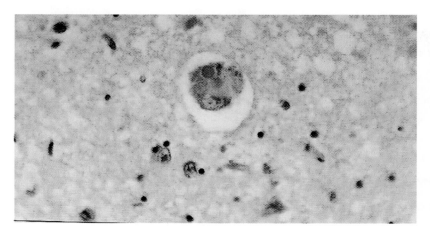

Fig. 9.11. Photomicrograph of a Lewy body (hematoxylin–eosin stain).

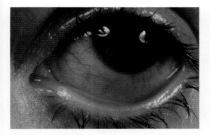

Fig. 10.2. Episcleritis (courtesy of Mr. P. Hamilton).

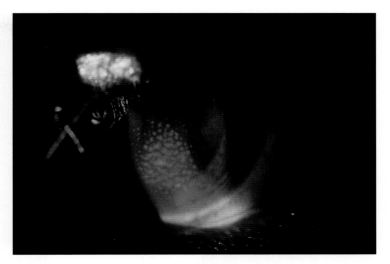

Fig. 10.3. Keratic precipitates (courtesy of Professor M. Stanford).

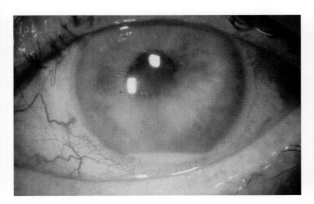

Fig. 10.4. Hypopyon (courtesy of Mr. P. Hamilton).

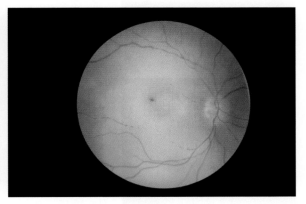

Fig. 10.9. Central retinal artery occlusion (courtesy of Mr. P. Hamilton).

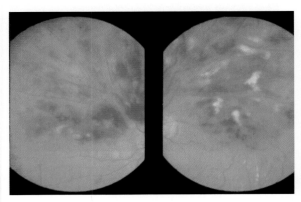

Fig. 10.10. Branch retinal artery occlusion with cotton wool spots (courtesy of Mr. P. Hamilton).

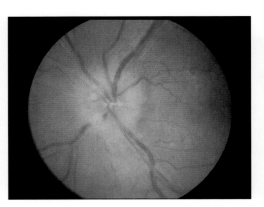

Fig. 10.11. Swollen optic disk (courtesy of Mr. P. Hamilton).

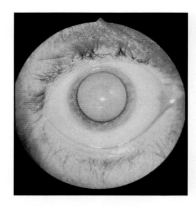

Fig. 10.12. Cataract (courtesy of Mr. P. Hamilton).

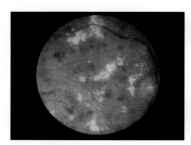

Fig. 10.14. Diabetic retinopathy with hemorrhages and exudates (courtesy of Mr. P. Hamilton).

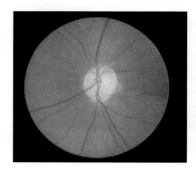

Fig. 10.15. Optic atrophy (courtesy of Mr. P. Hamilton).

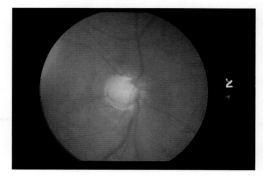

Fig. 10.16. Cupped optic disk (courtesy of Mr. P. Hamilton).

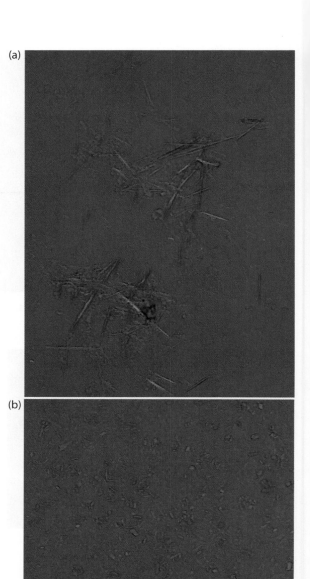

Fig. 11.2. Examples of synovial fluid crystals under polarizing microscopy. Sample from a tophus. The crystals lie within leukocytes aspirated from a swollen joint. (a) monosodium urate in gout (b) calcium pyrophosphate in pseudogout.

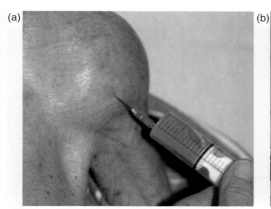

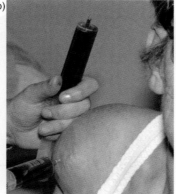

Fig. 11.4. Shoulder aspiration
(a) purulent synovial fluid in septic arthritis
(b) blood in hemarthrosis.

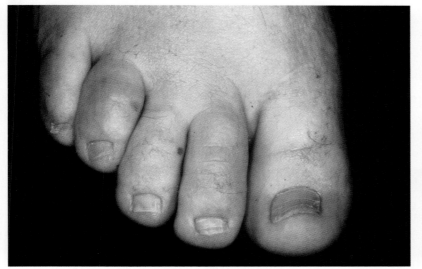

Fig. 11.11. Dactylitis (sausage) fourth toe in psoriatic arthritis.

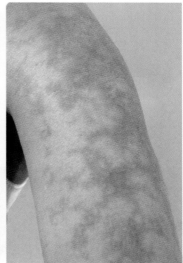

Fig. 11.14. Severe blotchiness of the skin (livedo reticularis) in a patient with SLE.

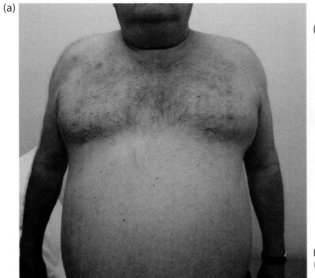

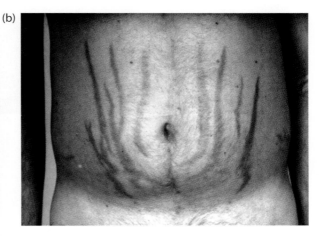

Fig. 12.3. (a) Central obesity, Proximal muscle wasting, (b) Characteristic highly colored striae of Cushing's syndrome.

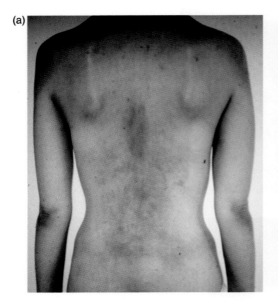

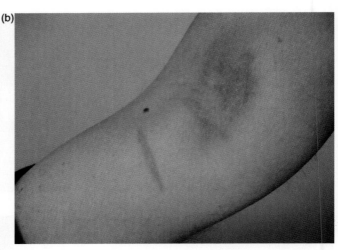

Fig. 12.9. (a) Patchy pigmentation in a patient with newly diagnosed Addison's disease. This patient had lost 20 kg in weight, had severe postural hypotension, a serum sodium of 122 and potassium of 7.8 mmol/l. Note the pigmentation over the pressure points on the elbows. (b) Pigmentation in a scar of a patient with Addison's disease.

Fig. 12.10. Vitiligo of the hands in a patient with Addison's disease.

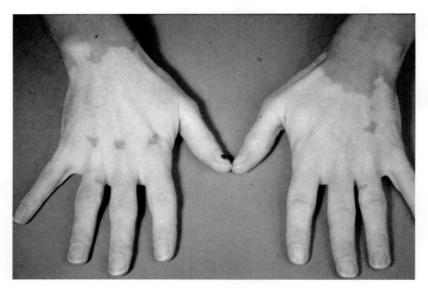

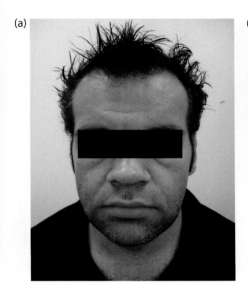

(a)

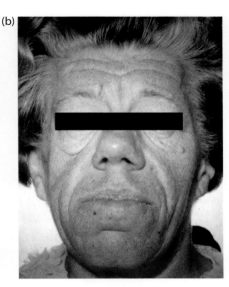

(b)

Fig. 12.16. (a), (b) Facial features of two patients with acromegaly showing generalized coarse features due to thickening of the soft tissues. There is particular enlargement of the nose, lips, and mandible (prognathism) in patient (b).

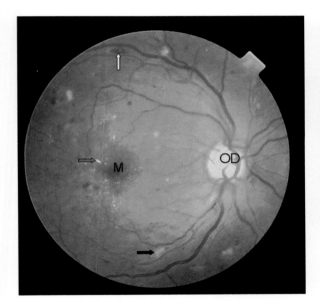

Fig. 12.17. Retinal photograph showing pre-proliferative retinopathy. OD = optic disk, M = macula, top arrow = intra-retinal hemorrhage, middle arrow = hard exudates, bottom arrow = cotton wool spot of retinal ischemia.

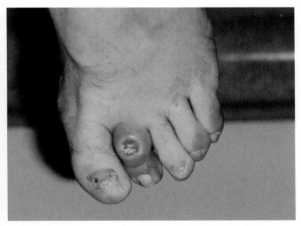

Fig. 12.18. Typical neuropathic ulcer in a patient with diabetes due to peripheral sensory neuropathy and deformity of the toe resulting in pressure on footwear and ulceration. There is swelling and redness of the toe indicating infection.

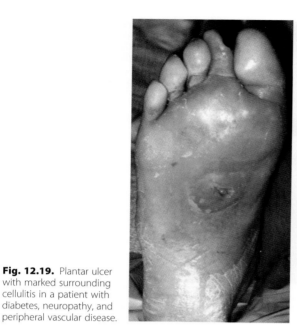

Fig. 12.19. Plantar ulcer with marked surrounding cellulitis in a patient with diabetes, neuropathy, and peripheral vascular disease.

Fig. 12.20. Dry gangrene of the first and third toes in a patient with diabetes, peripheral neuropathy, and peripheral vascular disease.

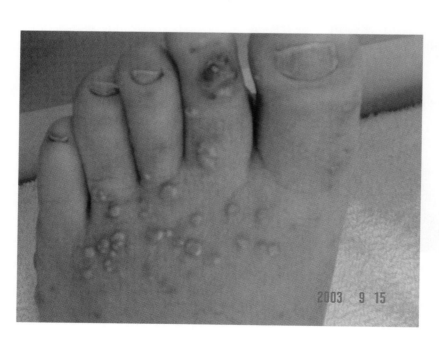

Fig. 12.22. Eruptive xanthomata on the feet of a patient with severe hypertriglyceridemia.

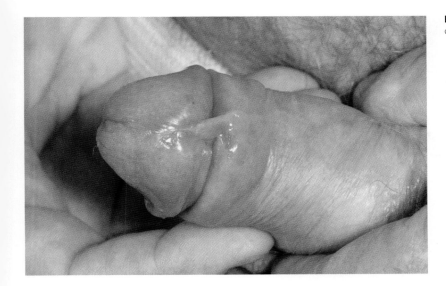

Fig. 14.5. Primary infection characterized by syphilic chancre.

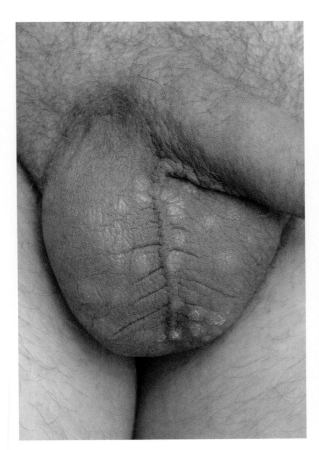

Fig. 14.6. Secondary syphilis: papulo-squamous lesions on scrotum.

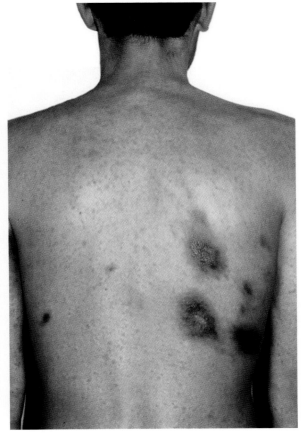

Fig. 14.13. Kaposi's sarcoma (KS) on back.

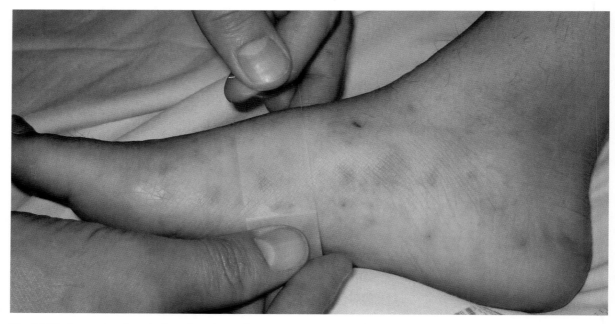

Fig. 15.10. A purpuric rash on the foot of a patient with meningococcemia. Typically, the rash does not blanch on pressure, as demonstrated with the glass slide.

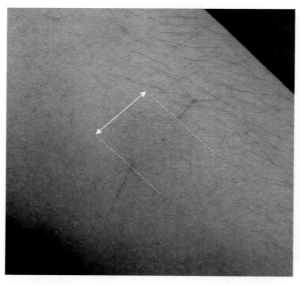

Fig. 15.12. A positive Mantoux skin result, 48 hours following a 2U intradermal injection of purified protein derivative into the flexor aspect of the forearm. The amount of skin induration (not erythema) was measured at 22 mm. (The ball-point pen marks, which have been used to delineate the extent of induration, can also be seen.)

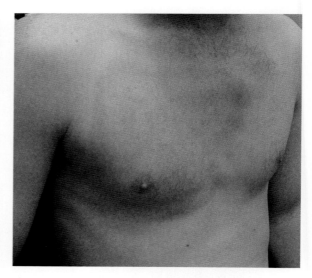

Fig. 15.13. The characteristic rash of Erythema migrans in a patient with early Lyme disease. Eight weeks before this developed, the patient had been walking through forested areas in Scotland and afterwards had discovered ticks attached to the skin on his chest. He was treated effectively with oral doxycycline.

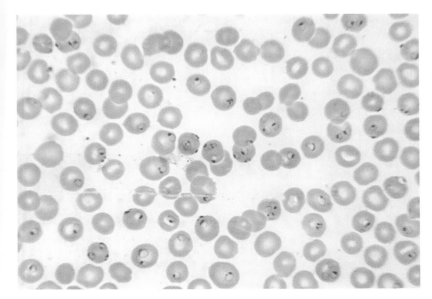

Fig. 15.17. A thin film showing multiple "ring forms" or trophozoites of *Plasmodium falciparum* within red cells. Some red cells contain more than one parasite, which is a unique property of this species of malaria parasite.

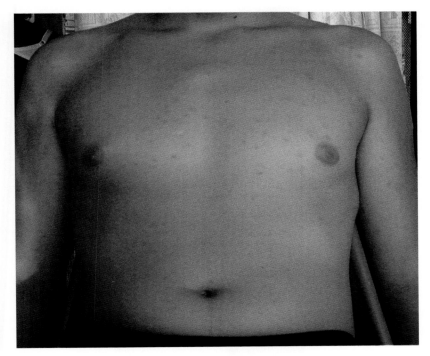

Fig. 15.18. A young boy presented with fever, conjunctivitis, and this maculopapular skin rash. Whilst on a family holiday in Sardinia a couple of weeks before, he had been removing ticks from a dog. Boutonneuse fever (*Rickettsia connori*) was diagnosed clinically and later confirmed by serology. He was treated with doxycycline and made an excellent recovery.

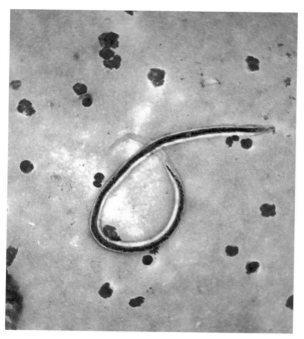

Fig. 15.19. A stained blood film taken from a patient at midnight showing microfilaria of *Wuchereria bancrofti*. The patient was from Guyana and presented with chyluria secondary to megalymphatics of the thighs and pelvis.

(a)

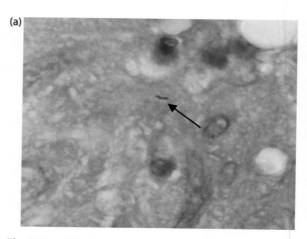

Fig. 15.21. (a) Daily temperature chart from an African patient with an FUO. (b) Disseminated tuberculosis was eventually diagnosed following a bone marrow biopsy, which revealed a granulomas containing acid-fast bacilli, indicated by the arrow.

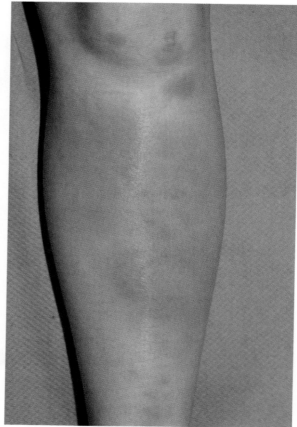

Fig. 16.2. Erythema nodosum.

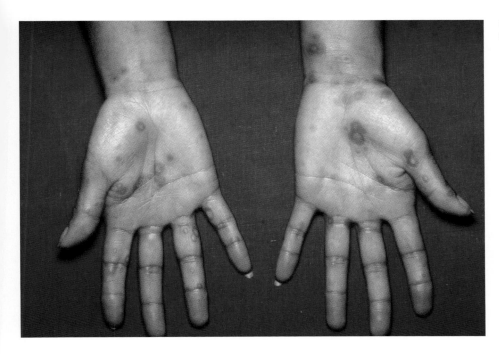

Fig. 16.3. Target lesions of erythema multiforme.

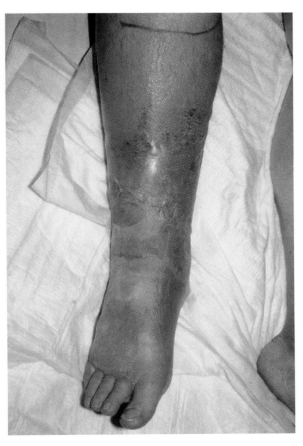

Fig. 16.4. Cellulitis.

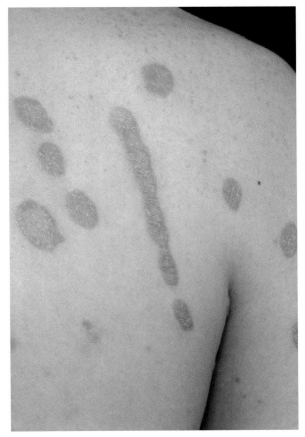

Fig. 16.6. Red, raised, well-demarcated patches of psoriasis exhibiting the Koebner phenomenon.

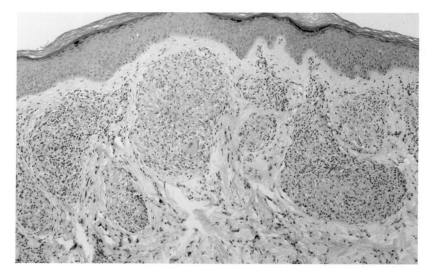

Fig. 16.8. Sarcoidal granulomas in the dermis.

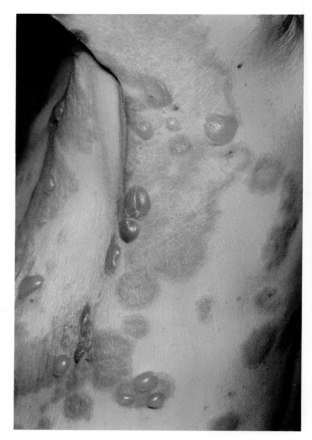

Fig. 16.9. Bullous pemphigoid.

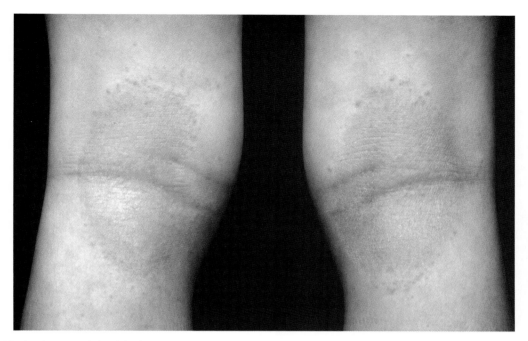

Fig. 16.11. Atopic eczema behind the knees.

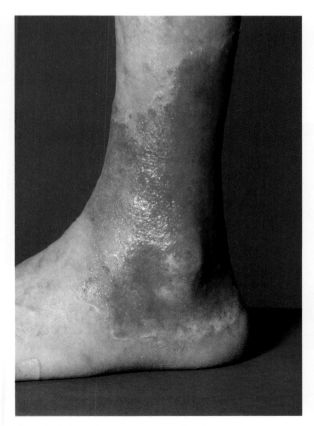

Fig. 16.12. Weeping venous eczema in gaiter area.

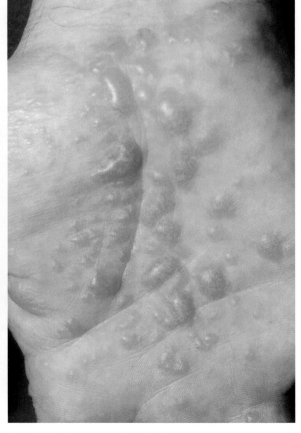

Fig. 16.14. Pompholyx: idiopathic hand eczema.

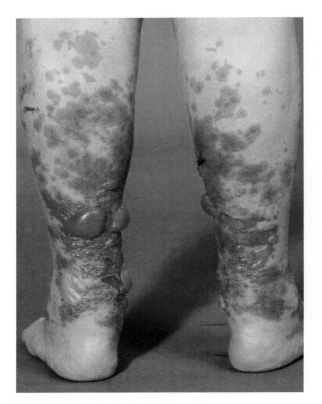

Fig 16.17. Severe leukocytoclastic vasculitis.

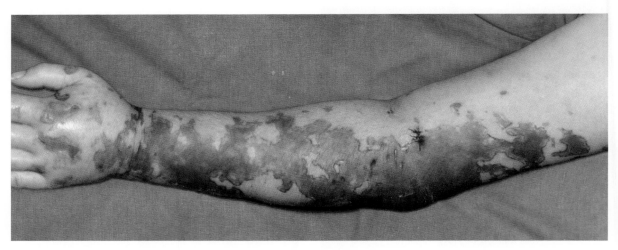

Fig 16.18. Purpura fulminans in acute meningococcemia.

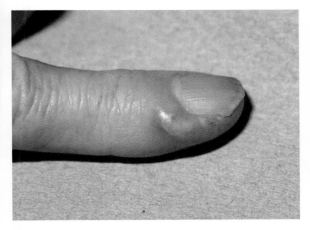

Fig 16.26. Acute paronychia.

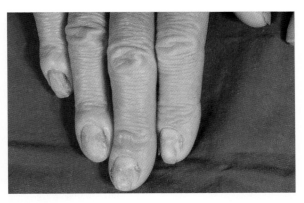

Fig 16.27. Chronic paronychia.

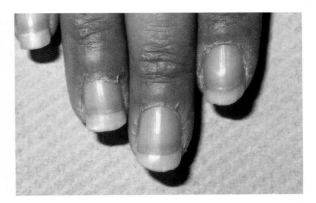

Fig 16.30. Nail fold hemorrhages and papules on the knuckles typical of dermatomyositis.

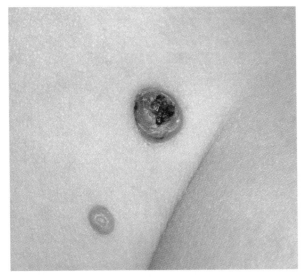

Fig 16.33. Small and giant molluscum contagiosum lesions showing umbilication.

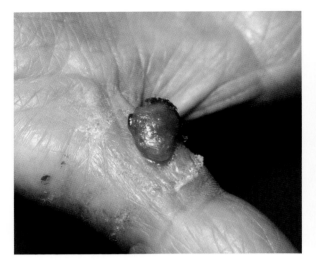

Fig 16.35. Pyogenic granuloma.

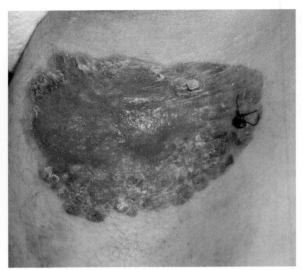

Fig 16.36. A large patch of Bowen's disease.

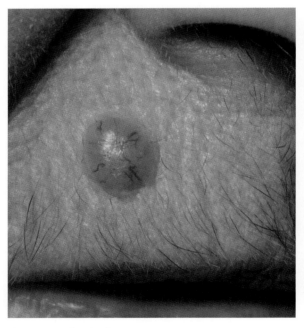

Fig 16.37. A basal cell carcinoma.

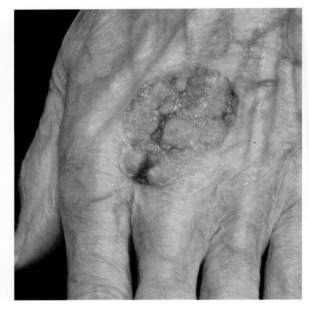

Fig 16.38. Squamous cell carcinoma on dorsum of hand.

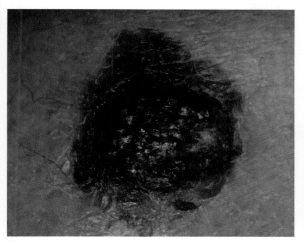

Fig 16.39. Nodular malignant melanoma arising from a superficial spreading component.

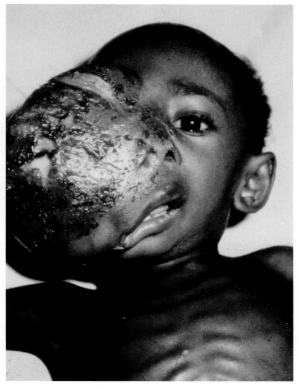

Fig. 17.5. Child with African type Burkitt's lymphoma presenting with a mass arising from the jaw. Other common sites include the abdominal viscera, particularly the kidneys. This variant rarely affects the lymph nodes, spleen, or bone marrow in contrast to the endemic, sporadic, non-African variant.

Fig. 17.7. Widespread lymphadenopathy involving the cervical and axillary nodes in a patient presenting with chronic lymphocytic leukemia.

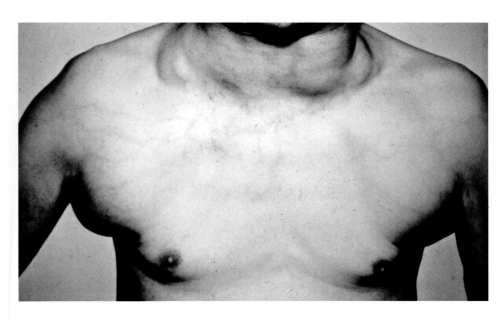

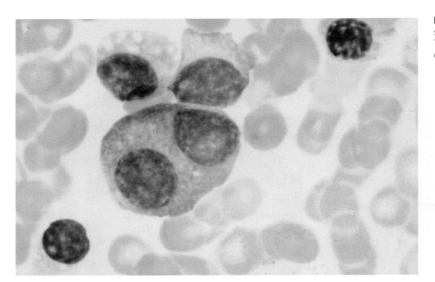

Fig. 17.9. Bone marrow aspirate showing abnormal binucleate plasma cell. The nucleus is eccentrically placed in the cell and has an open chromatin pattern.

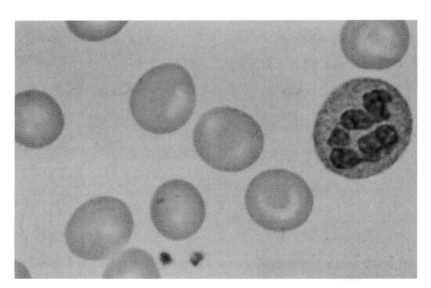

Fig. 17.15. Photmicrograph of a a hypersegmented neutrophil and target cells taken from a patient with liver disease and vitamin B12 deficiency. Target cells can also be seen in hemoglobinopathies (S & C), thalassemia, hypercholesterolemia, and post-splenectomy.

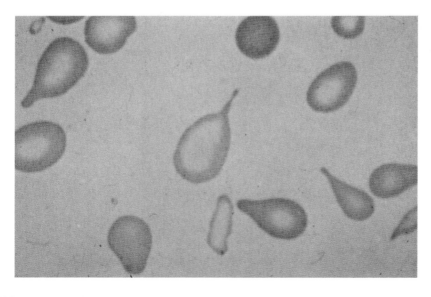

Fig. 17.16. Tear drop cells commonly seen in bone marrow fibrosis, megaloblastic anemia, iron deficiency, and thalassemia.

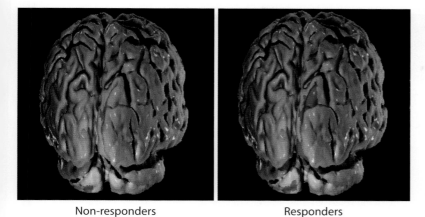

Fig. 18.4. Functional magnetic resonance images of dementia subject (left) and normal subject (right). The image distinguishes differences in brain activity on stimulation. (Image: Professer SHD Jackson, King's College, London.)

Non-responders   Responders

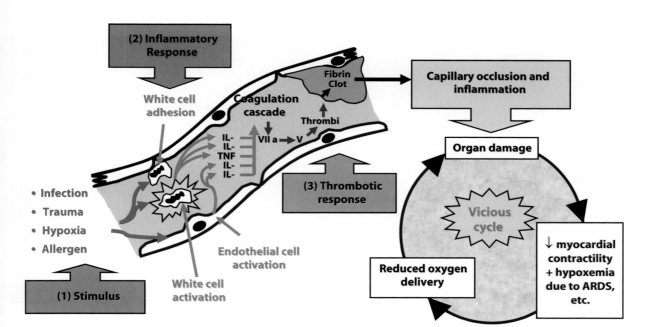

Fig. 19.9. The pathophysiology of shock.

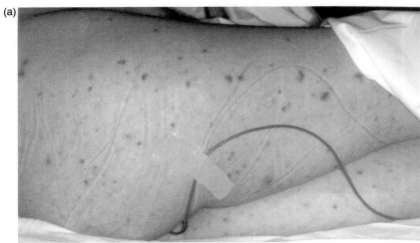

(a)

Fig. 19.12. Early and late rashes of meningococcal meningitis.

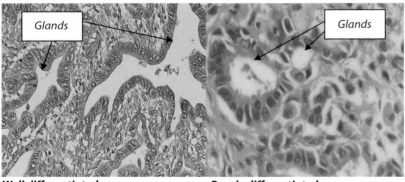

(b)

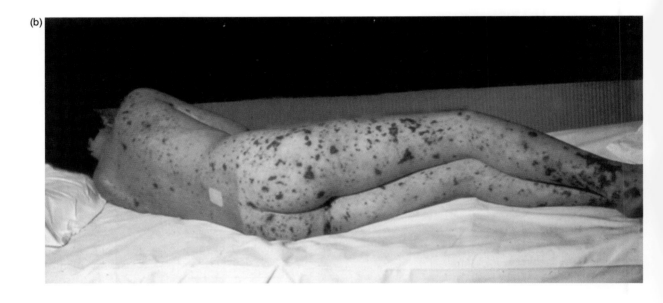

Glands

Glands

Well differentiated

Poorly differentiated

Fig. 20.7. Adenocarcinoma of the esophagus.

Table 14.3. Management of vaginal discharge

	Presentation	Diagnosis	Notify partner	Treatment
Physiologic	Discharge varies with menstrual cycle	On history	–	Reassure
Candida (thrush)	Itching/soreness	Clinical – can confirm with culture	–	Topical imidazole or single dose oral triazole
	External dysuria	If recurrent exclude diabetes mellitus		
	Dryness or lumpy discharge			
Bacterial vaginosis	Fishy smelling discharge, often recurrent	Creamy discharge without inflammation	–	Avoid douching or disinfectants
		pH >4.5		Metronidazole 400 mg bd 5 days
Trichomonas vaginalis	Profuse discharge with soreness	Green/yellow discharge, often frothy	+	Metronidazole 400 mg bd 5 days
		Genital inflammation	++	

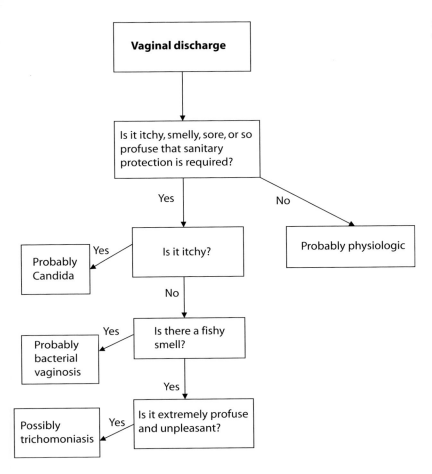

Fig. 14.2. Flow chart to show likely causes of vaginal discharge.

Recurrent BV may be caused by intrauterine increases the contraceptive devices, douching, and bathing in agents such as antiseptics, detergents, bath oils, and using vaginal deodorants.

BV increases the risk of pregnancy complications and pelvic inflammatory disease.

Pathology
Bacterial vaginosis is caused by a reduction in normal vaginal lactobacilli and their replacement by *Gardnerella vaginalis, Mycoplasma hominis*, and mixed anaerobes.

Investigations
The Amsel criteria. **Three** of these four features are required:
(1) Homogeneous gray/white discharge
(2) Fishy smell on adding 10% potassium hydroxide (positive amine test)
(3) Vaginal discharge pH >4.5
(4) "Clue cells" on immediate or stained microscopy of vaginal fluid; these are normal epithelial cells that appear stippled due to bacteria adhering to them.

If cultured appropriately, a high vaginal swab may show the presence of *Gardnerella vaginalis* and mixed anaerobes.

Management
Avoidance of vaginal douching or the use of antibacterial agents in bathwater and of oral, or topical metronidazole and clindamycin. Treatment of BV in pregnancy with clindamycin may reduce preterm delivery, but metronidazole seems to be ineffective. Asymptomatic women only require treatment if pregnant.

Treatment of male partners is unnecessary.

Outcome
The initial response to treatment is good in 70%–80%, but despite avoidance of exacerbating factors up to 30% of women experience recurrent symptoms within months.

Candida
Commonly known as thrush, it is caused by *Candida albicans,* a yeast. It forms part of normal vaginal flora and is only rarely sexually transmitted. It is the commonest cause of vulvo-vaginitis.

Clinical features
• Itching, accompanied by soreness.
• Lumpy white "cottage cheese" discharge or "dryness."

Table 14.4. Factors precipitating/exacerbating candida infection

Warm, damp environment	Nylon underwear, tights
	Hot, humid climate
Hormonal	Pregnancy
	Pre-menstrual
	Steroid treatment
Alteration in normal flora	Broad-spectrum antibiotics
Glycosuria	Diabetes mellitus
	Pregnancy
Immunodeficiency	HIV infection
	Malignancy
	Immunosuppressive drugs

• Painful sexual intercourse (superficial dyspareunia).
• Sore micturition (external dysuria).
• Vulvo-vaginal edema, erythema, and superficial fissuring of the vulval mucosa.
• Penile itching and maculo-papular rash in men, often accompanied by superficial fissuring.

Epidemiology
Candida species are ubiquitous, with spores being found in the mouth, bowel, vagina, and the skin of normal people.

Pathology
Fifty percent of women carry candida as harmless commensals (Table 14.4).

Investigations
A clinical diagnosis can be made by Gram stain with identification of Gram-positive spores and pseudohyphae, and confirmed on culture in a medium such as Sabouraud's or inoculated on a dry Swab and transported in Stuart's medium.

Management
First-line treatment is imidazoles, e.g. clotrimazole intravaginally as pessaries or creams. A single oral dose of a triazole, e.g. fluconazole (except in pregnancy), use of cotton rather than nylon underwear, the avoidance of tight clothing, and lubrication during intercourse also help. Male partners are treated only if symptomatic or they have penile erythema.

Outcome
Recurrent candidiasis is at least four symptomatic episodes in the preceding 12 months. General measures

are then important, and initial treatment is continued for 6 months.

Trichomoniasis

Trichomonas vaginalis (**TV**) is a flagellated protozoal parasite that causes profuse, offensive vaginal discharge in 70% of infected women, but is frequently asymptomatic in men.

Clinical features

- Unpleasant, abundant discharge with soreness; pruritus, superficial dyspareunia, dysuria, and involvement of the groins and legs.
- A profuse yellow frothy discharge.
- Labial erythema and swelling are common and the cervix displays punctate erythema (strawberry cervix).
- *T. vaginalis* infection in pregnancy is associated with adverse outcomes such as preterm delivery and low birth weight.
- Males may have symptoms of urethritis, but usually present only as asymptomatic partners of infected women.

Epidemiology

TV is an unusual cause of vaginal discharge in the UK, but more common in other populations such as in sub-Saharan Africa. Although considered a sexually transmissible infection, the organism can survive chlorination. Pools and damp towels account for some cases.

If symptomatic, the incubation time is usually 1–2 weeks, although asymptomatic infections can become symptomatic if an additional infection becomes superimposed. Once acquired, it can persist for years until treated. Occasionally, trichomoniasis is implicated as the cause of urethritis in a man.

Pathology

T. vaginalis infects the genitourinary tract specifically and has been isolated from almost all of its constituent parts. The resulting inflammation is superficial but often severe, and can result in contact bleeding.

Investigations

The motile organisms can be visualized in 60% by immediate microscopy of secretions taken from the posterior fornix in a drop of saline, a "wet prep." Culture is considered to be the gold standard but is not always available. Sometimes *T. vaginalis* is diagnosed as an incidental finding on cervical cytology. The false-positive rate is 30%.

Management

Short systemic course of metronidazole. Partner notification is important and abstinence is advised until sexual partners are treated.

Outcome

Treatment is effective in >90% of cases. Five percent of isolates have some metronidazole resistance, and treatment of these can be difficult.

Lumps and spots

Physiologic
Coronal papillae
Fordyce spots
Anogenital warts
Human papillomavirus
Molluscum contagiosum
Folliculitis
Insect bites
Sebaceous cysts

Patients commonly present with lumps or spots they have found in the genital area (Table 14.5).

History	Examination
Onset: sudden or gradual	Distribution of signs
Age, gender	Size and number
Site	Swelling, redness
Single/multiple	Appearance
Static/increasing/resolving	Texture/consistency
Pain/itching	
Spots elsewhere on body	
Sexual history	
Anyone else affected?	

Anogenital warts

Anogenital warts develop following infection with human papillomavirus (HPV). Not all who are infected develop visible warts. They seldom cause physical symptoms but patients find them disfiguring and distressing.

Clinical features

- One or more lumps in the anogenital area, gritty and slightly itchy. Common sites are vulva and penis, but they may appear elsewhere in the anogenital area or on other sites including the mouth.

Table 14.5. Likely diagnosis of genital lumps based on mode of presentation

	Days	Weeks	Months
Painful/ uncomfortable	Folliculitis/ boils Lymphocele (penile) Carcinoma		
Itchy	Scabies Insect bites		
Asymptomatic			Warts Molluscum contagiosum
Physiological "spots"	Fordyce spots (men and women): In men coronal papillae (pearly penile papules), in women vulval micropapillae		
		Sebaceous cysts	Condylomata lata (syphilis)

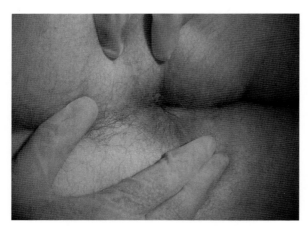

Fig. 14.3. Perianal warts.

- Perianal warts in heterosexuals are not usually linked to anal sex (Fig. 14.3). Warts higher in the anal canal are usually secondary to penetrative anal sex and more common in men who have sex with men.
- Warts on the mucosa are soft and fleshy. On dry hairy skin keratinised.

Epidemiology

Eighty percent of people are exposed to HPV, 10% harbor the virus, but only <1% have warts at any time. Incubation is 3–12 months. HPV is readily transmissible: 50%–70% of partners go on to develop warts. There are over 100 HPV genotypes. A third specifically infect the genital tract. Most are caused by types 6 and 11, but occasionally result from types linked to hand and foot warts (1, 2 and 4). HPV 16 and 18 are considered to confer high risk of genital cancers.

Warts may develop in previously asymptomatic HPV carriers following alteration of immunity as in pregnancy, when they can be resistant to treatment but resolve spontaneously following delivery.

Pathogenesis

HPV (types 16 and 18) has been linked to cervical intra-epithelial neoplasia (CIN), a precursor of cervical carcinoma, as well as intra-epithelial neoplasia of the vulva, vagina, and penis, which may precede squamous cell carcinoma of these areas.

Visible warts develop when normal progress from basal keratinocyte to superficial shedding of dead keratinocytes is disrupted. The infected keratinocytes remain viable for longer and there are alterations in intracellular adhesion properties causing the skin to become thicker and "heaped."

Investigations

Diagnosis is based on physical appearance. HPV typing of warts is not routine, but in atypical cases biopsy should be undertaken.

Management

Advice and implications for patient and partner(s) should be supplemented with written information, and condoms encouraged.

Treatments mostly involve destruction of affected skin:

- Cryotherapy (usually with liquid nitrogen).
- Topical podophyllotoxin (a chemical agent that attacks rapidly dividing cells) is most effective in soft, non-keratinized warts.
- Imiquimod is an immune response modifying agent that can also be effective.
- Minor surgery – curettage or excision.
- Cautery – usually with a "hot loop" but can be performed with laser.

Prevention

An HPV vaccine is effective against most common types of genital warts, and cervical cancer. It is for use primarily in females between ages 9 and 26.

Outcome

Most spontaneously resolve but this may take years. Within a few months of presentation, spontaneous resolution occurs in 10%–20%. With treatment, this increases to 90%. Between 20 and 40% recur. The chance of clearance is 60%.

Molluscum contagiosum (MC) is a poxvirus causing skin lesions sometimes confused with warts, but usually self-limiting.

Clinical features

- Immunocompetent young sexually active adults, small (<5 mm) spots in the genital area.
- Discrete pearly papules, smooth but usually umbilicated.
- Larger extra-genital lesions, for example on the face, can occur in immunocompromised people, for example, HIV infection.

Epidemiology

Incubation is 3–12 weeks. There are two peaks, amongst children via close physical contact, and in young sexually active adults.

Pathology

Molluscum contagiosum is a DNA virus, a member of the poxvirus family.

Investigations

The diagnosis is clinical. Electron microscopy shows poxviruses.

Management

Spontaneous regression is the norm in the immunocompetent. Treatment accelerates regression and is preferred. Podophyllotoxin can be used for home treatment whereas clinic treatments include cryotherapy, simple expression of the lesional contents, or piercing with an orange stick dipped in iodine or phenol. Contacts need not be traced, but ideally should be examined.

Outcome

Individual lesions regress spontaneously within 2–3 months, but total clearance often takes longer because of auto-inoculation. Spontaneous clearance is often preceded by inflammation of the lesion. Lesions recur in 15%–35%.

Fordyce spots

Sebaceous glands beneath the skin surface, visible in areas where the skin is thin and mobile, such as genitals and lips. The tiny white papules are more prominent when the skin is stretched. They occur in 80% of the population and are only visible post-puberty. They do not require treatment.

Coronal papillae

A normal variant, which can cause considerable anxiety amongst young men, especially as they may be confused with warts. They consist of multiple small pointed/smooth lesions in a band encircling the glans adjacent to the coronal sulcus. No treatment is required.

Vulval micropapillae

Normal variants, visible on the medial aspect of the labia minora where they can appear as delicate conical projections. They appear translucent and are shiny in appearance. Treatment is reassurance.

Genital ulcers, sores, and rashes (Fig. 14.4)

Genital herpes simplex
Syphilis
Tropical ulcer disease
    Chancroid
    LGV
    Donovanosis
Scabies
Pubic lice

History	Examination
Duration of symptoms	Distribution of signs
Age, gender	Size and number
Site(s)	Appearance
Single/multiple	Induration
Static/increasing/resolving	Any lesions elsewhere?
Pain/itching	
Are they recurrent?	
Systemic symptoms?	
Sexual history	
Travel history	

Herpes simplex virus (HSV)

Herpes simplex infection is a common cause of recurrent painful genital ulceration, although many

409

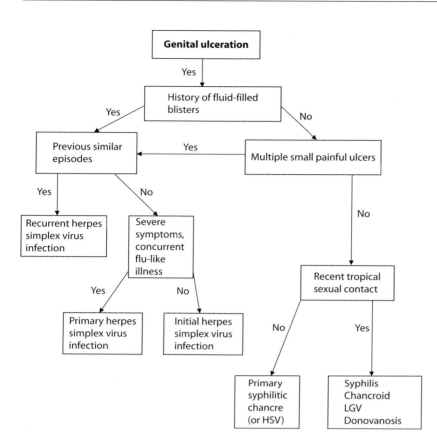

Fig. 14.4. Flow chart for likely diagnosis of genital ulceration found on examination.

infected individuals have no or minimal symptoms and are unaware of their infection.

Clinical features

- The initial episode of genital herpes is more severe than subsequent events. Painful, multiple small blisters, ulcers, which often merge with loss of the epithelium over a wider area. Localized tender (usually inguinal) lymphadenopathy. Flu-like symptoms from viremia.
- Complications may arise in immunosuppression: meningitis, acute retention of urine, and widespread dissemination.
- Recurrent episodes are shorter and less severe with a prodrome, of pain or tingling in the affected area or pain in the back and/or legs.
- Neonatal infection is rare but potentially fatal.

Epidemiology

There are two types, HSV-1 classically causes oro-labial sores (cold sores) and HSV-2 is associated with genital infection. Genital herpes related to HSV-1 infection is increasing, especially amongst young people. The seroprevalence of both types of HSV increases with age; other risk factors include female gender, years of sexual activity, and multiple lifetime sexual partners. Condoms are partially protective.

Pathology

Following primary infection, HSV becomes dormant in the affected dorsal root ganglia. It may reactivate spontaneously or due to external stimuli, which may be systemic, such as pyrexia, or local, such as trauma to the affected epithelium. This results in recurrent infection, which may be asymptomatic or symptomatic.

Investigation

Acute infection is diagnosed by demonstrating viral material in samples taken firmly from the lesion base. Tissue culture for HSV is widely available, but is less sensitive than nucleic acid amplification techniques.

Management

Treatment of an initial episode is acyclovir. This should be started on clinical grounds, rather than waiting for investigations. Symptomatic treatment includes topical lignocaine and oral analgesia. Antiviral treatment of recurrent infections has only limited effect on reducing symptom duration and is not necessary for mild or infrequent recurrences; symptomatic treatment with salt bathing is helpful as is counseling.

Episodic treatment, started within hours of recurrence, may abort an attack. Recurrences more than six times a year justify prophylactic acyclovir.

There is no evidence that topical acyclovir reduces severity, but some claim it aborts recurrence if used during the prodrome.

Outcome

HSV-2 recurs on average four to five times per year following initial infection, whereas HSV-1 recurs only once or twice a year. The frequency of recurrence diminishes over time. Most primary HSV infections are asymptomatic.

Syphilis

Syphilis is caused by infection with *Treponema pallidum*, a corkscrew-shaped bacterium or spirochete. It can be congenital or acquired; congenital syphilis is rare in industrialized countries as pregnant women are screened. Acquired syphilis is termed early if within the first 2 years of infection, and late beyond this time. Early syphilis may be **primary**, characterized by an ulcer called a chancre, **secondary** when there are systemic symptoms such as rash, or **early latent** after these two stages when there are no symptoms. Late syphilis may be **latent**, with no symptoms, or **tertiary**, with involvement of the nervous or cardiovascular systems, bone, or skin (Table 14.6).

Clinical features

Primary infection is characterized by a syphilitic chancre (Fig. 14.5), usually in the anogenital region, and associated inguinal lymphadenopathy. Classically a chancre is single, painless, and indurated. Sixty percent are multiple, or painful due to secondary infection.

In **secondary syphilis** there is systemic involvement with malaise, generalized lympadenopathy, and a polymorphic maculopapular rash (Fig. 14.6). The rash often affects the palms and soles and is usually

Table 14.6. Presentations of syphilis related to time after infection

Weeks	Months	Years
Primary ulcer chancre)		
STS often negative	Secondary syphilis	
	Rash	
	Generalized symptoms	
	STS positive	Latent disease
		STS positive but no symptoms
		Neurologic disease
		Cardiovascular disease
		Gummatous disease

non-itchy. Diffuse or patchy alopecia, nail pitting, and white patches termed "snail track ulcers" on mucous membranes. In the intertriginous regions, especially the anogenital area, the lesions can become hypertrophied and form highly infectious raised plaques. The eyes, liver, and bone can be involved.

Latent syphilis is called **early latent** if diagnosed serologically within the first 2 years of infection, or **late latent** if diagnosed beyond this time.

Prior to widespread use of antibiotics, **tertiary syphilis** developed in 40% of those infected, usually years later. Late stage disease commonly presents in one tissue, usually neurologic, cardiovascular, or gummatous skin and bone disease.

Neurosyphilis

The three main presentations of symptomatic **neurosyphilis** can overlap.

- Brain involvement results in progressive dementia, termed **paresis**.
- Involvement of the dorsal columns of the spinal cord result in **tabes dorsalis**, characterized by paresthesiae, ataxia, and paroxysms of stabbing pain, called lightning pains. The sensory defect can result in Charcot degeneration of joints and plantar ulceration.
- **Meningovascular** involvement results in meningeal symptoms such as headache and dizziness, and cerebrovascular disease resulting in hemiplegia, aphasia, ocular palsy, optic neuritis, or root pains. The characteristic associated pupillary abnormality is the

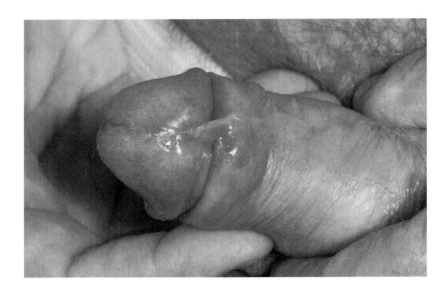

Fig. 14.5. Primary infection characterized by syphilitic chancre.

Argyll-Robertson pupil: the pupil constricts on accommodation but not to light.

Cardiovascular syphilis

Results from endarteritis, with replacement of elastic tissue of the aorta with fibrous tissue. Consequences include angina, aortic valve incompetence, proximal aortic aneurysm, and sometimes conduction defects.

Gummata

Inflammatory nodules that can be single or multiple. They occur anywhere, but most commonly in skin and bone. In the skin they are a painless, punched out ulcer, but multiple smaller gummata can co-exist. They heal centrally with scarring remaining active at the peripheries. In bone, local destruction results in perforation of the palate or nasal septum. Deformation of the tibia creates a characteristic "saber" appearance.

Syphilis co-infection in HIV can cause unusual features and progress more rapidly.

Early **syphilis in pregnancy** can result in miscarriage, stillbirth, or congenital infection; the risk is highest if the mother develops secondary syphilis whilst pregnant, and diminishes over subsequent years. **Congenital syphilis** can present within the first months of life or later. Congenital syphilis is readily prevented by treating women immediately after diagnosis, checking partners, and ensuring that potentially affected children are followed up.

Yaws is a treponemal infection caused by *Treponema pertenue*, which is identical to *T. pallidum* and

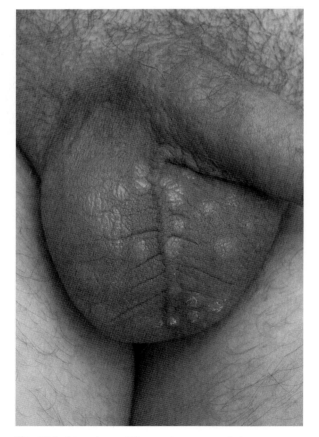

Fig. 14.6. Secondary syphilis: papulo-squamous lesions on scrotum.

causes the same serologic reactions. It is prevalent in tropical communities where it is transmitted by skin-to-skin contact. It can result in skin and bone disease, but not cardiovascular, neurologic, or congenital problems. A patient with positive syphilis serology from a yaws endemic area who has scars suggestive of old yaws should receive full treatment to cover the possibility of coincidental syphilis.

Epidemiology

Syphilis was rare in industrialized countries, but has recrudesced in homosexual men and heterosexual men and women.

The incubation period is 9–90 days (usually 2–4 weeks). Secondary infection follows after a further 6–12 weeks if primary infection is untreated. Historically, 60% with untreated syphilis were unaffected by late sequelae and 40% developed late disease. The natural history today is altered by the widespread use of antibiotics, and symptomatic late disease is rare.

Pathology

In late syphilis there is an inflammatory reaction with lymphocytic and plasma cell infiltration and endarteritis. This results in tissue destruction and compensatory fibrosis.

Gummata are characterized by an endarteritis with localized tissue destruction and fibrosis. They are non-infective.

Neurosyphilis results from direct infection by *T. pallidum* or associated endarteritis.

Investigations

The diagnosis of early syphilis is made by finding *T. pallidum* in lesions or infected lymph nodes by dark field microscopy in the clinic setting, by the direct fluorescent antibody (DFA) test, or by PCR (polymerase chain reaction).

Serologic tests for syphilis – termed STS – may be negative in primary syphilis but positive within 2 weeks. Diagnosis of syphilis has major implications for the patient and a positive test should always be repeated.

Antibodies detected in such tests may be non-specific or specific. Non-specific tests such as the VDRL (Venereal Diseases Research Laboratory) or RPR (rapid plasma reagin) detect an antilipoidal antibody denoting active treponemal infection, but may be falsely positive following any acute febrile illness, vaccination, autoimmune conditions, and even pregnancy. Specific tests include the EIA (treponemal enzyme immunoassay) and TPHA (*Treponema*

pallidum hemagglutination assay); they are usually positive in secondary, latent, or tertiary syphilis.

If neurosyphilis is suspected, examination of the cerebrospinal fluid (CSF) is recommended. Histology may be necessary to confirm gummata

Management

Treatment is penicillin by injection in doses to maintain therapeutic levels for 7–10 days in early infection and 17 days in late infection. A 28-day course of doxycycline is used in penicillin allergy. Tetracyclines are contraindicated in pregnancy; erythromycin or azithromycin can be used to treat the mother, but they do not cross the placental barrier well and so the neonate requires treatment with penicillin.

The Jarisch-Herxeimer reaction occurs within hours of treatment, and is a response to endotoxins exposed when treponemes are killed. It is a flu-like illness, more common, but seldom severe, in early syphilis. It can be serious if it is centered around focal lesions – the heart, nervous system, or placenta. Severe Herxeimer reactions are unusual, because so many with late disease have received antibiotics for other conditions. Steroid cover should be started if there is concern about crucially sited lesions.

Early syphilis is infectious and recent partners need to be notified. Late syphilis is not infectious, but long-term partners require assessment. Patients should receive oral and written information about the diagnosis, and be offered tests for other STIs including HIV.

Outcome

The outcome of treated early syphilis is excellent; response can be monitored by a fall in the titer of non-specific serologic tests such as VDRL. The levels may remain detectable indefinitely despite adequate treatment. Prognosis following treatment of late symptomatic disease depends on the underlying pathology; for example, in paresis treatment may delay or arrest progression but dementia does not reverse (Table 14.7).

Tropical ulcer disease

These infections are endemic in some tropical areas but are usually only seen in the UK when imported from abroad by the patient or, less commonly, a recent sexual contact. The travel history should include details of any sexual exposure abroad. Contact with prostitutes carries an especially high risk.

413

Table 14.7. Summary of acute STI management

Infection	Incubation	Symptoms	Investigation	Treatment	Contacts
Gonorrhea *Neisseria gonorrhoeae*	2–10 days	Purulent discharge or asymptomatic	Gram-positive coccobacillus confirmed by culture	[1]Cefixime 400 mg stat or ciprofloxacin 500 mg stat (if sensitive)	2/52 symptomatic 3/12 asymptomatic
Chlamydia *Chlamydia trachomatis*	10–21 days	Purulent discharge or asymptomatic	Obligate intracellular bacterium, NAAT or EIA or culture	Doxycycline 100 mg bd for 7 days or azithromycin 1 g stat dose	4/52 symptomatic 6/12 asymptomatic
Molluscum contagiosum	Average 2–8 weeks	Pearly smooth lesions	Physical appearance	Cryotherapy or podophyllotoxin or none	None
Warts *Human papilloma virus*	weeks–1year+	Warty growths	Appearance+/– biopsy	Cryotherapy or podophyllotoxin	Check current partners
Trichomoniasis *Trichomonas vaginalis*	7–14 days	Vag discharge Urethritis/balanitis Asymptomatic	Microscopy	Metronidazole 400 mg bd 5 days or oral tinidazole	Check current partners
Primary syphilis *Treponema pallidum*	9–90 days	Ulcer	Clinical and serology RPR/VDRL, NAAT	IM penicillin is first line	3/12

Notes:
NAAT = Nucleic acid amplification test.
EIA = Enzyme linked immunoassay.
[1] = consult microbiology for current advice.
If no partner in above periods trace last one regardless of time.

Chancroid
Clinical features
Genital ulcers are usually shallow and painful, with undermined edges and bleed to touch. Unilateral painful inguinal lymphadenopathy usually develops a few days after ulceration; the nodes can develop into abscesses called buboes in 25%.

Epidemiology
Chancroid is most common in poor communities in tropical and subtropical areas. The incubation period is short, usually 3–5 days.

Pathology
Chancroid is caused by the gram-negative bacterium *Haemophilus ducreyi*, a fastidious organism, which can be difficult to culture.

Investigations
Samples from ulcers and fluid aspirated from buboes can be Gram stained and examined for *H. ducreyi*. Culture in blood-enriched medium with carbon dioxide enrichment. Further investigations will depend on local availability and microbiologic advice should be sought; DNA amplification techniques are the most sensitive diagnostic methods, but are not widely available.

Management
A single dose of ciprofloxacin or a 7-day course of erythromycin is effective. Local hygiene is important in preventing secondary infection, and fluctuant buboes should be aspirated. Health education and partner notification are important.

Outcome
The outcome with early treatment is good, although treatment failure is more common in the uncircumcised and the immunocompromised.

Lymphogranuloma venereum (LGV)
LGV is a sexually acquired lymphatic infection with specific serovars of *Chlamydia trachomatis*.

Clinical features
- The first sign of infection is the primary lesion, a painless erosion, ulcer, or papule in the genital area. Penile lesions are generally overt, but internal lesions resulting from receptive vaginal or anal intercourse may not be noticed.
- Regional lymph nodes become enlarged and tender 1–6 weeks later. They may spontaneously regress, or become matted, with the development of a multilocular bubo and subsequent suppuration.

- Constitutional symptoms may be present; these include pyrexia, rigors, sweats, nausea and vomiting, myalgia, and arthralgia.
- If rectal, it can present with symptoms such as tenesmus, proctalgia, bloody diarrhea, and peri-anal discharge following receptive anal sex.

Epidemiology

LGV is endemic in some tropical areas such as parts of sub-Saharan Africa and South-East Asia. It was rare in industrialized countries until the recent outbreak in men who have sex with men. Infection of the rectal mucosa can mimic inflammatory bowel disease in presentation and even histology. Up until this outbreak, most infections presenting in the UK were acquired abroad.

The incubation period is usually 2–5 days but may be up to 30 days.

Pathology

LGV is usually caused by infection with one of the three invasive serovars of *Chlamydia trachomatis*, L1, L2, or L3.

Investigations

Scrapings taken from suspected primary lesions or pus aspirated from swollen lymph nodes can be analyzed using the NAAT test initially for the *Chlamydia* group. Alternative older methods of staining samples and examining them microscopically for inclusions, or tissue culture, can be attempted. Serologic tests for *Chlamydia* group antigens usually become positive during the first month following infection; if there is doubt a rising titer is diagnostic. The serology is non-specific and where positive can be caused by "non-trachomatis" chlamydiae.

Management

It is important to differentiate LGV from syphilis and other causes of lymphadenopathy. Treatment is weeks of tetracycline or erythromycin and aspiration or drainage of any fluctuant buboes. Partners should be notified.

Outcome

With early treatment, resolution is usual within 3–6 weeks, although this may be delayed by co-existent HIV infection. Surgical repair may be required in late cases with fistulae.

Donovanosis (granuloma inguinale)

Donovanosis is a progressive infection resulting in ulcers or granulations in the genital area and surrounding skin.

Clinical features

- The primary lesion is one or more papules which progress to become painless ulcers or granulomas.
- Regional lymphadenopathy with abscess formation follows.

Epidemiology

Donovanosis is found in some tropical countries, for example, India, the Caribbean, South Africa, Zambia, and Vietnam.

Pathology

The causative organism is now termed *Klebsiella granulomatis*, a fastidious organism which is hard to culture.

Investigations

Scrapings or biopsy material from involved tissue are stained and examined microscopically for Donovan bodies, the intracellular inclusions caused by *Klebsiella granulomatis*.

Management

Treatment with azithromycin or another effective antimicrobial should be continued for at least 3 weeks, and recent partners also assessed and offered treatment.

Outcome

Untreated infections may resolve spontaneously or slowly progress, with a wide range of potential complications including hemorrhage, genital lymphedema, and malignant change.

Scabies

Scabies is caused by infestation with the skin mite *Sarcoptes scabei*, acquired as the result of prolonged close bodily contact (even holding hands) or via bedding or clothes that are infested. It causes severe pruritus, especially at night.

Clinical features

- Papules and burrows may be found on the skin; the latter are ridges 5–15 mm long and are pathognomonic. Common sites affected are the hands, especially between the fingers, the wrists, the elbows, and the genital area. Facial involvement is rare in adults.

- Itching results from sensitivity to mite allergens, and may not develop for several weeks. It can be intense and create secondary eczema.
- Norwegian scabies is a variant presentation occurring in people who are immunocompromised. The lesions are crusted and contain many mites, which are highly infectious.

Epidemiology

Scabies is transmitted as the result of close bodily contact, either sexually or within a household or institution. The mite requires about 15 minutes to transfer from one host to a new host, so holding hands is a recognized mode of transmission, but shaking hands is too brief to permit transmission.

Pathology

The female mite burrows into the skin to lay eggs, leaving a burrow up to 1 cm long. Larvae hatch from the eggs which migrate laterally, forming papules in the skin as they mature.

Investigations

The diagnosis is usually made clinically, but can be confirmed by finding mites or eggs in scrapings from burrows examined by light microscopy.

Management

- Anti-scabetic agents such as permethrin or malathion should be applied to the entire skin surface below the neck and left for at least 12 hours, usually overnight, before washing off.
- Clean clothing should then be worn and bed linen changed; potentially infected items should be washed at a high temperature ($>50°$). Sexual and close contacts should also receive treatment.
- Pruritus can persist for several weeks despite successful treatment; symptomatic treatment with crotamiton cream and/or antihistamines may be helpful.

Pediculosis pubis

Pubic or crab louse infestation is a cause of itching in the region of the pubic hair.

Clinical features

- Patients may be asymptomatic or complain of intense itching in the pubic region, occasionally they may have noticed insects, eggs (nits), or bleeding from the bites or from scratching.
- The partner(s) may also be symptomatic.

Epidemiology

The infestation is transmitted by close bodily contact, with an incubation period ranging from 5 days to a few weeks.

Pathology

The crab louse, *Pthirus pubis*, infests the coarse hairs of the pubic area and other hairy areas of the body, and occasionally the eyelashes, but spares the head hair. It has crab-like claws, adapted specifically to grasp pubic hair. Each female lays about 50 eggs (nits), which adhere to the hairs.

Investigations

Lice or nits can usually be seen without magnification, although a hand lens is helpful. Low-power microscopy can confirm the diagnosis if necessary.

Management

An effective pediculicide lotion such as malathion 0.5% should be applied to all body hair, including facial hair if necessary, and left overnight before washing off. The application can be repeated 3–7 days later.

Current and recent sexual partners should also be examined and treated.

Outcome

Persisting nits may be dead and so their presence does not necessarily imply treatment failure; they can be removed with a nit comb. If lice persist, an alternative pediculocide should be used.

Human immunodeficiency virus (HIV)

HIV is a virus which, untreated, slowly destroys the body's immune system, resulting in fatal immunodeficiency termed AIDS (**acquired immune deficiency syndrome**). HIV is sexually transmissible, the risk of transmission is high when other sexually transmitted infections are present. The global epidemic affects 40 million people, of whom two-thirds live in sub-Saharan Africa and over 3 million die each year. Those dying are commonly young adults who form the economically active sector of resource-poor countries; their deaths leave behind orphans and contribute to destitution in their communities. HIV is now treatable, but drugs are expensive and available to a minority worldwide.

Clinical features

Early $\rightarrow$ **Latent** $\rightarrow$ **Symptomatic** $\rightarrow$ **AIDS**
$\longleftarrow$ **8–10 years on average** $\longrightarrow$

Early HIV

- About one-third of people infected with HIV develop symptoms around the time of seroconversion – a seroconversion illness. The symptoms of fever, lymphadenopathy, pharyngitis, or rash are non-specific and it is therefore rare to identify HIV at this early stage. It is in the first 3–6 months that infectivity is highest.
- The infection usually then enters a latent stage. In the majority the disease progresses over an average of 8–10 years, with a steady decline in immunity as measured by the CD4 count. Some individuals notice persistent generalized lymphadenopathy (PGL), with nodes of more than 1 cm at more than one extra-inguinal site, persisting more than 3 months. Most appear healthy, are unaware they have HIV, and so may transmit the infection.
- About 2%–5% of people with HIV do not progress, or progress very slowly, and are termed **long-term non-progressors**.

Symptomatic HIV

- Symptoms can be due to the virus, or to immunosuppression.
  - Direct effects of HIV include fatigue, malaise, sweats, weight loss, diarrhea.
  - Early (non-AIDS) conditions suggesting immunosuppression include oral candida (thrush), hairy leukoplakia, zoster infection (shingles), and rashes such as seborrheic dermatitis.

AIDS

AIDS has developed with characteristic conditions such as *Pneumocystis carinii* pneumonia or Kaposi's sarcoma, usually when the CD4 count falls below 200. The aim of management is to prevent AIDS developing by identifying HIV early and starting treatment before immune deterioration.

Individual presentations are considered below.

When to consider HIV infection?

Laboratory tests

  ↓ platelets

  ↓ lymphocyte count

  ↑ immunoglobulins

  ↑ plasma viscosity

Symptoms

  lymphadenopathy

  night sweats

  weight loss, diarrhea

Infections

  hepatitis B/C = risk factors

  oral candida

  recurrent pneumonia

  zoster in a young person

  tuberculosis

More than 90% of people with HIV will have at least one of the following risks:

- Men who have sex with men (MSM).
- Unprotected sex with individuals from endemic areas.
- Injecting drugs and sharing equipment/needles, or a partner that has.
- Sub-optimal medical care, with contaminated equipment or unscreened infected blood transfusion.
- Sex workers and clients who do not use condoms.

Transmissibility

HIV can be transmitted by blood or genital secretions. Urine, vomit, saliva, and feces are low risk unless contaminated with blood (Fig. 14.7).

The ability of an individual with HIV to infect another depends on:

(1) The stage of infection – the risk is greatest in early and late stages when levels of HIV in blood and genital secretions are highest.

(2) Access to susceptible cells – sexual intercourse is the route of acquisition worldwide for over 75%. The risk is highest for the receptive partner, and increases in the presence of other sexually transmitted infection or trauma.

Pathology and mechanism of problem

HIV exists in two forms, HIV-1, which is responsible for >98% of HIV infection worldwide, and HIV-2 which is endemic in parts of West Africa, but is less transmissible and pathogenic.

Both are retroviruses with the ability to convert their own RNA into DNA, using an enzyme called reverse transcriptase. The new DNA is integrated into host cells causing persistent infection and production of new RNA viruses.

HIV attaches to cell surface receptors and then crosses the cell wall. The main receptor is the surface

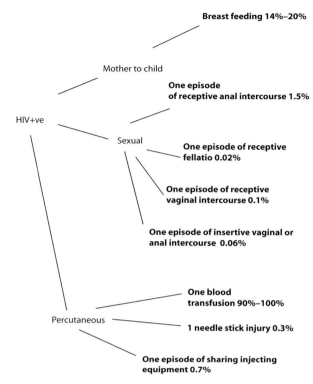

Fig. 14.7. Estimated risk of HIV transmission.

protein CD4 on T-helper lymphocytes. HIV infection results in depletion of CD4 bearing lymphocytes, causing reduced cell-mediated immunity together with other immune phenomena, such as uncontrolled antibody production resulting from inability to control B lymphocyte activity.

The progress of HIV infection is monitored by counting the absolute numbers of CD4 lymphocytes and their proportion of the total. The normal range is 700–1100. On average, it takes 8–10 years to progress from HIV infection to AIDS. This can be accelerated by:

Age over 35 years

Symptomatic seroconversion illness

Genetic make-up

Poor nutritional status

Co-existing systemic illnesses

- Initially, there is a rapid decline of CD4 cells coinciding with a burst in viral activity; this state of high viral load and low CD4 are not seen again until the late stages. It is possible, but rare, to develop AIDS soon after infection.
- During latent infection the CD4 count rises from its early nadir. The viral load drops as the virus comes under partial control of the immune system.
- In the later stages the decline in CD4 accelerates and may be associated with an exponential increase in viral load (Table 14.8).

Investigations

HIV antibody test Finding antibodies to HIV in adults or children over age 18 months indicates persistent infection with HIV. Babies born to mothers with HIV may have passively acquired maternal antibodies, and extra tests to identify the viral genetic material are needed to determine infection.

Modern HIV antibody tests usually become positive within 1 month of infection, although it can take 3 months. The period between infection and test positivity is termed the window period when an infectious state coincides with lack of diagnosis. Blood donors are asked about risks and if necessary asked not to give blood. All positive antibody results should be confirmed by another technique on the same sample, and another fresh sample tested to eliminate the possibility of labeling error.

Historically, there were psychologic and ethical issues linked to testing for what used to be a fatal and untreatable condition. Since 1996 the availability of effective therapy in industrialized countries has transformed the prognosis.

There are overwhelming advantages in detecting HIV before the immune system is weakened. With treatment the viral activity is controlled and the immune system can reconstitute. There remains no cure, but treatment now means that HIV is chronic rather than fatal.

Viral load: quantification of the viral load provides an indication of infection activity and a crude assessment of the rate of progression.

Viral resistance assays: Approximately 5%–10% of new infections are with HIV strains that have pre-existing resistance mutations that make certain drugs less effective.

CD4 count: in health, CD4 counts of 700–1100 cells/μl and a CD4% of >50% are normal. It is unusual for HIV-related symptoms to develop if the CD4 count is above 500 cells/μl, or for AIDS defining conditions to appear until counts drop below 200 copies/μl.

Table 14.8. Symptoms and their association with CD4 count and disease

	CD4>500/l	CD4>200/l	CD4<200/l	CD4<50/l
Shortness of breath, fever and cough	Bacterial pneumonia and TB		PCP	
Confusion				Cerebral lymphoma
				Cryptococcal meningitis
			Toxoplasma encephalitis	
			PML	
				CMV encephalitis
				HSV encephalitis
				Neuro syphilis
			HIV encephalopathy	
Focal neurology		Cerebral thrombosis	Toxoplasma encephalitis	
				Cerebral lymphoma
Vision				CMV retinitis
Diarrhea			HIV enteropathy	
			Protozoal infection	
			Treatment SEs	
Skin	Maculopapular rash	Wart/molluscum contagiosum Kaposi sarcoma		
	Primary HIV	Seborrheic dermatitis		
		Psoriasis		
	Increased skin allergy reactions to medication			

Management

HIV testing If a patient has symptoms suggestive of HIV infection, they should be encouraged to be tested, especially if risk factors are present. Informed consent is essential and the pre-test discussion or written information provided should include the following points:

(1) Effective treatments for HIV infection
(2) Risk factors for infection
(3) The window period
(4) What would happen if someone is found to have HIV
(5) Negative HIV tests do not affect chances of life insurance or mortgage.

HIV teams can offer counseling and support following an HIV diagnosis made within or outside their service.

Antiretroviral therapy There are currently over 20 licensed drugs for the treatment of HIV infection, from five main classes:

Nucleoside analogs: used as nucleic acid building blocks that cause the growing viral RNA to end prematurely; the curtailed viral particles are unable to induce infection.

Non-nucleoside reverse transcriptase inhibitors: inhibit the viral RNA chain by blocking reverse transcriptase.

Protease inhibitors: block the final cleavage of viral proteins required for the outer viral coat.

Fusion inhibitors: interfere with the fusion of the virus envelope to the cell wall thus preventing the introduction of viral DNA to the cell and preventing infection.

Integrase inhibitors: block integration of the DNA transcript into the host genome.

Drugs are used in combinations of three, generally including drugs from at least two of the above classes, as single agents permit the development of resistance. HIV treatment is initiated when the CD4 count is between 250 and 350, but can be recommended earlier if the patient is symptomatic, older, or there is rapid CD4 decline. Therapy may be delayed if there is doubt over the patient's commitment to therapy, as excellent adherence is crucial. The drugs produce few side effects (Fig. 14.8).

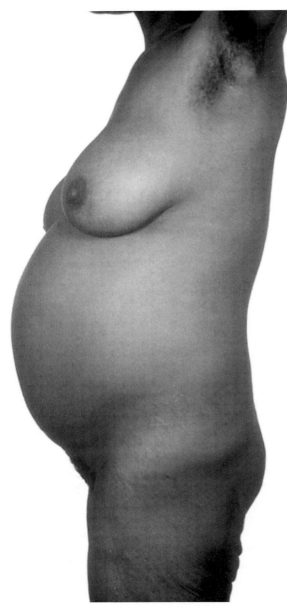

Fig. 14.8. Fat redistribution: a side effect of some antiretroviral drugs.

Mother-to-child transmission Without interventions about 13%–42% of mothers will pass on HIV to their babies, about half at delivery and about half during breast feeding; with optimal treatment this can be reduced to 1%. Where interventions are available, all pregnant women should be strongly recommended to have an HIV test.

Without treatment most transmission takes place around the time of birth, although it can occur earlier, and is associated with:

- High viral load and advanced disease
- Vaginal delivery, especially if prolonged and/or associated with breaches in the baby's skin, for example by the use of a scalp electrode
- Breast feeding

The following interventions contribute to reducing HIV transmission to 1%:

- Antiretroviral medication (one to three drugs) given to the mother during pregnancy and labor, and to the child for 1 month post-delivery
- Normal vaginal delivery is acceptable assuming an uncomplicated vaginal delivery is anticipated and treatment has resulted in an undetectable viral load. If these conditions are not met, elective Cesarean is indicated
- Formula feeding

Outcome

The advances in drug treatment (highly active anti-retroviral therapy – HAART) since 1996 have resulted in a sharp decline in the numbers of people dying from HIV, but there are still a significant number of people with undiagnosed HIV who present at a late stage with AIDS defining conditions.

With complete adherence to HAART, the viral load should become undetectable and the CD4 count steadily increases. The prognosis is promising, but may yet become complicated by the toxicity of long-term medication.

Sadly, effective treatment is currently unaffordable and unavailable for the vast majority of people infected worldwide. Without HAART, even patients who receive appropriate treatment for AIDS-defining illnesses die within an average of 2 years. In less resourced settings, death within 6 months of developing AIDS is usual.

Symptoms and their underlying causes include those in other chapters of this book but in HIV the following causes need special consideration.

Respiratory complications of HIV (Fig. 14.9)

Pneumocystis pneumonia (PCP) is the most common AIDS-defining condition in the developed world.

Clinical features

PCP is characterized by progressive shortness of breath associated with a non-productive cough and fever. On examination, there is usually tachypnea

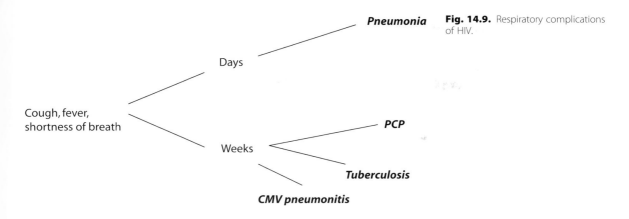

Fig. 14.9. Respiratory complications of HIV.

Cough, fever, shortness of breath

Days — **Pneumonia**

Weeks — **PCP**

Weeks — **Tuberculosis**

CMV pneumonitis

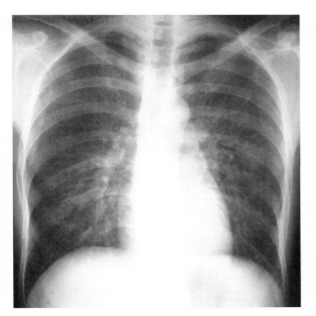

Fig. 14.10. Early *Pneumocystis* pneumonia (PCP).

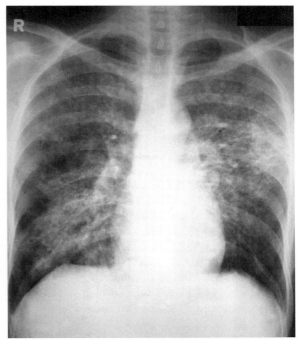

Fig. 14.11. Late *Pneumocystis* pneumonia (PCP).

at rest, but otherwise little to be found; oximetry, if available, may show hypoxia at rest and characteristically following exertion.

Investigations

Chest X-ray and arterial blood gases are needed at baseline followed by bronchoscopy with bronchoalveolar lavage (Figs. 14.10 and 14.11).

Management

High dose cotrimoxazole, initially intravenously, for a total of 21 days. Prednisolone should be added if the pO_2 is <8.5 on air, positive pressure ventilation may be needed. Secondary prophylaxis with cotrimoxazole is required until the CD4 count exceeds 200. Primary prophylaxis is indicated in all those presenting with a CD4 count less than 200.

Outcome

Following PCP there is usually permanent damage to the lungs; bullae can develop at the lung peripheries. When HAART is commenced, some patients develop immune reconstitution syndrome, characterized by an apparent worsening of inflammation and gaseous exchange.

Bacterial pneumonia is more common in people with HIV regardless of stage.

421

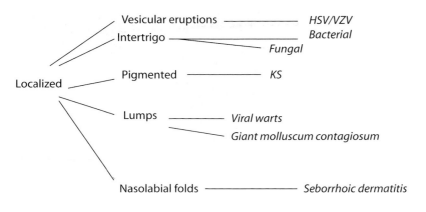

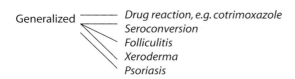

Vesicular eruptions ——————— *HSV/VZV*

Intertrigo ———————— *Bacterial*

Fungal

Pigmented ——————— *KS*

Localized

Lumps ——————— *Viral warts*

Giant molluscum contagiosum

Nasolabial folds ——————————— *Seborrhoic dermatitis*

Generalized ————— *Drug reaction, e.g. cotrimoxazole*
Seroconversion
Folliculitis
Xeroderma
Psoriasis

Fig. 14.12. Skin complications of HIV.

Tuberculosis: TB is an AIDS defining condition. The level of suspicion needs to be high in HIV. If the CD4 is greater than 350, there is no need to commence HIV treatment.

Skin complications of HIV (Fig. 14.12)

Seroconversion The rash of seroconversion occurs in a minority of individuals about 14 days after infection, presenting as a diffuse morbilliform rash mimicking a drug rash. At this stage, the HIV antibody test is usually negative.

Seborrheic dermatitis is a common condition but becomes worse or may develop de novo. Treatment is with topical ketoconazole or miconazole and topical steroids.

Psoriasis can develop de novo or worsen. The population prevalence is 2%, and 5% in HIV.

Kaposi's sarcoma (KS)

A multicentric tumor which is an AIDS-defining condition.

Clinical features

KS lesions present as firm purple to brown/black macules or nodules (Fig. 14.13). They may cause lymphatic obstruction and associated peripheral edema, and affect the gut and lungs (Fig. 14.14).

As well as its association with HIV, it also exists in an endemic form found in the Mediterranean, Jewish, and African populations.

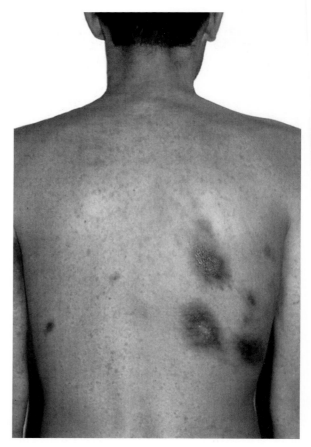

Fig. 14.13. Kaposi's sarcoma (KS) on back.

The diagnosis is often made clinically, but if there is any doubt biopsy should be carried out.

Management
The superficial skin lesions usually resolve with HAART alone, but when there is visceral involvement systemic chemotherapy may be required.

Outcome
Excellent provided that effective antiretroviral treatment can be introduced.

Intertrigo
Superficial bacterial and fungal infections are more common.

Vesicular eruptions
Herpes simplex and herpes zoster (shingles) both become more common as immunosuppression increases. Both respond well to oral acyclovir.

Oral disease

White plaques on palate and buccal mucosa	*Oral candida*
Corrugated white lesions on sides of tongue	*Oral hairy leukoplakia*
Pigmented lesions palate/gum	*Kaposi sarcoma*
Erosion of gums dental decay	*Gingivitis*
Large, painful, persistent ulcers	*Aphthous ulceration*

Oral candida (thrush) is common and associated with immunosuppression. It presents as white plaques on the buccal mucosa and on the hard and soft palate. Dysphagia in the presence of oropharyngeal candida is almost invariably caused by esophageal candida. It is an AIDS-defining illness (Fig. 14.15).

Treatment of oral candida is with topical agents such as amphotericin lozenges or nystatin oral suspension. Esophageal candidiasis requires systemic treatment with an azole.

Oral hairy leukoplakia (OHL) indicates underlying immunosuppression. It is caused by a chronic viral infection with Epstein-Barr virus. It presents with corrugated white plaques along the sides of the tongue and sometimes the buccal mucosa. It is asymptomatic and does not require treatment.

Oral aphthous ulceration can be severe resulting in painful dysphagia. This can impede nutrition and fluid intake. Topical steroid treatment can be used.

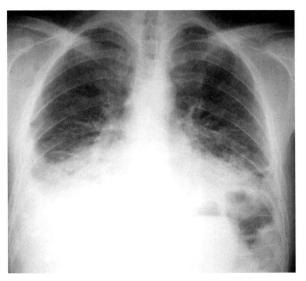

Fig. 14.14. Kaposi's sarcoma (KS) involving the lungs.

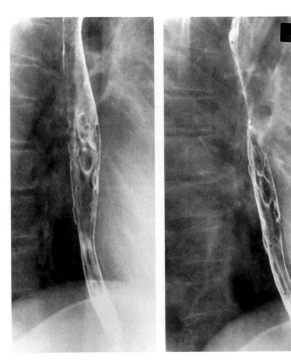

Fig. 14.15. Barium swallow showing esophageal *Candida*.

Diarrhea associated with HIV (Fig. 14.16)
Clinical features
A history of foreign travel or oro-anal sex may suggest an infective cause. Protease inhibitors are the antiretroviral agents most likely to cause diarrhea.

423

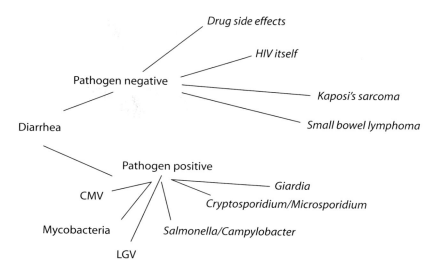

Fig. 14.16. Diarrhea associated with HIV.

Cryptosporidium/Microsporidium and *Giardia lamblia* are intestinal protozoa associated with self-limiting diarrhea in immunocompetent individuals, but the diarrhea can be prolonged in the immuno-compromised.

LGV is transmitted by receptive anal sex and there have been dramatic increases in incidence in men who have sex with men since 2003.

Pathology

Occasionally, despite extensive investigation, no cause other than HIV infection is found; the small bowel architecture is usually abnormal with reduced villous height decreasing absorption, and there may also be autonomic nervous system damage.

Investigations

At least three and ideally six stool samples taken on different days should be sent for microscopy for cysts, ova, and parasites, for culture, and for *Clostridium difficile* toxin. Blood cultures for bacteria and myco-bacteria should also be taken in febrile immunocom-promised patients.

Endoscopy and multiple biopsy of the duodenum or colon may be needed especially to exclude Kaposi tumor.

If LGV is suspected, then chlamydia NAATs should be performed.

Management

Specific treatment should be given for any pathogen identified.

In the absence of an identifiable cause, HAART usually leads to resolution, and if due to treatment drug substitution is usually possible.

Outcome

The outcome of treatment for specific infections is good provided the underlying HIV infection is also treated. HIV-associated diarrhea can persist despite HAART.

Neurologic problems and HIV (Fig. 14.17)

Imaging of the CNS by MRI or CT scan with gado-linium contrast is needed to differentiate a mass from meningitis. MRI is required to visualize the cerebel-lum and optimize images of lesions which might be missed on CT (Fig. 14.18).

In the absence of a mass lesion a lumbar puncture is needed, and the subsequent investigations (Fig. 14.19).

Cryptococcal meningitis

Cryptococcal meningitis is a severe life-threatening disease affecting those with advanced HIV, usually with CD4 <100/ul.

Clinical features

The presentation may be subtle, 10% having no symp-toms and one-third having no neurological history. The majority have headache and fever, some with nausea, vomiting, confusion, or mental slowness. Overt meningism occurs in less than half. Occasionally, *Cryp-tococcus neoformans* also affects non-meningeal sites such as the lungs or skin.

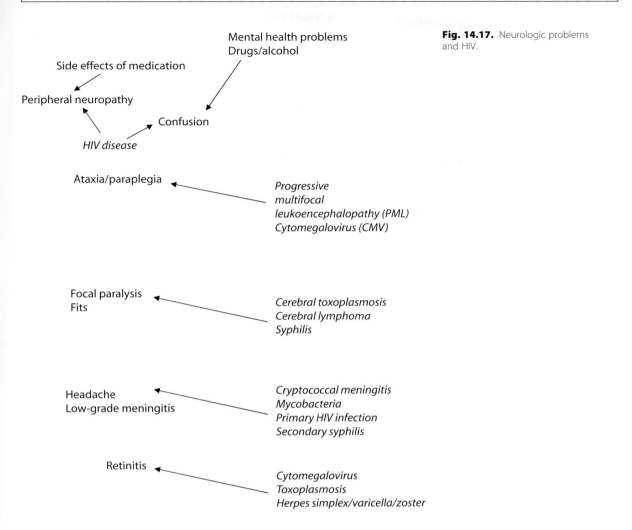

Fig. 14.17. Neurologic problems and HIV.

Epidemiology

Cryptococcus neoformans appears to be ubiquitous and enters the body usually through the lungs.

Investigations

Indian ink staining of the CSF frequently demonstrates the fungal spores, which grow in culture. Antigen can be detected in blood or CSF. Falling titers reassure that treatment is working but they can remain elevated at low levels for years.

Management

Intravenous liposomal amphotericin B and flucytosine followed by maintenance secondary prophylaxis with fluconazole and HAART. Very high CSF pressures may necessitate daily CSF drainage or a ventriculo-peritoneal shunt to preserve optic nerve function.

Toxoplasmosis

This is the commonest cause of focal cerebral lesions in HIV.

Clinical features

Toxoplasma encephalitis may present acutely with fits or insidiously with focal neurological deficits. The patient may be disoriented, and progress to coma if untreated.

Epidemiology

Toxoplasma gondii is a protozoon that seldom causes symptoms in immunocompetent people, but

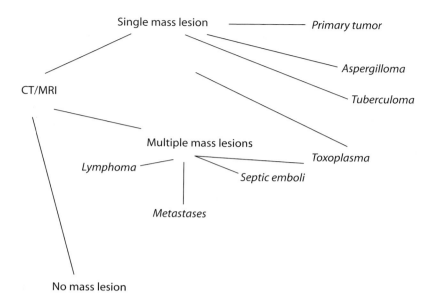

Fig. 14.18. MRI/CT imaging to differentiate mass from meningitis.

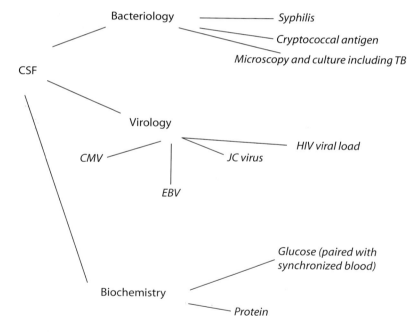

Fig. 14.19. Some of the tests frequently needed on CSF samples from HIV-positive patients.

with advanced HIV disease, it causes symptomatic neurologic disease.

Investigations
Brain imaging usually demonstrates more than one space-occupying lesion, with ring enhancement if contrast medium is used. LP is contraindicated, and in any case the CSF is not revealing because the lesions are within the brain substance. Brain biopsy is not routinely indicated, but considered when response to treatment is slow.

Management
Treatment is with sulfadiazine, pyrimethamine, and folinic acid followed by HAART.

Outcome
The outcome is good if treated early.

Cytomegalovirus (CMV) retinitis

This is a common cause of blindness in people with advanced HIV disease, usually with a CD4 count <50 cells/µl.

Clinical features

A common initial presentation is the development or worsening of floaters, blurred vision resulting from macula involvement, or a field defect. Fundoscopy with pupil dilatation is essential to demonstrate opaque white areas of retinitis interspersed with red hemorrhagic areas, an appearance likened to pizza.

Epidemiology

CMV retinitis is usually a reactivation of latent CMV in someone already infected. CMV is a common viral infection, especially in the groups of people at highest risk of being infected with HIV infection.

Investigations

If the appearance is consistent, treatment would be started on this basis alone. Additional investigations may include plasma CMV quantification.

Management

Ophthalmic advice should be sought. Treatment is ganciclovir, usually intravenously, followed by HAART. Vitreous implants have been developed, which permit local treatment and the avoidance of systemic exposure.

Outcome

The outlook can be good if CMV retinitis is treated before significant retinal damage. Extensive retinal disease is irreparable.

Further reading

www.hpa.org.uk Website of the Health Protection Agency, which provides current epidemiological information about STIs and HIV in the UK.

www.bashh.org Website of the British Association for Sexual Health and HIV, includes management guidelines for STIs.

www.aidsmap.co.uk NAM website, which provides general and clinical information about HIV, including treatment and care.

Klausner J, Hook EW, *Current Diagnosis and Treatment of Sexually Transmitted Diseases*, McGraw Hill, 2007.

Pattman R, Snow M, Handy P, Sankar K, Elawad B, *Oxford Handbook of Genitourinary Medicine, HIV and AIDS*, Oxford University Press, 2005.

Contents

with fever have infection but not all with infection have a fever. In this chapter the focus is principally on infectious causes of a febrile illness. The clinical approach to the febrile patient is outlined in Table 15.1 and discussed below. Assessment starts with noting whether infection is likely to have been acquired in the community or in hospital. Although the history and examination are pre-eminent, initial investigations may also provide clues to diagnosis. Taking all of these into account, the clinician frequently has to decide whether or not to give empiric treatment. The possibility that a non-infectious process could underlie a patient's febrile illness sometimes needs to be entertained, particularly if investigation fails to reveal a pathogen or source of infection.

What is the context? Community- or hospital-acquired infection?

This fundamental question helps to narrow the focus on the likely causative organisms. Figure 15.1 shows how commonly encountered pathogens are distributed according to where they are most frequently acquired. Community-acquired organisms invade healthy individuals and may result in life-threatening disease. The bacteria in this group often produce toxins or other factors responsible for their virulence. In comparison, many hospital-acquired organisms only tend to cause disease in susceptible individuals with other illnesses or impaired defenses. For example, these bacteria may make use of intravenous lines or catheters to invade the body and often lack well-defined virulence factors. Some organisms are important causes of both hospital- and community-acquired infections but when acquired in hospital are more likely to be resistant to standard antibiotics, e.g. methicillin-resistant *Staph. aureus*. Although most viruses are community acquired, some are highly transmissible between patients and staff alike and can cause hospital outbreaks.

Introduction

Fever is defined as an elevated core body temperature – due to natural circadian variation, the normal range is between 35.6 °C in the morning and 37.7 °C in the evening. The majority of patients

Are there any clues from the history for the likely source?

The patient's **age** is helpful when considering the likely cause, particularly if a virus is suspected (Fig. 15.2). Viruses cause many of the classic diseases of childhood, especially the rash syndromes. Vaccination has massively reduced the incidence of many but measles, mumps and rubella, for example, are still seen in unvaccinated adults. The increase in primary infections from herpes simplex virus, cytomegalovirus and Epstein-Barr virus in teenagers is from transmission through kissing and sexual activity. Neonatal human immunodeficiency virus (HIV) infection results from maternal transmission and later (HIV) from sexual activity. Influenza occurs in all age groups but the elderly are more vulnerable. Reactivation of varicella

zoster infection acquired in childhood (chickenpox) may also manifest as "shingles" with advancing age.

"**Drenching**" **night sweats** with fever that prompt a change of bedclothes or sheets may occur in tuberculosis or lymphoma. **Rigors** (shivering) frequently accompany the presence of bacteria in the bloodstream (bacteremia). Illness **duration** is important because few infections cause symptoms for more than 2–3 weeks, e.g. tuberculosis. Prolonged fevers are dealt with in the section on "fever of unknown origin." **Organ-based symptoms** usually direct the clinician to a likely source of infection (e.g. cough in pneumonia) but often there are no localizing features. It is necessary to seek specific **exposure risks** (Fig. 15.3) and it is vital that a **travel history** be taken, including time spent abroad and date of return. It is usually unhelpful to enquire about bites from mosquitoes or flies but **tick bites** are an exception because they are associated with specific infections, e.g. Lyme disease. These are painless and therefore often pass unobserved but patients may recall removing ticks from skin (or even their pet dog). Contact with **animals**, particularly scratches and bites from pets, may be significant and in some cases, these involve **occupational** and **recreational risks** (Table 15.2). Recreational risks include outdoor activities such as camping or walks in forests or heathland, where ticks live. Hobbies or sports may also be involved, for example leptospirosis following **water contact** in canoeists. **Recent contacts**, especially with **children** with rashes (e.g. viral exanthemas), gastro-intestinal illnesses (e.g. rotavirus), or a sore throat (e.g. group

Table 15.1. The clinical approach to the febrile patient

- What is the context? Is the patient from the community or already in hospital? *(Fig. 15.1)*
- Are there any clues in the history?
- What is the patient's age? *(Fig. 15.2)*
- Is there a history of relevant travel? *(Figs. 15.14 and 15.15)*
- Are there any other specific exposure risks? *(Fig. 15.3, Table 15.3)*
- Are there any clues on physical examination?
- Is there a skin rash? *(Fig. 15.4)*
- Is there lymphadenopathy? *(Fig. 15.5)*
- Is the patient immunocompromised and how? *(Fig. 15.6)*
- Are there any clues from the investigations? *(Fig. 15.7)*
- Does the patient require <u>urgent</u> antimicrobial treatment? *(Table 15.4)*
- Could there be a non-infectious underlying cause? *(See section on FUO)*

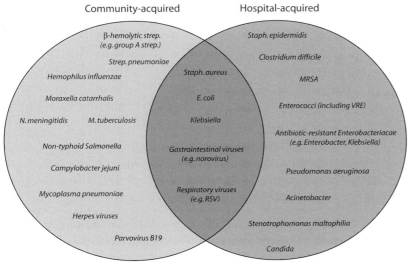

Fig. 15.1. Common causes of community- and hospital-acquired infection.

Community-acquired

β-hemolytic strep. (e.g. group A strep.)
Strep. pneumoniae
Hemophilus influenzae
Moraxella catarrhalis
N. meningitidis   M. tuberculosis
Non-typhoid Salmonella
Campylobacter jejuni
Mycoplasma pneumoniae
Herpes viruses
Parvovirus B19

Staph. aureus
E. coli
Klebsiella
Gastrointestinal viruses (e.g. norovirus)
Respiratory viruses (e.g. RSV)

Hospital-acquired

Staph. epidermidis
Clostridium difficile
MRSA
Enterococci (including VRE)
Antibiotic-resistant Enterobacteriacae (e.g. Enterobacter, Klebsiella)
Pseudomonas aeruginosa
Acinetobacter
Stenotrophomonas maltophilia
Candida

MRSA, methicillin resistant Staph. aureus; VRE, vancomycin-resistant enterococci; RSV, respiratory syncytial virus

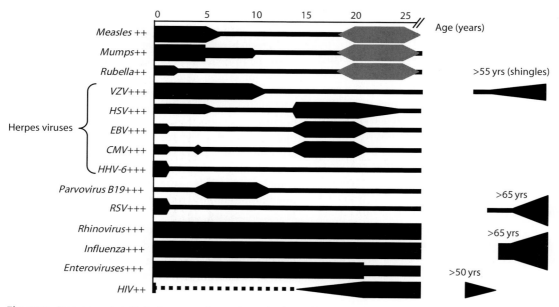

Fig. 15.2. Frequency of viral infections according to the patient's age. Herpes simplex virus (HSV), cytomegalovirus (CMV), Epstein–Barr virus (EBV), varicella zoster infection (VZV), human herpes virus-6 (HHV-6), respiratory syncytial virus (RSV), human immunodeficiency virus (HIV). A susceptible cohort of young adults (gray) that were not vaccinated against MMR (measles, mumps, and rubella) are shown in gray. Thickness of line indicates frequency (i.e. thicker means more frequent). +++ - very common; ++ - less common.

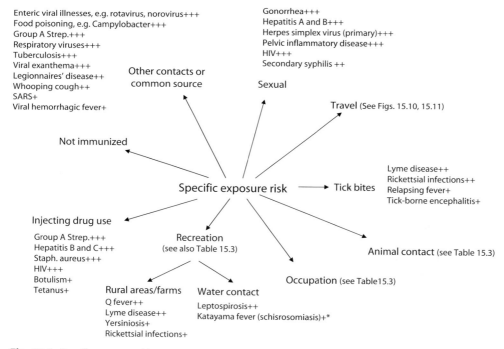

Fig. 15.3. Specific exposure risk. +++ - very common; ++ - less common; + - rare; * - non-endemic.

A streptococcus) are occasionally useful. It is unrewarding to enquire in detail about what a patient with a gastrointestinal infection has eaten but a **common source** may be suspected if a cluster of similar cases occurs simultaneously, e.g. *Campylobacter* after a barbecue. A **sexual history**, which includes assessment of **HIV risk**, should also be taken in a sensitive manner. A **drug history** is important since any medication can

Table 15.2. Infections causing fever associated with animal contact

Infection	Animal and transmission route	Exposure risk and comments
Anthrax	Herbivores (e.g. cattle, goats). Most commonly via skin contact with wool, hair and hide. Inhalation more rarely	Handling imported animal skins from endemic areas (tanners). Extremely rare in UK
Avian influenza (H5N1)	Chicken, ducks and geese. Inhalation	Poultry farmers. Bird markets. SE Asia but spreading?
Brucellosis	Mainly cattle, also camels, goats, and sheep. Consumption of unpasteurized dairy produce	Farm and abattoir workers, veterinarians, laboratory workers. Not endemic in UK
Capnocytophaga	Dog bites and scratches	Pet owners
Cat-scratch fever	Bites and scratches from kittens and feral cats	Pet owners
Histoplasmosis	Inhalation of dust contaminated with bird or bat droppings	Construction/agricultural workers in endemic areas of USA. Poultry farmers in and S. America. Spelunkers
Leptospirosis	Rodents. Exposure to water contaminated with infected urine	Farmers, sewer workers, veterinarians. Water sports
Pasteurellosis	Cat bites and scratches. Dogs also, less commonly	Pet owners
Psittacosis	"Sick" birds (especially parrots). Inhalation	Pet owners
Plague	Wild rodents (e.g. rats, squirrels, prairie dogs, etc.). Flea bites	Hunters and farmers. Laboratory workers. Not endemic in UK
Q fever	Cattle, sheep, and goats. Inhalation	Farm and abattoir workers, meatpackers. Rural exposure during calving or lambing season
Rabies/Lysaviruses	Commonly dog bites but also bites from cats and wild carnivores e.g. bats, foxes, and racoons	Wildlife biologists, hunters, and trappers
Rat-bite fever	Rat bite or scratch. Ingestion of contaminated food or water	Pet owners
Non-typhoid *Salmonella*	Reptiles (lizards, snakes, and turtles), chicks, and ducklings. Oro-fecal transmission	Pet owners
Tularemia	Small mammals (e.g. rabbits). Contact with infected animal fluids/blood, biting arthropods, contaminated food/water	Hunters and trappers. Northern hemisphere including USA (not endemic in UK)

cause fever and immunosuppressive therapy may predispose to opportunistic infections. The **past medical history** may indicate relapse of a previous condition (e.g. acute cholecystitis) and underlying **immunodeficiency** should be considered with recurrent, severe, or unusual infections. Since some bacteria adhere to **implants or prostheses** (e.g. heart valves, vascular grafts, and prosthetic joints), the presence of these materials should be noted. Recent **hospitalization** and, in particular, **instrumentation** (e.g. vascular or urinary catheterization) may also point towards a hospital-acquired infection. A history of **immunization** makes some conditions less likely but adults frequently do not accurately recall childhood vaccinations (Table 15.3). Vaccine-induced immunity may also wane and not all are highly effective, e.g. BCG does not prevent tuberculosis in adults. It is important to recognize that although many with tuberculosis do not have a contact history, they frequently come from a **country or ethnic group** where tuberculosis is common. **Family history** is important in the rare inherited febrile disorders, which are covered in the section on fever of unknown origin.

Are there any clues from the physical examination?

The **temperature chart** pattern does not generally provide a helpful clue to likely cause. Inspection of the **oral cavity** is particularly important. For example, tonsillar enlargement and pharyngitis may indicate infection with group A streptococcus or a viral etiology. Vesicles and ulcers may suggest viral infections (e.g. herpes simplex, varicella zoster, and enteroviruses), "snail track" ulcers occur in secondary syphilis and aphthous ulcers in Crohn's disease and HIV infection. Oral thrush and hairy leukoplakia on the tongue are also associated with HIV infection and Koplik's spots on the buccal mucosa are pathognomonic of measles. In hospitalized patients, venous cannula sites should be inspected for evidence of infection. **Splinter hemorrhages** or new or changing regurgitant **murmurs** indicate infective endocarditis.

Skin rash accompanies many febrile illnesses, especially the viral exanthemas of childhood. These are not always obvious and a search over the body should be in

431

Table 15.3. Immunization schedule

Disease (vaccine)	Age	Comment
Diphtheria/tetanus/pertussis/inactivated polio vaccine/ *H. influenzae* type B, meningococcal type C	2, 3, and 4 months	Primary course (three doses). 1 month between each dose
Measles/mumps/rubella	12 to 15 months (any age over 12 months)	First dose
Diphtheria/tetanus/pertussis/inactivated polio vaccine measles/mumps/rubella	3 to 5 years	Booster dose Second dose
Tuberculosis	10 to 14 years and neonates from high risk groups	
Diphtheria/tetanus/inactivated polio vaccine	13 to 18 years	Booster dose

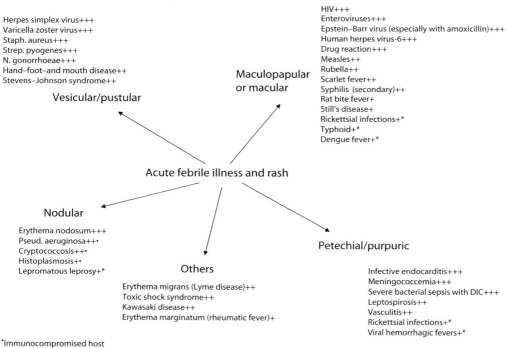

Fig. 15.4. Acute febrile illness and rash. +++ - very common; ++ - less common; + - rare; * - non-endemic.

good light. Recognition of the **petechial** rash of meningococcemia demands urgent treatment. Important causes of specific types of rash are shown in Fig. 15.4 and include some non-infectious conditions that may present with fever. **Lymphadenopathy** should be sought at all sites, including the axillas. Regional lymphadenopathy occurs when there is a localized infection and generalized lymphadenopathy occurs in disseminated infections (Fig. 15.5). Palpable **splenomegaly** is associated with a diverse range of infectious and non-infectious diseases, e.g. glandular fever, infective endocarditis, malaria, and lymphoma. Abnormal signs in **specific organ systems** (e.g. chest signs, jaundice, arthritis) are covered elsewhere.

Is the patient immunocompromised and how?

If the host immune response is impaired, infections are more severe and organisms that usually do not cause disease in healthy indviduals may become **opportunistic pathogens**. Understanding the type of immunodeficiency helps predict the organism susceptibility (Fig. 15.6). Hospital-acquired infections

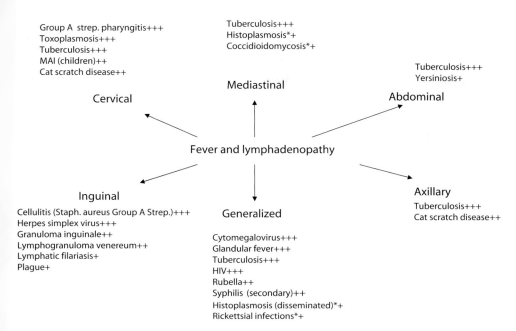

Group A strep. pharyngitis+++
Toxoplasmosis+++
Tuberculosis+++
MAI (children)++
Cat scratch disease++

Tuberculosis+++
Histoplasmosis*+
Coccidioidomycosis*+

Tuberculosis+++
Yersiniosis+

Cervical

Mediastinal

Abdominal

Fever and lymphadenopathy

Inguinal

Generalized

Axillary

Cellulitis (Staph. aureus Group A Strep.)+++
Herpes simplex virus+++
Granuloma inguinale++
Lymphogranuloma venereum++
Lymphatic filariasis+
Plague+

Cytomegalovirus+++
Glandular fever+++
Tuberculosis+++
HIV+++
Rubella++
Syphilis (secondary)++
Histoplasmosis (disseminated)*+
Rickettsial infections*+

Tuberculosis+++
Cat scratch disease++

Fig. 15.5. Infectious causes of fever and lymphadenopathy. +++ - very common; ++ - less common; + - rare; * - non-endemic.

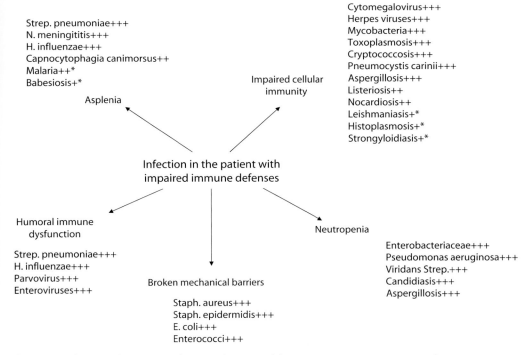

Strep. pneumoniae+++
N. meningititis+++
H. influenzae+++
Capnocytophagia canimorsus++
Malaria++*
Babesiosis+*

Cytomegalovirus+++
Herpes viruses+++
Mycobacteria+++
Toxoplasmosis+++
Cryptococcosis+++
Pneumocystis carinii+++
Aspergillosis+++
Listeriosis++
Nocardiosis++
Leishmaniasis+*
Histoplasmosis+*
Strongyloidiasis+*

Asplenia

Impaired cellular immunity

Infection in the patient with
impaired immune defenses

Humoral immune dysfunction

Neutropenia

Strep. pneumoniae+++
H. influenzae+++
Parvovirus+++
Enteroviruses+++

Broken mechanical barriers

Enterobacteriaceae+++
Pseudomonas aeruginosa+++
Viridans Strep.+++
Candidiasis+++
Aspergillosis+++

Staph. aureus+++
Staph. epidermidis+++
E. coli+++
Enterococci+++

Fig. 15.6. Infection in the patient with impaired immune defences. +++ - very common; ++ - less common; + - rare; * - non-endemic.

commonly occur where **natural mechanical barriers are breached** (e.g. bacteremia may result from vascular or urinary catheters and ventilator-associated pneumonia via endotracheal tubes). **Asplenia**, which occurs in sickle cell disease or following splenectomy, is a risk for severe infections involving capsulated bacteria (e.g. *Strep. pneumoniae*) and red cell parasites (e.g. malaria). This is because the spleen produces

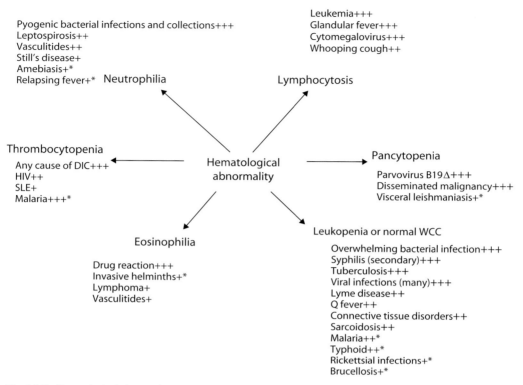

Neutrophilia
- Pyogenic bacterial infections and collections+++
- Leptospirosis++
- Vasculitides++
- Still's disease+
- Amebiasis+*
- Relapsing fever+*

Lymphocytosis
- Leukemia+++
- Glandular fever+++
- Cytomegalovirus+++
- Whooping cough++

Thrombocytopenia
- Any cause of DIC+++
- HIV++
- SLE+
- Malaria+++*

Hematological abnormality

Pancytopenia
- Parvovirus B19Δ+++
- Disseminated malignancy+++
- Visceral leishmaniasis+*

Eosinophilia
- Drug reaction+++
- Invasive helminths+*
- Lymphoma+
- Vasculitides+

Leukopenia or normal WCC
- Overwhelming bacterial infection+++
- Syphilis (secondary)+++
- Tuberculosis+++
- Viral infections (many)+++
- Lyme disease++
- Q fever++
- Connective tissue disorders++
- Sarcoidosis++
- Malaria++*
- Typhoid++*
- Rickettsial infections+*
- Brucellosis+*

Fig. 15.7. Hematological abnormalities. +++ - very common; ++ - less common; + - rare; * - non-endemic; Δ - associated with a low reticulocyte count.

antibody to polysaccharide antigens and clears opsonized and non-opsonized organisms from the circulation. **Impaired humoral immunity** (e.g. myeloma or congenital antibody deficiency) increases susceptibility to pathogens cleared by the antibody response. Patients with **neutropenia** (e.g. acute leukemia or post-chemotherapy) are unable to prevent local infections spreading into the bloodstream. Common sources of neutropenic sepsis include the mouth, skin, lung, and colon, which are reflected in the types of organism causing invasive infection in this group. The **impaired cellular immunity** of HIV infection, lymphoma or bone marrow transplantation predisposes to intracellular pathogens and reactivation of latent infections (e.g. tuberculosis and herpes viruses).

Are there any clues from the investigations?

Initial investigations can sometimes provide helpful clues (Fig. 15.7). Bacterial infections are more frequently associated with a **neutrophilia**. However, this is not invariably the case and **leukopenia** can be a feature of severe or overwhelming bacterial sepsis.

The total white cell count is often not significantly elevated in viral infections but a **lymphoctosis or "atypical" lymphocytes** may be seen on a blood film and are common in glandular fever. **Inflammatory indices**, such as the C-reactive protein (CRP) and erythrocyte sedimentation rate (ESR) are more elevated in bacterial than viral infections but are not dependable. **Thrombocytopenia** is a feature of disseminated intravascular coagulation (DIC), e.g. in severe bacterial sepsis, and is also common in malaria and some viral infections. Varying degrees of **renal** and **liver impairment** may reflect multiorgan failure in severe sepsis and/or point to specific infections (e.g. leptospirosis). **Pancytopenia** may be associated with malignant marrow infiltration but also characteristically occurs in some infections, e.g. advanced HIV, leishmaniasis, and parvovirus B19. Other investigations are described under "fever of unknown origin."

Does the patient require urgent antimicrobial treatment?

A difficult decision is whether to give empiric antimicrobial treatment to a febrile patient. Withholding

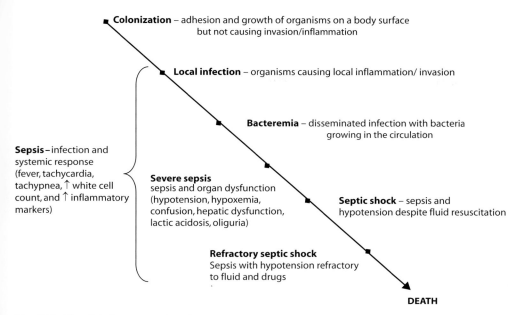

Colonization – adhesion and growth of organisms on a body surface but not causing invasion/inflammation

Local infection – organisms causing local inflammation/ invasion

Bacteremia – disseminated infection with bacteria growing in the circulation

Sepsis – infection and systemic response (fever, tachycardia, tachypnea, ↑ white cell count, and ↑ inflammatory markers)

Severe sepsis
sepsis and organ dysfunction (hypotension, hypoxemia, confusion, hepatic dysfunction, lactic acidosis, oliguria)

Septic shock – sepsis and hypotension despite fluid resuscitation

Refractory septic shock
Sepsis with hypotension refractory to fluid and drugs

DEATH

Fig. 15.8. The clinical spectrum of sepsis.

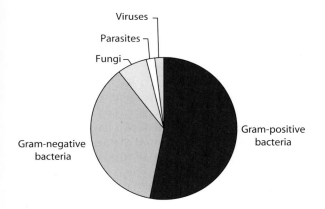

Fig. 15.9. Main pathogens involved in septic shock.

Viruses

Parasites

Fungi

Gram-negative bacteria

Gram-positive bacteria

Table 15.4. Features of severe sepsis where empiric antibiotic treatment may be indicated

- Rigors
- Petechial or purpuric rash that may indicate meningococcal sepsis
- Cardiovascular features of septic shock (tachycardia and hypotension)
- Tachypnea (respiratory rate >20/min) or respiratory failure
- Impaired consciousness, neurological signs, or meningism
- Extremes of age
- Asplenia or any severe immunodeficiency (especially neutropenia)

treatment to await results may lead to irreversible deterioration while inappropriate treatment may mask the diagnosis and risk drug side effects. The **clinical spectrum** of bacterial infection extends from harmless colonization to hypotensive shock with multiorgan dysfunction and death (Figs. 15.8 and 15.9). Features listed in Table 15.4 indicate a need for urgent, empiric antibiotic therapy after obtaining appropriate cultures where possible (i.e. at least two sets of blood cultures). Maximum cover with "broad-spectrum antibiotics" should be given if the source is unclear and the patient is very unwell. However, community-acquired bacteria are frequently sensitive to standard antibiotics and an early first dose is critical. If hospital acquired,

it is often important to **remove or treat the source** (e.g. removal of infected vascular lines or wound debridement) and the possibility of antibiotic resistance should be considered. Prompt commencement of **general supportive treatment** such as adequate fluid resuscitation is also vital.

Endemic infections
Bacteria
All bacteria are classified according to morphologic appearance and color after Gram stain (Gram-positive organisms are dark purple and Gram-negative organisms are light pink). The classification is useful clinically since it gives an early clue to identity of organisms thus directing the antibiotic choice.

435

Gram-positive cocci
Staphylococcal infections:
Staphylococcus aureus
Clinical features

- Many isolates in wounds and ulcers are harmless colonization. However, *Staph. aureus* also commonly causes skin and soft tissue infections, e.g. cellulitis, boils, and wound infections. Fever and features of inflammation (erythema, swelling, heat, pain, and tenderness) distinguish significant infection from colonization.
- *Staph. aureus* bacteremia presents with fever, chills and rigors. Patients with intravenous catheters and iv drug users are at high risk. Signs of severe sepsis with shock include tachycardia, tachypnea, and hypotension.
- *Staph. aureus* infective endocarditis affects both native and prosthetic heart valves. Embolic phenomena such as splinter hemorrhages should be sought in addition to a new or changed heart murmur. Infections typically progress rapidly, resulting in heart failure from valve destruction.
- Staphylococcal toxic shock syndrome (TSS) is toxin-mediated and associated with tampon use in menstruating women. There is acute onset fever, diarrhea and vomiting, hypotension, confusion, myalgia, and a widespread erythematous rash. Multiorgan failure frequently develops. In survivors, the skin on the palms and soles peels away after 1–2 weeks.
- *Staph. aureus* is the commonest cause of septic arthritis and osteomyelitis.
- *Staph. aureus* infects prosthetic material implanted inside the body, e.g. joints, heart valves, and vascular grafts.
- Colonization of the bronchial tree is much commoner than true infection but *Staph. aureus* occasionally causes pneumonia, e.g. community-acquired pneumonia may arise as a secondary bacterial complication to influenza or measles. True hospital-acquired pneumonia is rare.
- Staphylococcal food poisoning is caused by ingestion of pre-formed enterotoxin. It results in vomiting and diarrhoea within 1–6 hours but not fever.

Epidemiology
Staph. aureus is regarded as normal human flora when cultured from skin, nasopharynx, vagina, and gastro-intestinal tract. Although colonization can be transient, the nasopharynx is a site of persistent carriage. Patients become colonized after physical contact with carriers. Methicillin-resistant *Staph. aureus* (MRSA) is an increasing problem acquired in hospital where healthcare workers transmit it on their hands. Invasive *Staph. aureus* infection is associated with intravenous lines and is hence more common on intensive care and renal units.

Pathology
Staph. aureus is a commensal organism, but it can produce life-threatening human infection. Invasive *Staph. aureus* infections most commonly occur through a break in the epidermis. If limited to the skin, cellulitis or an abscess may develop. However, if bacteria enter the circulation, organisms are seeded throughout the body resulting in complications such as endocarditis, septic arthritis, and osteomyelitis. Attachment to host cells or tissues ("adherence") is a key step in initiating these infections. In addition, *Staph. aureus* adheres strongly to prosthetic surfaces (e.g. joints, heart valves, vascular grafts) and some strains also produce a protective biofilm (see *Staph. epidermidis* below).

Staph. aureus secretes a number of enzymes and toxins implicated in pathogenicity. In menstruating women, TSS toxin-1 (TSST-1) is released by certain strains of *Staph. aureus* growing in absorbable tampons. TSST-1 is not processed and presented to T-cells in the context of the MHC class II molecules by antigen presenting cells in the usual way. Instead, TSST-1 directly binds to T-cell receptors with MHC class II molecules without need for the usual internal processing (termed a "superantigen"). This activates a much greater proportion of T-cells and stimulates massive release of pro-inflammatory cytokines resulting in multiorgan failure.

Staph. aureus contains transmissible plasmids responsible for secretion of beta-lactamase, an enzyme that inactivates penicillin.

Investigations
Bacterial swabs should be taken from skin lesions, wounds, pus, aspirates, and other body fluids. Infection rather than colonization causes neutrophil leukocytosis and raised inflammatory markers. Deep surgical samples or aspirates from sites that are normally sterile are relatively easier to interpret, e.g. *Staph. aureus* grown from a bone biopsy or joint aspirate indicates osteomyelitis and septic arthritis respectively. In contrast, positive cultures from skin

ulcers or sputum may simply reflect colonization. Blood cultures growing *Staph. aureus* always signify invasive disease and the tips of removed intravascular catheters should be cultured. Other investigations depend on clinical features and sites of infection. CT or radiolabeled white cell scans may reveal an occult focus of infection. MRI scans are especially good for identifying bone infection.

Management
Cellulitis and wound infections are treated with antibiotics, but collections of pus must be drained. Flucloxacillin has excellent anti-staphyloccal activity but alternatives include macrolides (e.g. clarithromycin) and tetracyclines (e.g. doxycycline). A major principle of treatment is removal of the source. For example, antibiotics frequently fail to sterilize infected heart valves and replacement is often the only option. Similarly, if intravascular lines are implicated, they should be taken out and tampons removed from young women with TSS. *Staph. aureus* bacteremia is treated for at least 2 weeks.

Invasive MRSA should be considered in colonized patients and/or those with hospital-acquired infections. Vancomycin or teicoplainin (glycopeptides) are effective but can only be given intravenously. Oral therapy can be complicated but options include linezolid as a single agent, or dual-therapy combinations (e.g. involving doxycycline, clarithromycin, trimethoprim and rifampicin). Infection control measures are essential to prevent MRSA transmission in a hospital setting. Healthcare staff should clean their hands before and after seeing patients. MRSA-colonized patients are usually moved to a single room and staff must wear gloves and aprons. For known carriers, skin decolonisation may be attempted with topical antiseptics or antibiotics (e.g. chlorhexidine body washes). Intranasal mupirocin is given to eradicate nasal carriage. Unnecessary vascular lines should be removed to reduce the risk of invasive disease.

Outcome
Mortality of *Staph. aureus* bacteremia is 10%. Other complications depend on whether or not there has been seeding to bone, joints, or heart valves, which occurs in 5%–10%. If left-sided infective endocarditis develops mortality is 20%–40%.

Staphylococcus epidermidis
Staph. epidermidis is a human commensal and the most common organism isolated from normal skin.

It is relatively avirulent and unlike *Staph. aureus* is coagulasenegative. When isolated in blood cultures it usually represents skin contamination. True bacteremias are frequently related to intravenous catheters and repeated isolation occurs in prosthetic valve endocarditis. Bacteria adherent to prosthetic surfaces release an exopolysaccharide biofilm (or "slime") that protects them from host immune cells and antibiotic penetration. Septic shock with hemodynamic compromise is rare and patients with *Staph. epidermidis* bacteremia appear relatively well. Antibiotic treatment is usually not required in immunocompetent hosts and removal of intravascular lines is sufficient.

Streptococcal infections
Group A Streptococcus or Strep. pyogenes
Clinical features
- Group A Streptococcus (GAS) commonly causes wound and skin infections, e.g. erysipelas and cellulitis.
- Necrotising fasciitis is a severe, rapidly progressive infection of the subcutaneous fascia with sparing of underlying muscle. The limbs are most commonly involved. Fever and severe pain are common presenting features. There may be few signs on the skin surface initially but pain is due to evolving deep infection. The infection rapidly spreads along fascial planes, with soft tissue swelling and marked erythema. If aggressive surgical treatment is not immediately undertaken, gangrene quickly develops and the condition is life threatening.
- GAS pharyngitis produces sudden onset sore throat, pain on swallowing, and fever. The pharynx is red, the tonsils are swollen, and exudates visible. Tender cervical lymphadenopathy is typical.
- Scarlet fever affects mainly children causing severe pharyngitis, high fever, and typical, punctate erythematous skin rash all over the body, except around the mouth (circumoral pallor). There is exudative tonsillitis with white coating on the tongue, through which red papillae protrude ("strawberry tongue"). Desquamation of skin on hands and feet occurs later.
- Streptococcal toxic shock syndrome is a severe condition diagnosed when there is sudden onset septic shock and multiorgan failure associated with infection caused by GAS (most frequently necrotizing fasciitis). Fever is usual and confusion

common. Multiorgan failure involves the lungs, liver, kidneys, and DIC. Skin desquamation may occur later.

- GAS occasionally causes septic arthritis and infective endocarditis, particularly in IV drug users.
- Rheumatic fever, acute glomerulonephritis, and arthritis are post-infectious, immunologic complications.

Epidemiology

Humans are the only host and transmission occurs from direct contact or aerosolized micro-droplets. Asymptomatic carriage (on mucous membranes e.g. nasopharynx or skin) is commoner in children (15%–20%) than adults (5%). Epidemics may occur in the community and in hospitals. Serotyping distinguishes different strains according to the particular M-protein expressed on the cell wall and certain strains are more closely associated with specific syndromes.

Pathology

Streptococci are divided into two groups according to whether they cause complete (beta) or incomplete (alpha) hemolysis on a blood agar plate. The beta-hemolytic streptococci are sub-classified into Lancefield groups A to O depending on cell wall antigens that are expressed. *Strep. pyogenes* is beta-hemolytic and belongs to group A.

Cell wall proteins and a number of secreted toxins, proteases, and other soluble factors are responsible for the hyper-virulence and invasiveness of GAS. The spread of cellulitis and necrotizing fasciitis is facilitated by release of proteases e.g. DNAse, streptokinase, and hyaluronidase. Pyrogenic exotoxins cause the rash of scarlet fever, and the toxin released in TSS is a superantigen (similar to staphylococcal TSST-1), which triggers an overwhelming pro-inflammatory T-cell response and multiorgan damage.

Investigations

Neutrophilia and elevated inflammatory indices. GAS may be isolated from throat swabs and skin. In necrotizing fasciitis and TSS, blood cultures are usually positive. Elevated antibody levels against streptolysin O (ASO titer) is indirect evidence of invasive GAS infection.

Management

All GAS isolates should be treated. Penicillin remains the antibiotic of choice and GAS is always sensitive.

Pharyngitis should be treated for 10 days since there is an increased risk of rheumatic fever with shorter courses. An antibiotic with anti-staphylococcal activity, e.g. flucloxacillin, is often given in the treatment of cellulitis since infections caused by GAS and *Staph. aureus* are often difficult to differentiate on clinical grounds. Necrotizing fasciitis is a surgical emergency. Extensive, early debridement of all devitalized tissue is essential. Clindamycin is given in addition to high-dose penicillin in the treatment of necrotizing fasciitis, since it may help to stop toxin production.

Outcome

Prognosis depends on the type of infection. Pharyngitis is often self-limiting after 3–4 days, but suppurative complications may be severe and include quinsy (peritonsillar abscess). Non-suppurative complications include rheumatic fever, which develops 2–4 weeks after untreated pharyngitis. Post-streptococcal glomerulonephritis can occur after any GAS infection with a nephrotogenic strain. Mortality of necrotizing fasciitis and streptococcal TSS are high (20% and >30%).

Streptococcus pneumoniae or the pneumococcus
Clinical features
Immunocompetent hosts

- Commonest pathogen isolated in otitis media and a major cause of sinusitis.
- Most common identifiable cause of community-acquired pneumonia and acute exacerbations of COPD.
- Commonest cause of meningitis in adults >30 years.

Immunocompromised hosts

- Invasive infections are more common with chronic illness, e.g. alcoholics and diabetics, or with heart, liver, kidney, and lung failure.
- Recurrent bacterial pneumonia is a common complication of HIV infection and bacteremia is more common in children with HIV infection.
- Specific risks include defective antibody or complement function, e.g. congenital antibody deficiency and hematological malignancies. Overwhelming infection occurs in asplenic patients.

Epidemiology

Strep. pneumoniae colonizes the nasopharynx without causing symptoms in 15% of adults and up to 40% of children. Carriage rates are highest where there is overcrowding or closed communities e.g. prisons and homeless shelters. Transmission is by respiratory droplets and colonization rates are highest in winter. Invasive pneumococcal infections tend to occur in infants, the elderly, and the immunocompromised.

Pathology

Strep. pneumoniae are alpha-hemolytic, Gram-positive, elongated cocci that associate in pairs (diplococci). The organism has an external capsule. There are over 80 serotypes according to antigens expressed on its surface. Cellular attachment and colonization of the nasopharynx precedes penetration of the mucosa and entry into the circulation. Pneumococci invade nearby structures from the nasopharynx, including the sinuses, Eustachian tubes, and bronchi. Meningitis can develop following direct spread from a nearby focus (e.g. mastoiditis) or following bacteremia from any cause (e.g. pneumonia).

The external capsule is central to the ability to evade phagocytosis by neutrophils. Clearance of the organism is associated with development of specific anticapsular antibodies, complement activation, opsonization of bacteria, and phagocytosis. Hence patients with humoral immune deficiency or without a spleen are susceptible to invasive pneumococcal infection. Pneumococci also produce several toxins (e.g. pneumolysin).

Investigations

Most have a neutrophilia and elevated inflammatory indices. Definitive diagnosis is made by culture of sputum, pleural fluid, CSF, or blood. Blood cultures may be positive in pneumonia (<20%) and meningitis (~80%). Urinary pneumococcal antigen can also be detected rapidly when organisms have reached the bloodstream.

Management

Where penicillin-sensitive pneumococci are isolated, the best antimicrobial treatment remains a penicillin, e.g. amoxicillin. Resistance is classified as "intermediate" (high-dose benzylpenicillin effective, except in meningitis) and "full" (benzylpenicillin ineffective). In the UK, intermediate resistance is common but full resistance is rare. Where fully resistant strains are common (e.g. Spain, South Africa and the USA), vancomycin is an alternative. Collections of pus require drainage, e.g. empyema or infected sinuses in patients with meningitis.

Immunization with pneumococcal vaccine gives good protection for many years against important serotypes and is recommended for those over 65 and susceptible individuals. Daily penicillin prophylaxis should also be given to asplenic patients.

Outcome

Pneumococcal infections can be very severe, not least because patients with invasive disease often have concurrent medical problems. The mortality of pneumococcal meningitis is double that of meningococcal meningitis (~20%) and more survivors have residual neurologic deficit.

Other streptococci

Viridans streptococci

The "viridans" streptococci are a group of organisms, (classified as either alpha- or non-hemolytic) that inhabit the mouth, upper respiratory tract, and bowel. Dental extraction or other trauma may allow them to enter the circulation. Bacteremia in immunocompetent hosts rarely results in significant disease apart from the following:

- Viridans streptococci (e.g. *Strep. sanguis* and *Strep. mitis*) are the commonest causes of infective endocarditis. The outcome is better than from other causes of bacterial endocarditis.
- *Strep. bovis* causes bacteremia and endocarditis, especially in patients with colonic neoplasms.
- *Strep. milleri* has a propensity for forming pyogenic collections, e.g. hepatic abscesses, abdominal collections, and empyema. Infections are more common in diabetics or immunocompromised hosts and following gastrointestinal surgery or trauma.

Group B streptococci

Group B streptococci colonize the vagina and rectum and are an important cause of peripartum infections, neonatal bacteremi, and meningitis.

Group C and G streptococci

Cause similar infections to GAS, such as pharyngitis and cellulitis.

Enterococci

Enterococci form most of the normal bowel flora. Being relatively avirulent, they tend to cause disease in patients with chronic illnesses, especially with intravascular lines or urinary catheters. Infections are acquired endogenously from the patient's gut or exogenously by spread between patients. *E. fecalis* and *E. fecium* are the commonest, causing:

- urinary tract infections
- line-related bacteremias

- intra-abdominal infections, often with other gut organisms
- prosthetic valve endocarditis, typically in elderly patients

Enterococci are naturally resistant to many antibiotics such as cephalosporins. Amoxicillin or nitrofurantoin may be effective in urinary tract infections. Antibiotic-resistant strains are increasing in intensive care and renal units, e.g. vancomycin-resistant enteroccci.

Gram-positive bacilli

Listeria monocytogenes (listeriosis)

Listeria monocytogenes is present in soil, sewage, rivers, and the gastro-intestinal tract of many mammals. Transmission is by ingestion of contaminated food. Listeria can multiply at $4\,^\circ$C, and soft cheeses, unpasteurized milk, and cold meats are commonly implicated. Risk factors include: neonates or age >70 years, pregnant women, and immunosupression, e.g. steroids and chemotherapy, diabetes, renal transplantation, and HIV infection. Pregnant women and immunocompromised hosts should avoid high-risk foods, e.g. raw meat or soft cheeses made with unpasteurised milk.

Meningitis and bacteremia are the commonest presentations. Listeria is the third commonest bacterial meningitis in adults. Bacteremia is non-specific with fever and myalgia, possibly preceeded by gastro-intestinal upset. Diagnosis is by isolation from blood or CSF. Treatment is high-dose amoxicillin plus gentamicin.

Actinomyctes (branching Gram-positive bacteria)

Nocardiosis

Ubiquitous organisms found in soil. Infection usually occurs by inhalation of contaminated soil particles. *Nocardia asteroides* is the commonest species and primarily a pathogen of the immunocompromised. Pulmonary nocardiosis is the commonest manifestation. Radiographic features include nodules, cavitation, and consolidation. The central nervous system is commonly affected in disseminated disease but spread to other organs can also occur. Diagnosis is by microscopy and culture. Trimethoprim–sulfamethoxazole is the drug of choice.

Actinomycosis

Actinomyctes are commensals of the oral cavity, gastrointestinal, and female genital tract. Human disease develops when the mucosal barrier is breached. Infections tend to be chronic, with a tendency to form fistulas.

- Cervicofacial disease follows dental procedures with pain and jaw swelling caused by osteomyelitis. Fever is variable but fistulas draining pus to the skin surface are common.
- Abdominal disease occurs after gastro-intestinal surgery, appendicitis, or penetrating injuries. The ileocecal region, is the commonest site following appendicitis with weight loss, fever, right iliac fossa mass, and cutaneous fistulas. Pelvic infections are associated with intrauterine contraception devices.
- Thoracic disease is caused by aspiration, especially in alcoholics. Fever, weight loss, and respiratory symptoms are typical. Radiographic imaging may show cavitating lesions. Spread into the pleural space, adjacent ribs, or chest wall may result in empyema, osteomyelitis, and cutaneous fistulas.

Diagnosis is microscopy and culture. Penicillin for 6–12 months is the drug of choice. Relapse is common.

Gram-negative cocci

Neisseria meningitidis or the meningococcus

Clinical features

- Symptoms of meningitis include: fever, rigors, headache, and vomiting. The patient may be confused or drowsy. Meningism and photophobia may be present but the classic feature is a petechial rash that evolves over hours and does not blanch on pressure (Fig. 15.10).
- Less commonly, patients present with fulminant meningococcal bacteremia (meningococcemia) without meningitis. There is septic shock with reduced consciousness and rapid progression to multiorgan dysfunction. Coagulopathy caused by DIC may exacerbate the petechial rash. Gangrene of the extremities may also develop.
- Rarely, some present over days to weeks with chronic meningococcemia. There is intermittent fever, joint pains, and rash, which may be maculopapular rather than petechial.

Epidemiology

Neisseria meningitidis is part of the normal oropharyngeal flora in 5%–15% of healthy children and adults. Most occur under age 5 years but there is a second peak between 15 and 19 years. Transmission is increased amongst closed or overcrowded populations. Meningococcal meningitis is the only type that causes epidemics. There are several serogroups with seasonal

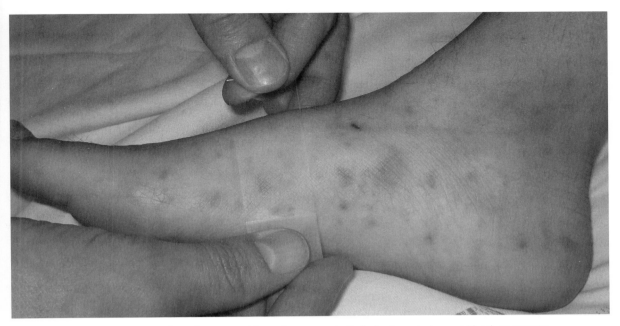

Fig. 15.10. A purpuric rash on the foot of a patient with meningococcemia. Typically, the rash does not blanch on pressure, as demonstrated with the glass slide.

patterns: group A, B, C, W, and Y135. Group A causes epidemics along the "meningitis belt" in sub-Saharan Africa during the dry season. Serogroups B and C cause most disease in the UK but the incidence of group C has fallen since the introduction of vaccination (there is no effective vaccine against group B).

Pathology

Gram-negative diplococci; transmission via respiratory route through infected droplets. In the majority there is no progression beyond asymptomatic carrier state. However, entry into the circulation may be facilitated by a concomitant upper respiratory tract infection. Once in the bloodstream, bacteria rapidly multiply and meningitis develops if bacteria penetrate the blood–brain barrier. Many features of severe sepsis are attributable to endotoxin, which triggers release of inflammatory cytokines (e.g. tumor necrosis factor-α and interleukin-1) that mediate endothelial wall damage, capillary leak, intravascular clotting, and myocardial dysfunction. In shock, poor perfusion produces tissue anoxia and organ damage, and as coagulation products are consumed by widespread clotting activation, the platelet count falls and DIC develops.

Investigations

Neutrophilia and inflammatory indices are raised. Diagnosis is by identification of *N. meningitidis* in blood or CSF. Where negative, PCR-based assays may be useful.

Management

Antibiotic treatment is started immediately after lumbar puncture in meningitis. However, if the patient has a typical rash and/or hemodynamic instability, antibiotics should be administered immediately. High dose IV penicillin or ceftriaxone is standard. Chloramphenicol is used when there is severe penicillin allergy.

Oral ciprofloxacin or rifampicin prophylaxis should be given to household and "kissing" contacts of meningitis cases. If group C is isolated, vaccination can be given.

Outcome

Complications include severe ischemic injury that may cause loss of fingers or toes. Brain damage or hearing loss may be permanent. Adrenocortical failure can occur in patients with fulminant meningococcemia (Waterhouse–Friederichsen syndrome). Mortality is up to 10% in Western countries but much higher in countries where modern intensive care facilities are not available.

Neisseria gonorrhoeae, or the gonococcus

N. gonorrhoeae causes infection of the genitourinary tract. In a small number of patients (<1%) gonococci invade the bloodstream. The manifestations of disseminated infection include:

- Septic arthritis involving a single joint.
- Polyarthritis (affecting the knees, ankles, and wrists), with fever, tenosynovitis, and a hemorrhagic, pustular skin rash.
- Perihepatitis (Fitz–Hugh–Curtis syndrome) results from direct extension of infection from the pelvis to the liver capsule.

Gram-negative bacilli
Enterobacteriacieae
Enterobacteriacieae are a diverse family of organisms (all Gram-negative bacilli) that produce a wide disease spectrum.

Clinical features
Immunocompetent host
- *Esherichia coli* (*E. coli*) is the leading cause of community- and hospital-acquired urinary tract infection.
- *E. coli* is the commonest cause of community- and hospital-associated bacteremia that may be associated with septic shock.
- Enterobacteriaceae are sometimes implicated in hospital-acquired pneumonia. Community-acquired pneumonia caused by *Klebsiella pneumonia* (Friedlander's pneumonia) is very rare.
- Several strains of *E.coli* cause diarrhea. Fever is typically absent in verocytotoxin-producing *E. coli* (e.g. *E. coli* 0157) that is responsible for severe colitis and hemolytic–uremic syndrome.
- Non-typhoid *Salmonella* and *Shigella* species cause fever and diarrhea (sometimes bloody). Enteric (Typhoid) fever is discussed later.
- *Yersinia enterocolitica* and, more rarely, *Y. pseudotuberculosis* cause fever, diarrhea and abdominal pain caused by ileitis and mesenteric adenitis lasting weeks. (*Y. pestis* is the cause of plague.)

Immunocompromised host In neutropenic patients there may be bacteremia with no obvious source.

Epidemiology
Found worldwide in soil, water, plants, and animal intestines. Some are normal commensals of the human gut that occasionally cause disease (e.g. *E. coli*, *Klebsiella*, and *Proteus* species), others are exogenous and frequently pathogenic (e.g. *Salmonella*, *Shigella*, and *Yersinia* species). Antibiotic-resistant Gram-negative bacteria are encountered in hospital and are emerging in the community. Transfer is often by hands of staff, and gut colonization with resistant organisms is assisted by antibiotic therapy that disrupts normal bowel flora.

Pathology
In the community, *E. coli* gains access to the bloodstream from the urinary or gastro-intestinal tracts, e.g. acute cholecystitis or pyelonephritis. In hospital, manipulation of urinary catheters and intravenous lines is frequently involved.

Some organisms are intrinsically resistant to penicillin by producing β-lactamase, e.g. *Klebsiella*. Others switch on β-lactamase production when exposed to antibiotics (e.g. *Enterobacter*). Genes conferring antibiotic resistance can be transferred on plasmids from one strain of bacteria to another, e.g. extended spectrum β-lactamases (ESBLs).

Investigations
Diagnosis is by Gram stain and culture from urine, blood, or other specimens.

Treatment
Most community-acquired Enterobacteriaceae remain susceptible to standard antibiotics. The choice depends on the source of infection. For example, cephalexin, trimethoprim, or co-amoxiclav are effective oral agents in uncomplicated urinary tract infections. Intravenous co-amoxiclav or cefuroxime can be used for pyelonephritis but if resistance is suspected or there is septic shock, IV gentamicin may also be given. If a gut source is suspected, metronidazole is added to cefuroxime to cover the anaerobes present in the bowel.

Outcome
Outcome depends on type of infection. Mortality from Gram-negative septic shock is significant.

Pseudomonas aeruginosa
Found ubiquitously in soil, water, and organic matter. Colonization of skin, gut and respiratory tract precedes infection. Serious infections typically occur in hospitalized patients with predisposing risk factors. Clinical syndromes include:
- Bacteremia associated with septic shock in neutropenic patients, especially with venous lines.
- Catheter-associated urinary tract infections.
- Skin infections in burns patients.

- Pneumonia in patients with endotracheal tubes, cystic fibrosis, or severe immunosuppression.

Pseudomonal infections may be life threatening in immunocompromised patients. Effective antibiotics include ceftazidime, ciprofloxacin, and imipenem.

Campylobacter jejuni

The commonest food-borne cause of diarrhea in the UK. Features include diarrhea (occasionally bloody), abdominal pain, and fever. The natural reservoir is the gastro-intestinal tract of birds and animals. Transmission is by eating undercooked meat (especially poultry), unpasteurized or "bird-pecked" milk on the doorstep, contaminated water, or from pets with diarrhea. Incubation is 2–5 days. Most simply require correction of fluid loss. Clarithromycin is required if symptoms persist.

Hemophilus influenzae
Clinical features

- Commonly causes otitis media and sinusitis.
- Common cause of exacerbations of COPD.
- Severe invasive infections occur in unvaccinated children <5 years (e.g. meningitis).
- Overwhelming infection in asplenic patients.

Epidemiology

H. influenzae is a Gram-negative bacterium that can be capsulated (serotyped A–F) or uncapsulated. It is found in the pharynx of carriers (80% of healthy people). Most severe infections involve H. influenzae type B but a conjugate vaccine has made carriage and hence its complications uncommon in the UK.

Pathology

Transmission is by airborne droplets or contact with respiratory tract secretions. Serum antibodies, the complement system, and the spleen are important for protective immunity against capsulated H. influenzae.

Investigations

Culture of appropriate specimens: sputum, blood, CSF, joint fluid.

Management

Sinusitis, otitis media, and COPD may be treated with oral amoxicillin, or macrolide antibiotics. Third-generation cephalosporins, e.g. ceftriaxone, are the choice for life-threatening type B infections in childhood. Asplenic patients should be vaccinated against H. influenzae type B.

Outcome

Outcome depends upon type of infection. Most respond well but severe type B infections in children can be life threatening.

Moraxella (Branhamella) catarrhalis

Gram-negative diplococcus that colonizes the nasopharynx of 1%–5% healthy adults. It has similarities to H. influenzae, causing otitis media in children and infective exacerbations of COPD in adults. Some strains are β-lactamase producing but it is usually susceptible to co-amoxiclav, macrolides, and cephalosporins.

Bordetella pertussis (whooping cough)
Clinical features

Predominantly affects unvaccinated children in the UK.

- Coryza, runny nose, mild fever, and dry cough ("catarrhal" stage).
- A week or so later the cough becomes more severe ("paroxysmal" stage). Paroxysms of uncontrolled coughing are followed by a characteristic inspiratory "whoop." Severe coughing can cause cyanosis, subconjunctival hemorrhage, or vomiting. Other complications include bacterial pneumonia, otitis media, and convulsions. The paroxysmal stage may last several weeks ("100-day cough").
- Adults with waning immunity occasionally have a mild infection.
- Incubation period is 7–14 days.

Epidemiology

Vaccine coverage reached 94% in 1995 and UK notifications of pertussis are <1000 cases/year.

Pathology

Highly infectious Gram-negative coccobacillus transmitted by aerosolized droplets.

Investigation

Culture from nasal swabs or antigen detection in nasopharyngeal aspirates. A blood lymphocytosis is sometimes present.

Management

Treatment is supportive. Erythromycin is used for treatment and prophylaxis of susceptible contacts.

Outcome

Although most recover, infections can be fatal. Pneumonia is the most common cause of death in children.

Legionella pneumophila (Legionnaires' disease)

Severe pneumonic disease caused by *Legionella pneumophila*. Seventy-five percent are sporadic and the remainder occur as outbreaks but the source is often not identified. Half are imported following foreign travel. Diarrhea, abdominal pain and confusion may appear more prominent than the pneumonic illness. Fatality is 15%. Non-pneumonic legionellosis ("Pontiac" fever) is a self-limiting flu-like illness.

Anaerobic bacteria (bacilli)

Clostridia

Large, Gram-positive, spore-forming, anaerobic bacilli. Widespread in soil, spores are hardy and survive for years.

Clostridium tetani (tetanus)

Clinical features

- Typically, there has been a "dirty" penetrating injury. Most cases develop 3 days to 3 weeks after the wound becomes contaminated with *C. tetani* spores.
- The most common presentation is generalized tetanus with muscle rigidity and violent muscular spasms, difficulty opening the mouth (trismus or "lockjaw"), spasms of facial muscles ("risus sardonicus") or neck and back ("opisthotonus").
- Localized tetanus is less common and produces rigidity and muscle spasms in the region of the wound.

Epidemiology

>700 000 deaths/year worldwide, mainly in developing countries. Tetanus is very rare in the UK.

Pathology

Spores germinate under anaerobic conditions present in a contaminated wound. Clinical features result from production of a neurotoxin called tetanospasmin, which irreversibly blocks neurotransmitter release by inhibitory neurons in the brainstem.

Investigations

The diagnosis is clinical.

Management

Human tetanus immunoglobulin is given to neutralize circulating free toxin. Wound debridement is important but sedation, intubation, and ventilation may be needed for spasms. Wound care prevents tetanus. Immunization lasts 10 years.

Outcome

Death occurs from respiratory failure and cardiovascular instability due to autonomic nerve involvement. With adequate intensive care facilities the death rate may be 10%–20%.

Clostridium botulinum (botulism)

Results from ingestion of pre-formed toxin in contaminated food such as home canned vegetables or cured meat. Less commonly, it follows in vivo production of toxin after wound contamination or gut colonization in infants. It is rare in the UK but commoner in USA and Europe. Wound botulism sometimes occurs amongst injecting drug users ("skin poppers"). Botulinum toxin inhibits release of acetylcholine at the neuromuscular junction, first causing cranial nerve palsies followed by symmetric, descending, flaccid paralysis. Autonomic dysfunction produces arrhythmias. Treatment is mainly supportive but antitoxin made from equine serum should be given early to prevent progression. In wound botulism, early debridement is vital and antibiotics have a secondary role.

Clostridium difficile

C. difficile is a hospital-acquired infection that affects debilitated or elderly patients who have received antibiotics. *C. difficile* colonizes the large bowel producing A and B toxins that cause diarrhea. Diagnosis is made by toxin identification in stool. Fever is common and blood neutrophilia typical. "Pseudomembranous" colitis (since necrotic plaques are characteristically seen on the mucosal surface of the colon) causes bloody diarrhea and may be life threatening, especially in the elderly. Treatment is with oral metronidazole or vancomycin. Relapse requiring re-treatment is relatively common.

Clostridium perfringens

Infection most commonly follows deep penetrating injury that compromises blood supply. This creates an anaerobic environment favoring growth of organisms introduced with the trauma. Bacterial toxins cause tissue necrosis and hypotensive shock. Gas production in deep tissues is seen on X-rays ("gas gangrene"). Treatment is extensive surgical debridement and penicillin, clindamycin, or metronidazole.

Gram-negative anaerobes

- Gram-negative anaerobes (e.g. *Bacteroides fragilis*) are part of the normal flora of the gastro-intestinal tract. Any infective process resulting from translocation of gut bacteria into the peritoneal cavity (e.g. bowel perforation or intra-abdominal abscess) therefore involves anaerobes. Whilst surgery is the most important treatment, metronidazole is given (combined with cefuroxime for endogenous Enterobacteriacae).

- Normal anaerobic flora in the upper gastro-intestinal tract can also cause pneumonia following aspiration or skin infection after human or animal bites.

- In the posterior pharyngeal space, *Fusobacterium necrophorum* can cause life-threatening infection, with fever, severe sore throat, neck swelling, and suppurative thrombophlebitis of the internal jugular vein (Lemière's syndrome).

Mycobacteria
Mycobacterium tuberculosis (tuberculosis)
Clinical features

- Ninety percent of infections are asymptomatic ("latent" infection).

- Three-quarters of symptomatic cases are pulmonary. Productive cough, hemoptysis, pleuritic chest pain, fever, night sweats, and weight loss are typical. Symptoms usually have been present for weeks by the time of presentation. A pleural effusion may indicate a tuberculous empyema.

- Lymphadenitis is the commonest extrapulmonary form, most frequently affecting cervical and mediastinal nodes. Constitutional symptoms are sometimes absent and patients may present with an enlarging lymph node mass. A discharging sinus or abscess on the skin surface may be present but, unlike a pyogenic collection, it is not tender, warm, or inflamed ("cold" abscess).

- Gastro-intestinal tuberculosis usually develops over weeks. There is typically fever, abdominal discomfort, and distension from ascites. Matted loops of bowel may be palpable.

- Cardiac tuberculosis causes pericardial effusion or constrictive pericarditis.

- Bone and joint tuberculosis most commonly affects spine or hips. Spinal infection starts with diskitis that spreads to adjacent vertebrae, eventually causing collapse and angulation of the spine (Pott's disease, Fig. 15.11). A paravertebra abscess may also develop adjacent to the infected spine. Joint infections are usually monoarticular.

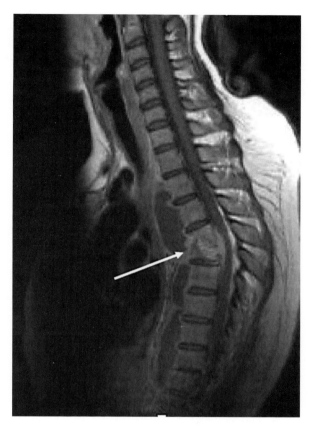

Fig. 15.11. An MRI scan showing a patient with spinal tuberculosis. Diskitis followed by destruction of the adjacent anterior vertebral bodies has resulted in collapse and kyphosis centered on T5 (shown by arrow). The spinal cord appears indented and an extensive paraspinal abscess is also seen anterior to the vertebral bodies.

- Tuberculous meningitis presents with headache, confusion and decreased consciousness over 1–3 weeks. Meningism and abnormal neurological signs may be present, especially third and sixth cranial nerve palsies. Discrete lesions in the brain ("tuberculoma") also occur.

- Genitourinary tuberculosis is rare. The presence of white cells in sterile urine may be early evidence of renal TB.

- Disseminated tuberculosis may present as fever of unknown origin since classic "miliary" shadowing may not be immediately evident on the initial chest X-ray. Choroid tubercles may be visible on the retina. The term "cryptic" TB is sometimes used when the site of infection is unknown.

Epidemiology
One-third of the world's population is infected with TB and 8 million new cases occur each year, the

majority in sub-Saharan Africa, the Indian subcontinent, and South-East Asia. Approximately 3 million die annually. In 90%, the host immune response is effective in containing but not eliminating the infection. Such "latent" disease is asymptomatic unless weakened host immunity results in disease reactivation. On a global scale, HIV infection is the most important risk factor. HIV-positive patients with latent tuberculosis have an 8%–10% annual risk of reactivation compared with a 10% lifetime risk in seronegative individuals. Extrapulmonary TB is also more common in immunocompromised hosts.

Pathology

Mycobacterium tuberculosis is a rod-shaped bacillus with thick cell walls rich in lipids, peptidoglycans, and arabinomannans. Bacilli are Gram-positive but not easily stained. However, they are colored red with a Ziehl–Neelson stain and are resistant to decolorization with acid or alcohol. Auramine stains are fluorescent and based on the acid-fast properties of the bacillus.

Transmission is by inhalation of aerosolized droplets. In the alveolar spaces, bacilli are phagocytosed by macrophages and survive by blocking maturation of the phagocytic vacuole into an acidic, hydrolytic compartment. The histologic hallmark of TB is "caseating" granulomas, which comprise a core of infected macrophages and monocytic cells, surrounded by CD4 lymphocytes. Interferon-γ secreted by CD4 lymphocytes synergizes with tumor necrosis factor-α produced by macrophages to enhance intracellular killing of bacilli. Although granulomas serve to seal off infected cells, activated macrophages also secrete proteases that damage host tissue. Caseating (literally "cheese-like") necrosis is thus seen inside granulomas microscopically. In >95% there is spontaneous recovery following primary infection. However, tubercle bacilli remain viable within granulomas and reactivation occurs when cell-mediated immunity is weakened. Most symptomatic disease, whether HIV-associated or not, results from this process. Disseminated or extrapulmonary infection results from hematogenous spread and is more common in children following primary infection or in the immunocompromised.

Investigations

Identification in body fluids, secretions, aspirates, or tissue samples by direct staining or culture. The diagnostic yield from sputum, pus, and tissue is good but microscopy and culture of CSF, ascitic, and pleural fluids are frequently negative. Organisms grow slowly in culture over several weeks and PCR-based assays are useful in rapidly differentiating *M. tuberculosis* from other mycobacterial species and can detect drug resistance at an earlier stage.

Tuberculin tests (Heaf or Mantoux) involve measuring delayed skin reaction in response to intradermal injection of purified protein derived from *M. tuberculosis* and provide indirect evidence of infection. A moderate response may indicate previous exposure to TB or to BCG vaccination. Strong, blistering reactions suggest active infection. Immunosuppression (from HIV infection, steroid therapy, malnutrition, etc.), sarcoidosis, and overwhelming TB itself, may produce false-negative reactions.

The characteristic chest X-ray appearance of pulmonary TB is intrathoracic lymphadenopathy with upper zone infiltrates and cavitation. In disseminated TB, multiple discrete opacities may be seen throughout both lungs. This pattern is sometimes described as "miliary" because the lesions look like millet seeds.

Management

It is advisable to obtain appropriate material for bacteriologic examination before starting antituberculous treatment. Treatment starts with the four first-line drugs: rifampicin, isoniazid, pyrazinamide, and ethambutol. Side effects include hepatitis (all), visual disturbance (ethambutol), and drug interactions (e.g. oral contraceptive, steroids, and anti-epileptic drugs). Pyridoxine is given to protect against isoniazid-induced peripheral neuropathy. After 2 months, rifampicin and isoniazid plus pyridoxine can be given alone if the isolate is fully drug sensitive. In most cases, 6 months' treatment is sufficient but longer courses are required with poor compliance, drug-resistance or central nervous system infections. The importance of full compliance needs emphasis and orange urine produced by rifampicin is a simple screening test for this. Supervised or directly observed therapy (DOT) should be considered if treatment compliance is likely to be poor. Steroids are given to limit inflammatory damage and subsequent fibrosis in tuberculous meningitis and pericarditis. Surgery may be needed, e.g. for loculated empyema or spinal disease with cord compression.

Immunization with BCG is given in some countries. Vaccination mainly prevents disseminated infections in children but does not protect against other forms of TB. The best prevention is early treatment of active cases. Newly diagnosed sputum

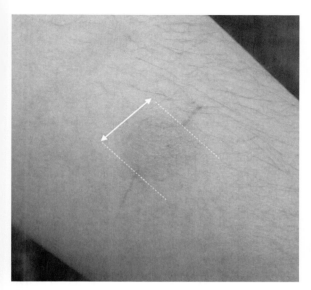

Fig. 15.12. A positive Mantoux skin result, 48 hours following a 2U intradermal injection of purified protein derivative into the flexor aspect of the forearm. The amount of skin induration (not erythema) was measured at 22 mm. (The ball-point pen marks, which have been used to delineate the extent of induration, can also be seen.)

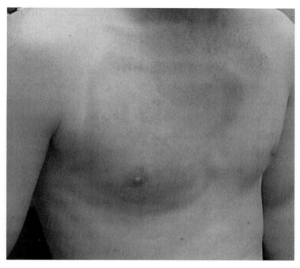

Fig. 15.13. The characteristic rash of *Erythema migrans* in a patient with early Lyme disease. Eight weeks before this developed, the patient had been walking through forested areas in Scotland and afterwards had discovered ticks attached to the skin on his chest. He was treated effectively with oral doxycycline.

smear-positive patients ("open" cases) are most infectious and should be isolated in a negative-pressure single room. Close contacts are screened with a tuberculin skin test and if symptomatic, with a chest X-ray .

Multi-drug resistant tuberculosis (MDRTB) is defined as resistance to both isoniazid and rifampicin. The treatment of MDRTB is complex and depends on the drug sensitivity pattern of the isolate. Patients must be admitted to a negative-pressure single room and treated with at least 5 effective drugs initially.

Outcome

Most, including HIV-positive patients, respond well to treatment and cure is expected with risk of relapse under 3%. However, disseminated infections can be rapidly fatal and survivors from tuberculous meningitis frequently have some permanent neurologic deficit.

Opportunistic (or atypical) mycobacteria

Opportunistic mycobacteria can be found in soil, water, animals, and birds. They are low-grade pathogens in humans and cause disease when immunity is weakened or undeveloped. For example, *M. kansasii*, *M. avium intracellulare* (MAI), *M. malmoense,* and *M. xenopi* cause pulmonary infections clinically and radiologically identical to TB. MAI also causes

lymphadenitis in children <5 years and disseminated infection in advanced HIV infection.

Spirochetes
Treponema pallidum (syphilis)
Secondary syphilis can produce a relapsing and remitting febrile illness, with or without a rash, and is notorious for mimicking other infections.

Borrelia burgdorferi (Lyme disease)
Clinical features
Transmission is by bites from an infected tick. Patients may recall removing ticks from their skin or have visited woodland and heathland areas. There are two stages to infection.

Early
- Within days the characteristic rash of erythema migrans develops at the site of the bite (localized infection). The classic appearance is a large, flat, well-demarcated, erythematous lesion with central clearing (Fig. 15.13).
- Malaise, fever, chills, arthralgia, myalgia, and headache represent disseminated infection. Cardiac conduction defects, meningitis, and cranial nerve palsies may occur. There is usually spontaneous resolution of these complications after several weeks or months.

447

Late

- "Late" Lyme disease develops months after the initial bite with chronic or recurrent arthritis, encephalopathy, and or polyneuropathy.

Epidemiology

First described in Old Lyme, Connecticut, USA. There are ~2000–3000 cases in the UK each year, especially involving visits to the New Forest, South Downs, Lake District, Exmoor, and Scottish Highlands. Peak times for tick bites are late spring and early summer.

Pathology

Borrelia burgdorferi is the causative organism that is present in tick (*Ixodes*) salivary glands. After the bite there is local multiplication of bacteria in the skin. Systemic symptoms represent dissemination of bacteria. Late Lyme disease is the result of chronic, persistent infection.

Investigations

Diagnosis is based on a characteristic illness with a history of exposure and positive serology.

Treatment

Oral doxycycline or amoxicillin for 2–4 weeks. Intravenous ceftriaxone may be needed for established disease involving the central nervous system.

Outcome

Excellent in most cases.

Leptospirosis
Clinical features

- Almost all have a recreational, occupational, or travel exposure risk that involves water or animal contact (especially rats). There is sudden onset high fever, headache, and myalgia. This lasts up to a week and in many there is no progression.
- The second phase may last 2–3 weeks. After a 48-hour remission, there is recurrence of fever with severe muscle pain, headache, red eyes, pneumonitis, and a maculopapular skin rash. Aseptic meningitis may also develop.
- In some, renal failure, deep jaundice, and hemorrhage develops in the second phase (Weil's disease). This runs a fulminant course with DIC and multiorgan failure.
- Incubation period is 7–14 days.

Epidemiology

Leptospirosis has worldwide distribution. There are approximately 60 cases in the UK annually. It is associated with farmers, sewer workers, veterinarians, and recreational activities involving water.

Pathology

Leptospira are excreted in the urine of many rodents, dogs, cats, wild mammals, fish, birds, and reptiles. Leptospirosis is caused by *Leptospira interrogans* that contains hundreds of serovars. Of these, *L. icterohaemorrhagiae* is most commonly pathogenic in humans and causes the most severe manifestation, Weil's disease. Organisms may remain viable in water or soil for weeks to months and human transmission occurs when bacteria enter through broken skin or mucous membranes.

Investigations

Neutrophil leukocytosis and very elevated inflammatory indices are typical. Renal and liver function tests are abnormal in Weil's disease. Creatine phosphokinase is sometimes raised indicating muscle inflammation. Diagnosis can be made by visualizing the organism in centrifuged urine by dark ground microscopy. Serologic tests and PCR-based assays on blood are more commonly used.

Management

All should receive treatment: oral doxycycline for mild cases and IV benzylpenicillin if severe.

Outcome

Most recover fully. In jaundiced patients, the clinical course can be fulminant with multiorgan failure, hemorrhage, and death in 10%.

Other bacteria
Bartonella henselae (cat scratch disease)
Clinical features

- 3–5 days after a cat bite or scratch, an erythematous, papular lesion develops on the skin. A week or so later, regional lymphadenopathy develops (axillary, cervical, and submandibular most commonly), which may persist for weeks to months and occasionally suppurate.
- If the conjunctiva is the route of entry, conjunctivitis and pre-auricular lymphadenopathy may develop (Parinaud's oculoglandular syndrome).
- Most cases are mild but fever, malaise, and myalgia may occur.

Epidemiology
Worldwide distribution. Transmission is from a bite or scratch from an infected cat, usually a kitten (fleas transmit the infection between cats). Most cases occur in children or young adults and many cat owners have serologic evidence of previous exposure.

Pathology
Bartonella are small, curved Gram-negative rods.

Investigations
Serologic tests or lymph node biopsy.

Management
Spontaneous resolution may take several weeks. Azithromycin may result in more rapid lymph node regression.

Outcome
Full recovery without long-term complications.

Coxiella burnetti (Q fever)
Clinical features
- A history of exposure to farm animals during the calving or lambing season may be obtained, but "urban" cases with no such risk are also reported.
- Symptoms are of an acute flu-like illness with pneumonia but many infections are subclinical.
- Infective endocarditis is the most common manifestation of chronic Q fever.
- Incubation is 7–30 days.

Epidemiology
Q fever affects wild and domestic animals (mainly cattle, sheep and goats), particularly in the Mediterranean Middle East. The name comes from "Query" fever, used to describe an outbreak of febrile illness in Australian abattoir workers in 1935.

Investigations
The white cell count is usually normal. Liver transaminases and bilirubin are often raised. Diagnosis is by serology.

Management
For acute infection, doxycycline for 2–3 weeks. Endocarditis requires treatment for 2–3 years.

Outcome
Most acute illnesses are self-limiting and resolve within a few weeks. Q fever endocarditis may be fatal.

Mycoplasma pneumoniae
Mycoplasma pneumoniae lacks a cell wall and is therefore resistant to penicillin. It causes "atypical" pneumonia, most commonly affecting children and young adults. It is best treated with macrolides or tetracyclines.

Chlamydia
- *C. pneumoniae* and *C. psittaci* can cause atypical pneumonia but many infections are mild or subclinical. *C. psittaci* is transmitted by the respiratory route after handling sick birds, especially parrots. However, only a minority give a history of bird contact.
- *C. trachomatis* causes genital tract infections and blindness in the developing world ("trachoma").

Viruses
Respiratory viruses
Common cold viruses
These cause self-limiting illnesses characterized by sore throat, sneezing, nasal discharge, congestion, and low-grade fever. Rhinoviruses are the commonest cause but coronaviruses, adenoviruses, respiratory syncytial virus, influenza, parainfluenza, and human metapneumovirus may also be responsible. Incubation is 1–3 days. Transmission is by airborne aerosol droplets or direct contact with nasopharyngeal secretions. Treatment is essentially symptomatic. Secondary bacterial infection may cause otitis media or sinusitis.

Respiratory syncytial virus
RNA virus best known for causing bronchiolitis in infants. It also causes pneumonia in the elderly, exacerbations of COPD, and severe pneumonia in immunocompromised patients.

Parainfluenza virus
The majority of illnesses are upper respiratory tract infections. It causes most acute laryngotracheobronchitis (croup) in young children and may also cause pneumonia in immunocompromised patients.

Influenza
Clinical features
- Abrupt onset fevers, chills, myalgia, malaise, sore throat, headache, and dry cough. Fever (>38 °C) usually lasts 3 days.
- Secondary bacterial pneumonia is common. Other bacterial complications include otitis media and sinusitis.
- Much rarer than bacterial superinfection is primary viral pneumonia, which develops rapidly

within the first 48 hours. Dry cough and increasing breathlessness are important symptoms. The chest X-ray shows bilateral infiltrates. Death may occur from progressive respiratory failure.

- In patients with underlying lung disease, e.g. COPD, respiratory failure may result.
- Incubation period is 1–3 days.

Epidemiology

There are two main strains, A and B. Influenza A (not B) infects many animal species but birds are the most important reservoir in nature. Influenza is highly infectious and transmitted in respiratory droplets and less commonly contact with respiratory secretions. All ages are affected, most commonly in winter.

Influenza A has been responsible for worldwide pandemics and regional epidemics. The virus has two surface antigens: hemaglutinin (H) and neuraminidase (N). Major change ("antigenic shift") gives rise to pandemics (every one to three decades), whereas minor changes ("antigenic drift") result in regional epidemics (every 1–3 years). In the 1918 pandemic, "Spanish flu" (H1N1) led to the death of over 20 million people worldwide. Since then, there has been "Asian flu" in 1957 (H2N2) and "Hong Kong flu" in 1968 (H3N2).

In 1997, a new strain arose in Hong Kong (H5N1) that was previously thought to affect only chickens, ducks, and geese ("Avian flu"). All 18 confirmed human cases had exposure to infected poultry and there were six deaths. Although non-pandemic, human-human transmission was subsequently reported. In 2009, "swine flu" (H1N1) originating in Mexico, caused the latest pandemic.

Influenza B causes epidemics as a result of antigenic drift but antigenic shift has not been observed and infections are less severe than A.

Pathology

Influenza is an orthomyxovirus. Inhalation and replication in the columnar epithelial cells of the respiratory tract produce inflammation, loss of cilia, and desquamation. Immunity involves the development of protective secretory and serum antibodies against the virus.

Investigations

Leukopenia is common. Viral antigens can be rapidly identified in nasopharyngeal aspirates by immunofluorescence and in throat swabs using PCR. Isolation of virus by culture takes longer. Paired serologic tests showing rise in specific antibody allows retrospective diagnosis.

Management

Uncomplicated cases are treated symptomatically. Neuraminidase inhibitors (e.g. oseltamivir and zanamivir) are active against both A and B. When influenza is known to be circulating within the community, treatment is recommended within 48 hours of symptoms to those at risk of severe infection.

Influenza vaccination is recommended for the elderly, patients with chronic respiratory, cardiac or renal disease, diabetes, and immunosuppression. Healthcare workers are also offered vaccination in the UK. Continuous monitoring of circulating viral strains is important for matching those prevalent in the community with those covered by the vaccine.

Outcome

Most recover spontaneously. The highest mortality is in the elderly and those with chronic illness.

Measles
Clinical features

- Fever, cough, coryza, conjunctivitis, and pharyngitis are present for the first 3–4 days. In the mouth, tiny white plaques pathognomonic of measles may be visible on the buccal mucosa (Koplik's spots). Around day 4, a maculopapular rash appears on the forehead. This spreads to the rest of the face and from head to feet over 2–3 days. Large areas become confluent and then fade away.
- Complications are more frequent and serious in adults and include pneumonia, otitis media, and meningoencephalitis (1 per 1000 cases).
- Incubation is 8–12 days.

Epidemiology

Worldwide distribution, predominantly children <5 years. One million children die annually in the developing world. Mass vaccination against MMR (measles, mumps, and rubella) was introduced in 1988 for children under 5 years, which has dramatically altered the epidemiology of these viruses in the UK. Infections are now occasionally seen in susceptible young adults who were not vaccinated (as they were too old) or received only one dose (see Table 15.2).

Pathology

Caused by a morbillivirus (RNA virus) belonging to the paramyxovirus family. It is highly infectious and respiratory droplets are the mechanism of transmission.

Investigations

The diagnosis is mainly clinical but confirmed serologically.

Management

Most require supportive care only. Immune globulin is given to susceptible contacts such as non-immune pregnant women, infants, and immunocompromised individuals. There is no link between vaccination and Crohn's disease or autism and parents should be encouraged to vaccinate their children.

Outcome

Most recover fully and immunity is life-long. Sub-acute sclerosing panencephalitis (SSPE) is a rare, late complication occurring after 1/100 000 episodes of measles and 1/1 000 000 vaccinations.

Mumps
Clinical features

- Many infections are subclinical.
- Classically, there is fever, headache, sore throat, myalgia, and tender enlargement of the parotid glands. Fever and swelling resolve over 1–2 weeks.
- Adolescents may present with epididymo-orchitis (usually unilateral) or meningitis (without parotid swelling).
- Pancreatitis, oophoritis, deafness, and arthritis may also occur.
- Incubation 17–19 days.

Epidemiology

Worldwide distribution, usually children and adolescents. Mumps was the commonest cause of viral meningitis in children before MMR. In the UK, there were only ~500 confirmed cases in 2002 but >8000 in 2004. Ninety percent were aged >15 years and inadequately vaccinated (see Table 15.2).

Pathology

Mumps is caused by a RNA virus belonging to the paramyxovirus family. Transmission is from respiratory droplets and direct contact with infected saliva.

Investigations

Diagnosis is clinical and confirmed serologically. Virus can also be cultured in CSF, saliva, or urine.

Management

Treatment is symptomatic, especially analgesia for orchitis, which may be severe.

Outcome

Recovery is usual. Sterility following epididymo-orchitis is uncommon. Encephalitis is rare but can be fatal.

Rubella, or German measles
Clinical features

- Subclinical infections are common.
- Adults may have a prodrome comprising pharyngitis, fever, headache, eye pain, cough, and myalgia. Following this, a fine, rose-pink maculopapular rash starts on the face and spreads distally within 24 hours. Post-auricular and sub-occipital lymphadenopathy is typical.
  The rash fades after 3 days but during this time polyarthralgia may develop and last several weeks.
- There is high risk of congenital rubella syndrome in non-immune pregnant women exposed to rubella. Features include: cataract, microcephaly, deafness, congenital heart defects, mental retardation, and diabetes. Risk to the fetus is greatest during first 12 weeks of gestation. Rubella is infectious 5 days before and 5 days after rash develops.
- Incubation is 16–18 days.

Epidemiology

Vaccination is effective and rubella is rare where vaccination is widespread (see Table 15.2).

Pathology

Highly infectious togavirus (RNA virus) spread by respiratory droplets. Immunity is life-long.

Investigations

Serology should be performed when suspected. During early pregnancy, all women are screened to establish their immune status.

Management

No specific treatment. If identified in non-immune pregnant women before 16 weeks gestation, termination may be discussed.

Outcome

Rubella is usually mild and recovery is the rule.

451

Herpes viruses

Herpes viruses are a family of DNA viruses. A characteristic of them all is the ability to produce life-long latent infection following primary infection.

Varicella–zoster virus (chickenpox)
Clinical features
Immunocompetent hosts

- Primary infection with varicella-zoster virus (VZV) results in chickenpox or varicella. In healthy children there is a mild febrile illness, characterized by pruritic, erythematous maculopapules, initially on the face and trunk (rarely palms or soles). The lesions progress through vesicular, pustular, and crusting stages over 3–4 days. New "crops" mean that appearance is usually at different stages of evolution. Scratching causes super-added bacterial infections.
- In adults, varicella is more serious. Life-threatening pneumonia may develop in smokers and pregnant women.
- Patients are infectious for 48 hours prior to the rash and until lesions have scabbed over (~5 days). Incubation is 10–21 days.
- Shingles is localized, painful rash, identical to that seen in chickenpox. The rash has a dermatomal distribution and never crosses the midline. It is usually present for a week.

Immunocompromised hosts
Disseminated infection occurs in immunocompromised patients. The rash may become hemorrhagic, and pneumonia, encephalitis, and hepatitis may develop.

Epidemiology
Ninety percent of adults have had chickenpox as children. VZV is highly contagious and the attack rate within a household is 90%.

Pathology
Transmitted by respiratory route or less commonly contact with vesicle fluid in chickenpox or shingles. After entry via the nasopharynx, there is viremic spread and sensory nerve root ganglia are the sites of VZV latency. When cell-mediated immunity wanes, particularly with advancing age, reactivation results in shingles. In patients with severely depressed cell-mediated immunity, for example, bone marrow transplant or lymphoma, reactivation may be disseminated and severe.

Investigations
Diagnosis is usually clinical. Scrapings from the base of vesicles may enable rapid identification by immunofluorescence or electron microscopy. Chest X-ray in chickenpox pneumonia shows small discrete opacities throughout the lungs, which may calcify after recovery. PCR analysis of CSF is useful in confirming VZV encephalitis.

Management
In children, no treatment is required apart from symptom relief and prevention of secondary bacterial skin infection. In adults with chickenpox, oral aciclovir or valaciclovir commenced within 24–48 hours of the onset of the rash may help to reduce the severity and duration of the illness. Early treatment of shingles also decreases the incidence of post-herpetic neuralgia. All immunocompromised patients and those with chickenpox pneumonia or encephalitis are treated with IV aciclovir.

Outcome
Childhood chickenpox has a good prognosis. Post-infectious cerebellar encephalitis may develop (1/6000 cases). Most deaths in immunocompetent adults are from pneumonia (<0.3%). Individuals with impaired immunity and neonates have a significant mortality if not treated promptly. After the dermatomal rash of shingles, pain may persist as post-herpetic neuralgia for months or years, particularly in the elderly.

Epstein-Barr virus (glandular fever)
Clinical features
Immunocompetent hosts

- Usually asymptomatic in children.
- In adolescents or adults it causes "glandular fever" or "infectious mononucleosis." There is a prodrome of fever, tiredness and malaise, followed by sore throat, fever, and lymphadenopathy. Exudative tonsillitis and petechiae may be visible on the palate. There may be generalized lymphadenopathy and splenomegaly. Maculopapular rash frequently develops when patients receive amoxicillin for a suspected bacterial infection. The illness usually resolves within 1–2 weeks but occasionally fever and fatigue may persist longer.

- Complications are extremely rare but include hemolytic anemia, severe hepatitis, splenic rupture, Guillian-Barré syndrome, and meningoencephalitis.
- Incubation is 2–6 weeks.
- EBV is also linked to malignancy, e.g. Burkitt's lymphoma in African children and nasopharyngeal lymphoma in China.

Immunocompromised hosts

- In HIV-infected patients, EBV is associated with nervous system lymphoma and Hodgkin's disease, as well as oral hairy cell leukoplakia of the tongue. In non-HIV infected individuals, there is a link with lymphoproliferative disorders, particularly B-cell lymphomas.

Epidemiology

EBV infects 90% of human beings and persists for the lifetime of the person. Fifty percent of children in Western countries are infected by the age of 5 years, but children in developing nations acquire EBV earlier.

Pathology

Contact with infected saliva, such as kissing, or via contaminated hands. EBV replicates inside local epithelial cells and B cells. Dissemination within infected B cells then follows. T cells become activated in response to the B cell infection, resulting in lymphoid hyperplasia and "atypical" lymphocytosis. Polyclonal antibodies, directed against viral antigens and a variety of non-viral antigens (so-called "heterophile" antibodies), are produced by B cells. These bind antigens present on sheep red blood cells causing agglutination, which forms a non-specific diagnostic test (Monospot or Paul Bunnell).

Investigations

Lymphocytosis and "atypical" lymphocytes are characteristic. Liver function tests show a slight transaminitis. The Paul Bunnell or Monospot tests are rapid but neither sensitive nor specific. Specific serology is available.

Management

Symptomatic relief.

Outcome

Usually an uneventful recovery. Although much cited link between EBV and chronic fatigue syndrome is not well established.

Cytomegalovirus

Clinical features

Immunocompetent hosts

- Most cytomegalovirus (CMV) infections pass without notice.
- Symptomatic infection is similar to glandular fever but rash is unusual ("CMV-mononucleosis"). Fever may persist for 2 weeks.

Immunocompromised hosts

- CMV develops within 3 months in transplant recipients. Sight-threatening retinitis, colitis, and encephalitis may occur in advanced HIV infection.

Congenital infection Occurs when mothers experience primary infection during pregnancy.

Epidemiology

Occurs worldwide. Fifty percent of adults have antibodies indicating previous infection.

Pathology

Transmitted in body fluids (blood, semen, cervical fluids, urine, and saliva). In transplant recipients, infection may result from an infected donor tissue. Reactivation of latent infection is the main reason for disease in HIV-positive patients.

Investigations

Atypical lymphocytes and lymphocytosis are common. Acute infection may be confirmed by specific serology. Detection of CMV antigen in body fluids (e.g. broncho-alveolar lavage) or viral DNA in the peripheral blood using quantitative PCR-based assays are also diagnostic.

Management

CMV-mononucleosis is self-limiting and does not usually require treatment. Intravenous ganciclovir, a nucleoside analogue of acyclovir that inhibits viral replication, is the drug of choice in the immunocompromised.

Outcome

In the immunocompetent, spontaneous resolution without any long-term sequelae is usual. However, CMV can be fatal in immunocompromised patients and retinitis can lead to blindness if untreated.

Herpes simplex infection

- Systemic features including fever are common in primary genital infection but less so in recurrent episodes.
- HSV is the commonest identifiable cause of viral encephalitis.

453

Human immunodeficiency virus

Seroconversion is frequently asymptomatic but many patients experience a febrile illness that may be associated with a maculopapular rash.

Parvovirus B19 infection

Clinical features

Immunocompetent hosts

- Commonly asymptomatic in children.
- In symptomatic children, erythema infectiosum begins with an erythematous rash on the cheeks (hence "slapped cheek syndrome"). Fever is unusual. The rash extends over 1–2 weeks and as it fades, has a lacy or reticular appearance on the legs.
- In adults, the rash may be absent but symmetric arthralgia involving the hands, wrists, and ankles may develop.
- A transient "aplastic crisis" may occur in patients with chronic hemolytic anemia, e.g. sickle cell disease.
- Incubation is 13–18 days.

Immunocompromised host

- Chronic infection can develop in immunocompromised patients (including HIV). This is characterized by persistent or recurrent episodes of anemia.

Congenital infection

- Fetal death may result if pregnant women become infected.

Epidemiology

Worldwide distribution. Most infections occur before middle age but especially in children aged 6–10 years.

Pathology

A DNA virus belonging to the Parvoviridae family. Transmission is by droplet inhalation or direct contact with respiratory secretions. It binds to red cell precursors in bone marrow causing reduced red cell production.

Investigations

Anemia with decreased reticulocytes is characteristic of aplastic crises. In immunocompromised hosts, specific antibodies may be absent but viral DNA can be detected by PCR.

Management

No specific treatment is available.

Enteroviruses (Cosackie and echoviruses)

Clinical features

- Most infections are subclinical or similar to the common cold.
- Enteroviruses are the commonest cause of viral meningitis, occurring mainly in adults.
- Pericarditis and myocarditis occur in young adults.
- Pleurodynia (caused by Cosackie B), also called epidemic myalgia or Bornholm disease (after the first description of an epidemic on a Danish island). Characteristic features are sudden fever, malaise, and severe chest pain caused by myalgia of the intercostal muscles ("devil's grip") lasting up to 2 weeks. Children and adolescents most commonly affected.
- Herpangina (Cosackie A) most commonly affects infants with sudden onset fever and sore throat. Small, painful ulcers or vesicles occur in the oropharynx.
- Hand foot and mouth disease (Cosackie A16) mainly affects young children, with vesicles on hands and feet, and mouth ulcers.
- In children, fever and maculopaplular rash can occur. This may resemble a glandular fever-like illness in adults.
- Poliomyelitis is described below.
- Incubation is 2–10 days.

Epidemiology

Highly contagious and found worldwide. Spread is by the fecal–oral route and humans are the only natural reservoir. Poor sanitation and overcrowding facilitate transmission.

Pathology

Enteroviruses belong to the picornavirus group ("pico-"; small RNA viruses). They are divided into three main subgroups (echoviruses, Cosackie viruses and polioviruses) and many serotypes. All infect the human gastro-intestinal tract and different disease manifestations result from tissue tropism of the serogroup involved.

Investigations

Diagnosis is usually by specific serology or PCR-based assays. Culture (e.g. from feces or throat swabs) can also be performed.

Management
No specific therapy.

Outcome
Most enteroviral infections, including meningitis and pericarditis, are self-limiting. Spontaneous resolution of myocarditis usually occurs but can lead to dilated cardiomyopathy.

Gastro-intestinal viral infections

Noroviruses
Noroviruses (also called "small round structured viruses" and "Norwalk-like viruses") are the most common cause of gastroenteritis in the UK. They typically cause profuse vomiting ("Winter vomiting" disease). The infective dose is low and transmission is via the fecal–oral route. Incubation is 12–48 hours. Outbreaks are common in semi-closed environments such as schools and hospital wards. Treatment is isolation and adequate hydration. Recovery is usual within 1–2 days.

Rotaviruses
Rotavirus is the most common cause of gastroenteritis in infants.

Hepatitis viruses A–E
Fever and other constitutional symptoms are common in the prodrome of hepatitis A but fever resolves by the time jaundice develops.

Systemic fungal infections
Fever is occasionally associated with invasive or disseminated fungal infections that particularly occur in the immunocompromised.

Candidiasis
Candida is ubiquitous in soil and commensal in the mouth, gastro-intestinal tract, and vagina. Most infections are local with mild symptoms, e.g. oral or vaginal candidiasis, and are caused by *Candida albicans*. Risk factors for disseminated candidiasis include: neutropenia, burns, indwelling central venous catheters, gastro-intestinal surgery, parenteral nutrition, and broad-spectrum antibiotic exposure. *Candida* in the bloodstream (candidemia) may be without symptoms but spread to almost all organs can occur resulting in microabcesses within the liver, spleen, kidneys, and brain. An ophthalmology assessment is needed in any candidemiac patient to exclude sight-threatening endophthalmitis. Rarely endocarditis

can also occur. Diagnosis of invasive candidiasis is by blood cultures and tissue biopsy. Disseminated candidiasis is treated with fluconazole (IV or PO) or amphotericin B (IV only).

Aspergillosis
Found worldwide, growing in soil and moist decaying vegetation, e.g. compost piles or stored hay. Human disease is acquired by inhalation and *Aspergillus fumigatus* is the commonest pathogen. Clinical disease results from either an allergic response to colonization (i.e. allergic bronchopulmonary aspergillosis) or invasive infection for invasive infection. Risk factors include: transplantation, neutropenia, AIDS, and high-dose corticosteroids. Pneumonia is the commonest manifestation and lung biopsy may be required to confirm the diagnosis. Nodular infiltrates are the commonest finding on chest X-ray, and CT scans show a characteristic "halo" pattern around the nodules. Dissemination to other organs (e.g. the brain) can occur and in severely immunosuppressed patients, fungus "balls" can grow in the sinuses and invade the orbit. Invasive aspergillosis may be rapidly progressive and fatal. Intravenous amphotericin or voriconazole are the drugs of choice.

Cryptococcosis
Cryptococcus neoformans causes cryptococcosis. It is present in soil and pigeon droppings and transmitted by inhalation. Risk factors for infection include HIV infection, steroid therapy, organ transplantation, leukemia, and lymphoma. *C. neoformans* is the commonest cause of meningitis in patients with advanced HIV infection. Diagnosis is by direct visualization of cryptococci in CSF stained with India ink and by culture. Antigen detection tests are also sensitive in CSF and blood. Treatment: IV amphotericin B, followed by fluconazole maintenance.

Protozoa
Toxoplasmosis
Clinical features
Immunocompetent hosts
- Only 10%–20% of acquired infections are symptomatic.
- Most symptomatic patients present with enlarged lymph nodes, often cervical. Malaise, sore throat, sweats, and low-grade fever may be reported.
- Chorioretinitis is a rare complication that mainly occurs in congenital infection.

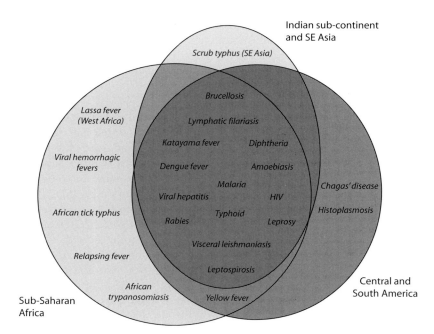

Fig. 15.14. Causes of fever in the returned tropical traveller.

Immunocompromised hosts Toxoplasmosis in the immunocompromised is serious.

- In advanced HIV infection (CD4 $< 100/\text{mm}^3$), toxoplasma encephalitis may present with fever, headache, confusion, focal neurologic deficit, and seizures. Brain CT shows typical "ring-enhancing" lesions.

- In organ transplant recipients, toxoplasmosis can cause multiorgan disease with encephalitis, pneumonitis, myositis, and hepatitis. Myocarditis occurs in cardiac transplant patients.

Congenital infection Congenital toxoplasmosis is acquired *in utero* when pregnant women become infected.

Epidemiology

Caused by the protozoan parasite *Toxoplasma gondii*, which is widespread and infects many animals. Cats spread it by shedding oocysts in their feces that remain viable in moist soil for months. Humans become infected by ingestion of food or water contaminated with oocysts or "cysts" found in undercooked or raw meat (mainly pork or lamb). Eighty percent of the French population have evidence of previous infection compared to 20% in the UK, where less raw meat is consumed.

Pathology

T. gondii exists in three forms: oocysts, tachyzoites, and cysts. If the host's cell-mediated immunity becomes compromised, bradyzoites are released from cysts and transform into tachyzoites which produce inflammation.

Investigations

Serology is the primary method of diagnosis.

Management

Immunocompetent adults or children usually require no treatment. Pyrimethamine and sulfadiazine are standard therapy in immunocompromised patients and afterwards, drug prophylaxis should be considered. Steroids are also given to reduce edema in cerebral toxoplasmosis.

Outcome

In most immunocompetent individuals, toxoplasmosis is self-limiting. In AIDS patients with cerebral toxoplasmosis, a rapid response to drug treatment is typical.

Tropical infections

Protozoa

Since many infections have a specific geographic distribution, an accurate travel history that details all countries visited is paramount (Figure 15.14). Travel to specific regions within a country are occasionally significant e.g. Lassa fever is transmitted only in parts of rural West Africa. Dates of travel

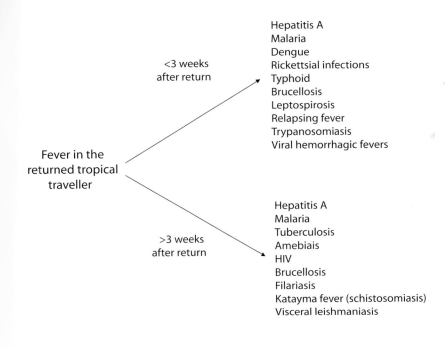

Fig. 15.15. Fever in the returned tropical traveller.

Fever in the returned tropical traveller

<3 weeks after return

Hepatitis A
Malaria
Dengue
Rickettsial infections
Typhoid
Brucellosis
Leptospirosis
Relapsing fever
Trypanosomiasis
Viral hemorrhagic fevers

>3 weeks after return

Hepatitis A
Malaria
Tuberculosis
Amebiais
HIV
Brucellosis
Filariasis
Katayma fever (schistosomiasis)
Visceral leishmaniasis

are essential since it possible to eliminate diseases from the differential diagnosis based on knowledge of the incubation periods of specific infections (Fig. 15.15). Falciparum malaria should never be forgotten in anyone developing fever within 3 months of return from an endemic area. TB, brucellosis, and visceral leishmaniasis typically cause a prolonged fever, and a history of recurrent febrile episodes may suggest "benign" malaria or filariasis. However, fever is not invariably present, e.g. non-invasive helminths are adapted to parasitizing human hosts without provoking significant inflammation. As before, specific exposure risk questions should be asked. For example, water contact is an important risk for leptospirosis (e.g. white water rafting) and swimming in the African lakes may result in Katayama fever (schistosomiasis). Visits to African game parks, walking in the bush, or riding horses are exposure risks for tick bites. A history of close contact with sick people is sometimes important, e.g. suspected viral hemorrhagic fever. Animal contact is also important, e.g. bird markets in Asia and avian influenza. Sexual risks should be considered in travellers. Vaccination against hepatitis A, typhoid, and yellow fever are usually effective but anti-malaria chemoprophylaxis is not failsafe and is frequently not taken with full compliance. Splenomegaly is present in diverse infections (e.g. malaria, typhoid, leishmaniasis, and tick typhus).

The white cell count is particularly helpful in the assessment of "tropical" fevers and eosinophilia is sometimes seen in invasive parasitic conditions. The blood film can be used to diagnose malaria in addition to several other febrile conditions including trypanosomiasis, filariasis, and relapsing fever (Fig. 15.15).

Malaria

Four species of malaria parasite infect humans: *Plasmodium falciparum*, *P. vivax*, *P. ovale*, and *P. malariae*. Falciparum is the most serious and can be fatal if not recognized. Non-falciparum infections are much milder and termed "benign" malaria.

Clinical features

- Fever occurs in all types of malaria, often with rigors and profuse sweating. Anemia, mild jaundice, and splenomegaly are also common.
- *P. vivax*, *P. ovale*, and *P. malariae* cause recurrent attacks with spontaneous remission. If untreated, relapses can occur for years.
- Falciparum malaria does not recur and usually develops within 3 months of return from an endemic country. Some infections progress rapidly to serious complications including: cerebral malaria, severe anemia, renal failure, non-cardiogenic pulmonary edema, and hypotensive shock.

- Falciparum malaria is more severe in young children, pregnant women, and those not raised in an endemic area. Severe infection also occurs in patients without a spleen.

Epidemiology

Malaria is the most important protozoal infection worldwide, distributed throughout many tropical and sub-tropical countries including the Indian sub-continent, South East Asia, Africa, and Central and South America. *P. falciparum* occurs in all regions but predominates in Africa. *P. vivax* causes the majority of the disease worldwide and is more common in the Indian sub-continent. *P. ovale* and *P malariae* transmission occurs mainly in Africa. Each year there are over 100 million cases and 1–2 million deaths from falciparum malaria. In Africa, the most severe disease is in children <5 years. Falciparum malaria is the most common species imported into the UK (>50%), between 1500 and 2000 cases every year result in 10–15 deaths. Resistance to antimalarial drugs is prevalent in some areas of the world.

Pathology

Malaria is transmitted by the bite of an infected female anopheline mosquito between dusk and dawn (1). "Sporozoites" from the insect's saliva enter the bloodstream and invade hepatocytes (2). Asexual multiplication then takes place in the liver and sporozoites develop into cyst-like forms called "shizonts" ("tissue schizogeny"). (*P. ovale* and *P. vivax* also have a dormant stage in the liver called the "hypnozoite", which reactivates to cause relapses) (3). When schizonts are mature, they burst releasing thousands of "merozoites" into the circulation, which invade red cells and mature into "trophozoites" (4). Further cycles of asexual multiplication involving red cell invasion, rupture, and merozoite release then follow ("blood schizogeny") (5). Some merozoites develop into male and female "gametocytes" that are ingested by a mosquito feeding on human blood (6). Sexual reproduction takes place in the mosquito gut, which completes the life cycle (7) (Fig. 15.16).

Central to the virulence of falciparum malaria is that, unlike the other species, shizogeny occurs in the deep capillaries. During parasite maturation a number of "knobs" appear on the surface of red cells increasing their tendency to adhere to capillary walls. Capillaries become occluded leading to poor tissue perfusion, hypoxia, and multiorgan damage. Non-cardiogenic pulmonary edema results from capillary wall injury and is made worse by iatrogenic overload with intravenous fluids.

The spleen becomes enlarged as it destroys parasitized red cells, causing anemia. Sickle cell trait is protective against *P. falciparum* infection, probably because parasitized red cells sickle and are removed from the circulation by the spleen. In contrast, patients with sickle cell anemia get more severe infections.

Investigations

Often there is anemia, a normal white cell count, and decreased platelets. Microscopy of "thick" and "thin" blood films is the standard method of diagnosis. A thick film formed by lysed red cells is better for detecting small numbers of parasites. However, when sufficient parasites are present, speciation is easier using a thin blood film smear, which is a single red cell in thickness (Fig. 15.17). The proportion of parasitized red cells can also be calculated in falciparum infections to give an indication of the parasite burden. At least three separate negative films are required to exclude malaria. Rapid, sensitive, and specific malaria antigen detection tests are also now available.

Management

Falciparum malaria Specific drugs include: quinine, mefloquine, atovaquone-proguanil, and artesunate compounds. Uncomplicated infections can be treated with oral agents. Intravenous quinine is indicated if there is vomiting or a severe/complicated infection, usually with a high parasitemia (>2%). Hypoglycaemia can result from malaria itself but quinine also stimulates insulin secretion and can cause arrhythmias. Patients receiving IV quinine therefore require regular blood sugar and ECG monitoring. Vigorous rehydration should be avoided as non-cardiogenic pulmonary edema can develop. An exchange blood transfusion is sometimes performed if there is very high parasitemia, e.g. >10%.

Benign malaria In most cases, chloroquine is effective against parasites in the blood but has no activity against latent forms in the liver. Primaquine is therefore given afterwards to eradicate hypnozoites. Glucose-6-phospate deficiency must be excluded to avoid hemolytic anemia caused by primaquine.

Prevention

Avoiding mosquito bites and full compliance with appropriate chemoprophylaxis.

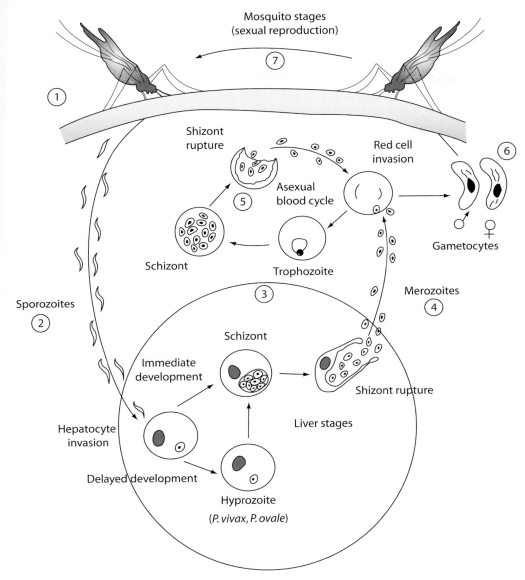

Fig. 15.16. Malaria life cycle.

Outcome

Full recovery is usual in benign disease. Cerebral malaria following falciparum infections may cause death or leave permanent neurologic damage in survivors.

Amebiasis

Clinical features

- In amebic dysentery, there is gradual onset diarrhea with blood and/or mucus. Fever is variable; fulminant colitis may develop.

- Amebic liver abscess may develop during the dysenteric illness or many years after leaving an endemic area, often with no preceding history of diarrhea. The liver is often tender and enlarged but jaundice is rare. Spontaneous rupture into local structures can lead to pericarditis, empyema, and peritonitis.

- Rarely, a chronic inflammatory mass may develop, particularly in the ileocecal region, from thickening of the bowel wall ("ameboma").

459

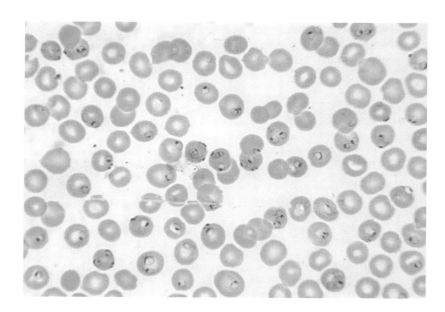

Fig. 15.17. A thin film showing multiple "ring forms" or trophozoites of *Plasmodium falciparum* within red cells. Some red cells contain more than one parasite, which is a unique property of this species of malaria parasite.

Abdominal pain and obstruction are the main features, sometimes with fever.

Epidemiology
Amebiasis is tropical in the sense that it is found in areas where sanitation is poor.

Pathology
Entameba histolytica is a protozoon ingested in food or water contaminated with "cysts." Following digestion, each cyst releases small amebae that develop into mature highly motile "trophozoites." In the majority, *E. histolytica* behaves like a gut commensal, harmlessly grazing on the colonic mucosa. It causes no symptoms and is excreted as cysts in the stool. Pathogenic strains occasionally become invasive and damage the mucosal wall causing dysentery.

Investigations
Neutrophil leukocytosis and very elevated C-reactive protein and ESR are universal. Microscopy of fresh stool in bloody diarrhea shows red cell ingestion by trophozoites and is diagnostic of invasive infection. In liver abscess ultrasound shows one or more lesions usually in the right lobe. "Amebic pus" obtained by aspiration is non-offensive in smell and described as looking like "anchovy sauce." Serologic tests are rapid, sensitive and specific.

Management
Metronidazole is the drug of choice but has no activity against amebic cysts. Diloxanide furoate is prescribed for 10 days afterwards to eradicate cyst carriage. Drainage is usually performed for large liver abscesses.

Outcome
Most forms of amebiasis respond to treatment but life-threatening complications such as abscess rupture can develop if untreated.

Leishmaniasis: visceral leishmaniasis (kala-azar)

Clinical features

Immunocompetent host
- Patients remain well until the disease is advanced. Fever may relapse and remit and the course is typically prolonged. Lymphadenopathy is variable but hepatosplenomegaly is common and the spleen can be enormous. In the later stages, there is weight loss and weakness with susceptibility to intercurrent infections.
- Incubation is 3–18 months.

Immunocompromised host
- Visceral leishmaniasis can develop as an opportunistic infection in HIV-positive individuals (CD4 count <200 cells/mm^3).

Epidemiology
Visceral leishmaniasis is found in India and East Africa (*Leishmania donovanni*), Latin America (*L. chagasi*), and the Mediterranean basin (*L. infantum*). It mainly affects children in Southern Europe and epidemics occur in India.

Pathology

Leishmania are intracellular protozoan organisms. The reservoirs of infection include dogs, rodents, and humans. Transmission is by the bite of female sandflies. Parasites multiply within macrophages at the site of the bite. If cell-mediated immune response is insufficient or impaired, parasites ("amastigotes") multiply until the infected macrophage ruptures, with dissemination to the liver, spleen, lymph nodes, and bone marrow. Pancytopenia occurs from marrow suppression. Parasites may persist in a subclinical, dormant state for many years until the host's immunity deteriorates (e.g. HIV infection) and infection reactivates.

Investigations

Direct diagnosis involves identifying amastigotes (2–4 µm in diameter) by microscopy from tissue samples such as bone marrow aspirate, liver biopsy, or splenic puncture.

Management

Intravenous amphotericin B and oral miltefosine. Spraying houses with insecticide to eliminate sandflies has been attempted.

Outcome

Untreated, visceral leishmaniasis is often fatal, usually from intercurrent infection. Response is determined by the host's cell-mediated immune response. Relapses are common.

Cutaneous leismaniasis

Infection is localized to skin usually as ulcerating lesions. Systemic symptoms are usually absent. Infections are acquired mainly in Central and South America, parts of Africa, India, and the Middle East. *Leishmania* species vary with geographic location. The vector is the sandfly.

Trypanosomiasis

Protozoal infection caused by three species of trypanosoma: two in Africa (*Trypanosoma brucei rhodesiense* and *T. brucei gambiense*) and one in South America (*T. cruzi*). African and South American trypanosomiasis cause different diseases and are very rarely imported into the UK.

African trypanosomiasis (African sleeping sickness)
Clinical features

- Transmission is by a tsetse fly bite. Incubation is 2 days to 1 month and the clinical course has two phase.

- A painful chancre initially at site of inoculation with regional lymphadenopathy. A relapsing and remitting febrile, influenza-like illness follows.
- After weeks or sometimes years (depending on the species), meningoencephalitis develops. This manifests as a dementia-like illness with excessive somnolence (hence "sleeping sickness"). Coma and death follow.

Diagnosis

Direct visualization of trypanosomes in a thick blood film or in stained aspirates from affected sites. Serologic tests are also available.

Treatment

Suramin is used in early infections but only melasoprol, a highly toxic arsenic compound, is effective in established meningoencephalitis.

Outcome

T. br. rhodesiense is fatal within 50 days of infection, whereas *T. br. gambiense* is sometimes self-limiting or runs a chronic relapsing and remitting course.

South American trypanosomiasis (Chagas' disease)
Clinical features

- Transmitted by infected feces of reduviid bugs, which are rubbed into bite wounds or mucus membranes. Transfusion of infected blood can also cause infection.
- Cutaneous edema at entry site or unilateral orbital edema if via the conjunctiva. There is fever and regional lymph node enlargement.
- Chronic complications (in ~25%) include dilated cardiomyopathy, cardiac conduction defects, megaesophagus, and megacolon.
- Incubation is 1–4 weeks.

Epidemiology

Southern USA to Argentina. Affects 20 million people. Most infections occur in children from poor, rural areas.

Pathology

Intense inflammatory infiltrates around trypanosomes damage muscle fibers and nerves causing the chronic complications.

Investigations

Diagnosis is by visualization of trypanosomes in blood and by serology. In Latin America, reduviid bugs are fed on a patient's blood and later examined for *T. cruzi* infection (xenodiagnosis).

Treatment
Nifurtimox for acute infections. There is no specific treatment for chronic infections.

Outcome
Acute infection can be fatal in the immunosuppressed and in young children. Heart failure is a consequent cause of death amongst young people in South America.

Bacteria
Typhoid and paratyphoid fevers (enteric fevers)

Clinical features
- Fever is the commonest symptom. Headache, abdominal discomfort, constipation, and dry cough are frequent.
- In the second week, signs become more apparent. The pulse may be disproportionately slow compared to fever ("relative bradycardia"). Splenomegaly may be present and "rose spots" (scanty pink macules that fade with pressure) may appear on the trunk.
- In the third week, confusion or a stuporose state may occur. Fatal complications may also develop, the commonest being gastro-intestinal hemorrhage and perforated bowel. Others include hepatitis, cholecystitis, pneumonia, encephalomyelitis, and abscess formation.
- Incubation is 14–21 days.

Epidemiology
Bacteria persist in the gallbladder or urinary tract of asymptomatic carriers who are the reservoirs of infection. Transmission is by the fecal–oral route via contaminated food or water. Enteric fevers are "tropical" because they are commonest where personal and environmental hygiene are poor. Typhoid is an imported infection in the UK.

Pathology
The causative organisms are *Salmonella typhi* and *S. paratyphi*, Gram-negative bacilli of the Enterobacteriaceae group. Following ingestion, they penetrate the mucosa of the small intestine and are transported to mesenteric lymph nodes. Organisms enter the bloodstream via the thoracic duct and secondary invasion of the bowel occurs via infected bile. Bacilli replicate in the intestinal lymph follicles of the terminal ileum (or Peyer's patches) and inflammation of gut lymphoid tissue leads to mucosal ulceration or perforation.

Investigations
White cell count is usually normal, but the C-reactive protein is usually considerably elevated. Culture of blood is the most useful but stool and urine may also be positive.

Management
Ceftriaxone is the empiric agent of choice until sensitivities are available. Ciprofloxacin can be given orally but resistance is common.

Outcome
If treated early, the outcome is good with occasional relapse. The persistent carrier state must be excluded after recovery, especially in food handlers.

Rickettsial infections
Intracellular Gram-negative bacteria. Several species cause human infection. Transmission is via arthropod vectors, e.g. ticks, mites, and lice.

Clinical features
- Many do not recall the original tick bite but a history of walking through long grass or "scrub" should be sought. A few days after the bite, a characteristic black "eschar" with secondary lymphadenitis develops. This is followed by fever, cough, conjunctivitis, lymphadenopathy, splenomegaly, and a generalized rash. The rash is usually maculopapular (Fig. 15.18) but may occasionally be petechial or even gangrenous.
- Different rickettsial species produce diseases of varying severity from mild and self-limiting to DIC and multiorgan failure.
- Incubation is 1–3 weeks.

Epidemiology
Table 15.5 shows the main rickettsial infections with their geographic distribution and arthropod vector.

Investigations
The white cell count is typically normal and thrombocytopenia is common. Specific serologic tests are used to confirm the diagnosis. Rickettsiae may be identified by immunohistochemistry and PCR in biopsy samples.

Management
Doxycycline or ciprofloxacin. Prophylactic measures to avoid tick bites.

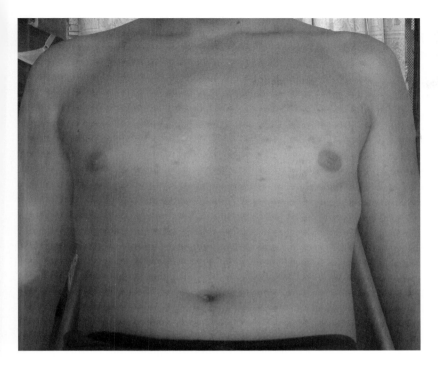

Fig. 15.18. A young boy presented with fever, conjunctivitis, and this maculopapular skin rash. Whilst on a family holiday in Sardinia a couple of weeks before, he had been removing ticks from a dog. Boutonneuse fever (*Rickettsia connori*) was diagnosed clinically and later confirmed by serology. He was treated with doxycycline and made an excellent recovery.

Table 15.5. Important rickettsial infections

Disease	Agent	Distribution	Transmission
Boutonneuse fever/African tick typhus	*R. connori*	Mediterranean, Africa, Asia	Tick bite
Epidemic typhus	*R. prowazekii*	Africa, Asia, Central and South America	Louse feces/broken skin
Murine ("endemic") typhus	*R. typhi*	Worldwide	Flea feces/broken skin
Scrub typhus	*R. tsutsugamushi*	Japan, S.E. Asia, North Australia	Mite bite
Rocky Mountain spotted fever	*R. rickettsii*	North, Central and South America	Tick bite

Outcome

This depends on the species. Rocky Mountain spotted fever and epidemic typhus are the most severe. Rocky Mountain spotted fever causes encephalitis and non-cardiogenic pulmonary edema with mortality up to 10%. If treatment is started early, the outlook is good.

Brucellosis

Clinical features

- A febrile illness that is often chronic, or relapsing and remitting, with sweats and malaise. Localizing features may be absent, but generalized lymphadenopathy or hepatosplenomegaly commonly occur.
- Large joint arthritis, sacroiliitis, and lumbar diskitis are the most frequent site-specific manifestations.

- Epididymo-orchitis, meningoencephalitis, brain abscess, and endocarditis are rare complications.
- Incubation is 2–4 weeks.

Epidemiology

Only a few countries, including the UK are brucellosis-free. Four species are human pathogens: *Brucella melitensis* (from goats, sheep, and camels), *B. abortus* (cattle), *B. suis* (swine) and *B. canis* (dogs). Transmission occurs through consumption of infected animals or milk products, contact with contaminated animal parts (e.g. placenta), and inhalation of infected aerosols. Unpasteurized dairy produce is the commonest source, especially milk, soft cheese, butter, and ice cream. It is an occupational disease in farmers and workers in abattoirs or microbiology laboratories.

Pathology

An intracellular Gram-negative bacterium. After entering the body, brucellae are taken up by macrophages, where some bacteria manage to survive within specialized compartments in the endoplasmic reticulum. Organisms are transported via the lymphatics to lymph nodes and the reticuloendothelial system and invade other organs via the circulation.

Investigations

Slight leukopenia with lymphocytosis. Mild hepatitis is common. Blood cultures and bone marrow cultures may be positive but diagnosis often rests on serologic tests. Liver biopsy may show granulomatous inflammation.

Management

Combinations of antibiotics that penetrate well into cells should be given for several weeks or months. WHO guidelines recommend doxycycline with either rifampicin or streptomycin.

Outcome

Responds well to antibiotic treatment. Endocarditis is the principal cause of mortality.

Relapsing fever

Clinical features

- Headache, fever and myalgia lasting for several days, followed by spontaneous remission for a similar duration before symptoms begin again. There may be as many as ten relapses and remissions depending on the species.
- Dry cough, hepatomegaly, splenomegaly, and lymphadenopathy are often present.
- Incubation is 3–18 days.

Epidemiology

Caused by two species of *Borrelia* bacteria (spirochetes). The reservoir of infection in louse-borne relapsing fever (*Borrelia recurrentis*) is humans, and infected fluids from the body louse (*Pediculus humanus*) are responsible for its transmission. Tick-borne relapsing fever (*B. duttoni*) is transmitted by bites from infected soft ticks in Africa (genus *Ornithodorus*) and the reservoirs are rodents and the ticks themselves. Louse-borne relapsing fever is associated with poverty, overcrowding, and poor hygiene.

Pathology

Borrelia multiply in the blood and the relapsing and remitting pattern results from the organism's ability to alter its surface antigen expression and evade the host immune response.

Investigations

Neutrophilia is typical. Diagnosis can be made by direct visualization on a stained thick blood film. Serologic tests are also available.

Management

Tetracycline, but treatment may be complicated by a systemic hypersensitivity reaction to killed bacteria, called the Jarisch–Herxheimer reaction.

Outcome

Tick-borne has more relapses but is milder than louse-borne relapsing fever. Untreated, louse-borne relapsing fever can cause multiorgan failure and has a mortality rate of 40% in epidemics.

Leprosy

Clinical features

- Subclinical disease is more common than overt infection. However, there is a spectrum of clinical disease, ranging from tuberculoid leprosy to lepromatous leprosy.
- In tuberculoid leprosy, there are well-demarcated, hypopigmented skin patches with loss of sensation to pain and temperature and thickened peripheral nerves, which are palpable.
- In lepromatous leprosy, there are widespread, erythematous nodular, macular, and plaque like skin lesions (erythema nodosum leprosum or ENL). There may be diffuse sensory loss, fever, and nasal congestion. Blindness may occur.
- Borderline leprosy is a mixed form of disease, which may shift either way along the continuum. Skin reactions can develop spontaneously or during treatment, and may be localized or generalized.

Epidemiology

Occurs in developing countries with a warm climate, e.g. Asia, Africa, and South America. The global prevalence has fallen from 12 to 1 per 100 000/year in the last two decades.

Pathology

A chronic granulomatous infection of the skin and peripheral nerves caused by *Mycobacterium leprae*. Transmission is by inhalation of bacilli in aerosols from patients with nasal discharge. The pattern of illness is principally determined by the strength of the cell-mediated immune response. In tuberculoid leprosy there is a vigorous, non-caseating granulomatous response involving skin and nerves with few detectable organisms. In lepromatous leprosy there are numerous bacilli and a diffuse inflammatory infiltrate with few granulomas.

Investigations

Diagnosis is from the presence of characteristic clinical features and histology from biopsy material, e.g. nerves and skin. Acid-fast bacilli can also be identified in skin smears.

Management

Depends on the clinical type but may include combinations of rifampicin, clofazimine, and dapsone, for months or years. Education is important since injury to anesthetic limbs may go unnoticed and cause neuropathic ulcers. Surgery may help claw hands and feet.

Diphtheria

Clinical features

- A gray-colored membrane develops in the pharynx following fever and sore throat. The patient is systemically unwell with fever and sweating. There is typically prominent cervical lymphadenitis and neck edema ("bullneck" appearance). Features of circulatory shock may be present.
- Breathing difficulty, myocarditis, and neurologic abnormalities may develop, including paralysis of palatal and ocular muscles.
- Incubation is 2–4 days.

Epidemiology

Epidemics occur in relatively poor and unvaccinated populations. Vaccine-induced immunity is not lifelong and there was a massive resurgence of cases in the former USSR during the 1990s.

Pathology

Corynebacterium diphtheriae is a Gram-positive rod transmitted by respiratory droplets. Release of an exotoxin is responsible for the epithelial necrosis, membrane formation, and edema, which may cause respiratory tract obstruction.

Investigations

Culture from throat swab, but treatment should not be delayed for microbiologic confirmation.

Management

Diphtheria antitoxin (hyperimmune horse serum) and erythromycin for 14 days. Children are routinely vaccinated.

Outcome

Death occurs in 10% of cases from respiratory obstruction and severe toxemia. In the later stages, cardiac and respiratory muscle failure may be fatal. Nerve paralyses eventually recover in survivors.

Anthrax

Clinical features

There are three clinical forms acquired from contact with infected herbivores (e.g. goats, sheep, cattle, and deer) or their hair, wool, and skin.

- Cutaneous anthrax accounts for 95%. A painless, black eschar develops at the site of bacterial entry with prominent surrounding edema.
- Inhalation anthrax has a rapid and fulminant course with chest pain, fever, cough, breathlessness, and circulatory collapse. Death rapidly follows.
- Gastro-intestinal anthrax is extremely rare and results from eating contaminated meat.
- Bioterrorism-associated anthrax has occurred in the USA.
- Incubation usually 1–7 days.

Epidemiology

Sporadic cases rarely occur in the UK and are sometimes occupational, e.g. working with imported animal hides. Outbreaks in the developing world occur in agricultural settings.

Pathology

Bacillus anthracis is a spore-forming Gram-positive rod. Spores can persist in soil for years. Cutaneous anthrax occurs by subcutaneous inoculation. Exotoxins are responsible for local edema and tissue necrosis. Inhalational anthrax occurs when spores enter the lungs and lead to hemorrhagic mediastinitis.

Investigations

Gram-stain, microscopy, and culture from the skin lesion. The chest X-ray may show mediastinal widening in inhalational anthrax.

Treatment

Penicillin, doxycycline, or ciprofloxacin are effective in cutaneous disease. Vaccination is recommended

465

for those handling dead animals and for laboratory staff.

Outcome

Treatment success depends on early recognition. Mortality is ~20% in cutaneous anthrax. Antibiotics have little impact on inhalational anthrax and most do not survive.

Plague

Clinical features

Transmission is from an infected rat flea bite.

- Following the bite, fever, chills, and exquisitely tender regional lymph node enlargement (buboes) develop, hence "bubonic" plague.
- Progressive dissemination via the bloodstream follows ("septic" plague).
- Localized pulmonary infection ("pneumonic" plague) via the bloodstream, or following inhalation of bacteria from another patient with "pneumonic" plague, causes extensive necrosis of the lungs and is rapidly fatal.
- Incubation is 1–6 days (shorter if via inhalation).

Epidemiology

Occurs throughout the world, particularly in Africa, Asia, and rural areas of the Western USA.

Pathology

Yersinia pestis, a Gram-negative coccobacillus belonging to the Enterobacteriacae.

Investigations

Gram stain and culture.

Treatment

Streptomycin or gentamicin. Vaccination is available for people at high risk.

Outcome

Ten percent of treated cases are fatal and over half of untreated patients die.

Cholera

Caused by *Vibrio cholerae*, a Gram-negative bacillus. Characterized by sudden onset profuse watery diarrhea with abdominal pain. Fever is not prominent. The diarrhea is toxin mediated and the consequent dehydration may be life threatening. Adequate fluid replacement is the mainstay of treatment.

Viruses
Arbovirus infections
Dengue fever
Clinical features

- Sudden onset fever, headache, musculoskeletal pain ("breakbone fever"). A generalized erythematous rash, like sunburn, develops. Recovery starts a few days after the rash appears.
- Occasionally, hypotension with or without hemorrhage develops 2–4 days into the illness (dengue shock syndrome or dengue hemorrhagic fever). Petechiae and bleeding from multiple sites can occur, e.g. hematemesis, hematuria, and epistaxis.
- Incubation is less than 7 days.

Epidemiology

Caused by a flavivirus, transmitted by mosquitoes (*Aedes aegypti*). 100 million infections occur annually. The highest burden is in South East Asia and South America, where most cases are in children.

Pathology

There are four virus serotypes. It is suggested that re-infection with a different serotype results in an antibody–virus complex that, instead of being protective, causes capillary wall injury, bleeding, and fluid leak. Coagulopathy from DIC is also a factor.

Investigations

Leukopenia and thrombocytopenia are common. Diagnosis is confirmed by serology.

Management

No specific treatment or effective vaccine. Hypotension and hemorrhage are treated with IV fluids and blood products.

Outcome

Most infections are self-limiting but immunity is short-lived. Hemorrhagic complications may be fatal if not treated promptly.

Yellow fever
Clinical features

- Most infections are subclinical or cause a mild febrile illness.
- In severe infections, there is fever, headache, and vomiting initially. Renal and liver failure, severe vomiting, gastro-intestinal hemorrhage, and shock follow.
- Incubation is <1 week.

Epidemiology

Occurs in Africa, Central and South America, but not in Asia.

Pathology

Yellow fever is a flavivirus- like dengue fever. Transmitted by *Aedes aegyptes* between monkeys and to humans. In populated areas, the mosquito may transmit the virus from infected people to other humans.

Investigations

Diagnosis requires a specialized laboratory to look for specific antibody. A liver biopsy (usually postmortem) shows mid-zone necrosis and "Councilman bodies."

Treatment

Treatment is supportive only. A live attenuated vaccine protects for 10 years.

Outcome

Florid infections are often fatal, but there is full recovery in survivors.

Viral hemorrhagic fevers

Viral hemorrhagic fevers are a group of acute viral infections that may result in hypovolemic shock and uncontrolled hemorrhage from multiple sites. Mortality rate is characteristically high. There is a risk of transmission to healthcare workers and suspected cases are usually admitted to high security infectious diseases units. There are strict guidelines about handling specimens and disposal of body waste. Incubation is up to 3 weeks.

Lassa fever

Caused by an arenavirus, first identified in Lassa, Nigeria. Causes several thousand deaths each year but many from endemic areas have serologic evidence of previous infection. The natural reservoir is the multimammate rat, and human infection is due to direct contact with infected rat urine. Treatment is mainly supportive, mortality is up to 50%.

Marburg and Ebola viruses

These belong to the filovirus family. Fruit bats are suspected to be the natural reservoir of Ebola. Marburg virus was first identified in 1967 in German laboratory workers exposed to blood or tissues from African green monkeys from Uganda. Mortality for both conditions is up to 90%.

Rabies

Clinical features

- Human infection is usually transmitted by rabid animal bite but infected saliva on broken skin or mucous membranes from licks and scratches presents a risk. Unprovoked animal bites are unusual and increase the suspicion of rabies.

- Incubation usually 20–90 days. The first sign is paresthesiae, itching, or pain at the inoculation site. Fever may also be present. After a few days, either "furious" or "paralytic" rabies develops.

- Hydrophobia is a cardinal symptom of "furious" rabies. Other features are spasmodic muscle contractions of throat, diaphragm, and respiration. Generalized spasms cause opisthotonus, and during attacks patients appear filled with terror. Spasms are precipitated by attempts to swallow fluids and blowing air onto the face ("aerophobia"). Other features include hypersalivation ("frothing at the mouth"), seizures, and episodes of extreme agitation. Death usually occurs within a week.

- In "paralytic" (or "dumb") rabies there is ascending, symmetric, or asymmetric flaccid paralysis, usually beginning in the bitten limb. Coma develops and death is inevitable.

Epidemiology

"Classic" rabies (RNA virus) is a lyssavirus. Closely related viruses found in bats produce an indistinguishable disease in humans. Almost all of the rabies deaths occur in the tropics but relatively few countries, including the UK, are free of classic rabies.

Pathology

Following the bite, there is local replication of virus in muscle and subcutaneous tissues. The virus travels along peripheral nerves towards the central nervous system. The length of the incubation period depends upon the distance the virus has to travel. In the central nervous system, encephalitis develops and the virus spreads widely to body tissues, including the salivary glands, back down peripheral nerves.

Investigations

The virus may be identified in body fluids and tissue by immunofluorescence, antibody response, and PCR. Rabid dogs and cats die within 10 days of biting so the diagnosis can be excluded if the animal remains healthy. Alternatively, the diagnosis can be made by examining the animal brain for classic dark-staining aggregates of viral protein within neurons ("Negri bodies").

Management

There is no treatment when clinical features develop. The focus is on prevention, especially by immunization. Rabies vaccine should be given to persons at risk, e.g. veterinarians, wildlife officers, and laboratory staff. Following a bite, the wound should be cleaned vigorously with soap and water and active immunization commenced. The aim of post-exposure prophylaxis is to stop the virus reaching the central nervous system by producing protective antibody.

Outcome

When rabies becomes clinically apparent, it is always fatal. Treatment is therefore purely palliative and intensive care merely prolongs life.

Poliomyelitis

Clinical features

- Most infections are asymptomatic or cause minor febrile illness (>95%).
- A small number of cases develop lymphocytic meningitis (~2%).
- Paralytic polio develops in <1%. Anterior horn cell infection in the spinal cord causes asymmetric, flaccid paralysis, with no sensory involvement. One or more limbs, or cranial nerves, may be affected.

Epidemiology

Poliomyelitis is on the verge of global eradication as a result of a worldwide vaccination initiative, but transmission still occurs in parts of Asia and Africa.

Pathology

Poliovirus is an enterovirus, transmission by the fecal–oral route.

Management

Treatment is supportive. The vaccine is given orally in either live or inactivated forms.

Outcome

There is rarely a full recovery following paralysis. Muscle wasting and limb deformity develop in the long term and respiratory failure may occur if there is respiratory muscle involvement.

Fungal infections
Histoplasmosis
Clinical features
Immunocompetent host

- The majority are asymptomatic or mild. Symptoms range from an influenza-like syndrome to severe respiratory illness with cough, fever, night sweats, and weight loss. Most symptoms resolve spontaneously within 10 days.

Immunocompromised host

- In individuals with underlying lung disease, e.g. emphysema, chronic pulmonary histoplasmosis causes a low-grade fever, productive cough, and malaise.
- Disseminated histoplasmosis occurs in patients with impaired cell-mediated immunity.

Epidemiology

Histoplasma capsulatum is a soil-based fungus associated with decaying bird or bat feces. The most endemic region is the Ohio and Mississippi river valleys in the USA where large flocks of starlings congregate. In South America, histoplasmosis is associated with chicken coops and bat caves.

Pathology

Infectious particles are inhaled. Cell-mediated immunity is required to control infection, and resolution occurs with the development of caseating and non-caseating granulomas.

Investigations

Serologic tests identify specific antibodies in blood. *H. capsulatum* antigens can also be detected in urine. Culture of clinical samples, e.g. sputum, CSF, or blood, is also diagnostic. In acute primary infection, hilar lymphadenopathy and patchy infiltrate may be seen on the chest X-ray. In chronic pulmonary infection there are upper lobe cavities, and in disseminated disease, there is scattered nodular pattern. A skin test is a valuable epidemiologic tool but less useful diagnostically.

Management

Most cases require no treatment, but itraconazole may be given to immunocompetent patients with symptomatic infections.

Outcome

In most cases a complete recovery is made without treatment, but disseminated disease in the immuno-suppressed may be fatal.

Other systemic fungi

Coccidiodomycosis (caused by *Coccidioides immitis*) is transmitted by inhalation of contaminated dust in dry desert climates. It is most common in the South-western United States and primarily causes a pneumonic illness. Disseminated infections can also cause meningitis.

Blastomycosis (caused by *Blastomyces dermatitidis*) has a similar distribution to histoplasmosis in the USA. It is associated with dust exposure and can cause acute or chronic infection of the lungs, skin, or bone.

Helminths
Trematodes (flukes)
Schistosomiasis (blood flukes)
Clinical features

There are three major species that infect humans with different geographic distributions: *Schistosoma hematobium*, *S. mansoni*, and *S. japonicum*.

- Transmission to humans requires contact with a fresh water source such as swimming in African lakes, e.g. Lake Malawi. Local dermatitis (or "swimmer's itch") may occur 1–3 days after free-swimming larvae (called cercariae) penetrate intact human skin.

- 6 weeks later a generalized hypersensitivity reaction called Katayama fever may occur. Typical features include fever, cough, wheeze, diarrhea, urticarial skin rash, and hepatosplenomegaly. This may be very severe but usually resolves spontaneously after a week or so.

- Months or years later, hematuria is the most common feature of chronic S. *hematobium* infection. In *S. mansoni* and *S. japonicum* infections, there are often few symptoms but intermittent bloody diarrhea and anemia may develop. The liver may also become enlarged and splenomegaly indicates portal hypertension.

Epidemiology

There are at least 200 million people with schistosomiasis. *S. haematobium* causes urinary schistosomiasis and is found in Africa and the Middle East. *S. mansoni* is also found in South America and the Caribbean. *S. japonicum* is found in China, Japan, the Philippines, and the Far East.

Pathology

Free-swimming cercariae are released from a specific fresh water snail that is involved in the fluke life cycle. After penetrating human skin, cercariae develop into adult flukes, which migrate in the venous system of either the mesentery (*S. mansoni* and *S. japonicum*) or urinary bladder (*S. haematobium*). Katayama fever is a systemic hypersensitivity reaction associated with the first release of eggs by mature flukes. The features of chronic infection are the result of granulomatous inflammation and fibrosis that form where eggs are deposited in either the bladder (in *S. haematobium* infection), or bowel and liver (in *S. mansoni* and *S. japonicum*). Heavy *S. haematobium* infection causes the bladder walls to become thickened and rigid over time with an increased risk of bladder carcinoma and obstruction. In heavy *S. mansoni* and *S. japonicum* infections, polypoid lesions develop in the colon, which tend to bleed. Liver fibrosis results in venous obstruction and portal hypertension.

Investigations

Eosinophilia is a common finding. Urine microscopy may identify red cells and eggs. Eggs may also be seen in bladder and rectal biopsy specimens. Serology is very useful, but remains positive for many years after successful treatment.

Management

Praziquantel is safe and the drug of choice for all species.

Outcome

Most infections that are treated before obstructive renal disease or portal hypertension develops respond well.

Other flukes

Other species of fluke cause liver (fascioliasis, clonorchiasis, opisthorciasis), lung (parogonamiasis) and intestinal (faciolopsiasis) disease in various parts of the world. Their life cycles also involve intermediate snail hosts and they are transmitted to humans that eat encysted cercariae attached to undercooked fish, crabs, or aquatic plants, depending on the species involved.

Nematodes (Roundworms)

Filariasis

Filaria are long slender worms. These include lymphatic filariasis, loiasis and onchocerciasis, which are transmitted by insect vectors. Only lymphatic filariasis causes an intermittent febrile illness.

Lymphatic filariasis

Clinical features

- Most are asymptomatic.
- Typical features are recurrent episodes of fever and chills associated with lymphangitis (pain, erythema, and tenderness over a lymphatic duct) and lymphadenitis. Attacks last a week or two and then spontaneously resolve.
- Recurrent lymphatic inflammation eventually leads to chronic lymphatic obstruction, gross lymphedema and massive overgrowth of the skin and subcutaneous tissues ("elephantiasis"). The legs and scrotum are most commonly affected.

Epidemiology

Lymphatic filariasis is caused by *Wuchereria bancrofti* and less commonly by *Brugia malayi*. *W. bancrofti* is found in Africa, the Indian sub-continent, South East Asia, and Central and South America. Most infections occur in Asia.

Pathology

Infective larvae are transmitted to humans by mosquitoes. These migrate to the lymphatic system and develop into adult worms (4–10 cm long), which cause sterile lymphangitis. Fertilized female worms produce microfilaria that infect the insect vector when feeding.

Investigations

Microfilaria may be seen on a blood film during early infections taken in the middle of the night (when mosquitoes bite) (Fig. 15.19). Eosinophilia is very common.

Management

Treatment is with diethylcarbamazine (DEC) over 2–3 weeks. Established elephantiasis can only be treated surgically.

Loiasis (Loa Loa)

Loiasis is confined to the forest areas of West and Central Africa, transmitted to humans by the bite of an infected horsefly or deerfly (*Chrysops*). Adult worms (~5 cm long) can survive in the subcutaneous

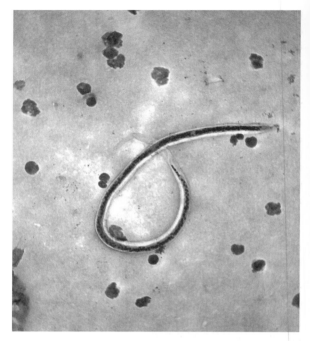

Fig. 15.19. A stained blood film taken from a patient at midnight showing microfilaria of *Wuchereria bancrofti*. The patient was from Guyana and presented with chyluria secondary to megalymphatics of the thighs and pelvis.

tissues of the human host for over 10 years but most infections are asymptomatic. Pruritic subcutaneous swellings (called "Calabar" swellings after a Nigerian town) appear transiently and, occasionally, patients may even see an adult worm migrating across their own conjunctiva ("eye worm"). Microfilariae produced by fertilized females may be seen on a blood film taken at midday. Eosinophilia is very common and serologic tests may be positive. Treatment is with DEC, as for lymphatic filariasis.

Onchocerciasis (Onchocerca volvulus)

Almost all cases are found in equatorial Africa, where ~20 million people are affected. "River blindness" is another name for this condition because the small biting blackfly (*Simulium damnosum*) that transmits infective larvae to humans breeds near rivers. Adult worms live in the tissues beneath the skin or coiled up in fibrous, subcutaneous nodules and may survive ~20 years in humans. Microfilariae produced by female worms migrate to the skin and eyes and are responsible for the disease manifestations. The commonest symptom is itching. Blindness results from an inflammatory response to microfilariae within the cornea and anterior chamber of the eye. Eosinophilia is common but microfilariae are absent from peripheral blood and there is no serologic test. The diagnosis is made by biopsy of a subcutaneous nodule or by direct visualization of microfilariae in a "skin snip" or in the eye, using a slit lamp.

Toxocariasis (*Toxocara canis*)

Caused by roundworm larvae that normally infect dogs (*Toxocara canis*) and less commonly cats (*T. cati*). Transmission is by ingestion of eggs passed in animal feces. Larvae hatch in the intestine, penetrate the gut wall, and migrate via the circulation to many organs in the body (called visceral larva migrans). This causes hepatomegaly, fever, and weight loss. Eosinophilia is common and diagnosis is by specific serology. Most infections are asymptomatic and recover without any treatment.

Trichinosis (*Trichinella spiralis*)

Trichinosis is distributed widely around the world and develops when undercooked meat containing the encysted larvae of *Trichinella spiralis* is eaten. Larvae spread to skeletal muscle where they burrow into muscle fibers. Fever with myositis, periorbital edema, and eosinophilia are typical features. There are specific serologic tests and treatment is albendazole.

Strongyloidiasis (*Strongyloides stercoralis*)

Strongyloidiasis is found widely throughout the tropics. The worms can live free in soil or as human parasites. Transmission occurs when larvae penetrate intact skin, e.g. walking barefoot. Adult worms (<3 mm long) live in the small intestine and females produce eggs that are passed with feces into the soil. Some larvae hatch in the gut, invade the bowel wall and migrate back to the small intestine via the liver and lungs. This "autoinfection" cycle means that strongyloidiasis can persist for decades.

Abdominal pain and diarrhea may occur and migrating larvae sometimes produce a transient skin rash (larva migrans) but most infections are asymptomatic. However, in the immunocompromised host, the autoinfection cycle can produce a "hyperinfection" syndrome, which may be fatal. Diagnosis is by serology or demonstration of larvae in small intestinal biopsies, sputum, and stool. Treatment is with ivermectin.

Other intestinal roundworms

Intestinal roundworms are the commonest helminth infections of humans and mostly affect children in tropical and subtropical regions of the world. These include ascaris (*Ascaris lumbricoides*), hookworm (*Necator americanus* and *Ancylostoma duodenale*), pinworm (*Enterobius vermicularis*), and trichuriasis (*Trichuris trichuria*). Transmission is by ingestion of eggs, usually hand to mouth. Mostly infections are asymptomatic or cause relatively minor symptoms without fever.

Cestodes (tapeworms)

Beef and pork tapeworms
(*Taenia saginata* and *T. solium*)

Adult tapeworms are ribbon-shaped worms that live in the small intestine and may grow to several meters in length. Transmission is by eating raw or undercooked beef or pork containing larvae in cyst form. Both beef (*Taenia saginata*) and pork (*T. solium*) tapeworms are common in Asia and Africa, but pork tapeworm also occurs in Central and South America. Most infections are asymptomatic or cause minor symptoms without fever. However, cysticercosis can develop if the eggs of *T. solium* are ingested in contaminated food or water. In the human intestine, larvae hatch from the eggs and invade host tissues. Cysts containing viable larvae that have reached the brain (neurocysticercosis) are a major cause of epilepsy in parts of South America.

Hydatid disease

Caused by *Echinococcus* species, canine tapeworms are found in domestic dogs, wolves, and foxes. Hydatid disease occurs worldwide, especially in rural, sheep-farming areas. Transmission is by ingestion of eggs excreted in dog feces. Eggs hatch into larvae, penetrate the bowel wall and migrate, most commonly to liver and lungs, where they form slowly expanding, cystic structures. Most infections are asymptomatic and fever is not a typical feature. Occasionally, a cyst may rupture causing anaphylaxis or disseminated infection. The diagnosis is by serology and characteristic radiographic appearances. Eosinophilia is not usually present until there is cyst rupture and suspected cysts should not be drained without careful consideration. Drug treatment is with albendazole but surgical excision is often also required.

Fever of unknown origin (FUO)

Introduction

FUO is defined as a body temperature of greater than 38.3 °C on several occasions for at least 3 weeks, the cause of which is not identified after 3 days of hospital investigation or two outpatient visits. This definition excludes over 95% of the infectious causes of a febrile illness that are treated successfully or self-limiting. Non-infectious causes must be considered, especially malignancy and inflammatory disorders and there are many "miscellaneous" causes. Figure 15.20 shows the diagnostic categories and their frequency. Important infectious and non-infectious causes are shown in Tables 15.6 and 15.7.

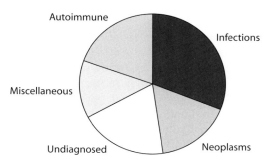

Fig. 15.20. Frequency of the categories of FUO.

Clinical features

The most important tools are a detailed history and careful physical examination. The duration is important since relatively few infections cause a fever lasting more than several weeks. In general, the longer the duration, the more likely that a non-infectious condition is the underlying cause. The history should include a thorough review of systems, e.g. weight loss may suggest malignancy, Crohn's disease, or TB. In the outpatient setting, it is important to establish whether or not the patient is truly febrile. Asking the patient to keep a chart of morning and evening temperature measurements, using an inexpensive electronic thermometer, is very useful. A family history should also be taken, the latter since some recurrent febrile conditions are hereditary, e.g. familial Mediterranean fever. If no cause is found, a full history and examination should be repeated since relevant facts are sometimes remembered and physical signs evolve over time. In addition, asking a colleague for their assessment can be very helpful since they bring a "fresh pair of eyes" to the problem.

Table 15.6. Important infections causing FUO

Bacteria	Viral	Fungal	Protozoal & Parasitic
Abscess (especially intra-abdominal)	Epstein-Barr virus	Pneumocystis jiroveci*	Toxocariasis
Bacterial endocarditis	Cytomegalovirus	Cryptococcosis*	Toxoplasmosis
Deep-seated focus (e.g. osteomyelitis)	HIV	Histoplasmosis*	Amebiais
Leptospirosis	Parvovirus B19		Lymphatic filariasis
Lyme disease			Visceral leishmaniasis*
Opportunistic mycobacteria*			Malaria
Q fever			Trichinosis
Rat bite fever			Trypansomiasis
Rickettsial infections (e.g. scrub typhus)			
Secondary syphilis*			
Trench fever (bartonellosis)			
Tuberculosis (extrapulmonary)*			
Typhoid			
Whipple's disease			
Yersiniosis			
Brucellosis			
Relapsing fever			

Note:
*Especially in HIV-infected patients.

Table 15.7. Selected non-infectious causes of FUO

Neoplastic	Rheumatological	Miscellaneous
Lymphoma	Adult Onset Still's Disease	Atrial myxoma
Leukemia	Ankylosing spondylitis	Autoimmune hemolytic anemia
Hepatoma	Behçet's disease	Castleman's disease
Hypernephroma	Cryoglobulinemia	Crohn's disease
Intra-abdominal carcinoma (e.g. colon, pancreas)	Giant cell arteritis	Cyclic neutropenia
	Gout and pseudogout	Drug fever
Metastatic carcinoma	Mixed connective tissue disease	Extrinsic allergic alveolitis
	Polyarteritis nodosa	Factitious fever
	Polymyositis	Familial Mediterranean fever
	Relapsing polychondritis	Other periodic fevers Hematoma
	Rheumatic fever	Kawasaki's syndrome
	Rheumatoid disease	Kikuchi's disease
	Sjögren's syndrome	Metal fume fever
	SLE	Pulmonary emboli
	Takayasu's aortitis	Sarcoidosis
	Wegener's granulomatosis	Seizures
		Thyroiditis

Epidemiology

The epidemiology of FUO depends upon the population of patients being investigated. Important factors include ethnic background, immune status, and age. Extrapulmonary or "cryptic" disseminated TB is one of the commonest causes of an FUO and patients are often from countries or ethnic groups where the infection is common. In HIV-positive patients with FUO, opportunistic infections are related to the CD4 lymphocyte count, e.g. *Pneumocystis jiroveci* pneumonia is rare with counts $>300/mm^3$. Neoplastic causes of fever, especially lymphoma, are also more common in this group. In neutropenic patients, fungal and bacterial infections are common causes of FUO, but the underlying disease, e.g. lymphoma, may also be responsible for a persistent fever. In the elderly, malignancy, temporal arteritis, chronic prostatitis, pulmonary emboli, drug fever, and tuberculosis are relatively more common. In young adults, SLE, Still's disease, and factitious fevers occur more frequently.

Pathology

Infections Silent foci of bacterial infection often take the form of intra-abdominal or pelvic collections, e.g. subdiaphragmatic and hepatic abscesses. Blood cultures in patients with bacterial endocarditis may initially be negative if one of the slow-growing HACEK (Gram-negative bacilli including hemophilius species) organisms are involved, or if the patient has received antibiotics. The culture-negative causes of endocarditis should also be considered in patients with a heart murmur, e.g. Q fever, bartonellosis, and brucellosis. Occasionally, EBV and CMV may cause a prolonged but mild febrile illness in younger patients.

Multisystem inflammatory diseases Adult Onset Still's Disease (AOSD) is the commonest rheumatologic cause of FUO and should be considered in adults with a classic triad of high fever, a transient ("evanescent") rash, and arthralgia. Pharyngitis is common and enlarged lymph nodes and splenomegaly may be felt. A neutrophil leukocytosis is typical in the blood and the serum ferritin is usually very high. However, there is no definitive laboratory test and other conditions with a similar clinical presentation need to be excluded.

The classical physical signs of giant cell arteritis are headache, jaw claudication, tender temporal artery and rarely, visual loss, but these may be absent. Fever is common and the inflammatory indices are usually very elevated (ESR >100 mm/h). Autoimmune and

473

connective tissue disorders can thus present with fever and no localizing features of note.

Malignancy Lymphoma is the commonest individual malignant cause of an FUO. Constitutional or B symptoms (weight loss, night sweats, and fevers) are present in a minority of patients with lymphoma. Others including liver metastases, renal cell carcinoma, and adenocarcinoma may also cause fever.

Miscellaneous Crohn's disease is an important cause and may present with weight loss, fever, and anemia, without pronounced gastro-intestinal symptoms. Sarcoidosis is a systemic disease most commonly affecting the lungs, eyes, and lymph nodes. A hematoma may cause unexplained fever, especially if there has been a retroperitoneal bleed or hemorrhage into the abdominal cavity. In factitious fever, patients may artificially warm the thermometer and this may be part of Munchausen's syndrome. Familial Mediterranean fever is a hereditary non-infectious condition that occurs in patients with Jewish, Turkish, Armenian, or Arab ancestry. It is characterized by recurrent attacks of fever with polyserositis (peritonitis, arthritis, and pleuritis) lasting for a few hours to days. The first attack occurs before the age of 20 years in 90% and is frequently misdiagnosed as appendicitis. It is one of four types of inherited syndromes transmitted as autosomal recessive or dominant. Other examples are Hibernian fever and Muckle-Wells syndrome.

Investigations

A list of routine tests and more specialized investigations is shown in Table 15.8. Raised inflammatory indices make factitious fever unlikely. Very high inflammatory markers (ESR >100 mm/h) are frequently seen in adult onset Still's disease, drug fever, endocarditis, giant cell arteritis, myeloma, and other malignancies. Mild liver function abnormalities occur in many causes of FUO including TB, viral infections, brucellosis, Q fever, Still's disease, and drug fever.

Abnormal findings on urinalysis may point towards a renal tract source but hematuria also occurs in endocarditis and vasculitis with kidney involvement. Three sets of blood cultures should be performed to increase the chance of isolating a systemic bacterial or fungal pathogen. Most serologic tests for infection and autoantibodies have a low diagnostic yield in the setting of an FUO. Serum should also be "saved" early in the illness so that an

Table 15.8. Investigation in the patient with unexplained fever

Basic

- Full blood count
- Blood film for malaria if appropriate travel history
- Electrolytes and liver function tests
- Inflammatory markers (ESR and C-reactive protein)
- Urinalysis, urine microscopy, and culture
- Blood cultures (at least two sets)
- Cultures from other sites where appropriate, e.g. stool, CSF, ascites, pleural fluid, joint fluid, etc.
- Chest radiograph

More specialized

- Paul Bunnell or Monospot test
- Auto-antibodies (e.g. rheumatoid factor, anti-nuclear antibodies), serum angiotensin converting enzyme
- Serologic tests depending on exposure risk, e.g. Q fever, brucella, leishmania, syphillis (and serum saved)
- HIV test if exposure risks present
- Tuberculin skin test
- Early morning urine collection if miliary or renal TB suspected
- Radiologic imaging (abdominal ultrasound, CT, or MRI scans)
- Echocardiogram
- Biopsy (bone marrow, lymph node, liver, skin, etc.)
- Radionucleotide scan?

increase in a specific antibody to a suspected pathogen may be demonstrated after a suitable interval. A malaria film should be performed in all with a history of relevant foreign travel and HIV testing with appropriate counseling should be done if there are risk factors.

The chest X-ray may reveal subtle miliary shadowing, but a CT scan may demonstrate significant lymphadenopathy, miliary nodules, or other lung lesions not evident on the plain film. Abdominal imaging (ultrasound or CT scanning) may reveal an occult collection, lymphadenopathy, or malignancy. Biopsy of any enlarged lymph node or abnormal skin lesions should be performed. Liver and bone marrow biopsies should also be considered when the diagnosis remains unclear. A bone marrow biopsy may be helpful in disseminated infections (e.g. TB, visceral leishmaniasis, typhoid, and histoplasmosis) and may help to exclude infiltrative or hematologic malignancies (Fig. 15.21). An echocardiogram to look for vegetations on heart valves should be performed if there is a regurgitant murmur or stigmata of infective endocarditis. With the advent of high resolution CT, radionucleotide scans have a controversial role but may still highlight an occult pyogenic collection.

(a)

(b)

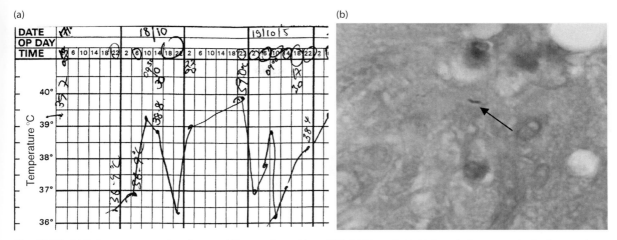

Fig. 15.21. (a) Daily temperature chart from an African patient with an FUO. (b) Disseminated tuberculosis was eventually diagnosed following a bone marrow biopsy, which revealed granulomas containing acid-fast bacilli, indicated by the arrow.

Treatment

Empiric courses of treatment with antimicrobials are generally ill advised unless the patient is unwell or severely immunocompromised, e.g. neutropenic. However, if empiric therapy is considered absolutely necessary, a full course should be given to prevent problems arising from suboptimal treatment, e.g. antituberculous therapy.

Outcome

The outcome depends upon the cause of FUO. In the undiagnosed group, the prognosis for the majority of patients is good and the fever usually resolves within a few weeks.

Further reading

British Infection Society www.britishinfectionsociety.org

Gillespie S, Bamford K, *Medical Microbiology and Infection at a glance*, Blackwell Publishing Ltd, 2007.

Health Protection Agency www.hpa.org.uk

National Centre for Infectious Diseases (USA) www.cdc.gov/ncidod/index.htm

The Royal Society of Tropical Medicine and Hygiene www.rstmh.org

Torok E, Moran E, Cooke F, *Oxford handbook of Infectious Diseases and Microbiology*, Oxford University Press, 2009.

World Health Organization www.who.int/en/

David McGibbon

Contents

Introduction

A consultation with a patient about a skin problem has three functions:

(1) To collect information via history, examination, and investigations and reach a diagnosis
(2) To respond to a patient's emotions
(3) To inform, educate, and facilitate a treatment intervention and/or a change of behavior to achieve self-reliance.

Arriving at the correct diagnosis after collecting all the appropriate data does not mean that the patient's skin condition will improve. Skin disease is often chronic, requiring indefinite compliance with treatment, and only if the doctor pays particular attention to (2) and (3) above is a patient likely to enjoy a continuing beneficial outcome.

Because dermatology is a visual subject, many believe one glance is enough for diagnosis. This is occasionally true, but most diagnoses rely on history and distribution of the rash.

Urticaria, for example, is almost always diagnosed on the history: so is polymorphic light eruption. These rashes have usually resolved by the time the patient is seen. Atopic eczema is diagnosed by its distribution and persistence and confirmed by examination. Recurring, itchy papules above the ankles in children usually mean insect bites.

From the history, construct a profile of the rash:

- When and where on the skin did it start?
- Do the spots come and go or come and stay?
- To where did it spread?
- Does it itch?
- What topical agents have been applied?
- What medications is the patient taking systemically?

In the majority this information provides the strongest clue to diagnosis. The occupation, personal, travel, and family history are of variable importance.

As well as constructing a profile for diagnosis obtain information to create a cameo of the current life-situation of the patient, so the former can be set in social context. Ask about relationships in the family and at work, economic status, social activities, and general lifestyle, and assess attitudes and responses to the rash. These factors may point to what has provoked a rash and to whether the patient's responses are normal. They also provide a guide to the logistics and likely success of treatment.

When examining the skin, observe from a distance the distribution and grouping pattern of the rash:

- Psoriasis tends to occur on elbows, knees, lower back, and scalp
- Atopic eczema in flexures
- Pityriasis rosea on the torso
- Nickel dermatitis on earlobes and wrists
- Polymorphic light eruption on light exposed areas
- Acne on face, chest, and back
- A linear pattern suggests external injury
- Symmetry suggests an endogenous cause

Then look close up and describe the lesions. All specialties are bedeviled by terminology, dermatology possibly the most.

Macule: a circumscribed area of skin different in color from its surrounding tissue

Papule: a small, solid elevation of the skin less than 0.5 cm in diameter

Wheal: a papule due to dermal edema

Nodule: a solid mass of the skin 0.5 cm or more in diameter

Plaque: an elevated area of skin 2 cm or more in diameter

Vesicle: a bubble less than 0.5 cm in diameter containing clear liquid

Bulla: a bubble more than 0.5 cm in diameter containing a liquid (clear, purulent, or hemorrhagic)

Pustule: a visible accumulation of pus (collection of neutrophils) in the skin (infected or sterile)

Erythema: redness due to vascular congestion or increased perfusion

Telangiectasia: visible dilatation of small blood vessels in the skin

Purpura: discoloration of skin or mucosa due to extravasation of blood

Petechia: a punctate, purpuric (hemorrhagic) spot 1–2 mm in diameter

Ecchymosis: macular purpura more than 2 mm in diameter

Scale: a flat plate or flake of stratum corneum

Crust: an accumulation of dried exudate, usually bacteria-rich

Atrophy: a diminution of tissue: epidermal, dermal, or subcutaneous

Sclerosis: an induration or hardening of the skin

Ulcer: a defect or loss of epidermis and some of the underlying dermis that heals by scarring

Erosion: loss of epidermis that heals without scarring

Tumor: an enlargement of the tissues by normal or pathologic material

Apart from defining the problem for the given patient circumstance, the second aim of the interview is to initiate a positive patient–doctor relationship. This is especially true for skin disease as the look of the skin is so important in social and sexual communication and behavior. The patient with skin disease suffers a diminution of self-image, which may be associated with self-disgust at the look of the skin, shame, guilt, or the feeling of being treated like a pariah. The resulting loss of self-esteem is very important in its daily effect on interpersonal relationships. Whilst taking the history, consciously assess the patient's responses to the illness and his or her way of coping with it. This provides an opportunity to react to these responses in a positive way, e.g. acknowledging the depth of anger or severity of disease so that feelings may be ventilated. In addition, except for infection with Herpes simplex and Herpes varicella zoster viruses, impetigo, scabies, and syphilis, always touch and palpate the rash, an action which will help the doctor–patient relationship and also help interpret the morphology.

The commonest investigation in dermatology is a skin biopsy, followed by the taking of bacteriology swabs for culture and sensitivity, skin scrapings for mycology examination and culture, patch testing for type IV hypersensitivity, and biopsy for skin immunofluorescence for diagnosing autoimmune blistering diseases.

Many skin diseases have an immunologic basis and an understanding of all four types of Gell and Coombs' hypersensitivity reactions is assumed.

There are over a thousand skin diseases and emphasis has been give to the commoner ones and the high-impact rarer ones. Each of the designated topics is preceded by an algorithm (Fig. 16.1).

Acute rashes

Most acute rashes (Fig. 16.1) especially in children are short lived and will resolve quickly. Many of these will be labeled as toxic erythema, expressed as a symmetric, erythematous, maculo-papular rash with itching or burning, resolving spontaneously within a few days. Most are likely to be an exanthema from a viral upper respiratory tract infection (an exanthema is a rash on the skin, an enanthema a rash on the oral mucosa). Treatment is reassurance and soothing topical applications in the form of emollient creams or calamine lotion. Other rashes are recognizable and need to be recognized not only because of the associated features or the necessity for treatment but also to demonstrate competence to the patient or relative.

Urticaria

If the individual components of a rash come and go within several hours (wheals) and they are intensely itchy, the diagnosis is likely to be mast cell degranulation giving rise to **urticaria** or **angiedema**. Mast cells may be degranulated in an immune or non-immune way. Ingested foodstuffs (e. g. nuts, shellfish, eggs), drugs (penicillin), or direct contact with natural rubber latex or animal dander from cats or dogs are all immune triggers, the cause and effect usually being recognized by the patient. Where the daily episodes of urticaria continue for longer than 6 weeks, no cause is recognized by the patient because the likely immune trigger is an autoantibody. Aspirin aggravates urticaria in a non-immune way and should be avoided. Ultraviolet radiation (UVR), heat, and cold may also trigger mast cells but the most frequent cause of these physical triggering agents is the shearing force from rubbing, which gives rise to dermographism. Overall, the commonest cause of degranulation is probably an upper respiratory tract infection.

Provided there is no tongue or intra-oral involvement to impair the airway, or anaphylaxis, treatment is straightforward using one of the low-sedating anti-histamines such as cetirizine, loratadine, or fexofenadine. Chlorpheniramine (piriton) is sedating and is only used for urticaria that is particularly severe at night or occurrence during pregnancy. On average, chronic urticaria takes 6 months to resolve with recurrences being not infrequent.

For a purpuric rash, see the section on purpura.

Erythema nodosum and erythema multiforme

Recognizable non-microbial rashes

Many rashes are recognizable particularly the non-microbial ones. **Erythema nodosum** produces tender, red lumps on the front of the lower legs 2 weeks after an insult (Fig. 16.2).

The individual lesions evolve over 3–4 weeks. A streptococcal sore throat and drugs are the commonest triggers. Sarcoidosis needs to be excluded if there is no obvious trigger or if new lumps continue to appear. Elsewhere in Europe *Yersinia* enterocolitis or coccidioidomycosis in California is more prevalent as a trigger. Primary tuberculosis is a much less likely cause in developed countries.

If a patient has target lesions symmetrically placed on the dorsum of both hands and feet, then **erythema multiforme** is diagnosed, with Herpes simplex being the most likely trigger (Fig. 16.3).

Drugs and other infections such as *Mycoplasma* should also be excluded. If there is extensive skin and mucosal involvement with oral and/or genital blisters or ulcers, particularly purulent conjunctivitis, then Stevens–Johnson syndrome is diagnosed, requiring expert treatment and systemic steroids.

Recurrent erythema multiforme is seen with recurrent Herpes simplex infection but also premenstrually. It is likely that the Herpes simplex virus, which is latent in the dorsal root ganglia of 98% of the population, is regularly activated but only travels down the nerves and reaches the skin if various factors are in play such as the premenstrual state, severe illness and fever, being tired, rundown or stressed, being immunosuppressed, or being exposed to UVR. Oral acyclovir, if given prophylactically, prevents attacks. It will abort an attack if given when the skin tingles and the vesicle first appears.

Toxic epidermal necrolysis (TEN) is an extreme variant of erythema multiforme where a few weeks after ingestion of a drug the patient becomes unwell. The skin goes bright red, blisters and is then shed from all over the body and there is extensive oral/mucosal ulceration. Recovery takes several weeks during which time infection may overcome and kill the patient. Drug-induced marrow failure, hepatitis, and renal failure further compromise survival. Treatment requires urgent referral to a specialist unit.

Pityriasis rosea is a distinctive exanthema, which is easy to diagnose. Most patients will have a herald

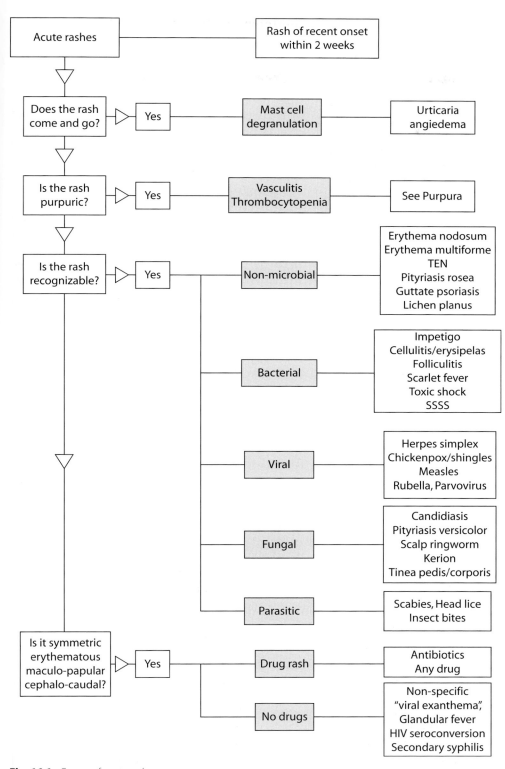

Fig. 16.1. Causes of acute rashes.

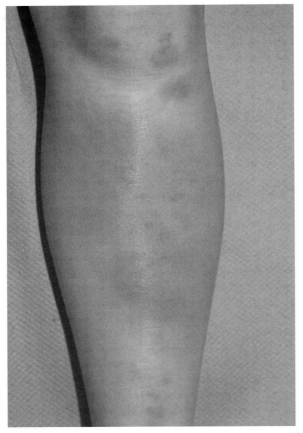

Fig. 16.2. Erythema nodosum.

patch, a lesion a couple of inches across coming out 2 weeks before an eruptive rash on the torso. The eruptive rash consists of oval, scaly lesions with the long axis of the oval following skin lines. Typically it evolves over a few weeks, stays for a few weeks, and then resolves over a few more weeks leaving no scarring but extensive post-inflammatory hyperpigmentation in a pigmented patient. No microbe has yet been identified as a cause, but it is likely to be microbial in origin. Topical steroids can reduce the symptoms if severe.

Guttate psoriasis can sometimes mimic pityriasis rosea. Two weeks after a sore throat in a susceptible individual, a patient develops small, well-demarcated red, scaly patches on the trunk, which may stay for several months. This is the typical appearance of the first expression of psoriasis in children. Usually it clears up after 6 months, resolution being aided with a course of ultraviolet light therapy.

Lichen planus can also come out in an eruptive way. There are three clues. The first lesions are often on the flexor aspects of the wrists. The second clue is the violaceous color. The third confirmatory sign is that individual lesions are flat topped (as seen with reflected light) as opposed to dome shaped.

Generally, although it may be drug induced, lichen planus is usually idiopathic, coming out of the blue. The oral and genital mucosa may be involved. Lesions persist for several months and the

Fig. 16.3. Target lesions of erythema multiforme.

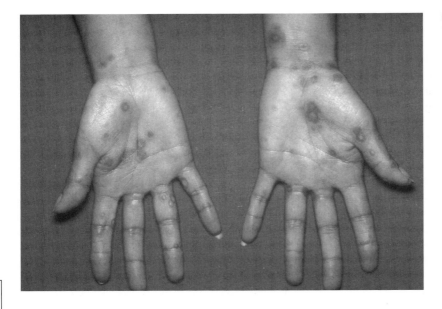

whole process usually takes a year before spontaneous resolution. Topical steroid ointments are helpful.

Infections and specific exanthemas
Recognizable rashes caused by bacteria

Impetigo is a bacterial infection of the stratum corneum, almost always staphylococcal, sometimes streptococcal. A virulent bacterium like *Staphylococcus* can infect normal skin, producing moist, stuck on crusts. It is common in children especially on the face. It is highly contagious and therefore advice should be given about measures to reduce contagion amongst the family, such as absence of physical contact and use of own flannel and towel. Specific treatment is flucloxacillin for 1 week. Topical hydrogen peroxide cream is useful for minor lesions.

Any skin rash can become superinfected (secondarily infected) with bacteria and, if impetigo fails to clear with routine treatment, it may be the patient has underlying eczema, scabies, head lice, or a fungal or viral infection.

Bacterial infection of the dermis is termed either **cellulitis** or **erysipelas**, the former being seen on the lower legs, and the latter on the face. Usually caused by *Streptococcus*, the microbe gains entry through the skin and the subsequent swollen, bright red area gradually expands over succeeding days as the infection travels locally through the skin. Blisters often follow (Fig. 16.4), despite the success of treatment with penicillin being clinically apparent by the loss of the bright red color, the diminishing edema as shown by appearance of wrinkles, and the falling fever. After one episode of cellulitis, further infections are much more likely. Particular care must be paid then to close common portals of entry such as a fissure in the toewebs or abrasions from toenails. Good foot hygiene and antifungal agents or even long-term antibiotics are necessary for some patients, especially if they are diabetic or have lymphedema.

If the *Streptococcus* happens also to be a microbe that secretes an erythemogenic toxin, then the skin will go bright red all over, starting on the face and then the trunk. However, *scarlet fever* usually comes from a streptococcal upper respiratory tract infection rather than anything local.

Staphylococci can also produce toxins eliciting a distant effect. Staphylococcal scalded skin syndrome (SSSS) is seen when a child becomes irritable, and develops a fever, then widespread erythema. The top layer of skin cracks and peels off in sheets leaving raw,

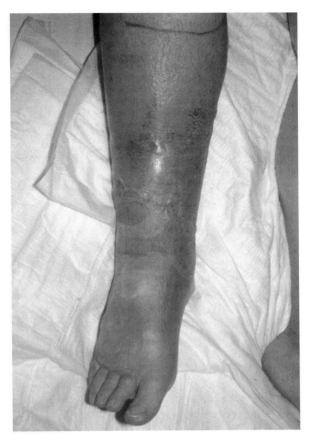

Fig. 16.4. Cellulitis.

tender areas underneath. This is all due to the toxin attacking the desmosomes of the stratum corneum causing it to be disrupted. Everything is over within a week. It is easily differentiated from toxic epidermal necrolysis as it does not cause oral ulceration. Flucloxacillin is the treatment of choice. Staphylococcal toxic shock syndrome is caused by a different exotoxin provoking high fever, scarlet fever-like rash, red palms and soles, vomiting, diarrhea, and hypotension.

Recognizable viral rashes

Primary infection with Herpes simplex is usually subclinical and the expression of a cold sore either peri-orally or genitally is evidence of the virus being activated as described above. Lesions contain millions of virions and are therefore contagious. Direct contact with another human skin may lead to superinfection of an atopic eczema, infection of a partner during intercourse, or infection of the newborn if the birth canal is involved.

Occasionally, an individual develops recurrent lesions away from the face or genitalia and the diagnostic clue is given by the history. Each episode is reproducible. The eruption comes out in the same area of skin each time, starting with tingling, becoming vesicular, resolving through crusting, and clearing up completely within 10 days without scarring. For infrequent, recurrent episodes, a course of oral acyclovir started immediately will shorten symptomatology. If the episodes are sufficiently frequent, daily prophylactic acyclovir is indicated.

The incubation period for **Herpes varicella zoster virus** (HVZV) infection (**chickenpox**) is 2–3 weeks after airborne droplet infection from a person with active disease. The child is often non-specifically unwell for a day, perhaps with a fever, before the itchy, papulo-pustules appear on the scalp and spread down caudally to the rest of the body. A cardinal sign is the umbilication of the early lesions sometimes with central necrosis and then crusting. Crops of new lesions appear amongst older ones over the next few days. Bullae and ulcers sometimes are seen in the mouth. Adults experience much more severe disease.

Systemic acyclovir makes little difference to the course of the disease in a normal healthy child. It is given to patients older than 12 years of age, any immunosuppressed, immunocompromised, or pregnant patient, or anyone at risk of pneumonia.

The virus has a tropism for spinal and cranial sensory ganglia and afterwards chickenpox lies dormant in these ganglia, occasionally reactivating. Intercurrent infection, stress, and local trauma perhaps interfere with local immune surveillance and allow the virus to reactivate, travel down a local nerve and appear in a dermatomal distribution characteristic of shingles. **Shingles** is seen with increasing frequency with age perhaps due to the declining immune function. In a younger patient HIV infection should be excluded. An aching, burning pain precedes the appearance of the rash by a few days. Occasionally, only erythema and a few papules are visible perhaps incompletely throughout the dermatome. Typically, clear vesicles appear which eventually become turbid, rupture and then crust. On average, the whole episode lasts 2–3 weeks. Four points need to be remembered:

(1) Individual lesions are infectious, traditionally until the crusts drop off. Therefore, patients need to be isolated from naive (previously unexposed to HVZV), immunosuppressed, or pregnant individuals.

(2) Involvement of the ophthalmic branch of the trigeminal ganglion requires expert eye care regardless of whether the nasociliary branch is involved or not.

(3) If the rash has spread outside the dermatome and/or if it is hemorrhagic in nature, underlying lymphoma should be excluded.

(4) The most important point is to try and prevent **post-herpetic neuralgia**, a crippling condition when it occurs. Any older patient with severe pain before or during shingles needs high-dose, oral acyclovir as soon as possible, perhaps with added systemic steroids to diminish local inflammation.

The incubation period for **measles** is 1–2 weeks, again following airborne droplet contact. The prodrome of coryza (runny nose), conjunctivitis, and barking cough (the 3 Cs) with fever and photophobia lasts for 3 or 4 days before the rash appears: the child is unwell. As with most rashes it starts on the head, on the face and behind the ears, and spreads downwards. The dark-red maculo-papules stay for 3–5 days.

Measles can be confirmed clinically 2 days before the rash appears by looking in the mouth for Koplik's spots. They look like large grains of salt with a red halo and are found on the buccal mucosa opposite the premolars.

With diminishing take-up of the MMR vaccine, the frequency of measles has increased, but the threat of **rubella** (German measles) during pregnancy is likely to mean that parents will continue to have their children immunized against this virus. Incubation period is about 2 weeks but both the prodrome and the exanthema tend to be milder than measles. A measles-like rash, perhaps with conjunctivitis, obliges a search for occipital and posterior auricular lymphadenopathy. This combination of exanthema and lymphadenopathy (and occasionally conjunctivitis) is also seen in Echo-, Adeno- and EB virus infections as well as rubella. It is mandatory to look for serologic confirmation of rubella by the presence of IgM antibodies. If positive, then contact screening is required to ensure the patient has not been in contact with anyone pregnant.

The same procedures should be gone through with suspected **parvovirus** infection, which also can produce fetal abnormality. It is also seen in children and usually presents with a characteristic exanthema of bright red macular erythema of the cheeks (slapped cheeks). This finding obliges a search for the diagnostic reticulate erythema found on the backs of arms and buttocks. Rubella and parvovirus infection can be complicated by a polyarthropathy/arthritis.

Recognizable forms of fungal infection

The yeast fungus *Candida* is a normal commensal of the gastro-intestinal tract, less frequently the oropharynx, and much less still in the vagina. Under the right conditions organisms can spread from these areas and cause skin infection. Moist, macerated skin as seen under pendulous breasts, in the groin, the axillae, and toewebs provides the right environment.

The presence of diabetes mellitus, steroid therapy, or immunosuppression encourages further growth. For these reasons, in men, candidal balanitis is a classic presentation for diabetes mellitus. The cardinal sign for all of these are the tiny, satellite papules or pustules just outside the advancing border of infection. Confirmation is straightforward by examination of skin scrapings for hyphae and mycology culture. Topical azole creams applied twice a day will cure after reversal of predisposing factors.

The *Malassezia* yeast, present on every adult's scalp, not only may trigger dandruff but when it grows in hyphal form on the trunk, produces **pityriasis versicolor**. As the hyphae grow on the skin, they interfere with melanin pigment formation, sometimes producing hypopigmented macules, sometimes hyperpigmented macules. These macules form asymptomatic patterns on the trunk of healthy young adults. Exposure to UVR during a holiday increases the contrast between infected and non-infected skin and leads a patient to believe that the rash was acquired when on holiday. The disease is common in humid countries and is also seen more extensively in patients on steroid treatment or in the immuno-compromised. A short course of oral azole therapy will kill the hyphae but the pigmentary changes take 6 months to reverse.

Dermatophytes are non-yeast fungi capable of living and multiplying in the outermost layer of the epidermis, i.e. in dead keratin. The term **tinea** denotes a dermatophyte infection, **tinea corporis** involving the trunk, **tinea capitis** the scalp, and **tinea pedis** the feet.

Over the last decade, highly effective antifungal creams have seen a big reduction in the frequency of tinea corporis and tinea pedis.

This reduction has been completely overshadowed by the development of endemic scalp **ringworm** in children in most large conurbations of the UK. This is because infection with the dermatophyte *Trichophyton tonsurans* spreads from human scalp to human scalp. Previously the commonest dermatophyte causing scalp ringworm was *Microsporum canis* and spread went from animal to human to animal and then back to human. The dermatophytes causing scalp ringworm invade the keratin of the hair shaft which then breaks off. Presentation is a scaly patch of scalp with broken hairs. Fungal infection stimulates inflammation, sometimes antigenically. Papules and pustules may be superimposed on this scaly patch. If the inflammation is particularly severe, a large, boggy swelling (kerion) with loss of hair may sometimes result.

In black children the disease is less obvious and any hair loss in a black child is ringworm until proven otherwise. Samples are best obtained using a sterile toothbrush brushed through the scalp and the bristles pressed directly into Sabouraud's growth medium.

Systemic therapy is needed to cure scalp ringworm so that the hyphae are eradicated from the hair shaft deep within the follicle. Standard treatment is oral griseofulvin 10–20 mg/kg for 6–8 weeks.

It is common to see ring lesions on the face, neck, or body or limbs of children with scalp ringworm or their siblings or their parents. The dermatophyte hyphae grow out concentrically from the site of infection. Usually, they produce scaling only but often the fungus generates inflammation and the rings become red and inflamed or even pustular. Skin scrapings for mycologic examination and culture are indicated. If **tinea corporis** is extensive systemic treatment is indicated, otherwise topical azole creams are enough.

In **tinea pedis** (athlete's foot) the wearing of socks and shoes increases the moisture content between the toewebs allowing dermatophytes to invade superficial keratin. This produces maceration, fissuring, and scaling between the toes; scaling over the whole of the plantar surface, or if the fungus is antigenic, ring-like patterns of secondary eczema on the soles or instep. Topical or systemic terbinafine will cure the infection but foot hygiene, reduction of maceration, and avoidance of communal baths and showers helps to prevent recurrence. In a diabetic, ischemic, or lymphedematous foot, meticulous foot hygiene is indicated to minimize the risk of streptococcal infection gaining entry from a fissure produced by fungal infection.

Nail fungal infection is discussed in the nail section.

Recognizable parasitic rashes

Pediculus capitis, the head louse, is adapted to travel through scalp hair quickly. Consequently, it can readily transfer to another scalp or can rush away to a part of the scalp that is not being examined. Fomites, i.e. brushes, hats, caps, and other head gear, are possibly more likely to spread the infestation through the nits rather than the adults as nits can hatch several days after being away from the host whereas the adult needs a regular blood meal. Nits are laid on hairs close to the scalp, they take 7–10 days to hatch and a nymph takes 8 days to mature. This cycle underlies the principle of applying shampoo and using a nit comb every 5 days for 3–4 weeks as a mechanical means of clearing the scalp. To minimize resistance, local advice should be taken as to which anti-louse compound should be used. Because head lice are endemic in schools, it is common, at the beginning of each term, to have a whole school search for and eradicate any lice in an attempt to minimize an endemic state.

The scalp itching is due to hypersensitivity and takes a few weeks to develop on first exposure. With age, this hypersensitivity diminishes and older child carers may be silent carriers of head lice. Therefore, the whole extended family needs to be examined.

Like the louse, the **scabies** mite is also host-specific for humans. Infection is spread by direct skin to skin contact though mites can live in infected bedding or clothing for a day or two. The mites burrow in the stratum corneum and favored sites include the sides of fingers, sides of hand, flexor wrist, axillary folds, nipple, genitalia and gluteal folds, and feet. The type IV hypersensitivity to fecal protein develops 1 month after contact. The first symptom is itching, often on the thighs and lower abdomen (itching from any cause is worse at night). Eczema then develops predominantly at sites of burrows but also in a generalized, micropapular pattern. In straightforward scabies the face is not affected. Some patients produce diagnostic nodules as part of their hypersensitivity response and these very typically occur on the genitalia, axillae, or trunk. In the index case of a family the diagnosis is often delayed because symptoms and signs take time to appear. When a second person develops the same problem the diagnosis becomes obvious.

Because of the long incubation period, individual contacts can be infected but asymptomatic. Therefore all close contacts of an infested person should be treated. Treatment consists of a cream or lotion applied to the whole skin except the scalp and central part of the face. Nails should also be cleaned and treated. Permethrin creams are the most effective topical agents.

Itching and secondary eczema tend to die down within a few days of treatment, aided by topical steroids. In atopic individuals post-scabetic eczema can persist for as long as 6 months. Sometimes it can be difficult to decide whether persistent symptomatology is post-scabetic eczema, inadequate treatment, or re-infection. Further treatment is often indicated.

Insect bites are straightforward to diagnose. An insect feeds leaving a grouped pattern of inflamed papules. Sometimes the pattern is linear along a border of tight clothing. In a child it is often seen above the ankle where mites from a cat or a dog have transferred to a different host after the animal has brushed up against the child's leg. It is common to find only one member of the family affected like this, usually with inflamed papules but sometimes with blisters.

As well as feeding off an individual, insects might inject a microbe of their own. Sandflies carry *Leishmania* organisms, ticks spread *Rickettsia* and *Borrelia*, mosquitoes carry malaria, and fleas and lice spread *Bartonella*.

Other acute rashes

Around 3% or 4% of hospitalized patients experience a cutaneous eruption due to **drugs;** 5% taking ampicillin for the first time will experience a skin rash. This is normally due to hypersensitivity to the side chain rather than true penicillin allergy but, to minimize future risk of anaphylaxis, the patient is labeled as penicillin allergic. Antibiotics are the commonest cause of these rashes in hospital and usually they are of minor import giving rise to itchy, maculo-papular rashes starting on the head and evolving in a cephalo-caudal direction, the whole lasting for a week or 10 days at the most.

Similar rashes can be triggered by an entero- or adenoviral upper respiratory tract infection, Ebstein Barr viral infection (glandular fever), or an HIV sero-conversion illness. If ampicillin is given to a patient with glandular fever the risk of rash rises to 95%. Treatment is supportive with cooling soothing creams or lotions.

Most drug eruptions are expressions of type I or type III hypersensitivity and many patients are on several drugs. As it takes 12 days or so for any hypersensitivity response to produce antibodies most drug eruptions on first exposure will come out 10–14 days after starting a drug. On second exposure, the rash will appear within 24–48 hours. The best help to incriminate a particular drug is to draw a time chart indicating when each drug was started and when the rash appeared. Some drug rashes, such as anticonvulsant-induced TEN, appear 3–4 weeks after starting the drug and yet others such as gold dermatitis take several months.

Secondary syphilis presents a few to several weeks after the primary chancre and is usually associated with mild systemic symptoms. The commonest pattern is a scaly reddish-brown maculo-papular rash on the face and then the trunk. It is not always non-itchy, and not every exanthema that appears on the palms and soles is syphilis, but these are indicators to take a sexual history, examine the oral cavity and genital mucosa, look for lymphadenopathy, and perform serologic tests for syphilis.

Chronic rashes

The definition for chronic rashes, i.e. present for longer than 4–6 weeks (Fig. 16.5), is somewhat arbitrary and by the time seen many of the acute rashes may well have persisted. The algorithm given for chronic rashes is self explanatory and assumes knowledge of urticaria, purpura, pigmentary change, and eczema.

Psoriasis

Definition

The hallmark of psoriasis is a persistent, red, raised (palpable) scaly spot, patch, or plaque. In the epidermis of this abnormal patch of skin, more keratinocytes than normal are being stimulated to divide. The epidermis therefore turns over much more quickly than normal and normal differentiation does not occur.

Epidemiology

Various factors are known to uncover or aggravate the psoriatic tendency:

(1) Psoriasis occurs in 2% of the population and its presentation is bimodal, under 20 years of age and over 50 years. There is a strong genetic influence in the younger age group, almost all give a positive family history, sometimes autosomal dominant, while the older group does not.

(2) Local trauma of various types induces visible psoriasis in the affected skin, the Koebner (isomorphic) phenomenon (Fig. 16.6).

(3) Streptococcal upper respiratory tract infection is the commonest trigger for guttate psoriasis.

(4) Stress is a difficult parameter to measure but it is well recognized that definite episodes of stress such as exams, marriage, divorce, or bereavement can all trigger or aggravate psoriasis.

(5) Psoriasis usually improves during pregnancy but may get worse. Flares can also occur at puberty and menopause.

(6) Ultraviolet radiation is used to treat psoriasis but a small percentage of patients get worse.

(7) Lithium is well recognized as triggering or aggravating psoriasis. The antimalarials, chloroquine and mepacrine, aggravate psoriasis less frequently.

Mechanisms

A suggested pathogenesis might be the exposure of a susceptible individual to a trigger, resulting in Th1 cell-mediated increased epidermal proliferation and altered epidermal maturation.

Clinical features

Gentle rubbing or scraping of the scaly psoriatic patch further accentuates the silveriness of the scale and further scraping uncovers pin-point bleeding points from the dilated capillaries in the papillary tips (Auspitz's sign). Psoriasis is itchy in some people. The pattern of skin involvement varies and may be: guttate (small drop); small to large plaque, usually extensor but sometimes flexural; annular or gyrate in pattern; studded with pustules or involvement of more than 90% of the skin (erythroderma). It is not uncommon for one site only to be affected, even for many years, e.g. scalp, natal cleft, nails, or glans penis.

Streptococcal upper respiratory infection in a susceptible individual may be followed 2 weeks later by guttate psoriasis. A monomorphic shower of small, pink, scaly spots, likened to raindrops on a dry pavement, is seen over the trunk and proximal limbs. The natural history is one of spontaneous remission over several months and treatment is geared to that response.

Plaque psoriasis typically affects the elbows, knees, lower back, and scalp. Why such extensor areas are picked out for involvement is unknown. Central or asymmetric healing of larger plaques on the trunk leads to annular or gyrate patterns.

Typically, the surface of flexural psoriatic patches shows no scaling, just a smooth, red, glazed or glistening surface. Sharply demarcated patches in the axillae, groin, natal cleft, popliteal or antecubital

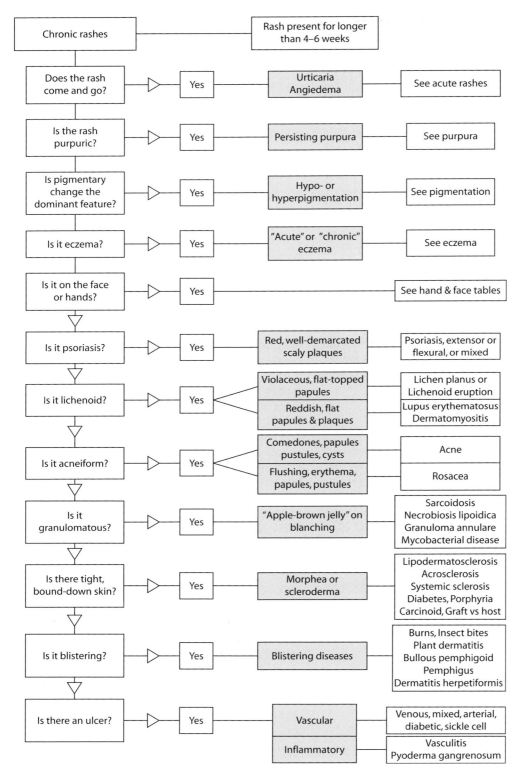

Fig. 16.5. Causes of chronic rashes.

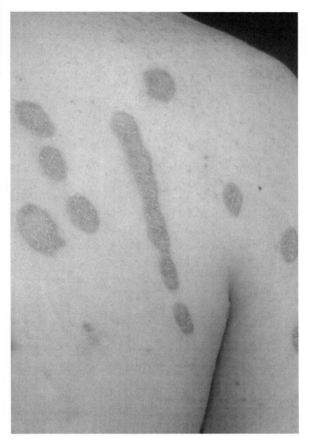

Fig. 16.6. Red, raised, well-demarcated patches of psoriasis exhibiting the Koebner phenomenon.

fossae, umbilicus, eyelid, or ear are suggestive. Patches are usually symmetric. Overlap does occur with seborrhoeic eczema, though in the latter case the patches are less well demarcated.

Small collections of neutrophils are commonly seen microscopically in ordinary psoriatic lesions but when they are large enough to be visible to the naked eye, pustular psoriasis is diagnosed and is seen in three forms:

(1) *Palmar–plantar pustulosis*

Only 10%–15% of patients with pustules localized to palms and soles have psoriasis elsewhere on the skin. Involvement of the thenar eminence and instep of middle-aged females is the commonest picture but other areas may be affected. Against a background of a well-demarcated red patch, milky, sterile pustules appear, rapidly drying into a brown macule. The disease persists for many years,

often aggravated by stress, and treatment is of marginal benefit.

(2) *Acrodermatitis continua of Hallopeau*

Sometimes the pustules also involve the tips of fingers and toes as well as palms and soles, again in middle-aged females. This pattern is more severe than the localized type and more likely to evolve into widespread pustular psoriasis.

(3) *Generalized pustular psoriasis*

Pustules may occur on any patch of chronic psoriasis but in the rare, severe, generalized form the disease may be fatal. Malaise and fever usher in angry, red areas of skin which may mimic cellulitis. Pustules appear at the edge of the erythema, then dry up fairly quickly, only for another cycle to start immediately or within a few days. A neutrophil leukocytosis is usual, fluid and electrolyte imbalance common, and the patient may succumb from secondary infection or renal problems. Systemic steroid therapy, or more especially steroid withdrawal, is a recognized trigger, as is methotrexate withdrawal and hypocalcemia. There is a greater frequency of joint problems than ordinary psoriasis.

The diagnosis of erythrodermic psoriasis is easy to make if there is a long history of chronic plaque psoriasis with slow evolution into more than 90% skin involvement, often through an intermediate angry or unstable phase. It is still straightforward in the generalized pustular pattern but no investigative tests discriminate it from other causes of erythroderma when the disease is of recent onset. Evolution into a non-erythrodermic pattern is the only dependable feature.

Nail involvement is present in up to 50%, including nail pitting, onycholysis, thickening of the nail plate (due to sub-ungual hyperkeratosis), and discoloration. The pits are usually variable in size and pattern as compared to those in alopecia areata. Onycholysis is defined as separation of nail plate from nail bed and is also seen after trauma, in fungal infection, thyrotoxicosis, and as photo-onycholysis. Nail changes may be present for years before psoriasis appears elsewhere. Local treatment is ineffective and systemic treatment not justified for psoriatic nail changes alone.

Psoriatic arthropathy may precede skin lesions by years.

Differential diagnosis

Reiter's disease is a psoriasis-like reaction triggered by urethritis or colitis and expressed as rupioid

Table 16.1. Treatments for psoriasis

First-line treatments	Second-line treatments	Third-line treatments	Fourth-line treatments
Topical: Vitamin A Vitamin D Steroid Tar Dithranol	Phototherapy: UVB TL01 PUVA In-patient therapy	Methotrexate Cyclosporin Retinoids	Anti TNFα

(barnacle-like) psoriasis on the soles and palms, a pustular, circinate balanitis, and psoriatic lesions elsewhere. Beta-blocker drugs may provoke a psoriasiform response with dry eyes. Occasional patients seem to oscillate between psoriasis and seborrheic eczema but usually in the latter the lesions are less well defined and covered with a moist scale. A single psoriasiform patch unchanged for years and unresponsive to treatment is likely to be Bowen's disease and biopsy is indicated.

Management

Conventional first-line treatment consists of a choice between the topical agents as listed in Table 16.1. Severe disease unresponsive to topical therapy is an indication for systemic therapy such as methotrexate. Expensive biologic response modifiers are reserved for individuals with severe disease unresponsive to third-line therapy.

In general practice topical steroids are the most common treatments, demand-led from the patient. They are convenient to apply, cosmetically acceptable, suppress the disease somewhat, and have, as far as the patient is concerned, few side effects. Topical steroids may produce skin atrophy and striae, make the skin less responsive to dithranol, and, rarely, may precipitate a pustular episode. Vitamin D creams are effective but more so and better tolerated if combined with a topical steroid.

In hospital practice, an attempt is made to keep dithranol or tar as the first choice. They are more effective but are inconvenient, smelly, stain clothes, and are more likely to irritate the skin.

Scalp psoriasis can be treated by whichever combination of the following triad works for a particular patient:

(1) a scalp application left on for 1–8 hours, followed by

(2) a washing out with shampoo, followed after drying by

(3) a steroid scalp application

Sunlight aggravates a small percentage of psoriasis patients but improves the vast majority. UVB (290–320 nm) exposure three times a week is effective alone, but may lead to burning in the short term and a carcinogenic effect in the long term, both side effects coming from the shorter UVB wavelengths below 310 nm. The optimal therapeutic wavelength appears to be around 313 nm (TL01) and may explain the success of treatment on the shores of the Dead Sea (400 m below sea level) where much of the natural UVB is filtered out by the aerosol of water vapor above it. Photosensitizers such as tar prior to exposure enhance the effect of UVB.

Psoralens are furocoumarins occurring naturally in various plants including celery, fennel, and fig. Contact with these plants may produce a pigmented, phototoxic eczema. Psoralen when combined with UVA phototherapy is known as PUVA, an effective treatment for psoriasis. The psoralen molecule gains entry into cells and inserts itself between adjacent pyrimidine bases. UVA wavelengths (320–400 nm) convert the non-covalent link into a covalent bridge between the strands of DNA, an effect likely to inhibit mitosis.

Psoralens can be applied topically or taken systemically, when the patient wears glasses for 24 hours to protect the eye from possible cataract formation. PUVA produces a 12-fold increase in skin cancer with reversal of the usual ratio of basal cell carcinomas to squamous cell carcinomas so an individual is restricted to a total of 200 treatments, a small number if the psoriasis is lifelong.

Methotrexate once a week usually provides good control of severe disabling psoriasis and associated arthropathy. Marrow suppression, hepatic fibrosis, and, rarely, diffuse interstitial pneumonitis are recognized complications.

Retinoids, derived from vitamin A, control the differentiation and proliferation of keratinocytes. They also have anti-inflammatory and anti-cancer properties. Etretinate is of most help in the pustular patterns of psoriasis and is also used with PUVA where it can reduce the total amount of UVA required for clearance. Side effects include teratogenicity, dry skin, and hyperlipidemia. Anti TNFα preparations: etanercept, infliximab, and adalimumab are all effective.

Outcome

Only 10%–15% of patients with psoriasis can expect a permanent remission from their skin disease. Guttate psoriasis has the best prognosis with the extensor pattern second. Only a third of patients with pustulosis of palms and soles are clear after 10 years.

Lichen planus or lichenoid eruptions

Lichen planus, the paradigm for lichenoid eruptions, is yet another skin expression of an immunologic response, that of T-cell mediated attack on keratinocytes. Lichen planus, diskoid lupus erythematosus, dermatomyositis, and graft versus host disease are all manifestations of this. Antimalarials, ACE-inhibitors, beta-blockers, gold, penicillamine, and thiazides may all trigger a lichenoid eruption.

Lichen planus usually starts on the flexor aspects of the wrists, spreading up the arms and, in a similar distribution, on the legs. Individual lesions are flat topped as opposed to dome shaped, best confirmed with reflected light.

Sometimes it erupts in a pityriasis rosea-like pattern on the trunk, or as an asymptomatic, lacy pattern on the buccal mucosa. It normally lasts 6–12 months and then remits spontaneously. An appropriate strength topical steroid is usually all that is required.

The classic color of lichen planus is violaceous but diskoid lupus erythematosus (DLE) occurring on the face as persistent, flat lesions is usually bright red. Long-standing lesions of DLE can show scaling, follicular plugging, scarring, and atrophy. This is particularly disfiguring in Afro-Caribbean skin where it produces hyper- and hypopigmentation and sometimes loss of tissue.

Lichen planus and DLE affecting the scalp destroy hair follicles and present as scarring alopecia.

Dermatomyositis presents as lesions over the knuckles and other extensor joints together with nail-fold telangiectases and hemorrhages. Although mostly an autoimmune disease, in 20% of adult patients it is a paraneoplastic sign and a search for underlying malignancy is warranted.

Acne and rosacea
Acne vulgaris
Epidemiology

Acne vulgaris affects the majority of adolescents at some time, 10% of them moderately severely with up to 5% of females continuing until the age of 40. A proportion of these will have polycystic ovary syndrome. Because androgens increase sebum excretion rates, androgenic steroid and corticosteroid therapy, androgen-secreting tumors, Cushing's syndrome, acromegaly, and congenital adrenal hyperplasia can all cause acne. Treatment is geared to the factors that contribute to the disease.

Clinical features

The two major factors of acne are narrowing of the pilosebaceous duct and hypertrophy of sebaceous lobules around certain follicles. Both are androgen dependent, some androgens being generated locally by the sebaceous glands, which are thus endocrine organs. It is uncertain why some follicles are targeted and others not and why most teenagers with acne eventually go into spontaneous remission.

With androgen stimulation, the wall of the follicular duct thickens and hypertrophies. Hypertrophied sebaceous glands secrete much more sebum and the follicle becomes distended. The dilated, partially blocked follicle is termed a microcomedone and allows for proliferation of *Proprionibacterium acnes,* a micro-aerophilic bacterium present in teenagers as a normal commensal. Further enlargement of the microcomedone results in typical blackheads (open comedones) and whiteheads (closed comedones). The latter occur where the whole of the duct has been blocked off, the duct then twisting like the neck of a balloon and atrophying, leaving a small cyst just under the skin.

Irritants and *P. acnes* antigens leaking out into the surrounding dermis can stimulate inflammation. Neutrophils migrate into the duct to appear as a superficial pustule or into the main part of the follicle to appear as a papule (Fig. 16.7).

More extensive inflammation and destruction of follicles results in large nodules and cyst-like lesions.

Scarring can occur with moderate acne but more so with cystic acne. Sometimes it is keloidal. In pigmented skin post-inflammatory pigmentation can occur with moderate acne and be just as debilitating.

Management

A teenager wants an instant cure for acne. The success of treatment lies in explaining the mechanism, that prophylaxis to prevent microcomedone formation during the acne-prone years is paramount, and that improvement occurs slowly over months.

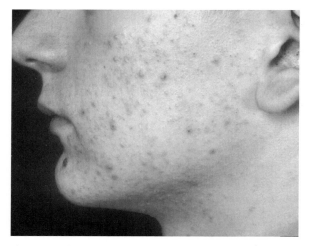

Fig. 16.7. Blackheads, papules, and pustules in acne.

Vitamin A creams normalize the follicular duct and have minor benefits on inflammation. They tend to dry and irritate and are poorly tolerated. Tolerance is improved by starting at weak concentrations or less frequent applications, building up to once a day application.

The next step is to reduce the *P. acnes* proliferation. If it can be tolerated, topical benzoyl peroxide delivers oxygen locally, reduces bacterial proliferation, and does not cause resistance. Otherwise topical antibiotics are indicated but *P. acnes* resistance is common and many topical antibiotics have become ineffective.

If papules and pustules are dominant, then systemic antibiotics are needed. The response is dose related, e.g. 1 gram of tetracycline or erythromycin per day for a minimum of 3 months.

Sunlight usually improves acne and a course of ultraviolet light therapy or the newer black light which reduces bacterial colonization can be helpful.

If moderate acne has not improved after 6 months of antibiotics, if there is obvious scarring or severe cystic acne, oral isotretinoin should be introduced early. Oral isotretinoin, a vitamin A derivative, also normalizes the follicular duct but its main effect is to shrink the sebaceous glands down and reduce sebum excretion. Isotretinoin has a variety of side effects and careful counseling and consent is needed. Pregnancy whilst taking isotretinoin has an even chance of fetal abnormality. Isotretinoin invariably produces dry lips and skin. Occasionally, it produces mood swings, depression, and a risk of suicide. Serum triglycerides may rise and should be monitored during treatment, which lasts approximately 6 months.

Isotretinoin will cure two-thirds of patients but some individuals with persistent acne, sometimes associated with polycystic ovary syndrome, may need two or three courses.

Except for punch excision of ice-pick scars, there is no good, guaranteed treatment of scarring. Dermabrasion and skin peels may improve the skin but risk post-inflammatory pigmentation changes which can persist.

Rosacea mimics acne by its similar expression of facial papules and pustules but is completely unrelated. Comedones are never seen. The cause is unknown. A typical presentation is a middle-aged female with years of frequent flushing and blushing. Persistent telangiectasia develops and then papules and pustules appear usually symmetrically on cheeks and forehead. Rosacea is sometimes asymmetric and occasionally associated with conjunctivitis if severe.

Standard treatment is to induce a remission with systemic tetracycline or metronidazole for 3–6 months and maintain it with topical metronidazole. Topical steroid applications may induce rosacea and should be avoided as should anything that provokes flushing.

Granulomatous eruptions

A granuloma is a collection of epithelioid cells (Fig. 16.8), part of the mononuclear phagocytic system. The stimulus can be an irritant such as keratin from a ruptured cyst or an undegradeable or self-perpetuating antigen. Clinically a persistent, painless rash is likely to be granulomatous if, when the skin is blanched, brownish translucent papules or nodules are visible. This is best exemplified by **sarcoidosis**, which affects the skin in 25% of patients. Apart from being a classical trigger for erythema nodosum, sarcoidosis may be expressed as a diffuse or localized granulomatous infiltrate. Diffuse infiltration in the nose and cheeks is termed lupus pernio. Localized papules or nodules occur usually at muco-cutaneous junctions, particularly on the nose or along the eyelid margin. Skin biopsy showing non-caseating granulomas confirms the diagnosis. Treatment of cutaneous lesions is unsatisfactory.

Necrobiosis lipoidica is yet another skin disease classically occurring on the shins. Sixty-four percent of patients have diabetes mellitus and it is seen in 1 in 200 patients with diabetes mellitus. The origin is uncertain and treatment is generally unhelpful. In **granuloma annulare** asymptomatic pearly papules are seen in children often in rings over joints. Usually diagnosed as ringworm these indolent papules also

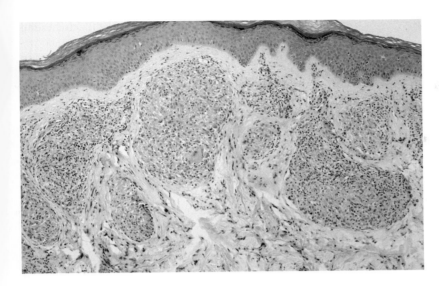

Fig. 16.8. Sarcoidal granulomas in the dermis.

demonstrate brownish translucency if firmly pressed. Parents want the reassurance of a diagnosis and the fact that it is not sinister.

Tight skin

If the rash exhibits tight bound-down skin where the epidermis cannot be pinched up between finger and thumb or cannot be moved freely on the underlying fascia, then a sclerodermal inflammatory response is operating. In scleroderma the process may involve hands, feet and face alone, so-called acrosclerosis, of which the CREST syndrome is a variant. If it involves the skin of the torso as well, it has a much more sinister prognosis. More commonly for dermatologists, individual localized patches or linear lesions of scleroderma are seen on trunk or limbs and this is termed morphea. In this systemic involvement is much rarer.

Acute **lipodermatosclerosis** is seen when venous hypertension promotes fibrosis in the subcutaneous fat. It can be quite painful and red and look cellulitic. The chronic form is responsible for the inverted champagne bottle leg seen in venous hypertension.

Blisters

The commonest causes of blisters are burns, insect bites, and plant dermatitis. This is especially true of poison ivy in the USA. Some individuals blister easily with insect bites, and certain strains of staphylococci may mimic this if causing bullous impetigo.

The autoimmune blistering diseases are examples of type II hypersensitivity. **Bullous pemphigoid** (Fig. 16.9) is seen in older patients and occurs because of the spontaneous occurrence of an autoantibody directed at proteins in the epidermal basement membrane. Ensuing inflammation lifts the epidermis off the dermis to give blistering. The whole process develops over several weeks starting with an itchy, erythematous, urticated rash on which big blisters develop, some of which may be hemorrhagic. The blisters are often seen around the thighs and pelvic girdle but may appear anywhere. Treatment is induction of remission with systemic steroids and maintenance with immunosuppressive agents.

Pemphigus vulgaris occurs in younger patients and usually starts in the mouth. Its spontaneous autoantibody is directed at the desmosomes of the keratinocytes which discohese and separate to produce fragile blisters. There is normally a several month history of chronic oral ulceration before fragile, quickly eroding blisters are found on the head and upper trunk. Treatment is similar to pemphigoid. Although **dermatitis herpetiformis** is associated with celiac disease, the source and target of the antibody is unknown. It is so itchy that the papulo-vesicles and blisters are normally scratched away by the patient. The rash is seen over joints, elbows, buttocks, knees, and scalp. It improves and can be cleared with a gluten-free diet, which patients don't usually keep to. In that situation dapsone is added in to keep them clear of rash and itch.

With all these autoimmune blistering diseases taking a skin biopsy and demonstrating the presence of the antibody through immunofluorescent techniques confirms the diagnosis.

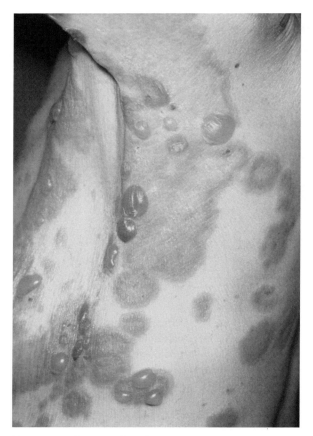

Fig. 16.9. Bullous pemphigoid.

Ulcerated lesions

Seventy-five percent of elderly patients with chronic leg ulcers on the lower leg will have venous disease alone. Perhaps 10% will have mixed arterial disease and perhaps another 10% will have pure arterial disease. Pain is not a particularly good discriminant in deciding between the three.

Venous ulcers are usually above the medial malleolus but may be lateral or occasionally below the malleolus. Normally there will be other concomitants of venous hypertension; hemosiderin staining, acute or chronic lipodermatosclerosis, and venous eczema. An important investigation is measurement of the ankle–brachial index (ABI), the ratio of systolic blood pressure in the leg to that in the arm. If the ratio is less than 1, then venous compression should not be employed because of arterial insufficiency. If it is greater than 1, then four-layer bandaging techniques will usually heal a venous ulcer. Hypertension, diabetes,

anemia, uremia, and poor nutrition all delay healing and should be excluded.

Diabetes can contribute to ulcers in a variety of ways, but if the ulcer is secondary to peripheral neuropathy then it is usually on weight-bearing areas on the sole of the foot or the big toe pad.

Inflammatory ulcers include chronic vasculitis and pyoderma gangrenosum.

In **pyoderma gangrenosum** a painful, rapidly expanding ulcer with a diagnostic bluish undermined edge appears on the leg. It is associated with a variety of conditions such as seropositive and seronegative arthritis, inflammatory bowel disease, paraproteinemia, and Behçet's syndrome. Most commonly it is idiopathic.

Treatment quickly reverses the diagnostic feature leaving a chronic non-healing ulcer. It is then the site that gives the best clue to diagnosis. Venous ulcers are in the gaiter area, arterial ulcers often on the foot itself, pyoderma lesions are usually away from these areas although may be close. A chronic, clean, granulating ulcer on the leg that shows no sign of healing may actually be a basal cell carcinoma (BCC) or squamous cell carcinoma (SCC) masquerading as a benign ulcer, and biopsy is indicated. Not all skin cancers have a heaped-up edge.

Eczema (Fig. 16.10)

Eczema is a difficult concept to understand and can only be defined in histologic terms: it is that inflammatory process expressed as spongiosis if "acute" and lichenification if "chronic", or any combination. Spongiosis refers to fluid between the epidermal keratinocytes and may be expressed as vesicles, small or large blisters, or weeping, i.e. "boiling over." In lichenification there is no spongiosis at all, but all layers of the epidermis are thickened or hyperplastic (increase in number of cells), anything from 50%–150% more than normal.

"Acute" and "chronic" in the context of eczema do not refer to a time course; any eczema can express itself first of all as lichenification and then perhaps become vesicular and wet and sticky if becoming acute. The terms dermatitis and eczema are used interchangeably. A classification and guide to eczema in general and to the hands and face in particular are shown in Figs. 16.10, 16.13 and 16.15.

The commonest type of eczema is **irritant**, seen most often on the hands. Exposure of the skin to

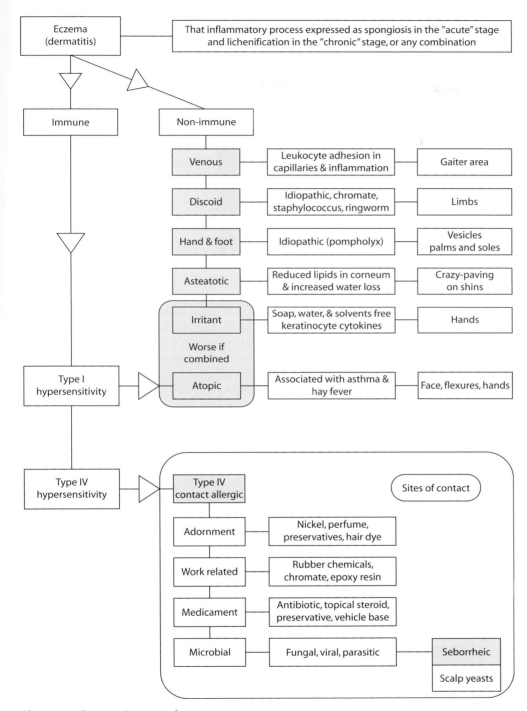

Fig. 16.10. Causes and patterns of eczema.

water and cleaning agents, i.e. solvents, dissolves the protective lipid from the superficial layers of skin allowing irritant molecules to penetrate into the epidermis causing keratinocytes to release inflammatory mediators. Too much hand washing can result in chapped, fissured finger webs which might eventually develop vesicles. In atopic patients the threshold is very much lower.

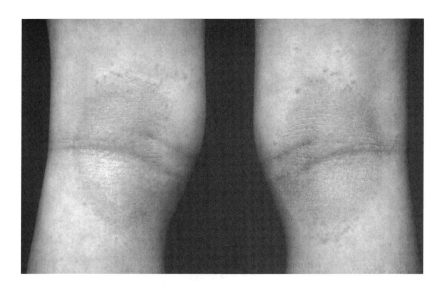

Fig. 16.11. Atopic eczema behind the knees.

Atopic eczema

Epidemiology

Fifteen to twenty percent of children have a tendency to **atopic** eczema. Although atopic eczema is classified as immune, the actual mechanism is uncertain as it does not always seem to be due to direct contact with allergens such as house dust mite on the skin. Known abnormalities include the atopic tendency for antigen responses to be diverted down the Th2 cell pathway with IgE and mast cell production, as well as reduced epidermal fillaggrin expression in 20%–30% of patients. Fillaggrin aggregates keratin filaments which contribute to the epidermal barrier. The resulting dry skin becomes much more susceptible to irritants and more permeable to microbes (*Staph. aureus*) and Th2 stimulating antigens. A chronically inflamed and scratched skin may then generate its own autoantigens. Therefore the primary abnormality may be a disordered epidermal barrier function.

Clinical features

There is usually a personal or family history of asthma or hay fever. In most individuals atopic eczema starts soon after birth on the forehead and cheeks as persistent, dry, rough skin and over time may progress to a different distribution such as the flexor joints (Fig. 16.11).

An extensor joint pattern is also seen in black children as are diskoid and follicular patterns. With pigmented skin though, the major problem is the untreatable discoloration from post-inflammatory hyperpigmentation.

Itching is a major feature of atopic eczema and can drive children into an itch crisis where the patient is consumed by a frenzy of itching. The skin very easily becomes impetiginized with *Staph. aureus* which might stimulate the eczema further.

The sudden eruption of small pustules on an eczema skin obliges the exclusion of superinfection with Herpes simplex which, if present, needs immediate systemic treatment as there is a risk of systemic involvement.

Management

The patient or parents should be provided with explanatory leaflets, videos, and the addresses and websites of self-help groups like the Eczema Society.

Patients should:

(1) Generally:
  (a) avoid dry (low humidity), dusty atmospheres, and extremes of temperature.
  (b) avoid wool next to the skin as it causes itch much more than cotton.
  (c) avoid contact with cold sores (Herpes) and impetigo (*Staph.*, occasionally *Strep.*).
(2) Minimize exposure to soap and water:
  (a) use a soap substitute (aqueous cream often stings, so avoid).
  (b) take a daily bath with added bath oil or emulsifying ointment creamed in warm water.
(3) Find the emollient that suits best and apply several times a day.

(4) Be maintained on:
  (a) ointments for chronic eczema and creams for weeping, acute eczema.
  (b) hydrocortisone-strength topical steroid preparations, with or without an antiseptic/antibiotic.
  (c) topical immuno-modulators such as tacrolimus or pimecrolimus.
(5) For an ITCH crisis patients can benefit from:
  (a) wetwraps: apply emollient or weak topical steroid to affected area, cover with one layer of wet tubular bandage, then a dry tubular bandage.
  (b) a short course of a stronger topical steroid.
  (c) systemic antihistamines to produce sedation.
(6) For an INFECTIVE crisis the doctor needs to:
  (a) exclude scabies and head lice infestation.
  (b) decide whether the infection is viral (Herpes simplex = Kaposi's varicelliform eruption) or bacterial (usually staphylococcal) and treat systemically.
(7) Poorly controlled patients might benefit from:
  (a) regular occlusive bandages (wet wraps).
  (b) dietary manipulation (avoidance of cow's milk protein).
  (c) a short course of systemic steroids.
  (d) hospitalization.
  (e) Chinese herbs (phytotherapy).
  (f) a reduction in mite exposure.
  (g) a course of UVB or PUVA (see psoriasis).
  (h) immunosuppressives (azathioprine or cyclosporin).

Outcome

Atopic eczema waxes and wanes throughout childhood, usually improving in the summer and flaring in the winter. Around 90% will have their skin back to normal by the age of 10 years.

The atopic tendency though is for life and eczema may reappear at any time, often on the face and hands and usually associated with stress.

Venous eczema is easy to diagnose as it occurs in the gaiter area of venous hypertension, sometimes floridly weeping but more usually in a sub-acute phase with wetness and scaling (Fig. 16.12).

It may be complicated, as any eczema, by the addition of type IV hypersensitivity from any cream or agent applied as a treatment, including topical steroids. Patch testing is a routine investigation.

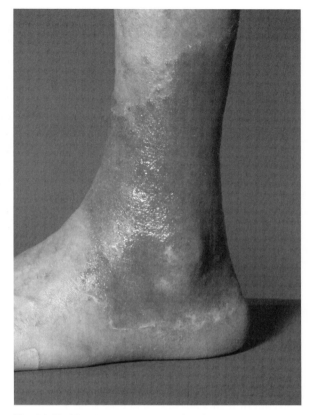

Fig. 16.12. Weeping venous eczema in gaiter area.

Treatment is topical steroids, with compression therapy if the ankle–brachial index is greater than 1.

Venous eczema illustrates another general principle, that of secondary spread. In venous eczema the rash starts on one gaiter area. After a time it may then appear at the same site on the contralateral leg. Then it may appear on both wrists and then higher up all four limbs. Finally it can come out on the trunk. Any eczema may spread away from the original area. For example nickel dermatitis may start under a bracelet on the wrist but then appear on the other wrist and up the arm without any direct contact with the metal there.

Diskoid eczema lesions on the limbs obliges the exclusion of ringworm as a trigger but usually no cause is found and mycology scrapings and culture are negative. Antibiotics and antiseptics often need to be added to the topical steroid applications to achieve better control. The eczema tends to wax and wane but persist.

Asteatotic eczema is really an effect of normal aging and not an eczema. A reduction with age in

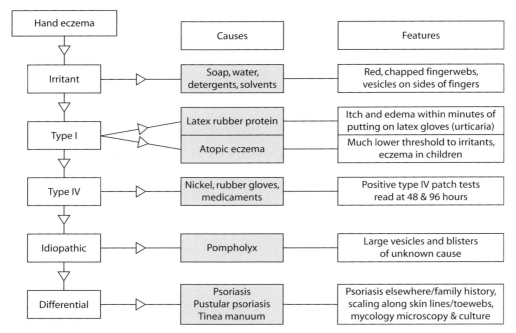

Fig. 16.13. Causes of hand eczema.

the quantity of water-rich lipid in the stratum corneum and on the skin surface means that the epidermis cannot retain water and tends to become very dry. Inflexibility in the stratum corneum leads to surface cracking like the crazy-paving pattern seen in a dried-up riverbed or lake. This is particularly evident on the shins of older patients and may become widespread. It is more evident with overwashing, in low humidity atmospheres such as air conditioning and during winter, or from the effect of fan heaters, e.g. in cars. Treatment is an acceptable emollient several times a day after reversal of triggering factors.

The commonest rash on the hands (Fig. 16.13) is an **irritant eczema**, especially in an atopic patient. Vesicles are much easier to see in the thicker epidermis of palms or soles, described by patients as bubbles. If particularly severe, the vesicles may become turbid and pustular, but this differs from pustular psoriasis where the lesions are pustular to start with and which then reabsorb to brown macules. In someone with persisting hand eczema, type IV hypersensitivity can be excluded by patch testing but foot eczema produced as a type IV response from fungal hyphal antigens in the stratum corneum must be excluded by mycology scrapings and culture and/or a trial of treatment.

In a patient with vesicular hand eczema who does not have an atopic tendency and in whom patch tests and mycology are negative, the diagnosis of **pompholyx** is made, i.e. idiopathic vesicular hand eczema (Fig. 16.14). Again emollients and topical steroids are the mainstay of treatment.

The cause of **eczema on the face** (16.15) differs with different ages. It is almost always atopic in children. During late adolescence seborrheic eczema appears for the first time and later type IV hypersensitivity becomes more important.

Seborrheic eczema is seen in 1%–2% of the population but is especially common in fairer skinned individuals. It tends to be bimodal affecting individuals in their 20s and 30s or 50s and 60s. The sebum excretion rate is not usually increased and the term seborrheic refers to a rash distributed where sebaceous glands are prevalent. The fact that treatment with antifungal agents alone improves most patients implies a causative role for the yeast *Malassezia*, a normal commensal of the scalp. A convenient pathogenesis might represent the eczema as being a type IV hypersensitivity response to antigens generated by the yeast. Seborrheic eczema is more common and more persistent in HIV disease.

Various patterns occur:

(1) Scalp and face: the patient usually has had a history of dandruff for several years with the redness and scaling occasionally spreading onto the eyebrow area, nasolabial fold, and ears. The

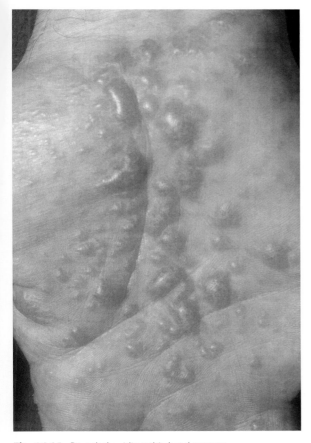

Fig. 16.14. Pompholyx: idiopathic hand eczema.

in the widespread seborrheic eczema seen in older patients.

Seborrheic eczema is also seen in infants and is commonly known as cradle cap.

Because type IV hypersensitivity eczema, also known as **contact allergic eczema**, involves an antigen on the skin, antigen-processing and transport to local lymph node, programming of memory T cells and then the subsequent effector pathway on antigen re-exposure, there is an assumption that most eczemas invoke this mechanism. This is not true but it is important to exclude as avoidance of the antigen (except for chromate in cement in building workers) will usually result in clearance of the eczema.

If a focused skin history starts with how long have you had the rash, the second question is where did it start? The rash of type IV hypersensitivity always starts where the antigen has first been in contact with the skin, which is not always obvious. Nickel dermatitis comes out on ear lobes from cheap metal earrings, at the umbilicus from a jeans stud, or at the wrist from a bracelet or watch. In perfume allergy the aerosolized perfume molecules affect sites such as the eyelids. Type IV allergy to rubber gloves may appear on the back of the hands and form a demarcated rash at the wrist. The chromate antigen is in cement and a hand and/or a diskoid eczema in a building worker is the norm.

Any cream, from whatever source, needs to contain preservatives, and though the risk is low, cream allergy, including the steroid ingredient, must always be considered, especially for resistant eczema.

Microbial proteins can be strongly antigenic. With scabies it is a fecal protein, with fungi the cell wall. Molluscum contagiosum infection can sometimes express a secondary eczema around individual lesions. As before the eczema appears at the site of infection and may then exhibit generalized spread.

Treatment for any eczema to some extent follows that of atopic eczema as described above. The patient must avoid triggering factors and use plenty of emollients, applied down the limbs and trunk. If applied up the limbs the application gets pushed into hair follicles and causes a secondary folliculitis. If the eczema is acute, wet and weeping, the skin may be soaked in soothing potassium permanganate solution for 15 minutes before applying an appropriate strength topical steroid cream. Potassium permanganate is an antiseptic and astringent (coagulates protein) which dries up the skin. It soothes and cools by evaporation of water off the skin. Chronic, lichenified eczemas are treated with emollients and appropriate

redness and scaling can then spread over the whole face. Blepharitis may be a particular problem.

Anti-dandruff shampoos containing selenium sulfide or other antifungal agents usually help. More severe expressions are treated as for psoriasis in the scalp.
(2) Petaloid lesions on the sternal area and upper back are uncommon but typical.
(3) Flexural involvement of axillae, groin, umbilicus, post-aural area and eyelids, and submammary areas can produce an intertrigo-like effect.

For the face, if topical antifungal agents alone do not control the rash then 1% hydrocortisone combined with antifungal agents is usually enough. As staphylococci can often superinfect seborrheic eczema, antiseptic applications or steroid/antibiotic combinations may also be helpful. The acute weeping form involving scalp or genital area may require systemic steroids. This form of treatment is often also needed

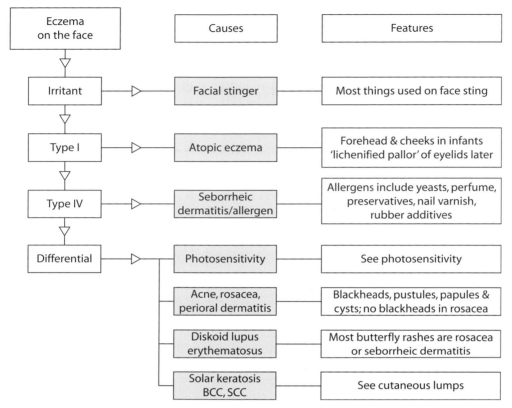

Fig. 16.15. Causes of eczema on the face.

strength steroid ointments. A balance has to be struck between the benefits of steroids and their ability to age and thin the skin if used long term. One percent hydrocortisone is safest but the object is always to minimize exposure. More than once daily application usually has no extra benefit. Tacrolimus is an alternative.

Purpura (Fig. 16.16)

The color of **purpura** (extravasated blood) is determined by the degree of extravasation, its level in the skin or subcutaneous tissue, and the different degradation products of hemoglobin. Deeper bruises and hematomas are usually blue; fresh, superficial hemorrhage is red, degrading over several days, perhaps through greens and yellows to brown (hemosiderin). A large ecchymosis of **senile purpura** stays red–blue for several weeks because of a delay in phagocytosis and degradation. **Purpura fulminans** is usually black.

Increased venous (capillary) pressure increases any tendency for hemorrhage. This is seen at its extreme where **venous hypertension** localizes hemosiderin staining to the gaiter area. Increased pressure in post-capillary venules increases the bleeding tendency of thrombocytopenia and helps localize the type III hypersensitivity circulating complexes responsible for leukocytoclastic vasculitis. Therefore the signs of vasculitis or thrombocytopenia are most commonly seen on the legs, buttocks, or where a venous tourniquet has been applied.

Purpura can also appear in a livedo or reticulate pattern on the skin. Again this is due to increased venous pressure but probably involving deeper, draining venules as well as the post-capillary venule. A broken livedo pattern is responsible for the angulated, geometric shapes purpura can exhibit.

Palpation of the purpuric skin shows two clinical signs, the diagnostic one of non-blanching but also whether or not individual lesions are palpable. The presence of bright red, small, non-palpable, purpuric lesions over the buttocks and lower legs is suggestive of **thrombocytopenia** regardless of cause. Examination of the retina is then mandatory. Hemorrhage may often be found on the oral mucosa as well. Severe

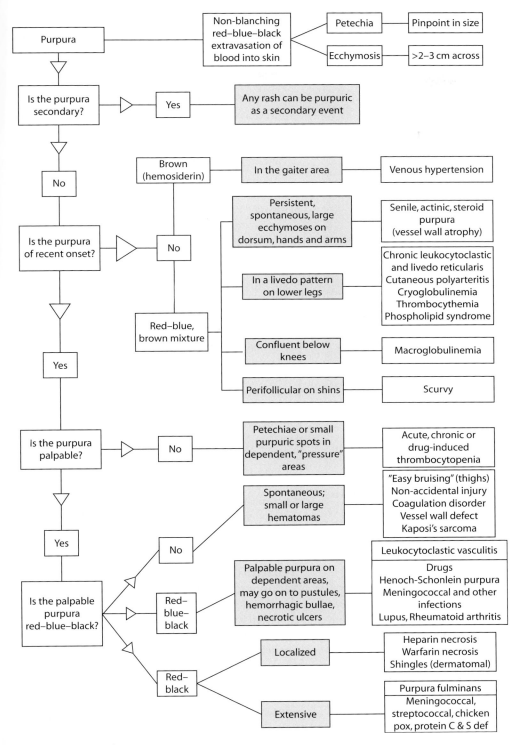

Fig. 16.16. Causes of purpura.

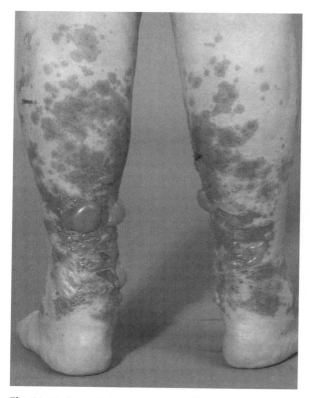

Fig. 16.17. Severe leukocytoclastic vasculitis.

thrombocytopenia can result in very extensive purpura. An immediate full blood count is indicated.

If the new lesions are bright red, palpable and on the lower legs this almost certainly means a **leukocytoclastic vasculitis** (Fig. 16.17) which might be triggered by microbes, e.g. *Streptococcus* or *Meningococcus*, hepatitis C drugs, proteins, or other antigens, including autoantigens. A skin biopsy would confirm the histologic presence of perivascular leukocytoclasis (broken-up neutrophil polymorphs), fibrin, and vessel wall damage. This type III hypersensitivity reaction pattern can go on to produce edema, pustules, hemorrhagic blisters, and ulceration. Typically, as for any type III hypersensitivity, the rash occurs 10–14 days after the trigger. The classic example is Henoch-Schönlein purpura 2 weeks after a streptococcal sore throat, and involving skin, joints, and gastro-intestinal tract. Occasionally, the purpuric rash of meningococcal infection is preceded by a transient maculo-papular blanching rash on the upper trunk.

No cause is found in 50% of patients with cutaneous leukocytoclastic vasculitis. The three important actions are:

(1) exclude a systemic vasculitis such as Wegener's granulomatosis, or connective tissue diseases such as lupus erythematosus.

(2) establish whether there is any internal organ involvement with vasculitis such as the kidney, joints, or eye.

(3) prevent skin ulceration through appropriate doses of systemic steroids. Skin ulcers secondary to vasculitis are painful, have a high morbidity, and may take a long time to heal.

Adolescent females often present with spontaneous, bluish bruising on the thighs, so-called **easy bruising**. Coagulation screens to exclude vitamin K or coagulation factor deficiency are usually normal as is a personal and family history of bleeding. A cause for easy bruising is not normally found. For linear or geometric-shaped bruising in a young child, it is necessary to exclude non-accidental injury. An asymmetric, bruise-like, papule or nodule, persisting for months, may be the first expression of **Kaposi's sarcoma** in an immunosuppressed individual.

The sudden onset of extensive, red–black purpura, often on limbs, following a microbial infection is termed **purpura fulminans** and is an emergency as limbs can be lost (Fig. 16.18). It may be associated with disseminated intravascular coagulation or protein C or S deficiency.

If localized, it might have appeared on breast or buttocks immediately at the start of warfarin therapy due to a consumption effect. Rarely, it is seen with heparinization, and even more rarely may represent necrosis throughout a dermatome if triggered by Herpes varicella zoster virus (shingles).

Pruritus (Fig. 16.19)

Pruritus is the sensation which provokes the desire to scratch and must be distinguished from other subjective sensations such as pain or burning.

The itch sensation may be triggered by both chemical and physical stimuli. Histamine, cowhage spicules (itching powder), and some proteolytic enzymes such as tryptase may trigger itching directly but many of these enzymes and various peptides (substance P) generate it indirectly by triggering histamine release from mast cells. Fibreglass promotes itch mechanically.

Itch is sensed by fine, free, unmyelinated nerve endings which carry histamine and protein receptors and trigger nerve impulses and release substance

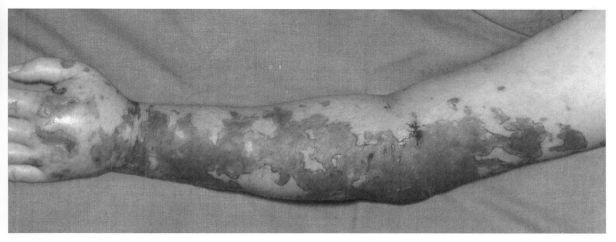

Fig. 16.18. Purpura fulminans in acute meningococcemia.

P locally. The latter is part of an autocrine loop stimulating adjacent mast cells to release TNFα which enhances receptor responsiveness on the nerve endings. Scratching or high frequency electrical stimulation may temporarily block the itch, analogous to the gate control theory for pain whereby simultaneous firing of large and small afferent fibers results in presynaptic inhibition of the smaller fiber. The itch of scabies is always said to be worse at night but this is true for almost every cause of itching. At night, the skin warmth and lack of other sensory input presumably allows more impulses to reach the cortex.

Patients respond to itch in a variety of ways. Itchy, urticarial rashes tend to be rubbed rather than scratched, usually with the finger pulp, atopic eczema patients use the nail tips to scratch, whilst patients with senile pruritus typically gouge out linear excoriations of skin on their upper shoulders and lower back. Persistent paroxysms of itching may well induce thickened skin expressed as lichenification, lichen simplex, or nodular prurigo.

Differential diagnosis

Where there is no defined rash, it is convenient to think of the causes, mechanisms and investigation of pruritus as outlined in Fig 16.19, although a defined cause may be found in only 20%–40% of patients.

Senile itch

Diagnosed after exclusion of other causes, this is by far the commonest and often intractable. Daily or twice daily applications of the preferred moisturizer usually suffice.

Systemic causes

Drug-induced pruritus is usually straightforward as the symptoms start soon after the drug has been prescribed, e.g. sulphonamides, ACE inhibitors, NSAIDs, interferon, chloroquine, bleomycin, morphine, or epidural opioid anesthesia. Others however like gold or quinine exhibit a delayed onset of several months.

On first exposure to the **scabies** mite no symptoms occur until 1 month has passed. The itch then starts (often on thighs and abdomen) and for several weeks signs of the secondary eczema may be minimal or related to the hands alone. Infestation with the head or pubic louse may present as a generalized itch although usually the itch is localized to the scalp or pubic area to start with. Persistent pruritus may be the presenting symptom of HIV infection. A light infestation with onchocerciasis may present with itching as the dominant feature. History of foreign travel may necessitate a filarial ELISA test and an eosinophil count.

Pruritus affects some 50% of patients with **chronic renal failure** and around 25% of patients on hemodialysis. Hepatitis C infection, primary biliary cirrhosis (PBC), cholestatic jaundice, pregnancy, the oral contraceptive, and cirrhosis are the major causes of pruritus caused by **hepatic disease**. Liver function tests and anti-mitochondrial antibody to exclude PBC are necessary investigations. If the cholestasis is irreversible, the return on treatments such as rifampicin, an enzyme inducer, or cholestyramine, a bile acid chelator, is poor.

Pruritus is present in 5% of patients with **thyrotoxicosis** and may be the presenting feature.

501

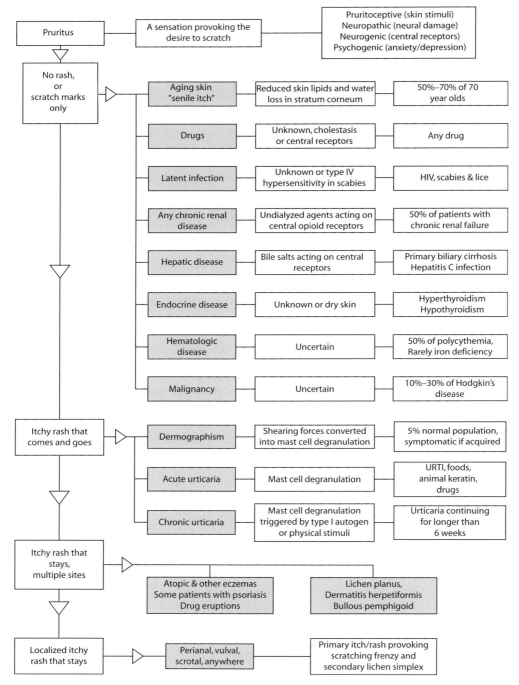

Fig. 16.19. Causes of pruritus.

Myxedema patients have dry, itchy skin. Itch in **diabetes mellitus** is due to candidal infection and probably never to the diabetes.

Fifty percent of **primary polycythemia** patients have pruritus, often triggered by a change in temperature.

Aspirin and paroxetine may relieve it. Iron deficiency is a rare cause of pruritus. Leukemia, myeloma, and paraproteinemia may all provoke itching. A full blood count, serum iron, and protein electrophoresis are necessary investigations.

Progressive, intractable itching with negative routine investigations requires a search to exclude **malignancy**, particularly Hodgkin's disease. Tabes dorsalis and multiple sclerosis may both trigger paroxysms of itching. Pruritus restricted to the nose may indicate a tumor of the floor of the fourth ventricle.

In florid cases of **dermographism** the wheals are easily visible but often they are not. When dermographism starts suddenly, drugs, upper respiratory tract infections, and stress are possible triggers. All patients with itching should be tested to see if they have a symptomatic triple response. **Water-induced (aquagenic) pruritus** is most commonly seen as a symptom of another cause of itching and as such is particularly common; sunlight, heat, and exercise are other triggers beside water. Some highly itchy dermatoses such as dermatitis herpetiformis may have minimal physical signs.

In the majority of cases a cause for the itch will not be found. Many of these patients will have their itching for several months and then it will resolve. In some stress and anxiety will be the cause. Rarely delusions of parasitosis will be associated.

Investigations
The history and examination are slanted to the above causes. The skin should be examined all over and hepatomegaly and lymphadenopathy excluded. A full blood count, serum iron, urea, creatinine, all electrolytes, liver function, antimitochondrial antibody, and thyroid function are routine, with the examination and investigations being repeated if the itch is intractable and progressive.

Management
Guidelines for pruritus treatment are much the same as for dry skin and eczema:
(1) Find and treat a specific cause if there is one.
(2) Avoid aggravating factors such as over-washing, strong detergents, dry heat, or irritant clothes.
(3) Replace moisture back into the skin with bath oil and regular use of moisturizers, including urea preparations.
(4) Prescribe specific topical antipruritic agents such as 1%–2% menthol in simple cream.
(5) Trial several different H_1 antihistamines alone or in combination with H_2 blockers until the right response is achieved.

Anogenital pruritus
Itch localized to the perianal area is very common, especially in males. Mucosal eversion and leakage of mucus leads to skin irritation and itching. Further scratching reinforces the cycle so chronic eczema ensues. Soothing hemorrhoid or local anesthetic creams might have triggered type IV hypersensitivity, necessitating exclusion by patch testing. Flexural psoriasis is occasionally itchy. Tinea cruris and erythrasma occasionally are the underlying triggers for itching and the physical signs may be masked by treatment with a topical steroid.

Pruritus vulvae may be linked to candidal or trichomonal vaginal infection, but if that is absent the itch is most commonly an expression of atopic eczema, psoriasis, or lichen sclerosus.

An itchy scrotum is usually thought of as psychogenic, persistent scratching and rubbing leading to gross lichenification.

Photosensitivity (Fig. 16.20)
Mechanisms
During passage through the earth's atmosphere, the sun's energy is reduced by one-third, partly from absorption by ozone. The spectrum then includes ultraviolet A (UVA, 320–400 nm), ultraviolet B (UVB, 290–320 nm), visible light, and infrared wavelengths.

The main acute effects of ultraviolet radiation (UVR) on normal skin are photosynthesis of vitamin D, sunburn, pigmentation (either immediate darkening or delayed pigmentation due to production of new melanin which takes several days), and diminished immune protection partly due to damaged Langerhans' cells. The chronic effects relate to premature aging (photoaging) and skin cancer (photocarcinogenesis).

A thinner ozone layer permits more of the shorter wave UVB through to sea level, which will result in greater sunburn, more tanning, more premature aging, more skin cancer, and more cataracts.

Differential diagnosis (Fig. 16.20)
Sunburn presents as erythema, pain and edema in previously un-tanned or lesser tanned areas. Dark-skinned Asian and Afro-Caribbean patients rarely suffer sunburn but they still can, and they do experience photosensitivity.

If a sun-induced rash develops as very itchy papules symmetrically in a few areas, minutes to hours after sun exposure, and lasts for a day or two, the rash is almost certainly **polymorphic light eruption**. Ten percent of all adult females are susceptible to this. It is likely to be a delayed hypersensitivity

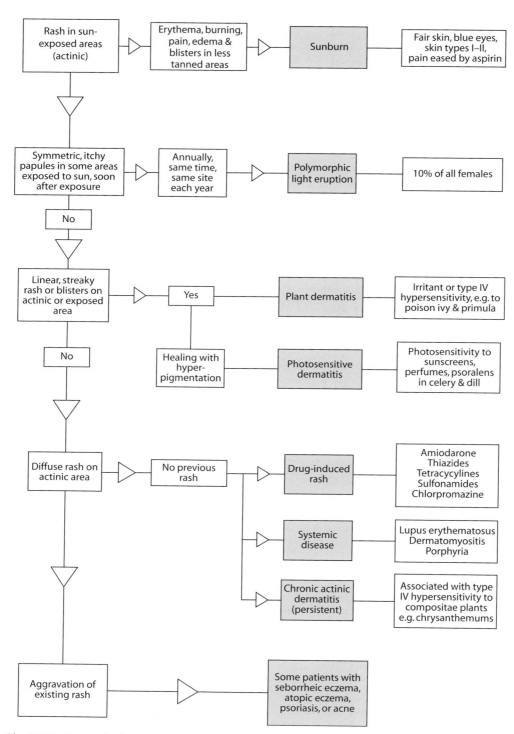

Fig. 16.20. Causes of rashes in sun-exposed areas.

response to a UVR-induced unknown antigen. It is reproducible in pattern and site, often coming out at the same time each year. Avoidance of UVR and protection via sunscreens is not usually effective and patients often need a low-dose course of UVB phototherapy to harden the skin up at the beginning of each spring.

Lupus erythematosus and **dermatomyositis** both need to be excluded as both can present with photosensitivity and little in the way of obvious rash.

If the rash comes out diffusely in light-exposed (actinic) areas, then the differential diagnosis lies between a choice of three. The rash may be **drug-induced** of which amiodarone, thiazides, and tetracyclines are the commonest triggers. It may be an aggravation of an existing rash of which seborrheic eczema, atopic eczema, psoriasis, and even acne are all possible. Or, finally, the rash may present as a persistent **actinic dermatitis** without any obvious trigger. If so the rash may well have been aggravated by airborne plant molecules landing on sun-damaged skin, being activated by light, and provoking an eczematous response. The chrysanthemum plant family is a common culprit. Avoidance of the plant does not reverse the process and patients often need long-term immunosuppression as well as sun avoidance and sun protection practices.

Plants such as primula can cause eczema on exposed areas without sunlight and others produce a streaky pigmented dermatitis on the back of the hands where plant molecules activated by UVR cause blisters followed by hyperpigmentation.

Porphyria usually presents first with increased skin fragility followed by blisters, usually on the backs of the hands. Long-term light exposure activates the porphyrins in the skin which have accumulated due to inherited partial enzyme deficiencies, being compromised further by alcohol intake, drugs such as estrogen, or iron excess in hemochromatosis.

Management

The standard treatment for all of these photodermatoses is to soothe the skin with cooling agents such as creams, not ointments, often with a topical steroid. Systemic steroids are sometimes required. Patch tests, photopatch tests, and solar simulator light testing can be used for confirmation if necessary. All patients need to be advised on UVR protection and the consequences of premature aging and skin cancer, both accelerated by smoking.

Protection from UVR is achieved through three methods: minimizing exposure at peak times, wearing hats and appropriate clothing, and sunscreens.

Skin can sense the warmth of infrared wavelengths immediately but can only sense UVR retrospectively from the damage produced. UVR transmission is greater: between 11am and 3pm during the day; in summer months; at higher altitude; nearer the equator; and where reflected from snow, sand or water.

Sunscreens act either through chemical means by absorbing UVR, or physical means by reflecting it. Sun protection factor (SPF) is a measure of how much longer than usual an individual can expose themselves to the sun before burning, i.e. SPF 15 means you can stay out 15 times longer. A sunscreen with SPF 15 confers 95% protection, provided it is put on thickly enough and applied half an hour before exposure and re-applied after swimming. A disadvantage with sunscreens is that individuals may stay out longer and expose themselves to more UVA, which might be just as detrimental in the long term. Some sunscreens protect against UVA and use the asterisk system depicted on the reverse of the bottle. Ideally all patients should be protecting against UVB and UVA.

Over-protection from UVR may result in inadequate vitamin D synthesis which is important not only in bone formation but may confer some protection against many internal cancers and inflammatory conditions such as Crohn's disease. Exposure of face and arms for 10 minutes at midday every day is thought to generate the vitamin D requirement.

Pigmentation (Fig. 16.21)

Melanin is manufactured in melanocytes positioned along the basal layer of the epidermis but whose dendrites extend up between keratinocytes, each servicing up to 40 keratinocytes with melanin-containing melanosomes. For a given skin site, all races have the same number of melanocytes and differences in color are related to the quality and quantity of melanin injected into the dependent keratinocyte. Melanosomes are packeted above the keratinocyte nucleus in an umbrella pattern, shielding it from ultraviolet radiation. Interference with this process or damage to either melanocytes or keratinocytes leads to various changes in pigmentation, see Fig. 16.21.

Secondary pigmentary changes

Mild damage to the epidermis will leave it paler, as seen on the face in children with **pityriasis alba**. Some

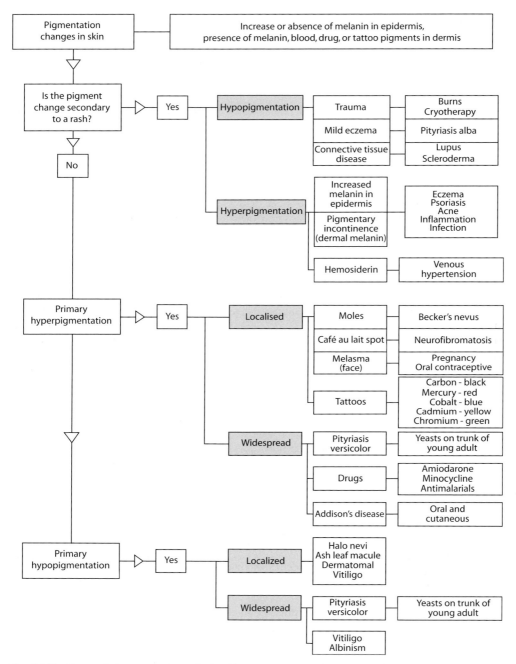

Fig. 16.21. Causes of pigmentary change in the skin.

diseases such as diskoid lupus erythematosus, lichen sclerosus, or scleroderma can produce complete depigmentation, though this might be more commonly seen after a burn or perhaps even from over-zealous cryotherapy.

It is more common for epidermal damage to result in hyperpigmentation. Either inflammatory prostaglandins stimulate melanization to make the epidermis darker or melanin pigment, having dropped down into the dermis after injury, stays phagocytosed in macrophages in the upper dermis for months to years, so-called pigmentary incontinence. The effect of incident light on this dermal pigment makes the skin appear darker. If the pigment is slightly deeper in the dermis, it will appear blue like a blue nevus or Mongolian spot, again through an effect of incident light and color reflection.

Primary hyperpigmentation

Ten percent of the population can have up to five café-au-lait macules, which are not always present at birth. To satisfy one of the diagnostic criteria of neurofibromatosis, individuals, if pre-pubertal, must have six or more café-au-lait macules greater than 5 mm. Pigmented moles are discussed under cutaneous lumps.

A large area of pigmentation over a shoulder area appearing during adolescence is diagnostic of Becker's nevus, a congenital abnormality visible from puberty, following androgen stimulation on susceptible melanocytes. Occasionally it is visible at birth.

A similar phenomenon, chloasma, albeit transient, occurs during pregnancy or oral contraceptive medication. Susceptible melanocytes on the face are stimulated by estrogens to give a reticulate pattern of pigmentation typical of pregnancy. Sun exposure is an important concomitant and sunscreens play a role in treatment.

Fashion trends have dictated an increase in tattooing in a variety of colors, patterns, and sites. A skin reaction in a tattoo might be indicative of allergy to the pigment but might also be a presenting sign of sarcoidosis at a site of trauma. The high concentration of paraphenylamine diamine in some henna tattoos leads to a very severe local reaction due to type IV hypersensitivity, occurring in tourists immediately after return from a holiday abroad.

Medication is a common cause of primary hyperpigmentation. Amiodarone produces pigmentation of the skin in sun-exposed areas in 10% of patients (photosensitivity in 75%). Minocycline pigmentation is also dose-related, appearing in scars, conjunctivae, and nail beds as well as the shins. Many of the drugs producing pigmentary change do so by deposition of drug products rather than melanin changes.

Addison's disease is a rare cause of generalized increased pigmentation with accentuation over joints, palmar creases, and on the buccal mucosa.

Primary hypopigmentation

A widespread, patterned, pale area of skin on the trunk of a young adult would suggest a diagnosis of pityriasis versicolor, an infection with the yeast *Malassezia*. The skin should be stretched and gently scraped to see if it scales easily and skin scrapings taken for confirmatory microscopy. Occasionally the yeast produces a hyperpigmented rash rather than hypopigmentation. Treatment is a short course of systemic itraconazole, although the pale areas of skin take several months to reverse. Recurrence is common and regular prophylaxis with antifungal shampoos to scalp and trunk suffices.

It is common to see pale areas of skin developing around individual moles, a halo nevus. This is an autoimmune effect directed locally against the mole which will disappear.

Generalized autoimmune attacks on melanocytes give rise to vitiligo, a familial condition present in up to 1% of the population. It starts as rounded macules which may eventually merge to give large areas of loss of color with convex, scalloped edges. Usually, the damage is enough to give permanent hypopigmentation. Whilst not as obvious in Caucasian skin, it is very obvious in Asian or African skin, particularly if in the acro-facial pattern on face and hands. Within those cultures the appearance has a tradition of stigmatization. Treatment is often not helpful. There is an increased risk of other autoimmune diseases, specifically thyroid disease.

Hair loss

Types of hair loss (alopecia) and associated features are depicted in Fig. 16.22. Patients are predominantly concerned with loss of hair from the scalp. Spontaneous loss from the body or face suggests alopecia areata (AA), hypopituitarism, or hypothyroidism, with AA the likeliest cause for loss of eyelashes.

Scarring alopecia

Certain diseases target and destroy individual hair follicles. **Diskoid lupus erythematosus** (DLE) and **lichen planus** can look similar clinically with well-demarcated areas of scarring in the scalp and loss of follicular ostia. Adjacent areas of scalp are often erythematous, scaly, and show follicular plugging. This sign comprises a collarette of scale sleeving the base of each hair. **Localised scleroderma** occurs in the scalp in a linear pattern with a scar running from vertex to forehead and down the nose, mimicking the distribution of a saber cut (coup de sabre). The importance of these three diseases is that they may occur in association with disease elsewhere, and thus help support a diagnosis, or in the scalp in their own right. Treatment is indicated to prevent extensive areas of scalp becoming permanently bald.

507

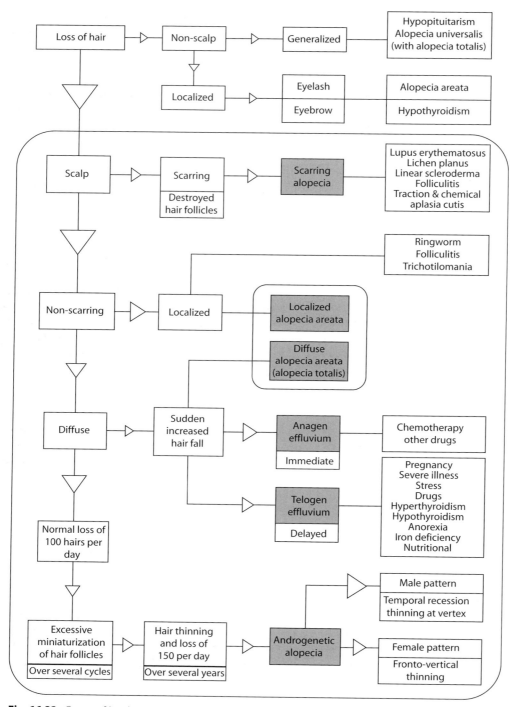

Fig. 16.22. Causes of hair loss.

Sustained tension on a hair converts it into a telogen hair. Further tension may convert it to a vellus follicle or initiate a folliculitis. The end result is apparent loss of hair. Someone having a ponytail for long periods loses hair round the edge of the scalp. Persistent, tight plaiting or rollers produce similar loss in different patterns. The alopecia is permanent.

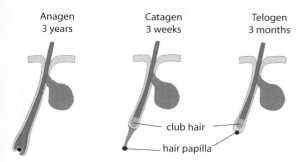

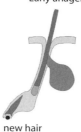

Anagen
3 years

Catagen
3 weeks

Telogen
3 months

Early anagen

club hair

hair papilla

new hair

Fig. 16.23. Hair cycle.

Anagen and telogen effluvium

Each scalp hair follicle grows a hair (anagen phase) for 3–5 years, Fig. 16.23. Then for 3 weeks it goes through a catagen phase before finally entering the resting, telogen phase which lasts up to 3 months. That follicle then grows a new hair which pushes out the spent one. Each follicle does this independently. Of the 100 000 hair follicles on the scalp, 5%–15% are in telogen at anyone time with the normal scalp losing 50–100 hairs a day.

Sudden diffuse hair loss is usually provoked by an abrupt interruption of the anagen growth phase of hundreds or even thousands of follicles at once.

If the "stress" provokes a severe interruption in normal growth, many anagen hairs will be shed almost immediately, so called **anagen effluvium**, e.g. within 1 week of starting chemotherapy. If the "stress" is less severe then many hairs will have their anagen phase stopped short much earlier than normal, be converted into telogen, and then be shed 3 months later, so-called **telogen effluvium**, e.g. 3 months after a severe illness. Or a combination might occur.

During pregnancy fewer hairs are shed, hair feels thicker and grows longer until the pregnancy ends, stressing the follicle. A few months after the birth all the hair that would have fallen out during pregnancy and often much more besides begins to be shed, much to the patient's dismay.

This situation goes on for several months then gradually diminishes. Clinical examination reveals diffuse hair thinning on the scalp but no scarring. A gentle pull will often bring away three to four hairs, the norm being zero to one. Pulling out a group of 20 hairs will show that more than 25% will have telogen roots.

The differential diagnosis is alopecia areata (AA) attacking random follicles diffusely all over the scalp instead of in localized patches. A diagnosis of AA is made by finding other features of AA, not always present.

In most situations the anagen/telogen effluvium will diminish within 6 months, taking another 6 months for the hair to thicken up again but often not to the original appearance.

Management involves explaining the "shock to the hair root," giving reassurance that not all the hair will be lost and that the majority will eventually grow back.

Occasionally for no obvious reason it will continue. If there is no obvious trigger, if the hair fall continues, or if regrowth is not occurring then attention needs to be paid to nutritional factors, endocrine factors, and drug or hormone causes. One cause of failure to rethicken is that the hair loss has uncovered the tendency to androgenetic alopecia.

Alopecia areata

Alopecia areata (AA) is a non-scarring alopecia that usually results in self-limiting areas of hair loss in the scalp. Prevalence is 0.1%–0.2% worldwide without any racial or sexual imbalance.

The anagen stage hair follicle is assumed to be an immune-privileged site which, if damaged for some reason, might expose epitopes that might stimulate an autoimmune response. Th1 lymphocytes then attack the hair bulb and damage it sufficiently to stop it from growing. The weakened shaft breaks off below the surface to produce the bald patch. In some follicles continuation of the telogen phase pushes the broken shaft above the surface to produce the diagnostic exclamation mark hair, 1–2 mm long. AA is the disease responsible in literature for patients going white overnight. In fact it usually happens over 2–3 weeks. For some reason the immune attack seems only to affect pigmented hair which then falls out, any graying or white hair is left behind, leaving the patient "white." When hair grows back it is often white first and then pigments later.

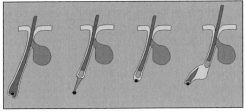
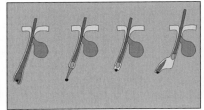
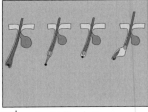

1st cycle. Terminal hair 2nd cycle 3rd cycle. Vellus hair

Fig. 16.24. Miniaturization of hair follicles over several years.

There is a family history in up to 15%, often associated with thyroid disease and other auto-immunity. Children and young adults are most affected. Patches may merge into each other, sometimes enlarging as others regrow. The scalp is a normal color with no scaling; just denuded of hair. The beard area may be involved as may eyelashes and eyebrows. If the whole of the scalp is involved, the condition is called alopecia totalis (AT). If the whole of the body is affected then it is alopecia universalis (AU). Fine nail pitting is also seen.

Differentiating AA from scarring alopecia is straightforward because the follicle mouths are still present. Care must be taken though with black children where scalp ringworm due to *Trichophyton tonsurans* masquerades as AA.

Most patients have less than 50% scalp involvement. Management involves reassurance that complete regrowth will have occurred within 6–12 months in 90%. Prognosis is worse in those with greater than 50% involvement, a history of atopy, or involvement of the hair margin on the neck. Topical steroids and topical minoxidil are often prescribed but are temporizing agents only. For severe and persistent cases regular application of an agent that induces type IV contact hypersensitivity brings some success but may provoke severe local or generalized reactions. If patients cannot be reconciled in some way to their baldness, wigs are often the only alternative.

Androgenetic alopecia

The effect of androgens on hair follicles is site specific. In pubic and axillary areas androgens at puberty stimulate the follicle to grow into terminal hairs. At the same time, the opposite is happening in the scalp. Over several cycles, these terminal hairs are being converted by these androgens back into vellus hairs (Fig. 16.24). The anagen phase becomes shorter resulting in more hairs being lost each day, and the follicle becomes smaller with successive cycles.

This genetically determined miniaturization of hair follicles is a secondary sex characteristic present in everybody to a greater or lesser extent. By the age of 30, 30% of white men will have some degree of **androgenetic hair thinning**, increasing to 50% at 50. It is four times more frequent in white men than black men. Ten percent of pre-menopausal women are affected and up to 70% by the age of 70.

The pattern of hair thinning differs between men and women although they may overlap. In men miniaturization results in thinning, then balding, starting at the temples and the crown, slowly expanding, eventually merging. In women thinning is the dominant component from the frontal hair margin to the crown with completely bald areas being rare.

Examination reveals a healthy scalp with thinning hair and bald areas in the pattern appropriate for the sex. Shorter, finer, miniaturized hairs are usually visible as well.

A negative family history of baldness does not preclude the diagnosis. Causes of anagen/telogen effluvium need to be excluded as androgenetic alopecia is so common the two conditions often present together. Rapid onset and progression of androgenetic alopecia with loss of frontal hairline should prompt measurement of serum testosterone to exclude an androgen-secreting tumor.

Topical minoxidil daily will give good regrowth in 15% and may delay progression. The treatment is life-long and discontinuation places the patient in the position they would have been if it had not been used at all. The cost of £1 per day is outside many people's budget.

Daily, oral finasteride blocks 5α-reductase and is very effective in men with little in the way of side-effects. Again treatment is life-long. It is not effective in women who need to use hairstyles and cosmetics to make their hair appear thicker.

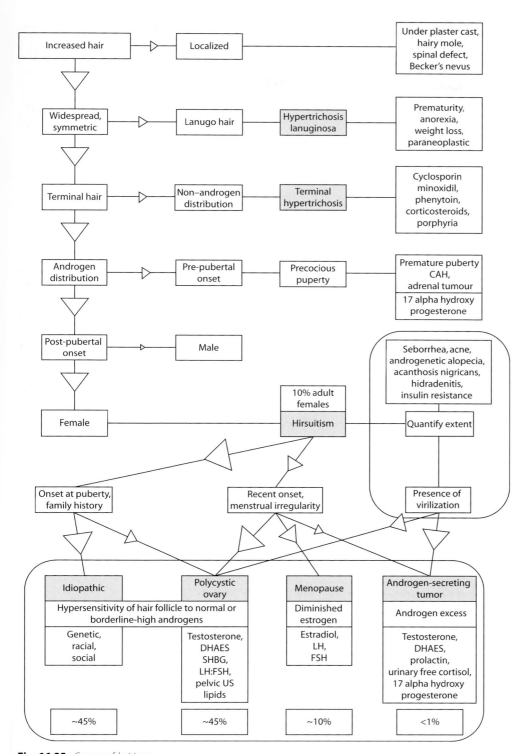

Fig. 16.25. Causes of hairiness.

Hirsutism and hypertrichosis

Unless destroyed by disease or a full-thickness burn, the distribution and number of hair follicles stays constant through life. Increased hairiness (Fig. 16.25), may occur from an increase in length of vellus hair (blond, soft and silky, lanugo-like) or an increase in the number of follicles growing terminal hair (thicker, stronger, containing melanin, and having a medulla, i.e. a central core). Hirsutism is defined as terminal hair growth in women in a distribution normally seen in men, and occurs in 10% of women in Europe and North America. If there is lanugo-like hair growth, or terminal hair growing in a non-androgen area, the condition is called hypertrichosis.

Hirsutism

Mechanisms

In females during puberty, androgens, including dehydroepiandrosterone (DHEA) and its sulfate (DHEAS), stimulate terminal hair growth in the pubic area and axillae. The degree of subsequent male-pattern hair growth is dependent on: the level of free androgens in the blood; the varying capacity in different individuals of 5α reductase activity in sebaceous glands to convert androgens to the more potent dihydrotestosterone (DHT); and the differing sensitivity of hair papillae to DHT.

Ninety-nine percent of circulating testosterone is bound to sex hormone binding globulin (SHBG). Small reductions in SHBG due to obesity allow for relative flooding of active, free testosterone. Serum testosterone and other androgen levels are measured to exclude androgen-secreting tumors but are normal or only borderline high in over 95% of hirsute patients.

Clinical features

The commonest expression of **hirsutism** would be the presence of terminal hair on: the upper lip; beard area; areolae, and the development of a male pubic pattern. Hirsutism may be quantified (11 body areas score 0–4) as a measure of response to treatment. Scores need to be seen in context of ethnic origin as females from the Mediterranean littoral and the Indian subcontinent score much higher than do women from East Asia, sub-Saharan Africa, and northern Europe.

Further androgenization may result in virilization expressed as: more hairiness, including chest and back; male pattern baldness; clitoral hypertrophy; voice changes and a muscular build; and other androgen-associated features such as seborrhea, acne, and insulin resistance.

Idiopathic hirsutism usually starts at puberty and develops slowly and steadily. Polycystic ovary syndrome (PCOS) may present in the same way, but a small proportion (1%–5%) of hirsute patients may have partial congenital adrenal hyperplasia.

Lanugo **hypertrichosis** may be seen: in premature babies; on the face as an expression of sudden weight loss (dieting, anorexia, bulimia); as a side-effect of drugs or as a paraneoplastic sign (lung, colon). Terminal hypertrichosis presents as excess hair in the non-androgen areas and is mostly drug induced, e.g. cyclosporin and phenytoin.

Investigations

Rapid, recent onset, especially with virilization, requires a search for an androgen secreting tumor (ovarian or adrenal). Prolactinoma presents with irregular periods, galactorrhea and hirsutism. Patients with Cushing's syndrome may well be hirsute. Fewer than 1% of hirsute patients will be found to have an endocrine tumor or pituitary disease. The majority of these patients with rapid onset will have PCOS.

Drug-induced hirsutism is most commonly triggered by anabolic steroids, corticosteroids, and phenothiazines.

Management

Television, film, and especially print media require female role models to have blemish-free skin, a full head of long hair, long eyelashes, perfect eyebrows, a small amount of pubic hair, but no hair anywhere else. This unobtainable ideal only aggravates the problem of increased hair. For some females, hirsutism is soul-destroying and it is important to reassure them they are still "normal" women and find some helpful treatment.

Physical methods Bleaching, plucking, shaving, waxing, and depilatory creams need to be repeated frequently as they do not destroy the hair follicle. Secondary folliculitis is a common side effect. Shaving does not increase hair growth; it produces uniform stubble that feels rougher than tapered hair of different length. Electrolysis destroys one follicle at a time, it is time consuming, expensive, painful, and may scar.

Laser treatment needs to be repeated over several cycles to be effective.

Pharmacotherapy Estrogens reduce ovarian androgen, raise SHBG, and compete for androgen receptors.

Dianette (a high-estrogen OCP with 2 mg cyproterone acetate) with 50 mg cyproterone acetate, a specific anti-androgen on day 5 to 15 of each cycle, produces some improvement. Cyproterone acetate produces feminization of a male fetus, thus pregnancy must be avoided.

Finasteride, used for benign prostatic hypertrophy, blocks 5α reductase. Its effect is mild and again may cause fetal abnormality.

Flutamide blocks the androgen P450 receptor and is reasonably effective but hepatitis, sometimes fatal, is a side effect.

Spironolactone has mild anti-androgen activity and is most useful for older women who might also be hypertensive.

In PCOS metformin is used for induction of ovulation and may be helpful for hirsutism. Eflornithine hydrochloride cream inhibits ornithine decarboxylase in hair papillae. Daily use for 8 weeks will usually diminish hair growth but it is licenced for use on the face only.

Nail disorders

Like hair, nail is a form of keratin growing out from a fold of skin. Like hair there are both cosmetic and disease considerations. The varnishing of nails produces minimal nail disability but the pushing back of the cuticle, which provides a waterproof seal between the nail fold and the nail plate, allows for entry of the usual insults and irritants in the form of water, solvents, and microbes. Excessive wetwork further retracts the cuticle. *Staphylococcus aureus* or *E. coli* infection can produce an **acute paronychia** (Fig. 16.26), which usually requires antibiotics and drainage.

Microbes are probably less important in **chronic paronychia**. Here there is thickening or bolstering of soft tissue all the way round the nail fold (Fig. 16.27). Repetitive irritant injury is the main cause perhaps with candidal superinfection. Avoidance of wetwork and protection with rubber gloves to allow reconstitution of the cuticle is the mainstay of treatment. Rarely sarcoidosis or lichen planus can mimic chronic paronychia.

Nail keratin is an appropriate medium for dermatophytes to colonize. Commonest in toenails, as the infection, **tinea unguium,** grows down the nail plate it produces yellowing, thickening, and onycholysis. Usually, several nails are affected. Ischemia and aging can produce the same appearance and it is mandatory to obtain mycology results from clippings before

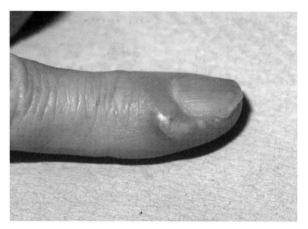

Fig. 16.26. Acute paronychia.

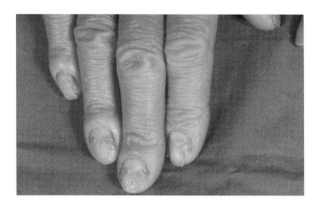

Fig. 16.27. Chronic paronychia.

embarking on a 3 month course of oral antifungal treatment such as terbinafine which has only a 70%–80% success rate.

Nail biting is the commonest injury to the nail. In children this can be minimized by the application of over the counter nail applications, which taste bitter. Blunt injury to the nail can result in a **subungual hematoma**. This is exquisitely painful and often needs to be drained under local anesthetic, providing instant relief from the throbbing pain. The appearance of a chronic subungual hematoma may mimic subungual malignant melanoma and if necessary a diagnostic nailbed biopsy through the nail is needed.

An **ingrowing toenail** may result from failure to cut right to the edge of the nail, leaving a spike that grows down into the skin or incurving of the nail. Many patients end up with surgical removal of the lateral margin. If ingrowing toenails are recurrent or

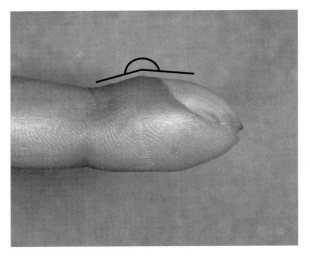

Fig. 16.28. Clubbing of nails showing the critical angle.

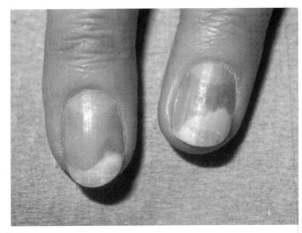

Fig. 16.29. Onycholysis.

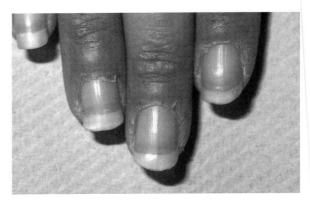

Fig. 16.30. Nail fold hemorrhages and papules on the knuckles typical of dermatomyositis.

disrupting life, surgical or phenolic removal of the nail is needed. An apparent ingrowing toenail with excessive granulation tissue may be drug-induced, either by HAART or retinoid therapy.

Examination of the nails can often reveal clues to previous or present systemic illness. Interference with growth in a single nail root will result in a transverse groove across the nail. This groove grows out with time and as the fingernails take about 6 months to grow out, the time of the original insult can be calculated. A symmetric transverse groove or **Beau's line** in all nails points to a systemic illness or chemotherapy, particularly taxanes.

In nail **clubbing** there is increased transverse and longitudinal curvature of the nail (Fig. 16.28). Soft tissue overgrowth under the base of the nail increases the angle between nail plate and nail fold from less than 160 degrees to over 180 degrees. Clubbing can be familial. Most acquired cases are related to pulmonary pathology such as fibrosis or lung cancer. Cyanotic congenital heart disease, infective endocarditis, cirrhosis, and inflammatory bowel disease make up most of the rest.

In **psoriasis** the nail grows quicker so that the nail plate may separate from the nail bed producing onycholysis (Fig. 16.29). Onycholysis may be produced by trauma, wetwork, fungal infection, and thyrotoxicosis as well as psoriasis. Tiny pits on the surface of the nail may indicate psoriasis or alopecia areata. Koilonychia (spoon-shaped nail plate) can be sign of iron deficiency but is often familial.

Nail-fold telangiectasia and hemorrhage is a distinctive feature of sensitivity to cold, CREST syndrome, systemic lupus erythematosus, and dermatomyositis (Fig. 16.30). The commonest cause of splinter hemorrhages is trauma. A thrombotic tendency, endocarditis, and trichinosis are much rarer causes.

In black individuals it is common to see pigmented streaks down the nails suggesting pigmented nevi in the nail matrix. This is much less frequent in a Caucasian population and a biopsy is indicated to rule out melanoma. Melanomas and squamous cell carcinomas can arise under the nail and there may be a long delay in diagnosis.

Cutaneous lumps
Benign lumps
Warty lesions
The term wart (Fig. 16.31), refers to a benign epithelial proliferation caused by the **human papillomavirus** (HPV). Verruca means the same thing but in

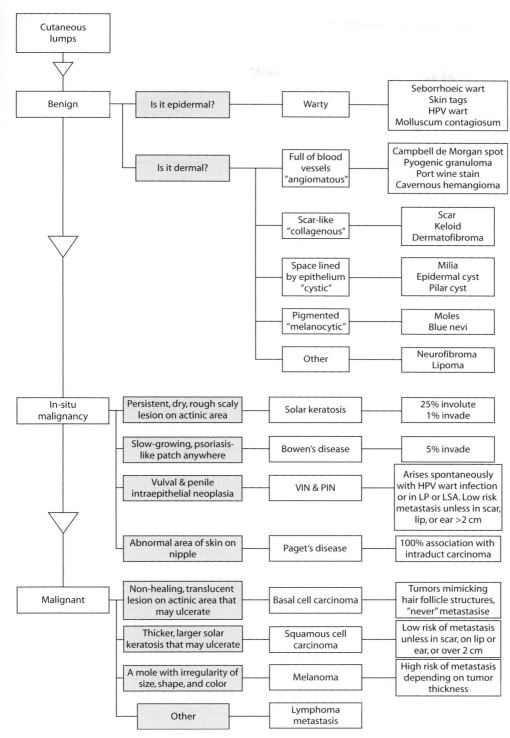

Fig. 16.31. Causes of cutaneous lumps.

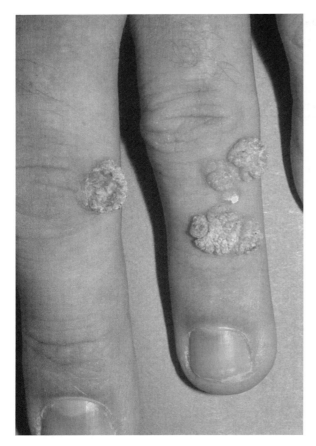

Fig. 16.32. HPV warts on fingers.

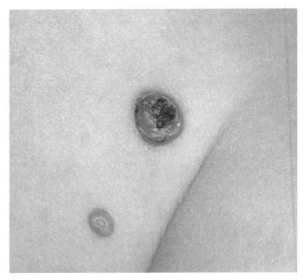

Fig. 16.33. Small and giant molluscum contagiosum lesions showing umbilication.

lay terminology is understood to be a viral wart on the sole of the foot. Wart and warty are also applied to clinically similar lesions not caused by HPV such as the seborrheic wart.

In HPV infection warty proliferation occurs after direct inoculation of material infected with the host-specific HPV into the epidermis (Fig. 16.32).

Walking on wet high-friction floors, shaving, nail-biting, thumb-sucking, or sexual intercourse provide for minor skin abrasion and a portal of entry.

Warts are seen in 10% of school-age children and with increased frequency in immunosuppressed patients. On the fingers they appear as skin-colored papules with a rough irregular surface. On the face they tend to be filiform (finger-like). On the feet they tend to occur on the weight-bearing surfaces mimicking corns. Occasionally, they cover a large area of the sole or heel and are called mosaic warts.

Two-thirds of warts resolve spontaneously within 2 years. Topical salicylic acid, used daily after the wart

has been rubbed or pared down, can achieve similar results in 3 months. Freezing with liquid nitrogen (cryotherapy) confers no more benefit than salicylic acid and is painful. For adults, cryotherapy, curettage if single, topical imiquimod, and intra-lesional bleomycin are used.

Infection with the **molluscum contagiosum** virus produces a different-looking wart (Fig. 16.33). The lesions are waxy, skin-colored umbilicated papules, found on the trunk and extremities in children. Each papule contains hundreds of virions which when shed can result in autoinoculation or infection of other children sharing baths or towels. The infection normally lasts 6–12 months until cell-mediated immunity clears the eruption spontaneously. In an adult it is usually on the face or, through sexual transmission, on the genitalia.

It is common in immunocompromised individuals, mostly on the face and beard area.

There is no specific treatment but cryotherapy is helpful in the adult. In HIV the infection usually clears when the CD4 count rises.

Seborrheic warts are benign epithelial proliferations occurring with increasing frequency with age. They are found on the skin where sebaceous glands are most dense, i.e. head and upper trunk. Often starting as light brown macules, they slowly thicken, become quite large, darken and sometimes are black (Fig. 16.34). They may itch and become erythematous and inflamed. Cryotherapy and curettage are standard treatments.

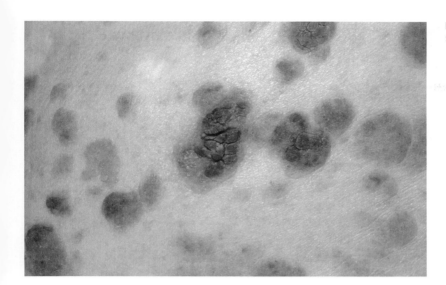

Fig. 16.34. Different expressions of seborrheic warts.

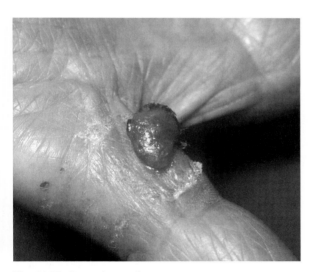

Fig. 16.35. Pyogenic granuloma.

Lumps in the dermis usually have the epidermis stretched over the top. A red-bluish color will usually denote the presence of blood in blood vessels. **Campbell de Morgan spots** are benign, small angiomas present in everybody as small bright-red dots on the trunk, they gradually enlarge with age.

A **pyogenic granuloma** is an uncontrolled, benign proliferation of primitive blood vessels in response to trauma. It is often crusted or covered with serous exudate (Fig. 16.35) and when knocked bleeds uncontrollably, a strong diagnostic pointer. It is benign and with time fibroses but that might take several months.

Treatment is curettage or excision ensuring destruction of the underlying feeding vessel to prevent recurrence.

Port wine stains and **cavernous hemangiomas** are developmental abnormalities of blood vessels. Port wine stains are present at birth and often become darker with age. Pulsed dye laser is very effective at diminishing the color and making camouflage creams more effective. Cavernous hemangiomas may be present at birth or appear on the skin in the first 2–3 months. They start as skin lumps, which go red, enlarge, and then fibrose and involute over several years. Laser treatment early on does not improve the eventual scar.

Many wounds heal with thick scars, which then involute, and it is impossible to say whether or not this will develop into a **keloid**. Scars and keloids are usually linear and skin colored although the early ones may be erythematous. Keloids can be very itchy. They are more frequent in Afro-Caribbean skin but also more frequent in all races over the sternum, deltoid area, and upper lip. Removal of benign skin lesions in these areas therefore needs good justification. Occlusion with steroid tape and silicone gel, intralesional injection with steroid, or excision followed by intralesional steroid and/or radiotherapy are standard treatments. The recurrence rate is around 50%.

Dermatofibromas are commonly seen as single or multiple lesions on the limbs of young females. They exist as a little button of fibrosis underneath the epidermis and if this button is pushed to one side the overlying epidermis is dimpled because it is tethered to the epidermis.

Dermatofibromas are benign and probably result from insect bites. If possible, excision is avoided, as scars on the convex surfaces of limbs tend to widen with age.

A **cyst** is a space lined by epithelium. **Milia** are tiny epidermal keratin cysts found on the cheeks sometimes after sun exposure. They arise in primitive hair follicles and can be enucleated with a sterile needle.

Most **epidermal cysts** arise secondary to acne on the face, neck, and back. They may become inflamed, swell up, and become tender from leakage of contents or secondary infection.

The term **sebaceous cyst** is a misnomer. They are derived from hair follicles and are lined by hair follicle epithelium and are thus pilar cysts. They are familial, autosomal dominant, and occur most commonly on the scalp and head. As with epidermal cysts, excision is more difficult if they have been inflamed.

The majority of **moles** appear on the skin during childhood and teenage years. During growth spurts they may appear for the first time, enlarge, or darken as part of their natural growth pattern. Ultraviolet radiation (UVR) is the major trigger to malignancy and moles should be protected, particularly from short bursts of burning sun exposure. A family history of **melanoma** is the strongest risk factor. Less strong are fair skin and blue eyes, multiple sun exposures during childhood, and previous radiotherapy and sunbed use. If a mole increases in area over 2 or 3 months, develops irregular or notched edges and irregular colors it needs expert assessment. Important features are highlighted in the ABCD screening classification (see below).

Neurofibromas are soft polypoid tumors developing during adolescence and young adulthood. The axillae should be examined for freckling and the skin for café au lait spots found in neurofibromatosis.

Lipomas are often familial and present as slowly growing lumps sometimes tender on limbs or trunk.

In-situ malignancy

There are various patterns of cutaneous *in-situ* epidermal malignancy each appearing slightly different. Histologically, the tumors remain confined to the epidermis and have not broken through the basement membrane.

Repeated exposure over 20–30 years to UVR can produce abnormal clones of keratinocyte-derived cells in the epidermis. These **solar keratoses** are persistent, dry, rough scaly lesions on an erythematous

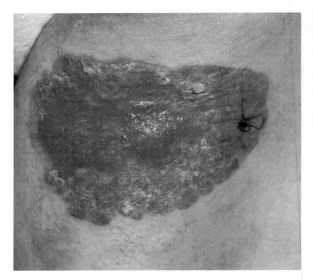

Fig. 16.36. A large patch of Bowen's disease.

background on face and other sun-exposed areas. They are better felt than seen. Many involute spontaneously and the risk of invasion is small. Cryotherapy or the application of 5-fluorouracil, imiquimod, or a non-steroidal anti-inflammatory cream are all useful methods of treatment.

A single psoriasis-like patch is **Bowen's disease** until proved otherwise (Fig. 16.36). This is a slightly different *in-situ* malignancy histologically where the epidermal cells are more dysplastic. This correlates with a slightly higher rate of invasion. There is sometimes some overlap between Bowen's disease and solar keratosis, especially on the legs of older women who have worn skirts all their lives and thus had their lower legs exposed to UVR. The best treatment is curettage because it is less damaging than cryotherapy and allows healing to occur much more quickly.

Vulval intraepithelial neoplasia (VIN) often goes with cervical carcinoma-in-situ and likewise might be associated with HPV infection. VIN might also arise in longstanding genital lichen planus or lichen sclerosus. Invasive carcinoma risk is high because it can spread rapidly to adjacent lymph nodes. Penile intraepithelial neoplasia (PIN) is more common in HIV. Both VIN and PIN treatment should be adequate to prevent invasion.

An abnormal area of skin localized to one nipple with redness, scaling, and perhaps discharge is **Paget's disease**. This *in-situ* intraduct carcinoma on the skin is always associated with an underlying intraduct

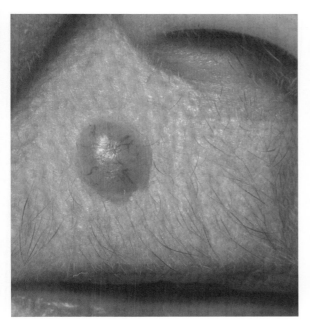

Fig. 16.37. A basal cell carcinoma.

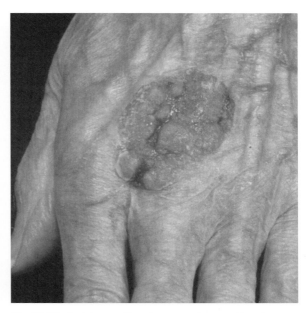

Fig. 16.38. Squamous cell carcinoma on dorsum of hand.

breast carcinoma. The differential diagnosis is atopic nipple eczema.

Malignant lumps

Basal cell carcinoma (BCC) is the commonest non-melanoma skin cancer. It is derived from keratinocytes and grows in patterns mimicking hair follicle structures. It occurs most commonly on the face and UVR exposure is the most important trigger. Individual lesions are translucent rather than pearly and show as non-healing lesions that gradually enlarge and may ulcerate (Fig. 16.37).

The translucent edge is lost if there is more stroma in the tumor and then the clinical edge does not correlate with the histologic edge and the lesion may look more like a scar. BCCs rarely metastasize but some infiltrate locally necessitating removal of large areas, validating the lay term " rodent ulcer."

Squamous cell carcinomas (SCC) are skin-colored and thicker and larger than a solar keratosis. As with BCCs they slowly and steadily enlarge and may ulcerate (Fig. 16.38). They have a much higher risk of metastasizing than BCCs, especially if they have developed in a chronic traumatized area such as a non-healing sinus, or are on a lip or ear, or are over 2 cm in size.

Small, well-demarcated BCCs can be treated with cryotherapy or curettage but standard treatment for BCC and SCC is excision with primary closure or secondary closure with a flap or graft.

Radiotherapy requires more hospital visits and produces a poorer scar that worsens with time. It is not used in younger patients.

Individuals with *in-situ* or invasive malignancy need standard advice to minimize sun exposure, self-check their skin, and stop smoking.

Renal and other organ transplantation has been associated with an increase of skin cancer because of immunosuppression. Ten to fifty percent of patients develop at least one skin cancer within 10 years of transplant. SCCs predominate and may become aggressive. Meticulous attention to sun protection with minimum immunosuppression is warranted.

Malignant melanoma

A tumor derived from melanocytes. Incidence world-wide has increased during the last 50 years and is 35 per 100 000 in Australia. It is one of the commoner causes of death in the 20–30 age group. The compulsion for a sun-tanned skin and the ease of travel are two main factors.

Melanomas may arise in a long-standing mole or *de novo*. They may start as a flat pigmented spot and then develop a nodule (Fig. 16.39) or arise as a nodule.

A convenient diagnostic aid for patient and doctor to decide whether a mole might be melanoma is the ABCD mnemonic:

519

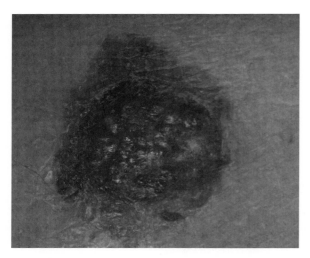

Fig. 16.39. Nodular malignant melanoma arising from a superficial spreading component.

(1) A is for asymmetry; one half should be the mirror image of the other half.
(2) B refers to border; irregular or notched margins are highly suspicious.
(3) C refers to irregularity of color.
(4) D refers to diameter; over 5 mm is the guideline.

This static guide does not take into account the fact that the mole is likely to have been steadily changing over recent months, the fifth important point.

The majority of melanomas exhibit these features as do many moles. Their importance is as a screening for referral to experts and early diagnosis. Breslow thickness is measured histologically from the stratum corneum to the deepest visible melanoma cell. The thinner the melanoma, the better the cure rate. Surgery is the only curative treatment. *In situ* melanomas excised with a 0.5 cm excision result in a 99% cure. Melanomas 1 mm thick are excised with a 1 cm excision producing 95% 5-year survival. Melanomas 4 mm thick are excised with a 2 cm excision margin with only 45% 5-year survival.

Prevention campaigns in the media and on the beach to emphasize sun protection and ABCD screening for early detection have reduced incidence and mortality in Australia.

Individuals who have had a melanoma need life-long monitoring of other moles and appropriate sun avoidance.

Further reading

Buxton P, Morris-Jones R. *ABC of Dermatology*, Wiley-Blackwell Publishing, BMJ Books, 2009.

Dawber R P, Sinclair R D. Hirsuties. *Clin Dermatol* 2001; **19**, 189–199.

Mann M, Berk D, Popkin D, Bayliss S. *Handbook of Dermatology. A Practical Manual*, Wiley-Blackwell Publishing 2009.

Twycross R, Greaves M W, Handwerker H, *et al.* Itch: scratching more than the surface. *Q J Med* 2003; **96**, 7–26.

Contents

Lymph node enlargement

Primary sites of production of lymphoid cells in humans are the thymus (site of T-cell production) and bone marrow (site of B-cell production), whilst secondary sites where cells are exposed to antigen and undergo proliferation and differentiation are the spleen, lymph nodes, and Peyer's patches in the small intestine. Reactive lymphoid tissue in the gut, skin, and respiratory mucosa occurs in response to infection or inflammation.

Clinical features

The differential diagnosis lies in infection, inflammation, and neoplasia. The age, occupation, and social circumstances of the patient are important clues to the underlying diagnosis, as are the character of the lymph node mass and the rate of growth. Pain is an unusual feature in lymphoma and there is a lack of associated signs of inflammation such as hyper-erythema and warmth. However, the rapid growth of tumor in a node may cause expansion and stretching of the lymph node capsule where nerve fibers are carried, or outstripping of new blood vessel formation, leading to cell death and necrosis, and pain from inflammation in the node. Inflammation and pain also occur secondary to pyogenic infection. An unusual, unexplained but well-described symptom in Hodgkin's disease is pain in nodes after drinking alcohol.

Examination provides important clinical clues to the etiology (Figs 17.1, 17.2). Nodes should be specifically sought around Waldeyer's ring and sites such as the epitrochlear, pre-auricular, and post-popliteal regions. An infective focus or primary tumor in the area drained by the node should be sought in localized lymphadenopathy. Lymphomatous nodes are usually rubbery and discrete, while those in metastatic spread from carcinoma are hard and matted. Lymph node enlargement secondary to local infection, e.g. a septic wound, is confined to the drainage site of the focus or may be generalized in systemic infections, e.g. glandular fever. These nodes are generally tender and "fleshy" to the touch and discrete unless the nodes have undergone frank suppuration, e.g. tuberculosis. Lymphoma is characterized by loco-regional or generalized lymph node enlargement.

Patients with early-stage lymphoma may have no systemic symptoms, but these may develop in more advanced disease with release of cytokines produced by the tumor. The symptoms are non-specific and take the form of weight loss greater than 10% of body weight in less than 6 months and fever and night sweats significant enough to require the patient to change their night wear or bed linen. These "B" symptoms are important because their presence is of important prognostic significance and they should be sought by direct questioning. Pruritis is a symptom that is often reported with lymphoma, but lacks prognostic significance.

On examination, evidence of involvement of other organs or end-organ damage should be sought to exclude non-malignant causes of the lymphadenopathy or evidence of more widespread disease. The presence of a butterfly rash over the face, lid-lag,

Fig. 17.1. Clinical algorithm.

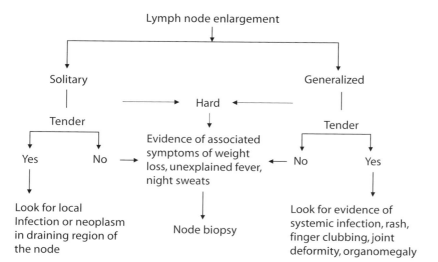

Lymph node enlargement

Solitary → Generalized

Tender → Hard ← Tender

Yes → No → Evidence of associated symptoms of weight loss, unexplained fever, night sweats ← No → Yes

Look for local Infection or neoplasm in draining region of the node

Node biopsy

Look for evidence of systemic infection, rash, finger clubbing, joint deformity, organomegaly

Patients presenting with an enlarged lymph node should be examined to assess whether it is localized or systemic, tender, or associated with other clinical symptoms or signs.

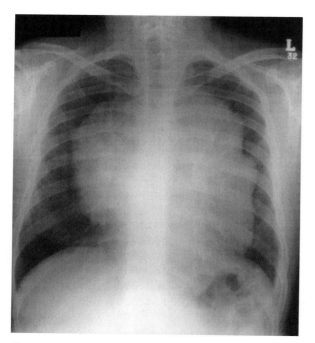

Fig. 17.2. Patient presenting with a cough and large anterior mediastinal mass on plain X-ray.

or finger clubbing may provide important clues for the underlying diagnosis of SLE, thyrotoxicosis, or bronchogenic carcinoma, respectively. Hepatosplenomegaly is a sign of advanced disease in lymphoma, although it is also seen commonly in many other disorders.

Pathology

Lymph nodes are composed of two types of lymphocytes, bursa derived (B cells) and thymus derived (T cells); the former sited in the germinal center and the mantle zone or cortex and the latter mainly in the paracortex (Fig. 17.3). The medullary cords are composed primarily of transformed lymphocytes and plasma cells. T and B lymphocytes develop from a common pluripotent stem cell under the influence of cytokines (Fig. 17.4). Normal T lymphocytes recognize an antigen as "foreign" and destroy it directly by the release of enzymes or indirectly by releasing cytokines that up-regulate other effector cell defense mechanisms. Normal activated B cells produce antibodies that bind to receptors on foreign cells and damage the cell through the activation of complement. Histologic diagnosis depends upon identifying the abnormal cell type and its distribution within the node architecture (Table 17.1). A variety of predisposing causes give rise to a disparate number of lymphoproliferative disorders (Table 17.2). Herpes and Epstein–Barr viruses are common human infections causing upper respiratory tract infection with sore throat and cervical lymphadenopathy. They are highly trophic for lymphocytes and are eradicated by a cytotoxic T-cell response that results in a persistent latent infection with the virus. HIV increasingly is seen as a predisposing cause of lymphoma. It can produce both T- and B-cell lymphoma and Hodgkin's disease.

Lymphoma produces a wide variety of histopathologic patterns dependent upon the type of lymphoma

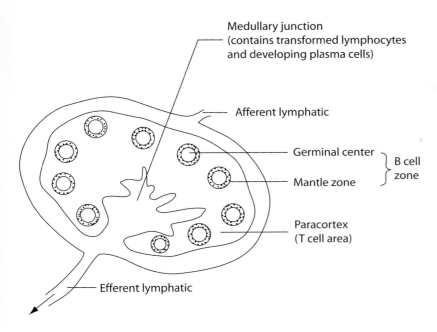

Medullary junction
(contains transformed lymphocytes
and developing plasma cells)

Afferent lymphatic

Germinal center ⎤
          ⎬ B cell zone
Mantle zone ⎦

Paracortex
(T cell area)

Efferent lymphatic

Fig. 17.3. Histologic section of normal lymph node. Lymph flows into the node through the afferent lymphatic and radiates through central sinuses to collect in the efferent lymphatic.

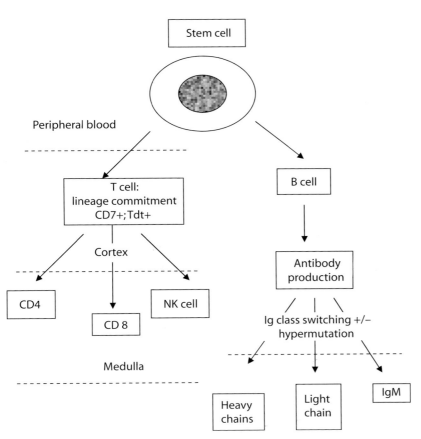

Stem cell

Peripheral blood

T cell:
lineage commitment
CD7+;Tdt+

B cell

Cortex

CD4

CD 8

NK cell

Antibody
production

Ig class switching +/−
hypermutation

Medulla

Heavy
chains

Light
chain

IgM

Fig. 17.4. T and B lymphocytes arise from a common stem cell precursor arising in the bone marrow and circulating in the peripheral blood. Stem cells enter the thymus and undergo rearrangement of the gamma/delta (*TCR1*) genes and subsequently the alpha/beta (*TCR2*) genes. Cells undergo positive and negative selection before passing into the thymic medulla and subsequently passing into the peripheral blood as mature T cells.

Table 17.1. Histologic features distinguishing a reactive and malignant lymphocytic infiltrate

Reactive infiltrate	Malignant infiltrate
<ul><li>Intertrabecular lymphocytes</li><li>Polymorphous infiltrate</li><li>Occasional germinal centers</li><li>Fibrosis unusual</li><li>Mixture of B/T cells</li></ul>	<ul><li>Peri −/+ intertrabecular lymphocytes</li><li>Homogeneous infiltrate</li><li>Germinal centers rare</li><li>+/− fibrosis</li><li>Predominance of B or T cells</li></ul>

Note:
Morphologic distinction between routine and malignant lymphocytic infiltrates may be difficult and should be interpreted in conjunction with the clinical features. Special stains, immunophenotyping, and cytogenetics analysis are helpful in making a definitive diagnosis.

Table 17.2. Causes of lymphadenopathy

Localized	
Infection	Pyogenic or non-pyogenic
	Syphilis, Chlamydia, Yersinia (granuloma inguinali when localized to the groin)
Malignant	Lymphoma
	Hodgkin's disease
	Non-Hodgkin's lymphoma
	Metastatic carcinomatosis, e.g. carcinoma of the stomach

Systemic

Infection		
Bacterial	Syphilis, Chlamydia, Yersinia (generalized in secondary infection)
	Cat scratch fever
	Tuberculosis
	Brucellosis
	Kikuchi's syndrome
Viral	Epstein–Barr virus (glandular fever)
	Cytomegalovirus
	HIV
	Rubella
	Adenovirus
Fungal	Histoplasmosis
Protozoal	Toxoplasmosis

Immunologic

Systemic lupus erythematosus
Rheumatoid arthritis
Sarcoidosis
Thyrotoxicosis

Reactive

Dermatopathic (secondary to skin disorders)
Kawasaki disease

Malignant

Non-Hodgkin's lymphoma
- B cell
- T cell
- NK cell
Hodgkin's disease
Chronic myeloid leukemia
Acute leukemia
Acute lymphocytic
Acute myeloid

process. Immunophenotyping of the node should be used to define the abnormal cell involved and confirm a clonal population of cells. Cytogenetic analysis is increasingly important to classify lymphoma and new technologies such as genomics and proteomics are producing disease "signatures," which are likely to be powerful tools in the future.

Investigations

A full blood count and blood film is mandatory in the investigation of lymphadenopathy. The white blood cell count may show a neutrophilia induced by a pyogenic infection or a lymphocytosis with atypical circulating lymphocytes in a lymphoproliferative disorder. Flow cytometry can identify the cause of lymphocytosis and may obviate the need for a node biopsy in CLL and other lymphoproliferative disorders. Cytopenias may be due to bone marrow infiltration in late-stage malignancy or secondary to immune destruction as a complication in autoimmune disorders. A biochemical screen will reveal renal or liver dysfunction, and elevation of lactate dehydrogenase (LDH), a ubiquitous enzyme found in all nucleated cells, is an important prognostic factor in lymphoma. Tissue culture and viral serology looking particularly for evidence of toxoplasmosis, cytomegalovirus, and herpes virus infections are important if infection is suspected from the clinical history. A lymph node biopsy with histologic immunophenotypic, cytogenetic, and molecular markers is needed to confirm the diagnosis of lymphoma.

Infection

The primary role of lymph nodes is to restrict the spread of infection. Infection may be focal or systemic and so the lymphadenopathy may be loco-regional or generalized. Pyogenic infection such as bacterial infection of a hand wound will produce epitrochlear node enlargement, or a treponemal infection inguinal lymphadenopathy. HIV or cytomegalovirus, on the other hand, will induce disseminated lymphadenopathy. In the history specific enquiry should be made of contact with animals (cat-scratch fever, toxoplasmosis)

Table 17.3. Etiology of lymphoproliferative disorders

Infection	
Helicobacter	[Malt lymphoma]
Epstein–Barr virus	[Burkitt's lymphoma]
HTLV-1	[Acute T-lymphoblastic lymphoma]
HHVS 8	[Castleman's disease]
HIV	[B- and T-cell high grade lymphoma]

Immunodeficiency

Hereditary
    Ataxia telangiectasia
    Common variable immunodeficiency
    Severe combined immune deficiency
    Wiskott–Aldrich syndrome

Acquired
    Post-organ transplantation
    Autoimmune disorders, e.g. Sjögren's syndrome
    Celiac disease

Note:
Most cases of lymphoproliferative disorders are unrelated to any predisposing cause, but infection and immunodeficiency are the most common causes when present.

Table 17.4. Lymphoma assessment

- Clinical examination
- Hematological evaluation
  - Hb
  - ESR
- Biochemical evaluation
  - LDH
  - LFT
- Bone marrow aspirate and trephine
- CT scanning

Note:
When assessing a patient with lymphoma for the extent of disease, account should be taken of clinical, pathologic, and radiologic measurements of the disease bulk.

and foreign travel (histoplasmosis, HIV). Common infections to exclude in the differential diagnosis of lymphadenopathy are shown in Table 17.3.

Microscopically, infection leads to discrete enlargement of the lymph node follicles with an inflammatory cell infiltrate and micro-abscesses if there is pyogenic suppuration. The node should be stained for the suspected organism (e.g. tuberculosis). The changes revert to normal with resolution of the infection.

Treatment should be directed at the underlying cause.

Autoimmune disorders

Patients are generally female and usually present in their 30s or 40s with generalized painless lymphadenopathy. There may also be a history of rash and joint pains, or swelling or ophthalmological disturbances. Specific enquiry should be made for systemic disorders such as joint problems, skin rashes, and ophthalmic problems. The diagnosis rests on clinical findings and serologic investigations. Lymph node biopsy is rarely necessary.

Lymphoma

Clinical features

The commonest presentation is with symmetric, painless lymphadenopathy. Constitutional symptoms of fever, weight loss, and night sweats imply a more advanced stage. Involvement of liver and spleen resulting in organomegaly occurs as the disease progresses; later, there may be bone marrow infiltration with myelosuppression and anemia causing lethargy, weakness, and shortness of breath. Any organ can be involved but skin tends to be associated more with T-cell lymphomas, whilst brain involvement is more frequent with HIV-associated tumors.

Epidemiology

The non-Hodgkin's lymphomas account for approximately 35% of all hematological malignancies with a crude incidence rate of 30 per 100 000 of the population. Malignant transformation may arise *de novo* or secondary to infection or immunosuppression (Table 17.13).

Pathology

Hodgkin's disease tends to spread from an initial focus through contiguous sites, but non-Hodgkin's lymphoma is less predictable. In the former, the disease usually starts in the left cervical region and spreads via neighboring nodal groups to involve the liver, spleen and, at a late stage, bone marrow. In follicular and small lymphocytic lymphomas, the bone marrow is involved early, but this occurs as a late event in diffuse high grade lymphomas.

Diagnosis

Initial investigations should be directed at establishing the diagnosis (Table 17.4) and subsequently staging the disease, which will inform decisions on optimum therapy and likely prognosis. Preliminary evaluation must include a full blood count, liver function test, calcium and phosphate, uric acid, lactate dehyrogenase, and urea and electrolytes. Some low-grade lymphomas secrete a paraprotein, and serum protein electrophoresis should be performed as this can be measured serially to assess response to treatment and monitor relapse.

Surgical node biopsy remains the preferred option to obtain histologic material for diagnosis, but if surgery is potentially difficult or a specimen needs to be obtained to confirm a previous diagnosis, a fine needle aspirate (FNA) may suffice. Non-specific findings from an FNA must be confirmed with an open biopsy where possible. The histologic specimen should be examined morphologically to recognize abnormalities of the lymph node micro-architecture and immunophenotypically using a panel of monoclonal antibodies to define the cell of origin. Other investigations include cytogenetics and molecular studies to monitor treatment and identify residual disease post-treatment. Rearrangements of the immunoglobulin or T-cell receptor gene loci lead to a number of non-random chromosomal breakpoints that may be etiologically responsible for the development or evolution of lymphoproliferative disease (Table 17.5).

Table 17.5. Genetic abnormalities in lymphoproliferative disorders

Numerical abnormalities	
Deletion	– 13q –
Amplification	– Trisomy 12 –
Mutations	
Activating	– ras
Inactivating	– rbl
Translocations	
Cyclin D1	– t(11:14)
BCL2	– t(14:18)
c–myc	– t(8:14)

Staging Defining the extent, or Ann-Arbor stage, of disease provides a prognostic parameter and informs therapeutic decision making, in particular whether or not local radiotherapy is appropriate, and the need for systemic treatment. Bone marrow involvement may be patchy, and increasing the number of aspirates can increase the positivity rate. A trephine biopsy is performed to define the architecture of the marrow and to aid the staging process, assess marrow reserve, and look for co-morbid marrow conditions that might compromise the use of chemotherapy. Patients are divided into three stages and further sub-divided into A or B, dependent upon the presence or absence of fever, night sweats, or weight loss (Table 17.6).

Imaging The recent development of new and improved radiologic and nuclear medicine imaging techniques has eliminated the need for surgical intervention to staged patients. Computerized tomography (CT) scanning of the head, neck, chest, abdomen, and pelvis should be performed to define the extent of lymphadenopathy and involvement of other organs. CT may fail to identify small volume nodal disease whilst splenic, hepatic, and extranodal disease may also be difficult to identify using CT. Positron emission tomography (PET) scanning is a functional study that measures the uptake of an isotope into the tumor and can be used to assess disease activity particularly in residual masses.

Prognostic factors

The International Prognostic Index (IPI) is a scoring system for non-Hodgkin's lymphoma utilizing the extent of disease, age, and performance status. Cellular variables such as bcl-2 expression, cell proliferation rate, p53 expression and mutation and bcl-6 rearrangements

Table 17.6. Ann-Arbor lymphoma staging system

Stage I	Localized to a single node or group of nodes
IE	One extralymphatic (E) organ or site
Stage II	Two or more lymph nodes confined to one side of the diaphragm
IIE	One extralymphatic organ or site (localized) in addition to criteria for stage II
Stage III	Two or more lymph nodes on both sides of the diaphragm
IIIE	One extralymphatic organ or site (localized) in addition to criteria for stage III
IIIS	Spleen (S) in addition to criteria for stage III
IIISE	Spleen and one extralymphatic organ or site (localized) in addition to criteria for stage III
Stage IV	Spleen and extranodal disease with or without lymph node involvement

Note:
Measurement of disease bulk as assessed by the stage of disease is a powerful prognostic indicator and is used to select whether local or systemic therapy should be delivered.

Table 17.7. Hodgkin's disease prognostic factor score

Score 1 for:
- Serum albumin <40
- Hemoglobin <10.5
- Male sex
- Stage IV disease
- Age >45 yrs
- WCC >15
- Lymphocytes <0.6 or <8% of WCC

Note:
In 1996 an international study group identified seven prognostic factors that predicted survival. The 5-year freedom from progression is directly related to the number of factors present and is 84% in patients with 0 factors and 42% for those with five or more factors present.

are likely to become more important in predicting outcomes. The Hasenclever Score is a similar system designed for Hodgkin's disease that identifies seven factors dividing patients into five prognostic groups by scoring 1 point for each of the factors identified (Table 17.7).

Classification

The classification of lymphoma has been changed repeatedly over 75 years, as new ways of identifying the cell of origin have become available. The WHO Classification designed in 1995 is currently the most widely accepted classification system (Tables 17.8 and 17.9).

Precursor cell neoplasms

These neoplasms arise from cells early in their ontogeny and are composed of the T- and B-cell lymphoblastic lymphomas and acute lymphoblastic leukemia (ALL).

The mature cell lymphomas/leukemias

The term "mature" identifies a cell that has progressed along the maturation pathway to an end stage cell and relates to the clinical behavior of the tumor. The histologic architecture of the node is a helpful indicator in identifying this type of tumor. The mature B-cell lymphomas can be divided into 11 subcategories based upon their different investigational characteristics.

Diffuse large B-cell lymphoma and Burkitt-like lymphoma

These are two clinical entities with markedly varied outcomes. High-grade lymphomas present as a nodal or extranodal mass that increases rapidly in size, sometimes over the course of days in Burkitt's lymphoma (Fig. 17.5), and may be associated with systemic symptoms of fever, sweats, and weight loss. Diffuse

Table 17.8. World Health Organization (WHO) classification of non-Hodgkin's lymphoma

B cell
- Precursor B cell
- Peripheral B cell
- Chronic lymphocytic leukemia/Small lymphocytic lymphoma
- Prolymphocytic leukemia
- Lymphoplasmacytic lymphoma
- Mantle cell lymphoma
- Follicular lymphoma
- Marginal zone lymphoma of mucosa associated lymphoid tissue (MALT) type
- Nodal marginal zone lymphoma with/without monocytoid B cells
- Splenic marginal zone lymphoma
- Hairy cell leukemia
- Diffuse large cell lymphoma
- Mediastinal (thymic); intravascular; primary effusion
- Burkitt's lymphoma
- Endemic; sporadic; immunodeficiency associated; atypical

T cell
- Precursor T cell
- Peripheral T cell
- T-prolymphocytic leukemia
- T-large granular lymphocytic leukemia
- Aggressive NK-cell leukemia
- T/NK-cell lymphoma
- Mycosis fungoides
- Sezary syndrome
- Angioimmunoblastic T-cell lymphoma
- Peripheral T-cell lymphoma (unspecified)
- Adult T-cell lymphoma/leukemia (HTLV−1+)
- Anaplastic large cell lymphoma
- Primary cutaneous anaplastic large cell lymphoma
- Subcutaneous panniculitis-like T-cell lymphoma
- Enteropathy-type T-cell lymphoma
- Hepatosplenic gamma/delta T-cell lymphoma

NK cell

Table 17.9. World Health Organization (WHO) classification of Hodgkin's lymphoma

- Lymphocyte predominant
- Classical:
  - Nodular sclerotic
  - Mixed cellularity
  - Lymphocyte depleted
  - Lymphocyte rich (nodular)

large B-cell lymphomas (DLBCL) may arise from transformation of an underlying indolent lymphoma, when the outcome is poor. Burkitt's lymphoma may be either the African variety seen commonly in children and young adults in association with EBV infection or the non-African form not associated with EBV and occurring in older patients.

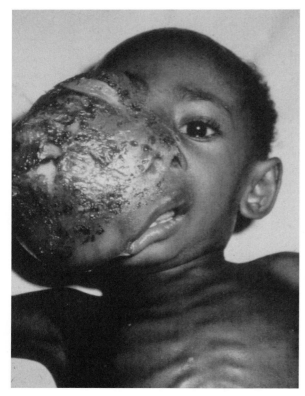

Fig. 17.5. Child with African type Burkitt's lymphoma presenting with a mass arising from the jaw. Other common sites include the abdominal viscera, particularly the kidneys. This variant rarely affects the lymph nodes, spleen, or bone marrow in contrast to the endemic, sporadic, non-African variant.

Morphologically, there is infiltration and destruction of the nodal architecture or other tissues by large lymphoid cells consisting of centroblasts and immunoblasts. The immunophenotype of diffuse large B-cell lymphoma is variable, indicating that this is a heterogenous group of tumors. Transformed follicle center lymphomas typically have a germinal center cell phenotype. The others have a post-germinal center phenotype being IgD, sIg, CD23, and CD5 negative.

Anaplastic large-cell lymphoma (ALCL)

This entity expresses neither B- nor T-cell markers and was previously defined on the basis of its cytology and the expression of CD30. The t(2;5) translocation has recently been identified giving rise to the expression of the anaplastic lymphoma kinase (ALK) protein. This variant tends to involve lymph nodes and extranodal sites in children and young adults and, although aggressive, carries a good prognosis with appropriate therapy. t(2;5) (ALK) negative cases do less well and may represent a different condition. Primary cutaneous anaplastic large cell lymphoma is ALK negative and closely related to the benign disorder lymphomatoid papulosis.

Hodgkin's disease

The cell of origin in Hodgkin's disease (HD) remains contentious, but recent evidence supports this being a B cell. It is sub-classified into lymphocyte predominant and classical variants that clinically behave differently. Classical HD is sub-divided into four sub-types that have different histo-morphologic characteristics (Table 17.9) and different clinical presentations.

Management

For early stage mature cell lymphomas without evidence of end-organ damage a "wait and watch policy" is advocated. Having established the need for therapeutic intervention the mainstay of treatment is radiotherapy for treating localized Stage I and Stage IIa disease, chemotherapy for more advanced disease. Chemotherapy describes a group of drugs that disrupt DNA replication and activate programmed cell death or apoptosis in tumor cells. Alkylating agents (e.g. cyclophosphamide, chlorambucil, melphalan) are effective in lymphoproliferative disorders either alone or in combination with other agents. The topoisomerase inhibitors, e.g. etoposide, interfere with the stability of the DNA helical structure during mitosis, resulting in the unraveling of the double helix and disruption of DNA replication. The antimetabolites, represented by methotrexate, are dihydrofolate reductase inhibitors that inhibit purine and pyrimidine synthesis. Newer purine analogs (e.g. fludarabine and cladrabine) have been used effectively in patients with low and intermediate grade lymphoma. Vincristine and vinblastine block the mitotic spindle during mitosis and are usually used in combination with other agents. Corticosteroids are active in the treatment of lymphoma and act by directly inducing programmed cell death by up-regulation of pro-apoptotic and down-regulation of anti-apoptotic cellular proteins.

The rapid expansion of our understanding of the pathogenesis at cellular, genetic, and molecular level has led to the development of novel approaches to treatment.

Outcomes

Outcomes for lymphoma vary between sub-types but have improved significantly in the last 25 years. Low-grade follicular lymphoma is probably incurable with conventional treatment, although reduced intensity allogeneic stem cell transplantation has improved disease-free survival and may be curative in a small selected population. Median survival for most patients remains at 7–8 years. Diffuse high-grade lymphoma progresses, untreated, over months but with intensive treatment is potentially curable. Early Stage I and II Hodgkin's disease carries a good prognosis with the 10-year survival being approximately 80%. More advanced stage disease has a less favorable prognosis, although 40%–50% of patients who are eligible for autologous stem cell transplantation achieve long-term disease-free survival and may be cured of their disease. The international prognostic score for advanced Stage III-IVB Hodgkin's disease predicts for progression and survival (Table 17.7).

Chronic low grade lymphoproliferative disorders

Normal B lymphocyte differentiation is characterized by progressive genetic and phenotypic changes with maturation from precursor cell to mature end-stage memory B cell or plasma cell. The different chronic leukemias/lymphomas arise from maturation arrest at different stages. A polyclonal increase in lymphocytes should be distinguished from a monoclonal infiltration by demonstration of immunoglobulin light chain restriction. The tumors arising at these different stages are defined by their immunophenotypic, genetic and molecular "signature" (Fig. 17.6).

Chronic lymphocytic leukemia (CLL)/small lymphocytic lymphoma (SLL)

This is a neoplasm of small round B, and in <10% of cases, T lymphocytes. The term small lymphocytic lymphoma is used to describe those cases that have morphologic and immunophenotypic features of CLL, but do not have circulating tumor cells.

Epidemiology
It is the commonest leukemia in Western Europe and the United States, but is rare in the Orient, being more common in men with a peak age incidence of 65 years. There appears to be an increased risk of disease in first-degree relatives of patients with this condition.

Clinical
Stage 0 disease presents with an isolated lymphocytosis, often identified by chance followed by lymph node enlargement as the disease progresses (Fig. 17.7). Occasional patients complain of fatigue, weight loss, and night sweats or may present with jaundice and symptoms of acute anemia if they develop the complication of autoimmune hemolytic anemia. Painless lymphadenopathy and progressive hepatosplenomegaly typically develop as the disease progresses with bone marrow failure and myelosuppression in the latter stages. Extranodal involvement of the skin, breast, and eye are reported. In 10% of patients the disease may progress to a high grade non-Hodgkin's lymphoma (Richter's syndrome), in 20% to a prolymphocytic leukemia phase, and in rare cases to a T-cell or NK-cell lymphoma. The median survival of such patients is significantly reduced.

Diagnosis
The disease is characterized by small monomorphic lymphocytic bone marrow infiltration and lymphocytosis in peripheral blood (Rai stage 0). As the disease progresses, lymphadenopathy (Rai stage 1), hepatosplenomegaly (Rai stage 2), anemia (Rai Stage 3), and thrombocytopenia (Rai Stage 4) develop. Patients

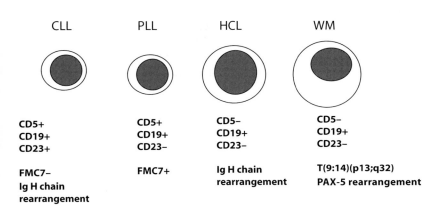

Fig. 17.6. B lymphocytes express different antigens at different stages of maturation. By using a panel of monoclonal antibodies, sub-types of lymphoma are defined according to the cell of origin.

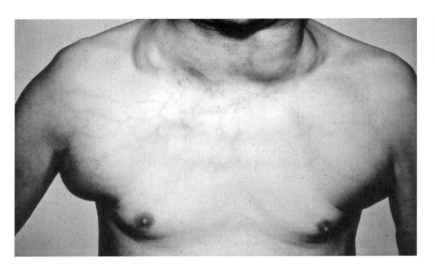

Fig. 17.7. Widespread lymphadenopathy involving the cervical and axillary nodes in a patient presenting with chronic lymphocytic leukemia.

should have a direct antiglobulin test, reticulocyte count, and liver function tests to identify the complication of hemolytic anemia. Characteristically, immunoglobulin production is reduced with hypogammaglobulinemia that makes patients susceptible to infection. Peripheral blood flow cytometry is performed to define a clonal population of B or T lymphocytes and distinguish this from infection. Prognostic molecular markers (e.g. ZAP 70) and chromosome abnormalities (e.g. del 17p) can identify patients likely to progress more rapidly and who may benefit from more aggressive treatment.

Treatment and outcomes

Treatment is not always required and should be offered only to people who are symptomatic or have evidence of disease progression, marrow failure, or complications such as hemolytic anemia. The disease generally follows an indolent course, but it is variable and is not curable with conventional treatment. Advanced disease stage and short tumor cell doubling times (<12 months) are predictors of poor outcome. Chemotherapy is indicated for advanced disease, end-organ damage, or complications such as hemolytic anemia.

Waldenstrom's macroglobulinemia
(see Immunosecretory disorders)

Prolymphocytic leukemia (PLL)
This extremely rare condition occurs in <5% of cases of lymphoma. The median age at presentation is 65–70 years with a slight preponderance of males.

There is a very high lymphocytosis in the peripheral blood, often in excess of $200 \times 10^9/l$, with bone marrow infiltration and little or no lymphadenopathy, but massive splenomegaly. The diagnosis is made from the morphologic features on the blood film, the immunophenotypic findings, and the cytogenetic abnormalities that allow it to be distinguished from mantle cell lymphoma.

Hairy cell leukemia (HCL)
This is also a rare lymphoma/leukemia. It occurs at a slightly lower median age than PLL with a marked male to female predominance of 5 : 1. In contrast to PLL, this condition presents clinically with leukopenia and splenomegaly. Morphologically characteristic medium-sized lymphocytes are found in the bone marrow and in small numbers in the circulation. The cytoplasm is abundant and associated with "hairy" projections from the cell wall that characteristically display no chromosome abnormalities.

Treatment
The major clinical problem for these patients results from the effects of anemia, thrombocytopenia, and leukopenia that result in recurrent infections, easy bruising, and bleeding. Splenectomy is effective for the majority of patients but, more recently, excellent responses are reported with the use of 2-chlorodeoxyadenosine (2-CDA) with some patients seemingly cured.

Abnormal hematology investigations
Patients may present initially without symptoms and be found to have abnormal hematology on routine screening. The further investigation of any abnormality will be dependent upon the clinical setting.

Table 17.10. Factors influencing the ESR

(1) Extent of red cell rouleaux formation
(2) Ratio of red cells to plasma (PCV)
(3) Plasma viscosity
(4) Laboratory technical factors
  - ambient temperature
  - bore of tube
  - dilution or otherwise of the blood
  - time over which the test is performed (normally 1 hour)

Note:
The rate of fall of red cells is dependent upon factors relating to the dispersion of red cells, viscosity of the plasma, and technical factors that are standardized in the different methods of estimation.

Table 17.11. History and examination in cases of a raised ESR

History	Examination
Onset and duration of symptoms	Bone tenderness
Visual disturbance	Fundoscopy: retinal hemorrhages
Cough/sputum	Chest signs
Headache	
Parasthesiae/carpal tunnel syndrome	Joint swelling/inflammation
Pain: site, e.g. bone, joint, muscle	
Weight loss (>10% body weight/6 mos)	Skin inflammation
Sweats/rigors	

Note:
A raised ESR may be caused by local or systemic infection, inflammation, or malignancy and evidence for this should be obtained from the history and examination.

High ESR

The erythrocyte sedimentation test (ESR) is a simple, empiric test that measures the rate of fall of red cells through the plasma. It is dependent on a number of interactive factors (Table 17.10) and the normal range is 0–5 mm in men and 0–7 mm in females. The international standard technique used is the Westergren method. The presence of anemia encourages rouleaux formation and alters the PCV that, in turn, accelerates the ESR. Other factors controlling rouleaux formation are fibrinogen, alpha 2, and gamma globulin concentrations.

The history and examination are important in the differential diagnosis of a raised ESR (Table 17.11). Particular attention should be paid to the presence of fever, systemic symptoms, and any local symptoms, in

particular pain (Fig. 17.8). The ESR is moderately raised with certain physiologic changes such as pregnancy and age (it may be raised to 20 mm in individuals over 60 years without obvious cause). In disease states it is a non-specific phenomenon, reflecting changes in plasma protein concentrations, and is of most use in following the course of a known disease. It can be exceptionally high (>100) in paraproteinemic states and polymyalgia rheumatica, whilst in infection, degenerative disorders, and malignancy the level only rarely rises to these levels (Table 17.12). Plasma viscosity is thought to better reflect disease severity than the ESR because it is more specific and is unaffected by sex or age.

Immunosecretory disorders

The immunosecretory disorders comprise a group of diseases characterized by the expansion of a clone of immunoglobulin secreting B cells. Immunoglobulins are glycoproteins secreted by plasma cells and late stage lymphocytes normally as a polyclonal response by the immune system in reaction to an infectious stimulus.

The immunosecretory disorders arise primarily in the bone marrow or, in a minority of patients, in extramedullary tissue and are defined by the type of heavy or light chain paraprotein component present (Table 17.13), the distribution of plasma cell infiltration in the bone marrow or other organs, and the clinical presentation. The diagnosis is suspected by the present of an abnormal paraprotein in the blood. An interesting, but rare, group of lymphoproliferative disorders is characterized by the presence of a diffuse increase of all the immunoglobulins (hyperglobulinemia) (Table 17.13), which is in contrast to the hypo-gammaglobulinemia that is seen in light chain myeloma and non-Hodgkin's lymphoma.

Monoclonal gammopathy of uncertain significance (MGUS)

This is a condition characterized by the presence of an isolated monoclonal paraprotein in the absence of a clonal population of lymphocytes, lytic bone lesions, or evidence of end-organ damage. The incidence of this condition rises steadily with age from 1% at age 50 years to 3% at aged 70 years. In approximately one-third of patients the paraprotein regresses and disappears over time, whilst in a further third the paraprotein levels remain unchanged and the patient will succumb to an unrelated condition. In the

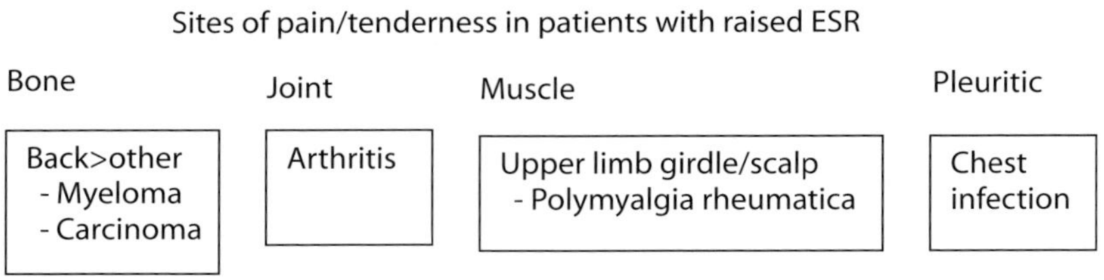

Sites of pain/tenderness in patients with raised ESR

Bone	Joint	Muscle	Pleuritic
Back>other - Myeloma - Carcinoma	Arthritis	Upper limb girdle/scalp - Polymyalgia rheumatica	Chest infection

Fig. 17.8. A raised ESR is a non-specific finding frequently associated with malignancy, inflammation, and infection. Malignancy commonly causes backache, whilst joint pain implies inflammation. Muscle and soft tissue pain is more commonly due to infection or immunologic disorders such as polymyalgia. Chest infection is a common cause of infection and pain is normally due to pleuritic inflammation.

Table 17.12. Causes of a raised ESR

Physiologic	Pregnancy (Oral contraception) Age Anemia
Infection	
Degenerative disorders	Rheumatoid arthritis
Malignancy	Multiple myeloma Waldenstrom's macroglobulinemia Carcinoma Lymphoma
Tissue necrosis? Inflammation	Myocardial infarction Polymyalgia rheumatica
Hypoalbuminemia	Nephrosis
Infusion of high molecular weight dextrans	

Note:
Changes in ESR may a useful indicator of underlying disease and can be used to monitor disease progression. A normal ESR does not exclude organic disease but most acute and chronic infective, degenerative, and neoplastic diseases cause changes in plasma proteins that raise the erythrocyte sedimentation rate.

Table 17.13. Variants of immunosecretory disorders by paraprotein type

Monoclonal gammopathy

IgG; IgA; IgD; light chains:
  Monoclonal gammopathy of uncertain significance (MGUS)
  Plasmacytoma of
  • bone
  • extramedullary plasmacytoma
  Multiple myeloma (MM)
  • Stable disease
  • Progressive disease
  • Free light chains (Bence-Jones protein)
  • Non-secretory
  POEMS – characterized by the presence of
  • Peripheral neuropathy
  • Organomegaly
  • Endocrine dysfunction
  • Monoclonal gammopathy
  • Skin rash
  Plasma cell leukemia (PCL)
  Primary amyloidosis (AL)

IgM
  Waldenstrom's macroglobulinemia (WM)
  Chronic lymphocytic leukemia (CLL)
  Non-Hodgkin's lymphoma

  Heavy chain disease
  • Gamma chain disease (Franklin disease)
  • Alpha chain disease
  • Mu chain disease (Mediterranean fever)

Polyclonal hypergammaglobulinemias
  Castleman's disease
  Angio-immunoblastic lymphoma
  Infection

Note:
Disorders associated with a paraprotein need to be distinguished from those producing a polyclonal increase in immunoglobulins.

remainder of patients the disease progresses to a lymphoproliferative disorder or myeloma with an actuarial risk of approximately 1% per annum. Patients frequently present with an unrelated condition and the abnormality will be detected during routine investigations.

Management

In the absence of disease progression or end-organ damage this condition should not be actively treated. Studies are ongoing to identify those patients at high risk of progression. Patients need to be reassured and monitored for evidence of increasing paraprotein concentrations, organomegaly, or end organ damage, which would lead to the initiation of treatment.

Multiple myeloma
Clinical features

Clinically, patients present with a spectrum of features. Often, there are non-specific symptoms of lethargy, anorexia, and weight loss. Frequently, patients

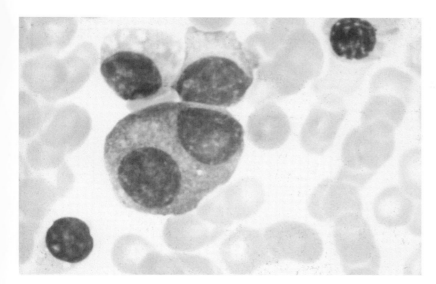

Fig. 17.9. Bone marrow aspirate showing abnormal binucleate plasma cell. The nucleus is eccentrically placed in the cell and has an open chromatin pattern.

will complain of signs and symptoms resulting from bone infiltration, marrow failure, and renal impairment or hypermetabolic syndrome. Back pain is frequent (80%), often with symptoms of cord or nerve compression and fractures through lytic lesions (Fig. 17.10), vomiting, and constipation secondary to hypercalcemia may all be presenting symptoms. Tiredness is commonly associated with metabolic disturbances secondary to renal impairment and anemia. Bone marrow failure may lead to bleeding and recurrent infection. Renal impairment is common and its pathogenesis multifactorial and includes infection, light chain deposition in the glomeruli, dehydration, hyperviscosity, and amyloid deposition.

Epidemiology
Myeloma is a plasma cell malignancy accounting for approximately 1% of all malignancies and 12%–15% of hematologic malignancies. Annual incidence varies in different populations; in the UK it is currently 4 per 100 000, but striking increases have been reported over the last 40 years. Less than 3% of cases occur under the age of 40 years and 70% are over 65 years. The incidence in black males exceeds white males by almost 2 : 1.

Pathology
This disorder is characterized by a neoplastic proliferation of plasma cells (Fig. 17.9) most often in the bone marrow, less frequently in an extramedullary mass most commonly around the nasopharynx. The other two features are the presence of a monoclonal protein

in the serum or urine and lytic lesions in bone. The differential diagnosis of a monoclonal gammopathy is shown in Table 17.13.

Investigations (Table 17.14)
Diagnosis depends upon identifying two of three major criteria:

- paraprotein in serum or urine
- plasmacytosis on bone marrow aspirate and trephine or a plasmacytoma
- lytic bone lesions on plain X-ray (Fig. 17.10) or MRI scan.

Both blood and urine are examined for the presence of a paraprotein because light chain myeloma will be missed in up to 15% of cases where kappa or lambda chains are excreted in urine and do not appear in the blood. Other investigations are directed at establishing the presence of end-organ damage or complications (Table 17.14) and defining prognostic factors (Table 17.15). Translocations of chromosome 14 are not uncommon, in particular with 11q13, 4p16, 8q24, and 16q23. The t(4:14) and del 13 are associated with a poor prognosis.

Management
Patients presenting with renal failure, hypercalcemia, or cord compression should be treated as a medical emergency. Many patients present with asymptomatic or smoldering disease and a paraprotein that is detected routinely that may remain quiescent for years. Such individuals should be managed conservatively

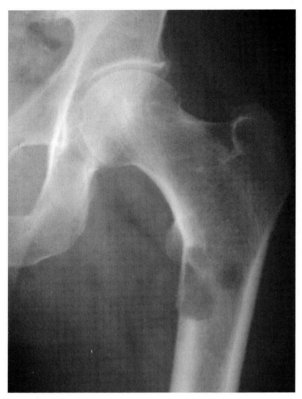

Fig. 17.10. Plain X-ray of femur demonstrating lytic lesions throughout the shaft of the femur and pelvis of a patient with multiple myeloma.

Table 17.14. Multiple myeloma: investigations

Hematologic	Imaging
FBC	Skeletal survey
BM aspirate and trephine	CT scanning
CRP	Magnetic resonance
Serum beta 2 microglobulin	PET scanning
Biochemical:	
Protein electrophoresis and quantitation	
24 hr urine collection for protein analysis	
S Ca/phosphate	
S Urate	
Urea and electrolytes	
Liver function tests	
S creatinine	
S albumin	

Notes:
Technetium bone scan is usually negative (unless there is a fracture) due to inhibition of osteoblast activity.
Investigations for multiple myeloma should be aimed at confirming the diagnosis by identifying a paraprotein in the peripheral blood or urine, plasmacytosis in the bone marrow, and lytic lesions in the skeleton. Hematologic and biochemical abnormalities should also be performed to identify evidence of end-organ damage.

initially and followed up for evidence of disease progression.

Supportive care

Improved supportive care has had a major impact on outcome, improving quality of life, and increasing life expectancy at all stages of the disease. Pain control is important. Anemia can be managed with red cell transfusion or erythropoietin. Infection risk is increased through immunocompromise from disease and treatment with myelosuppressive drugs. Bisphosphonates inhibit osteoclast activity and are used to treat bone disease to reduce hypercalcemia and the risk of fractures. New generation bisphosphonates such as clodronate and zoledronic acid may also have anti-tumor activity.

Induction therapy

The introduction of melphalan as first-line therapy for myeloma more than 30 years ago increased life expectancy from 6 to approximately 36 months. Response rates for melphalan-containing combination

Table 17.15. Poor prognostic factors in multiple myeloma

Clinical
- Age >70 years
- Irreversible renal failure
- Lytic bone lesions

Laboratory
- Hemoglobin <10 gs/dl
- Serum albumin <30 g/l
- Serum beta 2 microglobulin >4mg/l
- Chromosome abnormalities
  Hyperdiploidy
    Trisomy 3, 5, 7, 9, 11, 15
  Non-hyperdiploidy
    Loss of 13q, 16q, 6q
    Translocations
      t(4;14)(p16:q32)
      t14;16)(q32:q23)
      t(6:14)(p21:q32)

Note:
Age, serum albumin, serum beta 2 microglobulin, and renal dysfunction are clinical factors that have consistently been shown to be associated with outcome. Patients fall into two main chromosome groups, hyperdiploid and non-hyperdiploid, that define standard and poor prognostic risk groups, respectively.

regimens are 40%–60% but complete remissions are seen in fewer than 10% of patients. Complete remissions are reported in up to 30% of patients with high dose melphalan or combination chemotherapy and up to 50% with autologous bone marrow transplantation as consolidation treatment. Dexamethasone is useful, particularly for patients with renal failure where chemotherapy administration is compromised by impaired renal excretion.

At least three large international studies have now shown survival benefit for autologous stem cell transplantation in patients aged <70 years. However, patients continue to relapse and the procedure is not considered curative. Allogeneic bone marrow transplantation may be curative in a minority of patients aged <65 years who have an HLA identical sibling donor.

Outcomes
Despite a variety of treatment approaches, multiple myeloma remains incurable. Approximately 15% of patients survive longer then 10 years. Outcome, however, is age dependent, median survival being 19 months in patients aged >65 years and 42 months for those <65.

Waldenstrom's macroglobulinemia
Clinical features
Patients may present initially for investigation with lymphadenopathy or hepatosplenomegaly. Alternatively, they may present with constitutional symptoms, cytopenias(s), or symptoms attributable to the monoclonal protein, e.g. hyperviscosity syndrome, cryoglobulinemia, amyloidosis, or autoimmune phenomena such as peripheral neuropathy and cold agglutinin disease.

Pathology
This is a lymphoplasmacytic lymphoma found in association with an IgM paraprotein.

Epidemiology
It is rare below 50 years and increases in incidence with age.

Investigations
A lymph node biopsy, bone marrow aspiration, and trephine and immunoglobulin electrophoresis and quantitation should be performed to define the disease. A CT scan is used to delineate the extent of lymphadenopathy. Plasma viscosity should be measured to identify hyperviscosity. Cytogenetic studies are normal.

Treatment
Asymptomatic patients with normal or low plasma viscosity (<4) may be monitored expectantly. The standard primary therapy for patients with symptomatic WM has been chemotherapy with alkylating agents with or without steroids. The purine analogs fludarabine and cladribine are used increasingly and the chimeric anti-CD20 antibody, rituximab, has activity and is used in combination with chemotherapy.

Outcome
Overall survival varies between 60 and 106 months.

Heavy chain disease
This is a rare B-cell malignancy associated with the secretion of a monoclonal heavy chain with no associated light chain production. It can be missed because it may not produce the characteristic "spike" on conventional electrophoresis and requires immunoelectrophoresis or immunofixation to identify the paraprotein. Cases present as a variant of lymphoma so that gamma heavy chain disease has characteristics of lymphoplasmacytic lymphoma with lymphadenopathy and lymphocytic infiltration of the bone marrow, Waldeyer's ring, liver and spleen, plus associated autoimmune phenomena and eosinophilia. Alpha heavy chain disease resembles chronic lymphocytic leukemia whilst Mu heavy chain disease is a variant of mucosa-associated lymphoid tissue tumor (MALToma).

Polymyalgia rheumatica
This condition overlaps with giant cell arteritis, the two conditions sometimes occurring together.

Epidemiology
The median age at presentation is 70 years and the condition is rare below 50. It is more common in women, and Caucasians have a higher incidence than other ethnic groups.

Clinical features
Patients present with pain and tenderness of the upper limb girdle or less commonly the hips, whilst visual disturbances, headache, and scalp tenderness or soreness of the jaw are frequent complaints in giant cell arteritis. (See Chapter 11.)

Investigations
The diagnosis is suspected from the clinical history and examination and high ESR, usually >80 mm/h. A temporal artery biopsy showing the typical

changes of an inflammatory arteritis will confirm the diagnosis of giant cell arteritis. Steroids will induce complete remission and may be helpful in confirming the diagnosis.

Outcome

With the prompt institution of treatment symptoms rapidly respond. Loss of vision from giant cell arteritis may ensue if treatment is delayed.

Abnormal hemopoiesis

The hemopoeitic tissue contains multipotent, self-maintaining stem cells capable of undergoing proliferation and differentiation into functional blood cells that maintains the number of blood cells in the circulation. The blood-forming cells are found in the bone marrow in association with stromal cells and extracellular matrix molecules that together form the hemopoietic microenvironment. The interaction of hemopoietic cells and the microenvironment, through the secretion and presentation of growth factors and interaction of cellular adhesion molecules, modulates cell growth and survival and sustains and maintains hemopoiesis.

Cytopenia
Pathophysiology

Cytopenia, or reduced cell count, occurs due either to a reduction in cell production by the bone marrow or increased peripheral destruction. Normal hemopoiesis is under the control of cytokines, which, by binding to membrane cell receptors induce signal transduction and modulation of gene expression in the nucleus (Fig. 17.11) resulting in modulation of cell proliferation and survival.

Anemia

Erythrocytes transport and deliver oxygen to peripheral tissues bound to iron in the heme moiety of hemoglobin. The binding affinity of oxygen to hemoglobin is dependent on the oxygen tension in the arterial blood, temperature, pH, and levels of 2–3-bisphosphoglycerate and adenosine triphosphate (ATP). In anemia, erythrocytes produce more 2–3-bisphosphoglycerate, which decreases the oxygen binding affinity of hemoglobin A, releasing more oxygen into the tissues and thereby causing a shift in the hemoglobin–oxygen dissociation curve.

Clinical features

A careful history and examination should be taken to identify the cause of anemia (Table 17.16). The

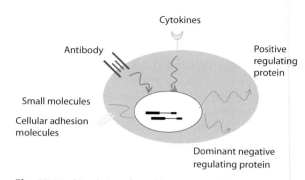

Fig. 17.11. Stimulation of a cell by an external factor requires binding through a membrane receptor and subsequent activation of a transcription pathway, and genetic modulation with the production of positive or negative regulating proteins. These changes result in the cell proliferating, apoptosing, or moving.

symptoms of anemia (Fig. 17.12) occur as a result of the compensatory mechanisms induced by oxygen deprivation, namely:

(1) Increased cardiac output resulting in a raised pulse, palpitations, headache, vertigo, dizziness, and tinnitus. Severe anemia may cause visual disturbances due to retinal hemorrhage, cotton wool spots, and exudates.

(2) Increased respiratory rate and shortness of breath, and occasional pulmonary edema and dyspnea, secondary to anemia-induced raised pulmonary artery pressure.

Significant clinical symptoms tend to occur when Hb falls below 8–9 g/dl (Table 17.17). The speed of onset may modify the symptoms. Acute blood loss induces sweating, vasoconstriction of the mucous membranes and skin causing pallor of the conjunctivae, lips, gums, and palmar creases. Anemia that develops slowly, such as that due to vitamin B_{12} deficiency, allows time for the patient to compensate by adjusting their activity and for physiologic adjustments in the cardiovascular system and oxygen dissociation curve, making patients tolerant of severe anemia. Co-morbid diseases, e.g. COPD, heart disease, may modify or exacerbate symptoms of anemia particularly in the elderly who are generally less tolerant of anemia.

Evidence of overt or covert bleeding should be sought and enquiries should be made into a family history of a bleeding diathesis (e.g. von Willebrand's disease). The most common source of blood loss is the GI, genital, and urinary tracts. Clinical evidence of iron or B12 deficiency should be specifically sought.

Table 17.16. History and examination in a patient with anemia

History	Examination
Family history	Evidence of organomegaly:
Travel history	Lymphadenopathy
Dietary history	Hepatosplenomegaly
Bleeding	Evidence of associated chronic inflammatory disorder: Joint swelling
Occupation Drug history	
Alcohol history	Evidence of iron deficiency:
	Angular stomatitis
	Sore tongue
Symptoms:	Nail ridging/koilonychia
• Bone/joint pain	Evidence of B12/folate deficiency:
• Polyuria/nocturia	Peripheral neuropathy
• Association with food/ drugs/weather	Circumoral parasthesiae
• Parasthesiae	Evidence of bleeding:
	Petechiae/ecchymoses
	Evidence of immune disease:
	Vitiligo
	Evidence of autoimmune disorder:
	Skin rash
	Joint disruption
	Thyroid dysfunction
	Evidence of hemolysis:
	Jaundice
	Growth or bone defects

Hepatosplenomegaly may develop due to compensatory extramedullary production of RBC in primary marrow failure or secondary to sequestration into the liver or spleen as in myeloproliferative (e.g. CML) or lymphoproliferative (e.g. NHL) disorders.

Causes
A low Hb concentration may arise as a result of failure of red blood cell production, premature red cell removal from the circulation, or impaired hemoglobin production (Fig. 17.13).

Investigations
In many instances the cause of anemia can be deduced from assessment of the quantitative cell count, the reticulocyte count, and examination of the blood film. Examination of a bone marrow aspirate and trephine is required in more difficult cases and specialized hemolysis, hemoglobinopathy, and hemorrhagic investigations may be needed (Fig. 17.14).

Iron deficiency
Clinical features
A history should be sought of blood loss from the GI or urinary tracts and in women the genital tract, e.g. menorrhagia. Symptoms of iron deficiency include sore tongue, angular stomatitis, and brittle ridged nails or koilonychia. In chronic, severe cases patients may complain of dysphagia secondary to the development of a post-cricoid esophageal web (Paterson-Kelly-Brown or Plummer-Vinson syndrome), which resolves with successful treatment of the iron

Fig. 17.12. Symptoms and signs of anemia.

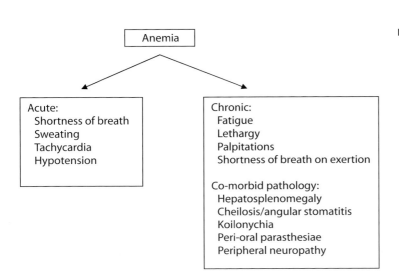

Table 17.17. Anemia due to red cell disorders

Red cell disorders

(1) Bone marrow failure (decreased RBC production):

Congenital	• Fanconi's anemia
	• Kostmann's
Acquired	• Drugs
	• Deficiency states
	Vitamin B12
	Folate
	Iron

(2) Hemolysis [Increased RBC destruction]:

Immune:	• Drug induced
	• Lymphoproliferative disorders
	• Paroxysmal nocturnal hemoglobinuria
	• Cold hemagglutinin disease
	Acute
	Chronic

Non-immune membrane abnormalities

	Hereditary spherocytosis
	Hereditary eliptocytosis
	Stomatocytosis
Infections:	• Malaria
	• Bacterial infection
	Clostridia
	Bartonella

Mechanical:	March hemoglobinuria
Chemical:	Benzene
Other:	• Zieves syndrome
	• Vit E deficiency
	• Enzymopathies
	Pentose phosphate pathway:
	G6PD
	Glutathione reductase deficiency
	GSH deficiency
	Catalase deficiency
	Embden–Myerhof pathway
	• *Hexokinase deficiency*
	• *Pyruvate kinase deficiency*
	NADH methemoglobin reductase deficiency

(3) Impaired hemoglobin production:

Hemoglobinopathies:

	• Sickle cell disease (HbSS)
	• Thalassemia syndromes
	• Hemoglobin C disease (HbC)

Deficiency states

	• Iron
	• Vitamin B12/folate

deficiency. Children with severe deficiency may develop pica (a compulsion to eat dirt or paint) or pacophagia (a craving for ice). Because iron is needed in virtually every cell in the body to support enzyme activity, deficiency is associated with fatigue and lethargy, which may be out of proportion to the degree of anemia.

Epidemiology
Iron is the commonest nutritional deficiency in the world.

Pathology
Iron is distributed throughout the body in both storage (hemosiderin (300 mg) and ferritin (700 mg)) and metabolically active (2 g in hemoglobin and 500 mg in myoglobin and enzymes) pools. A small amount of approximately 3 mg of iron is available in a transport pool. Iron is absorbed from the duodenum and upper jejunum and is dependent both on the form in which it is eaten (iron from meat being better absorbed than that from green vegetables), and on interactions with other foodstuffs which affect the bioavailability of iron (e.g. tannins in tea and bran reduce absorption whilst vitamin C increases absorption). Only 10% of available iron is absorbed from the diet, although this can be modulated by the intestinal mucosal cells in an as-yet undefined manner. Iron is transported from the intestine to the bone marrow, placenta, or liver parenchymal cells by the transport protein, transferrin. After binding via specific membrane receptors, the molecule is endocytosed and transferred to the mitochondria and then into protoporphyrin to become heme, the transferrin being extruded and recycled for further use. Iron that is not utilized in hemoglobin or enzymes is stored either as insoluble hemosiderin in the bone marrow macrophages or liver Kupffer cells or as a soluble form, ferritin, in spleen macrophages, bone marrow, serum, or liver hepatocytes.

Iron deficiency may result from inadequate or inappropriate dietary intake or increased iron requirements, impaired absorption, or excessive iron loss through bleeding. Increased physiologic requirements occur during the first 2 years of life, the adolescent growth spurt and in women during pregnancy, or as a result of menorrrhagia. Deficiency occurs with upper bowel malabsorption syndromes such as celiac disease and after intestinal surgery. The commonest source of blood loss is the gastrointestinal tract, due to gastric or duodenal erosions and ulceration often exacerbated

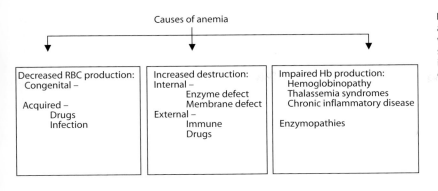

Causes of anemia

Decreased RBC production:
 Congenital –

 Acquired –
  Drugs
  Infection

Increased destruction:
Internal –
  Enzyme defect
  Membrane defect
External –
  Immune
  Drugs

Impaired Hb production:
 Hemoglobinopathy
 Thalassemia syndromes
 Chronic inflammatory disease

 Enzymopathies

Fig. 17.13. Clues to the cause of anemia should be sought by ascertaining whether the red blood cells are of normal size and identifying whether the anemia is an isolated abnormality or involves other hemopoietic cells lines.

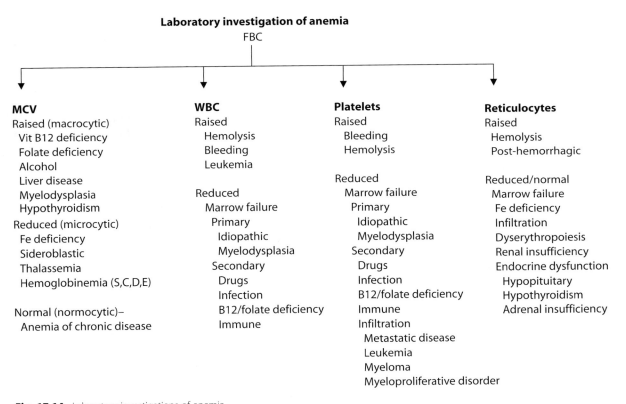

Laboratory investigation of anemia
FBC

MCV
Raised (macrocytic)
 Vit B12 deficiency
 Folate deficiency
 Alcohol
 Liver disease
 Myelodysplasia
 Hypothyroidism
Reduced (microcytic)
 Fe deficiency
 Sideroblastic
 Thalassemia
 Hemoglobinemia (S,C,D,E)

Normal (normocytic)–
 Anemia of chronic disease

WBC
Raised
 Hemolysis
 Bleeding
 Leukemia

Reduced
 Marrow failure
  Primary
   Idiopathic
   Myelodysplasia
  Secondary
   Drugs
   Infection
   B12/folate deficiency
   Immune

Platelets
Raised
 Bleeding
 Hemolysis

Reduced
 Marrow failure
  Primary
   Idiopathic
   Myelodysplasia
  Secondary
   Drugs
   Infection
   B12/folate deficiency
   Immune
   Infiltration
    Metastatic disease
    Leukemia
    Myeloma
    Myeloproliferative disorder

Reticulocytes
Raised
 Hemolysis
 Post-hemorrhagic

Reduced/normal
 Marrow failure
 Fe deficiency
 Infiltration
 Dyserythropoiesis
 Renal insufficiency
 Endocrine dysfunction
  Hypopituitary
  Hypothyroidism
  Adrenal insufficiency

Fig. 17.14. Laboratory investigations of anemia.

by the use of aspirin and non-steroidal anti-inflammatory drugs. Another important but much less common source of iron loss is the genitourinary tract where iron can be lost due to chronic intravascular hemolysis (e.g. paroxysmal nocturnal hemiglobinuria, microangiopathic hemolytic anemia due to mechanical damage by heart valves, intravascular mechanical trauma due to the rare hemoglobinuria).

Diagnosis
A low serum ferritin defines iron deficiency, but it is an acute phase reactant which may be spuriously elevated and results need to be interpreted in the clinical context. Absence of iron in the bone marrow can be used to confirm the low iron status. Progressive changes in the peripheral blood occur as iron deficiency increases, initially with a fall in the MCV and/or MCH,

539

Table 17.18. Causes of macrocytosis

Alcohol
Vitamin B12 deficiency
Folate deficiency
Liver disease
Drugs
- cytotoxic agents
- azathioprine
- zidovudine
Hypothyroidism
Myeloma
Myelodysplasia
Reticulocytosis
Acquired sideroblastic anemia
Chronic obstructive airways disease
Aplastic anemia
Congenital dyserythropoietic syndromes
Lesch–Nyhan syndrome

Table 17.19. Causes of megaloblastosis

Nutritional	Iron deficiency
	Vitamin B12/folate deficiency
Malabsorption	
Gastric	Intrinsic factor deficiency
	Gastrectomy
Ileal	Celiac disease
	Crohn's disease
	Ileal resection
	"Blind loop" syndrome
Drugs	Phenformin
	Methotrexate
	Trimethoprim
	Alcohol
Other	Congenital dyserythropoiesis
	Erythroleukemia
	Sideroblastic anemia

hypochromic, microcytic red cells in the blood film, and a reduced MCHC.

A rectal examination should be performed to look for bleeding, melena, or masses as a potential source of blood loss.

Treatment

Anemia should be treated with iron replacement given to correct the anemia and replenish iron stores and treatment of the underlying abnormality. Intolerance of oral iron or failure to absorb it from the gastro-intestinal tract can be overcome with parenteral therapy.

Macrocytic anemia

Macrocytosis describes a raised mean red cell volume (MCV).

Attention should be given to the dietary, alcohol, and drug history (Table 17.18). A full blood count and examination of a blood film should be performed to look for evidence of reticulocytosis, hypersegmented neutrophils ("right-shifted"), and poikilocytosis, very often in association with a mild to moderate decrease in platelets and less commonly a decreased leukocyte count. An analysis of the vitamin B12 and folate status, thyroid function, liver function, and an autoantibody screen should exclude other common causes of macrocytosis. A bone marrow aspirate and trephine with cytogenetic analysis is important to look for evidence of a clonal disorder (e.g. myeloma or myelodysplasia) and the presence of megaloblastosis. The latter finding implies the presence of a congenital

or acquired deficiency of vitamin B12 or folate disorder (Table 17.19).

Vitamin B12 deficiency

Anemia develops slowly, allowing patients to adapt to the low hemoglobin with few symptoms. Patients may present with a sore tongue, peripheral or perioral parasthesiae, and signs of other autoimmune disorders such as vitiligo, thyroid, or adrenal deficiency. Severe vitamin B12 or folate deficiency may induce psychiatric disturbances and infertility. A search should be made for evidence of associated conditions that may give rise to vitamin B12 deficiency such as skin rash (dermatitis herpetiformis).

Investigations

Once B12 or folate deficiency has been established, further investigations are indicate to establish the cause:

Autoantibody screen – anti-gliadin antibodies (celiac disease)

Bone marrow aspirate and trephine

Endoscopy

The Schilling test requires administration of IV vitamin B12 to saturate body stores, followed by the oral radioactive vitamin B12, given initially without and subsequently with intrinsic factor. A 24-hour urine collection identifies the excretion of radioactive B12. This cumbersome test has been superseded by serologic testing (see above).

Table 17.20. Causes of anemia of chronic disease

Chronic infection
  Tuberculosis
  Osteomyelitis
Chronic inflammation
  Rheumatoid arthritis
  Connective tissue disorders
Renal failure
Malignancy
  Carcinoma
  Lymphoma

Treatment

This consists of treating the underlying disorder (e.g. celiac disease) and replacement with vitamin B12 weekly for 6 weeks to replenish stores and 3-monthly thereafter, or folic acid 5 mg daily by mouth. If treatment is given without knowledge of the vitamin B12 level, it should be given in combination with folic acid to avoid the precipitation of neurologic damage. Blood transfusion is not normally required and should only be given with caution.

Anemia of chronic disease

The hematologic changes seen in this disorder are manifested by an isolated normochromic/normocytic (or hypochromic) anemia that returns to normal with resolution of the underlying condition.

Diagnosis

Characteristically, the blood picture shows a normochromic/normocytic anemia. Plasma iron, total iron binding capacity, and saturated iron binding capacity are all reduced, whilst bone marrow macrophage iron and plasma ferritin are both increased. These findings are consistent with defective handling of iron at a molecular level resulting in abnormal hemoglobin production. The causes are shown in Table 17.20.

Management

The management of the anemia of chronic disease should be directed at the treatment of the underlying disease.

Sideroblastic anemia

Clinical/complications/differential

Patients present with a mild to moderate, isolated anemia, and symptoms related to this.

Pathology

This is a condition characterized by dyserythropoietic anemia with variable hypochromia in the peripheral blood and excess iron in the marrow, which contains large amounts of erythroblasts with cytoplasmic iron granules arranged around the nucleus ("ring sideroblasts"). Ring sideroblasts may be present in small numbers in a wide variety of clinical disorders, but large numbers indicate sideroblastic anemia. The primary congenital condition is unusual, occurring primarily in males in childhood or early adolescence. The primary acquired condition is a form of myelodysplastic syndrome accounting for 10%–12% of all myelodysplastic cases and occurring primarily in older patients. The congenital form has a hypochromic, often microcytic picture, the acquired form is characterized by a dimorphic blood picture. A secondary form of the condition occurs with abnormalities of B6 metabolism (e.g. anti-tuberculosis chemotherapy, celiac disease, and alcoholism) or conditions associated with disturbance of heme synthesis (e.g. lead poisoning, alcohol, and porphyria).

Management

Initial management is treatment or removal of any underlying cause. The congenital form may respond to pyridoxine. Transfusion should be reserved for those individuals who are symptomatic with hemoglobin below 8–9 g/l. A small percentage of patients with the acquired condition will transform to acute leukemia, and hemopoietic stem cell transplantation is reserved for selected individuals.

Pure red cell aplasias

These are rare disorders. The congenital form, Blackfan Diamond syndrome is associated with developmental disorders including skeletal abnormalities, congenital heart defects, and renal abnormalities. The acquired condition is either primary idiopathic, autoimmune, or secondary and may be transient to infections such as parvovirus, CMV, HIV, or B19 virus. In 50% of subjects it is associated with a tumor, which is most commonly a thymoma and less frequently CLL or solid tumors. Other secondary causes to exclude are systemic lupus erythematosus, myasthenia gravis, and rarely riboflavin deficiency.

Diagnosis

This is made by identifying a severe normochromic, normocytic anemia with a low reticulocyte count (<1%), with a normal platelet and white cell count.

The bone marrow is normocellular but with absent erythroblasts.

Treatment

This is of the underlying cause or, in those where no cause can be identified, steroids or immunosuppressants.

Outcome

Fewer than 20% of patients remit spontaneously and patients with a thymoma will respond to thymectomy. Relapse is not unusual but responds to repeated treatment with immunosuppressants. In a small percentage of patients it is reported to evolve into aplastic anemia or acute myeloid leukemia.

Hemolytic anemia

Hemolytic anemia arises from premature destruction of circulating red blood cells either in the circulation or in the reticulo-endothelial system.

Clinical features

A family history or the country of origin may suggest the underlying diagnosis. Symptoms in childhood would indicate a congenital disorder. A drug history and the existence of any underlying disease may also provide important indicators of the etiology. Jaundice may be a sign of hemolysis and the presence of splenomegaly, cyanosis, or any associated illness may be related.

Investigations

Investigations initially should confirm the presence of hemolysis with hyperbilirubinemia and a raised LDH. A raised urobilinogen and low haptoglobins are seen in chronic hemolytic states, and urinary hemosiderin is suggestive of intravascular hemolysis. A full blood count, differential, and blood film are essential to look for evidence of the underlying cause such as spherocytes, microangiopathy, or malaria parasites. The presence of Heinz bodies indicates drug intoxication, chemical poisoning, or unstable hemoglobin, e.g. Hb Koln. An indirect and direct antibody test (DAT) should be performed to demonstrate antibody in the plasma or bound to the cell membrane. The reticulocyte count is normally raised in hemolysis. The causes of red cell hemolysis are shown in Table 17.21.

Non-immune mediated hemoglobinopathies

The hemoglobinopathies are inherited disorders due to either a quantitative or qualitative defect of hemoglobin synthesis.

Table 17.21. Causes of hemolysis

Acute:	• Infection	• Mycoplasma
		• Malaria
		• Clostridia welchii
		• Viruses
	• Drugs	
	• Chronic lymphocytic leukemia	
	• Burns	
	• Paroxysmal nocturnal hemoglobinuria (PNH)	
	• Mechanical:	
	• Disseminated intravascular coagulation (DIC)	
	• Thrombotic thrombocytopenia (TTP)	
	• Cardiac valves	
	• March hemoglobinuria	
	• Toxins:	
	• Snake venom	
Chronic:	• Acquired	• Systemic lupus erythematosus (SLE)
		• Idiopathic
	• Congenital	• Hemoglobinopathies
		• Sickle cell disease
		• Thalassemia
		• Red cell membrane defects
		• Hereditary spherocytosis
		• Hereditary elliptocytosis
		• Red cell metabolic defects
		• G6PD deficiency
		• Pyruvate kinase deficiency
		• Vascular abnormalities/hemangiomas

Quantitative defects : thalassemia

Pathology

The thalassemic disorders are caused by an imbalance of globin chain synthesis and are classified according to which globin chain is synthesized at a reduced rate. Alpha thalassemia is an autosomal recessive disorder resulting from a deficiency of alpha chains with the accumulation of gamma chains (hemoglobin Barts (gamma$_4$)) in the fetus and beta chain tetramers (hemoglobin H (beta$_4$)) in adults. There are four loci for alpha globin chain production. If only one locus is affected the outcome is a silent carrier with no signs of the disease. Two loci will cause a mild asymptomatic hypochromic, microcytic anemia, whilst three loci results in the production of hemoglobin Barts and hemoglobin H, both of which have reduced oxygen-carrying capacity and result in anemia and splenomegaly. If four loci are affected, there will be no alpha chain production which is incompatible with life because Hb F cannot be formed and death results usually in the 24th–26th week of pregnancy from hydrops fetalis.

Beta thalassemia is due to a deletional or non-deletional mutation of the gene on chromosome 11. A single gene mutation results in a clinical condition known as beta thalassemia minor (or trait) and a two-gene mutation causes beta thalassemia major or Cooley's anemia. A further condition, beta thalassemia intermedia, is characterized clinically by a less severe form of anemia. In beta thalassemia, the excess alpha chains attach to the red cell membrane causing membrane damage and hemolysis. Mutations may result in either no beta chain production (beta^0) or partial beta chain production (beta$^+$).

The delta globin chain is required for adult hemoglobin A2 production, which makes up approximately 3% of all adult hemoglobin. The hetereozygous state is asymptomatic, but is important to define for counseling because, when inherited in the double heterozygous state with beta thalassemia trait, it can obscure the diagnosis.

Clinical features

Patients present with signs and symptoms of anemia, the severity of which is dependent in alpha thalassemia on the number of loci deletions or mutations as described above.

Patients with both beta genes deleted present with signs and symptoms of severe anemia and evidence of extramedullary hemopoiesis such as bossing of the skull, loosening of the teeth, and hepatosplenomegaly, plus evidence of hemolysis and iron deposition producing darkening of the skin, hypopituitarism, and diabetes mellitus. Beta thalassemia trait is often identified as a mild hypochromic anemia, frequently mistaken for iron deficiency.

Epidemiology

Thalassemia is probably the commonest genetic disorder worldwide being spread throughout the Mediterranean and Middle East, Indian sub-continent, and South East Asia, although the incidence does vary. Alpha thalassemia is particularly common in the Far East and South-East Asia but uncommon in Africa and rare in northern Europe. Interestingly, the distribution of beta thalassemia appears to be associated with the distribution of malaria and may protect against this parasite by inhibiting its growth.

Management

Currently, the mainstay of management for the thalassemias is supportive care with red blood cell transfusions and prevention of iron overload by the regular administration of iron chelator agents such as desferrioxamine; vitamin C should be given to aid chelation. Patients should be vaccinated against Gram-positive cocci such as pneumococci because of the risk of overwhelming infection.

Allogeneic stem cell transplantation has been used successfully in selected patients with beta thalassemia with limited success, and there is extensive research into the development of oral iron chelators.

Qualitative defects

These are normally due to a single substitution of an amino acid in the hemoglobin chain resulting from a single base change in the gene.

Sickle cell disease

Pathology

The sickle cell mutation arises from the substitution of a thymidine for an adenine group at the sixth codon of the beta gene (GAG to GTG).

Clinical features

The predominant signs and symptoms arise as a result of vaso-occlusive complications, manifested most commonly as painful crises, often in the small bones of the hands and feet (hand–foot syndrome), or presenting as acute chest syndrome with chest pain and hypoxia, particularly in early life. Later in life, involvement of the long bones is common and abdominal crises occur secondary to occlusion of the small vessels of the mesentery and abdominal viscera. Infection secondary to hyposplenism needs to be excluded as patients often present with low grade fever. Occlusive episodes in the central nervous system can present with hemiparesis, seizures, or dysphasia, whilst renal occlusion produces hematuria, which needs to be differentiated from infection. Priapism is common in males. Hematologic crises occur independently of vaso-occlusive episodes. These take the form of aplastic crises, hemolytic crises, or acute splenic sequestration presenting as medical emergencies. Leg ulcers are common and may become intractable causing damage to underlying tendons. Papillary necrosis may cause hyposthenuria, and microthrombi in the retina may result in infarction and visual impairment.

On examination, patients may be in great distress from painful crises and be unable to move an affected limb. They often have a low-grade temperature, hypotension, or dehydration. The spleen should not be palpable and, if it is enlarged, should raise the possibility of splenic sequestration or an associated hemoglobinopathy, such as beta thalassemia.

543

Epidemiology

The highest prevalence of hemoglobin S is in tropical Africa, but it occurs with less frequency in the Middle East and in parts of India, where it follows the old slave trade routes.

Management

Painful bone crises should be managed by removing the patient from precipitating causes, keeping them warm, administering oxygen, correcting dehydration with intravenous fluids, and treating concurrent infection. Localized swelling or tenderness in a limb requires X-rays to exclude underlying osteomyelitis. Pain must be controlled as appropriate, but frequently requires opioids. Pethidine should be avoided because of its addictive qualities. Hemolytic crises should be managed with immediate transfusion of packed red cells.

Exchange transfusions in association with plasma exchange may be needed to treat acute stroke, and long-term transfusion support reduces the risk of recurrent neurologic problems. Allogeneic stem cell transplantation is appropriate in selected younger patients with recurrent CNS complications and has met with limited success but remains a research tool.

Hydroxyurea has been shown to increase the levels of hemoglobin F, which improves clinical status by virtue of its increased oxygen carrying capacity, resulting in reduced transfusion need.

Other common hemoglobinopathies
Hemoglobin C

The homozygous state is normally asymptomatic, whilst the homozygous condition is associated with mild hemolysis and splenomegaly. It occurs in a similar population to sickle cell disease and the double heterozygous hemoglobin SC disorder is common and has a clinical course the same as sickle cell disease.

Hemoglobin D

This condition occurs particularly in northern India and is asymptomatic in the heterozygous and homozygous state. It travels on electrophoresis in the same position as hemoglobin S and may be missed unless agar gel electrophoresis is performed. It is important to identify this condition because, when it occurs in the double heterozygous state with hemoglobin S, it results in a severe form of sickle cell disease.

Hemoglobin E

This is common in South-East Asia. The heterozygous state may be mistaken for iron deficiency because it causes hypochromia and microcytosis with only mild or no anemia and target cells on the blood film. The homozygous condition induces a mild anemia associated with splenomegaly. It must be distinguished from hemoglobin C by agar gel electrophoresis.

Membrane defects: spherocytosis
Clinical features

Patients are normally asymptomatic but may present with anemia, jaundice, or splenomegaly or symptoms of gallstones with long-standing hemolysis. It is caused by a deficiency of spectrin, resulting in enhanced sodium efflux from the cell, a loss of red cell deformity, and hemolysis.

Epidemiology

Spherocytosis has autosomal dominant inheritance and is the commonest red cell membrane disorder.

Investigations

The diagnosis is made from the family history, examination of the blood film, and biochemical evidence of hemolysis. There is increased red cell osmotic fragility, and red cell spherocytes on microscopy.

Management

The anemia does not normally require treatment, but therapy may be indicated for complications such as folate deficiency, cholelithiasis, leg ulceration, and aplastic crises secondary to viral infections.

Chemical-induced red cell enzyme defects

Glucose 6-phosphate deficiency is the commonest red cell enzyme deficiency, resulting in increased susceptibility of hemoglobin to oxidative stress and the formation of cytoplasmic denatured hemoglobin or Heinz bodies when exposed to certain drugs, infection and, in some cases, broad beans (favism). It is an X-linked condition seen most commonly in Black, Asian, and Mediterranean races. Hemolytic episodes are self-limiting because reticulocytes have a higher G6PD content than mature cells, which limits and eventually halts the hemolytic process. Management should be directed at patient education to avoid precipitating factors known to cause hemolysis.

Other enzyme deficiencies are rare and require specialist laboratory investigations to confirm the diagnosis, and specialist care.

Methemoglobinemia

An acquired form of hemoglobinemia can be induced by drugs or oxidizing agents, such as organic nitrates or phenacetin.

The congenital form may arise either from a globin chain or enzyme defect. Globin chain defects affect the alpha or beta chain in the region of the Fe pocket which results in stabilization of iron in the ferric form resulting in methemoglobin (Met Hb). In both situations, the clinical effects include cyanosis. General health is usually good in the congenital form, whilst in the acquired form severe tissue hypoxia results from the failure of Met Hb to release oxygen to the tissues, and most patients present requiring urgent treatment of hypoxic symptoms.

Diagnosis requires a high index of clinical suspicion confirmed by spectrophotometric analysis for the abnormal hemoglobin. Mild cases may respond to large doses of vitamin C, more severe cases require methylene blue intravenously or an exchange transfusion.

Physical damage to red cells
Microangiopathic hemolytic anemia (MAHA)

This type of anemia arises from the mechanical destruction of red cells through a variety of mechanisms (Table 17.22).

The blood picture shows red cell fragmentation (schistocytes), poikilocytosis, and a raised reticulocyte count. Often, the platelet count is reduced. Treatment should be directed to correcting the underlying abnormality.

Table 17.22. Causes of microangiopathic hemolytic anemia

Thrombotic thrombocytopenic purpura (TTP)

Hemolytic–uremic syndrome (HUS)

Vasculitides

- Wegener's
- SLE
- PAN

Disseminated intravascular coagulopathy (DIC)

- Malignancy
- Pregnancy; hemolysis, elevated liver enzymes; low platelets (HELLP syndrome)
- Organ rejection
- Infection

Heart valve replacement

A-V malformations

March hemoglobinuria

Burns

Drugs – cyclosporin

Management

Hemolysis can be halted by removal from or treatment of the underlying cause.

Infection

Hemolysis may be exacerbated in patients with G6PD deficiency or any infection associated with splenomegaly but, in addition, certain infections have a propensity to initiate rapid red cell destruction with hemolysis. The most well-described world-wide is malaria. Although seen in all sub-types of the infection, it is particularly common with *P. falciparum*, inducing an acute and severe intravascular hemolysis with the passage of red or black urine ("black water fever"). Blood transfusion and renal support may be required with this dangerous complication. Other infections associated with hemolysis include *Clostridium welchii*, *Mycoplasma pneumoniae*, *Salmonella*, *Haemophilus influenzae*, Epstein-Barr virus and cytomegalovirus. Treatment should be directed at the underlying infection.

Immune mediated

Immune hemolysis is due to idiopathic or secondary production of autoantibodies directed against the patient's own red cells arising in association with a malignancy, lupus erythematosus, or infection. A direct and indirect antiglobulin test is mandatory if an immune etiology is suspected to detect the presence of autoantibodies, although false-positive and -negative reactions may occur.

Patients present with the signs and symptoms of hemolysis and care should be taken to identify any associated condition, such as a skin rash in systemic lupus erythematosus or lymphadenopathy in lymphoproliferative disorders.

The main causes of immune hemolysis are idiopathic or drug induced.

Idiopathic

This may develop insidiously or present acutely with sudden onset of jaundice and severe anemia. A search should be made for any history or signs of an underlying cause; significant splenomegaly should raise the suspicion of a lymphoproliferative disorder. The antibody is usually a warm reacting IgG, which coats the red cells and binds to Fc receptors on the reticulo-endothelium resulting in phagocytosis and red cell destruction.

Clinical

Patients present with symptoms of anemia and jaundice. Mild splenomegaly is usual. Investigations demonstrate evidence of hemolysis and there is frequently a neutrophilia.

Management

Hemolysis usually responds to prednisolone, starting in doses of 40–100 mg daily. Patients who fail to respond or relapse may need cytotoxic drugs such as cyclophosphamide and azathioprine.

Drug induced

A number of hemolytic mechanisms have been identified. Clinically, the hemolysis may occur abruptly or only after subsequent exposure to the offending agent. In these cases the drug forms a complex with the antibody (usually IgM in nature) and binds to the red cell membrane, activating complement, which is detectable by the direct anti-globulin test (DAT), and inducing hemolysis (the "innocent bystander mechanism"). Quinidine, rifampicin, antihistamines, chlorpromazine, probenecid, and melphalan induce this type of response. Alternatively, the hemolysis may occur over a long period, as is sometimes seen in patients receiving high doses of penicillin. In this situation the drug binds firmly to the red cell membrane and forms a hapten that elicits an antibody response (normally IgG) that binds to the red cell and leads to its removal by the reticulo-endothelial system. The DAT is positive for IgG. Other drugs eliciting a hapten response include cephalosporins, tetracyclines, and tolbutamide.

Management

Usually witholding the drug will halt the hemolytic process.

Another important cause of warm autoimmune hemolytic anemia is ABO incompatibility.

Cold hemagglutinin disease (CHAD)

This is precipitated by the development of cold agglutinating antibodies (acting most strongly at <20 °C) directed against anti-I on adult red cells or anti-I on cord red blood cells. These antibodies activate complement and are a cause of hemoglobinemia and hemoglobinuria. This condition is most often idiopathic, but may also be associated with infections such as *Mycoplasma pneumoniae* and Epstein–Barr virus (glandular fever), or arise secondary to B-cell malignancies.

Management

Patients should, where possible, keep warm so that hemolysis can be reduced to a minimum. CHAD secondary to infection is usually self-limiting.

Table 17.23. Causes of secondary polycythemia

Hypoxia	Inappropriate erythropoietin secretion
• High altitude	• Renal disease, e.g. hydronephrosis, cysts, carcinoma
• Cardiopulmonary disease	• Hepatocellular carcinoma
• Smoking	• Cerebellar hemangioma
• High oxygen affinity Hb	
• Methemoglobinemia	

Polycythemia

This term describes an excess of red blood cells and an increase in the red cell mass.

Epidemiology

The primary condition is rare occurring in approximately 1.5 per 200 000 of the population with a male predominance, and the maximum incidence is at age 50 years.

Pathology

A low erythropoietin level characterizes the primary condition, whilst secondary cases have excess erythropoietin production due to hypoxia or aberrant erythropoietin secretion, normally from the kidney or a tumor (Table 17.23). The hemoglobin is normally greater than 18 g/dl, the red cell count above 6×10^{12}/l, and the PCV above 0.55. The red cell volume can be measured using red cell isotope labeling and is greater than 36 ml/kg in men and 32 ml/kg in women. Bone marrow aspirate and trephine show hypercellularity with excess megakaryocytes and reduced or absent iron stores.

Conventional chromosome analysis is usually normal, although gene expression profiling may provide a molecular signature to assist with diagnosis in the future. Recently, a clonal mutation of the Janus kinase 2 (*JAK2*) gene has been described, which is present in >80% of patients with this condition. The constitutive phosphorylation of this gene leads to cytokine hypersensitivity, and has also been identified in other myeloproliferative disorders. It is hoped that identification of this mutation will lead to new therapeutic approaches to controlling this disease.

Clinical features

The primary form of the disease is associated with thrombocytosis, leukocytosis, and splenomegaly with symptoms related to the increased blood viscosity and hypermetabolism. Pruritis, made worse by warm water, can be a particularly distressing and difficult symptom to treat. Patients often have suffused conjunctivae, and plethora and hepatosplenomegaly occurs in up to 60% of cases. Uric acid is frequently elevated secondary to the hypermetabolic state and gout may occasionally be a presenting problem. Approximately 10% progress to acute myeloid leukemia. Thromboses and bleeding constitute the major causes of morbidity and mortality, although occurring in fewer than 1% of cases. Peptic ulceration is also reported.

Thrombocythemia (see Platelet disorders)
Chronic myeloid leukemia (see Leukemia)

White cell disorders
Leukopenia
Leukopenia refers to a reduced circulating white cell count affecting one or more white cell types. It is due to either bone marrow suppression or peripheral destruction. The normal adult total white cell count is 3.5×10^9–7.0×10^9/l but is significantly lower in Afro-Caribbeans.

Clinical
The history is important in identifying the cause of leukopenia and care should be taken to identify whether there has been any suggestion of a low count previously (e.g. FBC taken at the time of previous surgery or routine health check) and whether there are any symptoms related to leukopenia, such as recurrent or life-threatening infections occurring over a protracted time period, suggestive of a long-standing problem. Recent weight loss or fever suggests a systemic illness or underlying tumor. Pain is an uncommon symptom may occur secondary to bone infiltration (e.g. myeloma) acute leukemia or blastic transformation of chronic myeloid leukemia. Signs of a lymphoproliferative disorder or rashes associated with an auto-immune disorders (e.g. systemic lupus erythematosis) should be sought. Hepatosplenomegaly suggests peripheral consumption of white blood cells (Table 17.24).

Investigations
These should always include a full blood count and blood film to confirm the low white cell count and exclude spurious causes such as "clumping" of cells. A bone marrow aspirate and trephine will differentiate between a hypocellular marrow as in primary marrow failure and a hypercellular marrow secondary

Table 17.24. History and examination of patient with neutropenia

History	Examination
Drug history/Chemical exposure	Arthropathy
Recent infection (particularly viral)	Rash
Family history	Splenomegaly
Foreign travel (e.g. malaria)	Oral ulceration/infection
Bleeding	Bruising
Weight loss	Bone tenderness

Note:
The normal range for neutrophils is lower in Afro-Caribbeans than in Caucasians. The commonest cause in a hospital population is drugs. Evidence should be sought for infection and other findings of marrow failure.

to infiltration with abnormal cells or excess white cell precursors associated with peripheral consumption. Other investigations should look to define an auto-immune cause or evidence of recent viral or bacterial infection.

Causes of neutropenia (Table 17.25)
Drugs and chemicals
Chemotherapy-induced leukopenia is dose dependent, but most drugs have been reported to be associated with myelosuppression. The onset may be acute due to an idiosyncratic reaction to protein-bound drug or slower due to neutrophil hypersensitivity. Susceptibility to drug-induced agranulocytosis may be enhanced by the presence of genetic variants of drug-detoxifying enzymes as is sometimes seen in slow acetylators given sulfasalazine. Specific questioning should ask about sedatives, tranquilizers, analgesics, and anti-inflammatory intake. Chemical exposure may occur from occupational exposure or hobbies (e.g. model-making or gardening) or secondary to hair dyes or cosmetics.

Where a drug can be identified, it should be stopped if appropriate. If the leukocyte count does not recover promptly, granulocyte colony stimulating factor (G-CSF) should be administered. Patients with evidence of infection should be treated vigorously with appropriate parenteral antibiotics.

Myelodysplastic syndromes
This term defines a group of related disorders characterized by abnormal maturation and morphology in the bone marrow and mono-, bi-, or tri-lineage cytopenias in the peripheral blood.

547

Table 17.25. Causes of neutropenia

Marrow failure:	Congenital:	• Familial	
		Kostmann Syndrome	
		Schwachman-Diamond	
		Dyskeratosis congenita	
		Racial variation	
	Acquired:	• Infection: Bacterial	• Typhoid
			• Brucellosis
		Viral	• Influenza
			• HIV
			• Measles
			• Cytomegalovirus
		• Drug induced	
		• Immune: Systemic lupus Erythematosus	
		• Vitamin B12 deficiency	
		• Alcoholism	
		• Myelodysplasia	
	Cyclical		
Peripheral destruction		• Splenomegaly from any cause	
		Felty's syndrome	
		Portal hypertension	
		Lymphoproliferative disorder	
		Tropical splenomegaly	

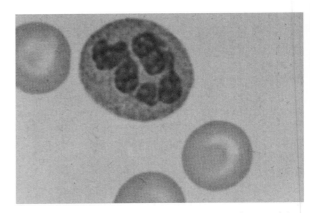

Fig. 17.15. Photomicrograph of a hypersegmented neutrophil and target cells taken from a patient with liver disease and vitamin B12 deficiency. Target cells can also be seen in hemoglobinopathies (S & C), thalassemia, hypercholesterolemia, and post splenectomy.

Epidemiology

The crude incidence of the disease is approximately 7 per 100 000 of the population.

Clinical

Patients present with insidious onset of tiredness and malaise with mucosal bleeding from the nose and gums due to thrombocytopenia. Leukopenia is associated with recurrent infection, particularly respiratory infections and oral and vaginal thrush. The differential diagnosis must include megaloblastic anemia, aplastic anemia, chronic myeloid leukemia, acute myeloid leukemia, and myelofibrosis.

Investigations

These should include a full blood count and differential, serum B12 and folate levels, bone marrow aspirate and trephine, and chromosome studies.

Management

Supportive care is with blood and platelet transfusions and prophylactic antimicrobials. A minority of patients benefit from growth factors, but curative treatment requires the use of intensive combination chemotherapy and allogeneic hemopoeitic stem cell transplantation in selected patients.

Infection

This is most frequently seen with viral infections, e.g. HIV, infectious mononucleosis. The mechanism is most probably due to neutrophil damage by the infectious agent and sequestration in the RE system. Other viral infections frequently associated with neutropenia include chickenpox, measles, rubella, influenza, and dengue fever. Bacterial infection normally induces a leukocytosis but neutropenia is associated with brucellosis, typhoid and paratyphoid, bacillary dysentery, and malaria. Severe overwhelming infection may be associated with leukopenia and is a poor prognostic sign.

Deficiencies

Leukopenia, often in association with other cytopenias, may be induced secondary to a deficiency of vitamin B_{12} (Fig. 17.15) or acutely in folate deficiency as seen in patients in intensive care not given folate supplementation.

Immune

White cell destruction may be induced by anti-leukocyte antibodies that may occur in isolation or in association with other immune anemias and thrombocytopenias. A mild to moderate form of immune neutropenia is reported in neonates due to the transplacental passage of iso-immune maternal IgG anti-neutrophil antibodies.

Treatment need only be initiated if there is evidence of recurrent life-threatening infection. Steroid therapy may be effective or, in severe or refractory cases, immuosuppressives and plasmapheresis are of potential value.

Hypersplenism

Splenic enlargement from any cause (e.g. Felty's syndrome, tropical sprue) may present with sequestration of cells and the premature removal of neutrophils from the circulation.

Congenital neutropenia syndromes

These constitute a number of disparate conditions with a spectrum of clinical presentations. The commonest form is benign familial neutropenia which is normally associated with only mild neutropenia, is more common in Afro-Carribean families, and does not require therapeutic intervention. Other forms may be associated with pancreatic and protein abnormalities (Kostmann's syndrome) and can be fatal unless treated aggressively. Another group of disorders is associated with constitutional and skeletal abnormalities (e.g. Shwachman–Diamond syndrome).

Leukocytosis

Leukocytosis is an elevation of the white cell count and can be due to involvement of one or more of the white cell lines or an excess of early progenitors or blasts. The commonest cause of leukocytosis is acute infection but inflammation, tissue damage, allergic reactions, and metabolic conditions need to be considered (Table 17.26). The initial approach to leukocytosis is to differentiate between a benign and malignant condition. The history should include a detailed evaluation of the family history, current medication, and environmental exposure.

Leukemoid reaction

Describes a rise in neutrophil count in association with the appearance of circulating blasts and white cell precursors (a "left shift"). This arises in the setting of severe infection such as pertussis, infectious mononucleosis, and tuberculosis. Hemoglobin and platelet counts are normal and, if secondary to bacterial infections, the neutrophils may contain increased cytoplasmic granulation and intracellular basophilic inclusions composed of agglutinated ribosomes (Dohle bodies). The white cell count resolves with resolution of the underlying cause.

Leukoerythroblastic reaction

Describes the neutrophilia that occurs in association with a left shift in the white cell series and circulating nucleated red cells. It occurs in response to marrow infiltration with fibrosis or tumor and, more rarely, secondary to hemolysis.

Table 17.26. Causes of neutrophil leukocytosis

Physiologic:	Pregnancy	
	Bleeding	
	Steroids	
Infection:	Usually bacterial and more rarely viral or protozoal	
Tissue damage:	Inflammation	• Arthritides
		• Inflammatory bowel disease
	Tissue damage	• Post surgery
		• Myocardial infarction
		• Bleeding, e.g. sub-arachnoid
		• Hemolysis
	Metabolic	• Gout
		• Pre-eclampsia
		• Diabetic ketoacidosis
	Allergic	
Myeloproliferative disorders:		• Chronic myeloid leukemia
		• Myelofibrosis
		• Primary thrombocythemia

Myeloproliferative disorders

These disorders share similar clinical features. All arise from a clonal mutation of a pluripotent stem cell that can transform to acute leukemia. Chronic myeloid leukemia (CML) is characterized by the presence of the Philadelphia chromosome, which may be identified in a minority of the other disorders that make up this group. Recently a molecular marker, JAK2, has been identified that is mutated in a significant proportion of myeloproliferative disorders (MPD).

Myelofibrosis

Clinical

This is a rare disorder that can present either in a chronic form or less commonly with acute onset similar to acute leukemia. The chronic form has a median age of onset of 60 years and is characterized by the insidious onset of tiredness and mucosal bleeding often with fever, left upper quadrant discomfort, and weight loss. Patients may present with anemia, neutropenia, and/or thrombocytopenia. The differential diagnosis includes infection, metabolic disorders, and autoimmune diseases.

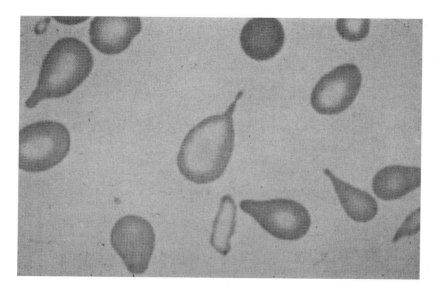

Fig. 17.16. Tear drop cells commonly seen in bone marrow fibrosis, megaloblastic anemia, iron deficiency, and thalassemia.

Investigations

These should include full blood count and differential looking for tear-drop cells (Fig. 17.16), liver function tests, LDH, bone marrow aspirate, and trephine and chromosome analysis. In primary myelofibrosis the trephine shows excess reticulin and fibrosis and abnormal, mononuclear megakaryocytes. Secondary fibrosis is induced by abnormal infiltration of the marrow (e.g. metastatic carcinoma, lymphoma) and infection (e.g. tuberculosis). Monosomy 7 may occur in myelodysplasia and a t(1:21)(1p3q13) abnormality would support a diagnosis of acute megakaryocytic leukemia.

Treatment

Treatment of primary myelofibrosis is supportive in the first instance. Interferon alpha has been given with varying success, whilst the judicious use of oral chemotherapy agents early in the disease may reduce the spleen size enough to reduce the effects of hypersplenism and clinically improve the signs and symptoms of anemia. In a proportion of patients the condition will progress to acute leukemia.

> Lymphocytosis (See Table 17.27)
> *Eosinophilia (Table 17.28)*
> *Polycythemia (see Red cells)*
> *Chronic myeloid leukemia (see Leukemia)*

Leukemia

Leukemia is a tumor of hemopoietic precursor cells arising from the bone marrow. It is classified as chronic or acute defined by the speed of clinical progression. The World Health Organization (WHO)

Table 17.27. Causes of lymphocytosis

Viral infection	Epstein–Barr virus
	Hepatitis
	Cytomegalovirus
	Infectious mononucleosis
Chronic lymphocytic leukemia	
Other	Post splenectomy
	Vigorous exercise

Table 17.28. Causes of eosinophilia

Allergies	Myeloproliferative disorders
Skin disorders	Loeffler's syndrome
Parasitic infestation	Hypereosinophilic syndrome
Collagen disorders	Lymphoma

classification takes account of the importance of cytogenetics, immunophenotype, and molecular genetics in addition to histology.

Acute leukemia

Clinical features

Acute leukemias develop over weeks or, occasionally, days. Fatigue, weight loss, and fever are common presenting features, and symptoms and signs are primarily those of bone marrow failure. Anemia presents as lethargy and tiredness, shortness of breath, and congestive cardiac failure. Neutropenia is clinically manifested by infections (particularly bacterial chest

Table 17.29. Clinical features of different sub-types of acute leukemia

• Bone marrow fibrosis and failure	• M7 or megakaryocytic leukemia
• Gum swelling	• M5 or acute monocytic leukemia
• Renal tubular damage	• M4 or acute myelomonocytic leukemia
• Thrombosis/bleeding	• M3 or acute promyelocytic leukemia (APL)
• Organomegaly	• Chronic myeloid/lymphoid leukemia

Note:
Acute leukemia leads to the symptoms and signs of bone marrow failure but different sub-types give rise to specific clinical findings that identify significantly different outcomes or may lead to specific treatment or complications.

Table 17.30. Investigation of leukemia

Hematology	*Immunology*
FBC, blood film, reticulocytes	Autoantibody screen
Blood group, antibody screen, DAT	HLA typing
Coagulation screen	
Bone marrow aspirate and trephine	*Radiology*
Cytogenetics and immunophenotyping	Plain chest X-ray
Biochemistry	*Cardiology*
Urea and electrolytes	Electrocardiogram
Liver function tests	Echocardiogram if significant cardiac history
Serum calcium, phosphate, and urate	
Infection screen	*Other*
Blood cultures	Semen storage where appropriate
Hepatitis A, B, and C serology	Dental assessment
HIV I and II	
CMV	

Note:
The investigation of leukemia should be designed to confirm the diagnosis and identify infective foci, end organ failure, or specific complications.

or superficial wound infections, fungal infections of the oropharynx and vagina), and mucosal ulceration. Mucosal bleeding usually involving gums, nose, or uterus, ecchymoses, and petechiae are manifestations of thrombocytopenia. Certain sub-types of leukemia present characteristic features that affect treatment and outcomes (Table 17.29).

Epidemiology

Acute myeloid leukemia is the commonest adult acute leukemia accounting for 3 cases per 100 000 of the population annually. The median age at presentation is 64 years, frequency increases with age. Acute lymphoblastic leukemia has a biphasic distribution, being highest in children aged 4–6 years and young adults aged 25–35 years.

Etiology and pathogenesis

There is an association with pre-existing myelodysplasia, prior exposure to cytotoxic chemotherapy (particularly alkylating agents and epipodophyllotoxins), ionizing radiation, benzene, and constitutional chromosomal abnormalities (e.g. Down and Fanconi's syndromes). An association has also been made with smoking. The HTLV-1 virus (human T-cell leukemia virus) has been associated with a specific type of adult T-cell leukemia. Cytogenetic abnormalities are used to assist in diagnosis of sub-types, inform treatment decisions, and to help prognostication.

Investigations

Examination of the peripheral blood film and bone marrow demonstrates an excess of myeloid blast cells. Other investigations are required to identify co-existent myelosuppression, end organ damage, and infection (Table 17.30).

Management

Initial treatment is to treat sepsis and correct or support end-organ damage. Careful attention to fluid balance and urination, if necessary with a urinary catheter, is important.

Infection risk is particularly high for patients receiving immunosuppressants, e.g. steroid or ciclosporin, with chronic GvHD, or a previous history of tuberculosis or HIV. Common occult sites of infection are lung, indwelling catheters (*Staph. epidermidis*), perianal (*E.coli*, *Pseudomonas*, and *Klebsiella*) and periodontal (*Bacteroides*). Blood cultures should be taken prior to initiating antibiotics and the patient clinically monitored over 72–96 hours, and treatment altered in the light of the results of investigations.

Fungal infections are an important complication of hematologic malignancies particularly in those with prolonged, severe neutropenia, chronic antibiotic usage, and post stem cell transplantation. *Aspergillus* and other molds may be difficult to diagnose, resulting in delayed initiation of treatment and high mortality rates. *Pneumocystis carinii* pneumonia is seen most frequently in lymphoid malignancies and patients receiving long-term steroid or purine analogs (e.g. fludarabine and 2-CDA).

Respiratory syncytial virus and the parainfluenza viruses are common causes of morbidity and mortality in transplant units.. Reactivation of herpes type I virus infections, CMV, and HZV frequently arise with intensive myelosuppressive therapy. Clinically, patients present with pneumonitis, gastritis, esophagitis, weight loss, hepatitis, retinitis, hemorrhagic cystitis, vertigo, or graft suppression.

Treatment

Specific treatment is dependent upon accurate diagnosis and should be delivered in specialist centers with experience of treating these life-threatening conditions. Chemotherapy drugs are usually administered in combination and at high doses designed to kill the tumor cell and overcome resistance. Supportive treatment with antimicrobials, growth factors, and blood products has significantly improved the outcome for patients.

Outcome

Median survival in adult leukemia has risen during the last 20 years. Thirty to forty percent of patients aged less than 65 years, depending upon the type of leukemia, can now be expected to survive disease-free at 5 years and are likely therefore to be cured of their disease.

Chronic leukemia

Chronic lymphocytic leukemia/small lymphocytic lymphoma
(see Lymphadenopathy)

Chronic myeloid leukemia

This malignant transformation of a pluripotent bone marrow cell is characterized by a translocation of genetic material from chromosome 22 (the *bcr* gene), to chromosome 9 (the *abl* gene), resulting in the t(9;22)(q34;q11) Philadelphia chromosome and a *bcr/abl* fusion gene product. Five to ten percent of patients have a variant chromosome translocation or a cryptic translocation of chromosome 9q34 or 22q11. In CML the abnormal p210 protein produced by the *bcr* fusion gene is associated with increased tyrosine kinase activity and it is tempting but unproven to speculate that this has a causative role in this disease.

The disease can occur in childhood but median age at presentation is in the fifth and sixth decades. There are no known predisposing factors for this disease, although radiation has been implicated (e.g. nuclear bombing of Hiroshima).

Clinical features

Patients present insidiously with tiredness, fatigue, weight loss, and night sweats or gout secondary to a hypermetabolic state. The condition may come to light on routine FBC for an unrelated condition. The clinical findings include splenomegaly that may be massive, extending into the right hypochondrium with mild to moderate hepatomegaly. Patients may complain of fullness in the abdomen, easy satiety, or acute pain in the left hypochondrium secondary to splenic infarction. The disease presents in three stages:

Chronic phase: Clinically and hematologically stable over months or years.

Accelerated phase: A rising white cell count and excess blast cells in the bone marrow.

Blast phase: Overt leukemia with a blast cell count over 30% in the bone marrow, circulating blasts in the peripheral blood with thrombocytopenia and anemia.

Diagnosis

The finding of organomegaly, anemia, and bleeding in association with a blood film shows leukocytosis with basophilia, anemia and, often, a thrombocytosis in the chronic phase of the disease. The bone marrow aspirate is hypercellular with an increase in the myeloid series and a right shift. Increased fibrosis is seen on reticulin staining. Chromosome analysis demonstrates the Philadelphia chromosome and molecular marker studies the *bcr/abl* fusion gene. Biochemical abnormalities include a raised vitamin B12, serum urate and LDH, and a low ESR and neutrophil alkaline phosphatase (NAP) score (in contrast to infection).

Treatment

The chronic or "stable" phase may be associated with few symptoms and most people are able to lead a near normal life with no need for therapeutic intervention. After a variable time, this phase progresses to an accelerated phase, then to the blast (leukemic) phase and acute leukemia. Oral chemotherapy, e.g. hydroxyurea, is effective in controlling the elevated WBC and thrombocytosis in the chronic phase, but more intensive combination chemotherapy is needed as disease progresses to a more aggressive stage. The Philadelphia chromosome is rarely eliminated without recourse to hemopoietic stem cell transplantation.

Platelet disorders
Thrombocytopenia
Clinical features

Bleeding into the skin produces petechiae or ecchymoses, whilst mucosal bleeding produces GI or GU bleeding or epistaxis. Women of child-bearing age may present with menorrhagia. Retinal bleeding may cause impaired vision. Lymphadenopathy or hepatosplenomegaly is suggestive of a lymphoproliferative disorder and a skin rash of lupus erythematosus.

Pathogenesis

Thrombocytopenia arises either from a failure of production by the bone marrow, excessive removal from the circulation, or a combination of both. A spurious thrombocytopenia occurs when circulating giant platelets, in some congenital platelet disorders (Table 17.31), are mistakenly identified by automated counters as red blood cells leading to a falsely low platelet count. The cause of thrombocytopenia varies with age. In childhood, idiopathic immune thrombo-cytopenic purpura, marrow aplasia syndromes, and hematologic malignancies are more common. In adults HIV infection is one of the commonest causes but drugs, malignant infiltration of the marrow, and splenomegaly are other common causes (Table 17.31).

Investigation

A full blood count will confirm an isolated thrombo-cytopenia, whilst a blood film may identify giant platelets or red cell fragments if part of a consumptive thrombocytopenia. A bone marrow aspirate and trephine should be performed to examine cellularity, megakaryocyte numbers, and morphology and to exclude an infiltrative or primary marrow disorder. Other investigations include autoantibody and plate-let antibody screening to identify an immune disorder and microbiology to exclude infection, including HIV.

Treatment

Spontaneous or post-traumatic hemorrhage is an indication for therapeutic intervention. Platelet trans-fusions are effective in the acute setting to control hemorrhage and when peripheral platelet consumption or an immune etiology can be ruled out. Steroids, immunosuppressants, or splenectomy may be required for patients with immune thrombocytopenia with per-sistent or life-threatening symptoms. Intravenous IgG immunoglobulin is used to induce a temporary remis-sion to cover episodes of high risk such as dental extractions or surgical procedures.

Autoimmune thrombocytopenia

This condition occurs in children and adults. During childhood the onset may be abrupt, usually follows an acute viral infection, and resolves spontaneously over

Table 17.31. Pathogenesis of thrombocytopenia

Bone marrow failure

Congenital
  Fanconi's anemia
  Megakaryocytic aplasia (TAR syndrome)
  Wisco-Aldrich syndrome

Giant platelet syndromes
  May-Hegglin syndrome
  Epstein syndrome
  Chediak-Higashi syndrome

Acquired
  Drugs/chemicals
  Infection – HIV
  Deficiency syndromes, e.g. Vitamin B12, folic acid
  Uremia
  Alcoholism
  Bone marrow infiltration
    Malignancy
    Non-malignant

Peripheral destruction

Immune destruction
  Autoantibodies:
    Autoimmune thrombocytopenia
    Systemic lupus erythematosus
    Drug induced (hapten formation)
    Low grade lymphoproliferative disease
  Isoantibodies:
    Post transfusion
    Feto-maternal incompatability
Excess consumption due to intravascular damage:
    Disseminated intravascular coagulation
    Microangiopathic consumption
      Thrombotic thrombocytopenic purpura (TTP)
      Hemolytic–uremic syndrome (HUS)
      Prosthetic heart valves
Structural platelet disorders:
    Bernard–Soulier syndrome
Splenomegaly
Massive transfusion

4–6 months. In adults it is usually more insidious, preceded by infection in a minority of patients. In the majority of individuals it becomes chronic, although the severity of the thrombocytopenia may fluctuate.

Asymptomatic patients should be observed and treatment only initiated for significant clinical bleeding or prior to surgery or dental procedures. High-dose intravenous immunoglobulin induces temporary responses in 70%–80% of patients and is the treatment of choice to cover acute bleeding episodes or surgical procedures. Steroids are effective in most cases. Patients who fail to respond or develop resistance to

Table 17.32. Precipitating events causing DIC

(1) Hypoxia and acidosis

(2) Endothelial cell damage (cytokine or endotoxic shock)

(3) Exposure to tissue factor (following trauma)

(4) Exposure to proteolytic enzymes (snake venom)

Note:
Disseminated coagulation is caused by a wide variety of events that result in the release of cytotoxic compounds that induce widespread fibrin formation and the consumption of coagulation factors resulting in a combination of thromboses and bleeding.

steroids may benefit from the addition of immuno-suppressives or splenectomy.

Disseminated intravascular coagulopathy

This condition is seen as a complication following a number of disorders resulting in intravascular activation of the coagulation pathway with fibrin deposition and consumption of platelets and coagulation factors. Although hemorrhage is the dominant feature, thrombosis in the microcirculation can result in gangrene of the digits and extremities. The precipitating event is varied (Table 17.32).

Presentation is with acute fulminant bleeding or thrombosis, or as a more chronic condition, often secondary to malignancy, manifested by laboratory coagulation abnormalities and oozing from mucosal surfaces or intravenous sites.

Hemolytic–uremic syndrome/thrombotic thrombocytopenic purpura

This is a rare condition characterized by development of clots in the microcirculation, particularly brain and kidney, which results in the consumption of platelets. It arises as a result of the defective breakdown of von Willebrand factor (vWF) in the circulation due to a deficiency of an enzyme called vWF cleaving protease or ADAMT 13. This may be an inherited deficiency or later in life the development of an antibody that inhibits protease activity. In adults the condition may be precipitated by infection (e.g. some strains of *E. coli*), pregnancy (when it needs to be distinguished from eclampsia), or drugs (e.g. ciclosporine, quinine).

Patients present insidiously with fever, headache, and diarrhea and, as the platelet count falls, they develop bruising and bleeding. Later they develop confusion, focal neurologic signs, and seizures, and renal impairment with decreasing urine output. Progressive hemolysis is accompanied clinically by pallor and jaundice with increasing red cell fragmentation and thrombocytopenia on the blood film.

The diagnosis is made from the clinical features associated with a low platelet count, renal impairment, and red cell fragmentation.

Treatment

This is a medical emergency that requires replacement of the deficient vWF cleaving protease by transfusion of fresh frozen plasma or factor VIII, with or without the use of regular exchange transfusion. Red cell transfusions are sometimes given to maintain the hemoglobin, but platelet transfusions should be avoided as this may sometimes exacerbate the condition. Prognosis needs to be guarded with many patients showing a relapsing remitting course requiring frequent admissions and repeated treatment.

Thrombotic thrombocytopenic purpura

A rare condition caused by an inherited or acquired deficiency of ADAMTS-13.

Thrombocytosis

This condition is defined by an isolated rise in the platelet count above the upper end of normal. It may occur either as an isolated finding or as part of a myeloproliferative disorder with an increase in other blood cell numbers. Commonly, it is a reactive response to bleeding (e.g. post-operatively), inflammation (arthritis), malignancy, or following splenectomy when the count is usually $<1000 \times 10^9$/l and clinical complications are rare.

A history and examination for evidence of underlying infection, inflammation, or bleeding should be sought. Clinically, patients with reactive thrombocytosis are usually asymptomatic, although patients with a primary marrow disorder present with mucosal bleeding (gums, menorrhagia), or arterial (digital ischemia) or venous thromboses (mesenteric, portal, splenic, penile). Examination should identify skin purpura or tissue bleeding and should include ophthalmoscopic examination for retinal hemorrhage. Splenomegaly is unusual, but should raise the possibility of an underlying myeloproliferative disease.

Pancytopenia

This is characterized by low circulating red cells, leucocytes and platelets. It may arise from primary bone marrow failure or peripheral destruction or premature removal from the circulation. Primary bone marrow failure of all the formed elements is referred to as aplastic anemia; rarely, a single cell line is affected and just erythroid cells in pure red cell aplasia.

Table 17.33. Causes of bone marrow aplasia

Congenital
  Intrinsic stem cell defect
  Defect in bone marrow microenvironment
  Growth factor deficiency or defect

Acquired
  Infections:
  - Hepatitis
  - HIV
  - Parvovirus
  Drugs:
  - Chemotherapy
  - Azathioprine
  - Antibiotics
  - Antibodies – anti CD20
  Chemicals:
  - Benzene
  Irradiation

Clinical

In children it may be familial or congenital and often associated with skeletal defects, called Fanconi's anemia. In adults it is acquired and most commonly idiopathic but may also be associated with drugs or irradiation. Drug-induced aplasia is often dose related (e.g. chemotherapy) or idiosyncratic (e.g. phenylbutazone, tolbutamide, gold). Acute transient forms may be seen as a complication of infections, in particular viral infections (e.g. HIV, hepatitis A). Less severe aplasias occur in endocrine deficiencies such as myxedema, Addison's disease, and hypopituitarism.

Pathology

There is a reduction in one or more of the circulating hemopoeitic cells with reduced or absent hemopoeitic precursors in the bone marrow aspirate and trephine. Paroxysmal nocturnal hemoglobinuria (a red cell membrane protein defect) should be excluded by performing a Hams acidified serum test, testing for hemosiderin in the urine, and red cell immunophenotyping to detect the absence of CD55 and CD16.

Aplastic anemia

This is defined as pancytopenia with hypoplastic bone marrow. It is rare, accounting for 2–5 cases per million of the population. Patients with severe aplasia have a white cell count $<500 \times 10^6/l$ and platelets $<20 \times 10^6/l$. Reticulocytes are low as marrow does not respond to the erythropoeitic drive. The causes are shown in Table 17.33.

Paroxsysmal nocturnal hemoglobinuria
Clinical

A condition characterized by dramatic, episodic paroxysms of dark urine secondary to massive intravascular hemolysis precipitated by infection, surgery, and occasionally intravenous contrast medium. Patients have a propensity to venous and arterial thrombosis manifested as Budd-Chiari syndrome and pulmonary hypertension. Usually there is low grade hemolysis and iron deficiency secondary to urinary blood loss. Renal abnormalities include acute or chronic renal failure and tubular dysfunction. Patients may present with anemia, thrombosis, aplastic anemia, or acute leukemia.

Pathology

Red cells are sensitive to autologous serum complement because of the defective formation of glycosylphosphatidylinositol (GPI), which provides a membrane attachment anchor for proteins such as CD59, CD 58, CD16, and CD14. The loss of these proteins renders the cell sensitive to complement-mediated cell lysis and red cells, white cells, and platelets may be affected.

Diagnosis

Anemia can be macrocytic due to the reticulocytosis or microcytic hypochromic secondary to iron deficiency and an associated low white cell and platelet count. In the bone marrow there is erythroid hyperplasia. The urine should be examined for hemosiderin and may remain positive for up to 1 week after a hemolytic episode. A Ham's acid hemolysis and sucrose lysis test should be performed to demonstrate red cell sensitivity to complement and flow cytometry to detect the GPI.

Treatment

Patients who require red cell transfusion should be given washed cells to remove complement. Steroids have limited effect and patients with venous thrombotic complications should be anticoagulated. Patients should be monitored for evidence of transformation to aplastic anemia. Allogeneic stem cell transplantation is potentially curative and should be considered in selected patients.

Hemostasis

Hemostasis is the process whereby damaged blood vessels are repaired, but blood is maintained in a fluid state and blood flow re-established in a timely manner. It is system that coordinates the interaction between blood vessel endothelium, platelets, and coagulation factors to maintain a balance between the thrombotic and coagulation systems.

Thrombosis

Clinical features

Coronary artery thrombosis may induce sudden death, myocardial infarction, or unstable angina whilst cerebral ischemia can cause transient focal neurologic deficits or visual dysfunction or cerebral infarction with dense, permanent neurologic loss. Acute arterial obstruction causes a painful, cold, blue limb with absent pulses. Bowel thrombosis presents with an "acute abdomen" and rectal bleeding and should raise the suspicion of underlying myelofibrosis or malignancy.

Arterial thrombosis occurs as a result of atheromatous plaques or dislodgement of thrombi following myocardial thrombosis, atrial fibrillation, aortic aneurysm, infective myocarditis, cardiac valve disease or, rarely, a venous embolus may traverse a patent foramen ovale.

Venous thrombosis most commonly affects the limbs and pulmonary tree with pain, tenderness, swelling, pallor, and increased temperature of the affected limb. Acute pulmonary embolism presents clinically with chest pain, acute shortness of breath, hemoptysis, and, in severe cases, shock. Hepatic vein thrombosis is a common complication of myeloproliferative disorders.

A prothrombotic state should be excluded in patients with no predisposing conditions, recurrent thrombosis, and in patients under 40 years of age.

Epidemiology

The prevalence of prothrombotic conditions varies according to the population studied. The commonest inherited prothrombotic condition in Caucasians is protein C deficiency due to factor V Leiden mutation, occurring in up to 15% of the population but 5% in the Middle East and rare in Africans and Asians. Other conditions are significantly less common. The relative risk of thrombosis varies between different abnormalities.

Investigations

Initial assessment should establish whether or not a thrombus is present, the site of the thrombus, its extent, and whether it is localized or systemic, and whether there is any co-morbid contraindication to anticoagulation or anti-platelet therapy. Although a congenital cause of thrombosis is more likely in patients aged <40 years, in all patients a history should

Table 17.34. Factors predisposing to thromboembolism

Arterial	Venous	Arterial and venous
Smoking	Malignancy	Estrogens
Hypertension	Pregnancy	Primary polycythemia
Hypercholesterolemia	Trauma	Myelofibrosis
Diabetes	Surgery	PNH[a]
Lupus anticoagulant	Immobility	Behçet syndrome
Primary thrombocythemia	Nephrotic syndrome	Homocysteinuria
Atrial fibrillation	Prothrombotic states	
TTP[b]		

Notes:
[a]Paroxysmal nocturnal hemoglobinuria.
[b]Thrombotic thrombocytopenic purpura.
Pre-disposing causes of venous and arterial thromboses are different, although they occasionally overlap.

be taken to identify predisposing factors such as previous thrombotic events, a family history of thrombosis or sudden unexplained death, or recurrent fetal loss (Table 17.34).

Investigation of a prothrombotic disorder (Table 17.35) includes a coagulation screen, full blood count, urea and electrolytes, liver function tests, and plain chest X-ray. The platelet count is elevated in primary thrombocythemia and reduced in thrombotic thrombocytopenic purpura (TTP). Microangiopathy on microscopy occurs in TTP and disseminated intravascular coagulopathy (DIC) as a result of damage to red cells as they pass through fibrin strands laid down in the microvasculature following activation of thrombosis. Impaired renal function may suggest TTP or hemolytic–uremic syndrome (HUS). Paroxysmal nocturnal hemoglobinuria (PNH) predisposes to thrombosis. The investigation of a prothrombotic anomaly is indicated in patients presenting with thrombosis under the age of 40 years with no predisposing cause, a family history of thrombosis, females with a history of recurrent fetal loss, or unexplained recurrent thrombosis.

Treatment

Initial treatment should be directed at the thrombus and subsequently at removal or treatment of any underlying cause. Low molecular weight heparin should be given in the first instance and, once symptoms are controlled, the patient can be transferred to warfarin for long term control. Patients who have an

Table 17.35. Investigation of a prothrombotic state

Full blood count and film

INR/APTT[a]

Liver function tests

Urea and electrolytes

Fasting glucose/Hb A$_2$

Functional and immunologic assays of:

    Anti-thrombin III

    Protein C

    Protein S

    Plasminogen

Factor V Leiden

Prothrombin G202/OA mutation

Homocysteinemia

Antiphospholipid antibodies

ADAMTS13

CD55 and CD59

JAK2

Notes:
[a]INR = international normalized ratio; APTT = activated partial thromboplastin time.

irreversible underlying predisposition to thrombosis require long-term warfarin treatment. Thrombolytic therapy is indicated for life-threatening complications. Low-dose aspirin is frequently used in coronary artery disease prophylaxis and for the management of transient ischemic attacks. Other prophylactic measures include the use of TED stockings perioperatively and early mobilization and physiotherapy post-operatively.

Bleeding

The coagulation system is based on a cascade of reactions that have a number of negative feedback loops leading to the production of a fibrin meshwork that traps platelets, red cells, and white cells to form a stable plug at the site of vessel injury preventing further blood loss.

Clinial features

Clinical bleeding takes several forms. Bleeding from mucosal surfaces can cause menorrhagia, epistaxis, hematuria, hemoptysis, or malena. Continuous oozing of blood over a prolonged period is characteristic of platelet deficiency or dysfunction whilst bleeding into muscle, joint, or deep tissue, either spontaneously or following trauma such as dental extraction, is more characteristic of a coagulation disorder.

Platelet disorders: quantitative disorders
Thrombocytopenia (see above)
Qualitative disorders (Table 17.36)
Bernard Soulier disorder

This is an autosomal recessive disorder characterized by large platelets, a reduced platelet count when performed on an automated machine, and a defective collagen platelet test. Patients present young with purpura and occasionally catastrophic hemorrhage. Investigation shows that the platelets fail to express the glycoprotein Ib receptor responsible for platelet adhesion to collagen.

Coagulation protein disorders

These are congenital or acquired, quantitative or functional, but clinically the syndromes associated with them are identical. A rare cause of acquired coagulation defects is the development of protein inhibitors. The coagulation disorders are rare diseases affecting 1–2 persons per 10 000 of the population but vary with geographic (5–6 times more common in South America), social (inbreeding in Amish community), and religious factors (large families).

Congenital coagulation factor disorders: factor VIII (hemophilia) and factor IX (Christmas disease) deficiencies:

These are the commonest coagulation disorders accounting for approximately 1 per 10 000 and 1 per 1000 of the population, respectively. They are X-linked recessive conditions, the gene for factor VIII being carried on the X chromosome. Up to 30% may be sporadic with no family history of disease.

Clinical features

Bleeding from the umbilical cord may be the initial presenting event, but more commonly bruising and hematomas occur and may be severe enough for the parents to come under suspicion of battering the child when they seek medical help. Others present early in childhood once the infant learns to walk and begins to knock into objects. Spontaneous bleeding, particularly into joints, causes acute pain, often presaged by parasthesiae in the joint, and chronic degenerative arthritis in the longer term. Bleeding into soft tissue such as the tongue may be life threatening and was a common cause of death prior to the introduction of factor VIII. Spontaneous or post-traumatic intracranial bleeding is potentially life threatening. Patients presenting with headache or loss of consciousness should be treated as a medical emergency and investigated with

Table 17.36. Causes of platelet disorders

Congenital	Acquired
Adhesion defects	Renal disease
Bernard Soulier	Drugs:
Von Willebrand's disease	Non-steroidals
Ehlers-Danlos syndrome	Chloroquine
Idiopathic	Prostaglandins
Defective ADP	Cephalosporins
Glanzmann's deficiency	Tricyclic
Afibrinogenemia	antidepressants
Release reaction	Dextrans
Wiskott-Aldridge	MPD[a]:
TAR[b]	Myelofibrosis
Chediak-Higashi	Primary polycythemia
Hermansky-Pudlak	Thrombocythemia
Gray platelet syndrome	CGL[c]
Cyclo-oxygenase deficiency	DIC[d]
Thromboxane synthetase	Scurvy
deficiency	
Membrane coagulant	
Platelet factor-3 deficiency	

Notes:
[a]Myeloproliferative disorder.
[b]Thrombocytopenia with absent radii.
[c]Chronic granulocytic leukemia.
[d]Disseminated intravascular coagulopathy.

CT scan or MRI, given large doses of factor VIII, and evaluated for surgery to evacuate any hematoma. Damage to the vertebral canal and peripheral nerve compression are potential problems, which need to be identified and managed urgently. Ilio-psoas bleeding may present as a mass needing careful investigation and conservative management. Bleeding post-dental surgery is a common presentation in less severely affected hemophiliacs. Characteristically, primary hemostasis is achieved at the clinic, but the following day the socket oozes from poor clot formation.

Investigations
Initially, a full blood count (FBC), liver function tests (LFT), specialized coagulation tests, viral studies, and appropriate imaging of any affected joint are needed (Table 17.37).

Pathology
Bleeding into the joint arises from the synovium producing an inflammatory response, synovial hypertrophy, and destruction of the articular joint surface. Repeated bleeds induce progressive fibrosis and fixation with loss of peri-articular muscle mass.

Treatment
Treatment should be managed through a specialist Hemophilia Center. Adequate quantities of factor VIII

Table 17.37. Investigation of coagulation disorders

Screening tests
INR
Activated prothrombin time
Thrombin time
Full blood count and film
Liver function tests
Urea and electrolytes
Skin bleeding time

Specialized tests
Coagulation factor assay
Factors II; VII; IX; X
Factors VIII; thrombin; fibrinogen
vWFR cofactor
vWF Ag
vWF multimers
Inhibitor screen
Platelet function tests

or IX are needed to control acute bleeding using the factor assays to monitor therapy. Pain control is crucial and longer-term management of joint complications with physiotherapy and orthopedic support are critical to the long-term management. Patients must be followed up for infectious complications such as hepatitis B and C, and human immunodeficiency viruses, that arise from the use of large quantities of human blood products.

Planned surgical interventions should be covered with prophylactic factor VIII infusions or in mild or moderate cases desmopressin (DDAVP, given pre-operatively may be enough to elevate factor VIII levels to cover the procedure.

Families should be counseled and a family pedigree identified using a family tree and DNA analysis. Antenatal diagnosis is available for those who request it, but is associated with significant fetal loss.

Factor VIII inhibitors may develop secondary to the use of coagulation factors or in patients with underlying malignancy. This poses a major therapeutic problem that may be treated with alternative sources of factor VIII, activated prothrombin complex concentrates, and/or plasmapheresis. In those in whom the inhibitor arises secondary to an underlying tumor, treatment of the malignancy may result in disappearance of the inhibitor.

Von Willebrand's disease
This is a common and heterogeneous coagulation disorder comprising a number of quantitative and qualitative sub-types of deficiencies of adhesive glycoproteins

required to bind platelets to endothelium and stabilize plasma factor VIII.

Epidemiology

The incidence is as high as $1:100$ but varies geographically, being reported in $120:100\,000$ in the Nordic countries but only $25–30:100\,000$ in the UK. It may be more severe in patients with blood group O.

Clinical features

Most cases are mild but bleeding may be severe in the homozygous state (Type III variant). Characteristically patients present with mucosal bleeding (e.g. epistaxis, menorrhagia) or easy bruising. Mild thrombocytopenia is seen in Type IIB due to spontaneous platelet binding and clearance from the circulation. Protracted bleeding following surgery or dental extractions is a common presentation and joint bleeding occurs with Type III disease and may be confused with hemophilia.

Investigations

Patients should be screened with an INR, aPTT, skin bleeding time, FBC, LFTs, and U&Es plus a coagulation screen. Specific diagnosis requires specialist investigation for von Willebrand factor cofactor (vWF Co), von Willebrand factor antigen (vWF Ag), and vWF multimers, factor VIII assay and platelet aggregation studies.

Pathology

vWF is a complex multimeric carrier protein produced and released by endothelial cells that binds factor VIIIc in the circulation. Deficiency or dysfunction of the von Willebrand factor is responsible for altered platelet adhesion to sub-endothelial collagen, failure to form the platelet plug, and impaired coagulation at the site of damage to the blood vessel wall. It is typically autosomal dominant but one sub-type is autosomal recessive; rarely it may be acquired. The acquired type is a quantitative deficiency of vWF caused by autoantiodies often associated with hypothyroidism or underlying malignancy.

Treatment

Intermediate purity factor VIII contains vWF, and higher concentrations are found in fresh frozen plasma and cryoprecipitate and can be given to correct the bleeding time prophylactically. The Weibel–Palade bodies in endothelial cells store vWF and administration of desmopressin facilitates its release which may be adequate prophylaxis in Type I disease without exposing patients to blood products.

Acquired coagulation factor disorders:
Liver disease

Factors II, VII, IX, and X are produced by liver parenchymal cells and require vitamin K for their production. Dietary deficiency of vitamin K (e.g. prolonged intravenous feeding, alcoholism) or impaired absorption (e.g. malabsorption, long-term antibiotic therapy), or failure of utilization (e.g. drugs, primary liver failure) all lead to defective production.

Clinical features

Mucosal bleeding, oozing from puncture sites, and skin bleeding are characteristic features. GI bleeding, which is not uncommon in liver disease, is exacerbated by the coagulapathy.

Investigations

Laboratory investigations generally show a prolonged INR and APPT, and specific factor assays are needed to identify the deficient factor(s).

Renal disease

Both acute and chronic renal impairment are associated with multifactorial bleeding disorders. Factor IX may be lost in patients with proteinuria secondary to nephrotic syndrome and loss of Factor X is associated with amyloidosis, whilst in chronic renal impairment, long-term antibiotic prophylaxis may result in vitamin K deficiency. Platelet abnormalities occur secondary to defective megakaryocyte production, and thrombocytopenia secondary to long-term heparin use during dialysis or consumption in HUS or TTP.

Disseminated intravascular coagulation (DIC) (see above)
Acquired inhibitors
Clinical features

Inhibitors occur in association with a malignancy or immuno-secretory disorders such as multiple myeloma or Waldenstrom's macroglobulinemia, secondary to autoimmune disorders or spontaneously in otherwise healthy individuals. The lupus anticoagulant arises in association with systemic lupus erythematosus and is frequently reported in pregnancy, malignancy, and normal individuals. The lupus anticoagulant is associated with recurrent thrombosis and miscarriages.

Pathology

The antibody is active against phospholipid.

Treatment

This should be directed at the underlying disorder plus steroids or other immunosuppressant.

Further reading

Essential Haematology, ed AV Hoffbrand, JE Pettit, PA Moss, 5th edn. Blackwell Publishing, Oxford, UK, 2006. An excellent introduction to clinical hematology for undergraduate and non-hematology specialists.

www. haematology.org Contains excellent photo micrographs for self-assessment and links to other hematology sites.

www. bcshguidelines.com The British Society of Haematology guidelines site that provides state-of-the-art guidance on all aspects of clinical and laboratory investigations and management of a wide range of hematological disorders.

Wintrobe's Clinical Haematology ed. GM Rodger, F Parashevas, J Foerster, BE Gladder, R Means, 12th edn. Lippincott, Williams and Wilkins, London, 2008.

The elderly patient

Mark Kinirons

Contents

Falls

Causes

Accidental (30%)	Tripping on pavement
Gait & balance deficits (20%)	Muscle, locomotor, nervous system diseases
Dizziness (10%)	Nervous, otologic, and miscellaneous disease
Drop attacks (10%)	Brainstem cerebrovascular disease
Dementia/Delirium (5%)	Alzheimer's/vascular/Lewy body dementias; delirium
Orthostatic hypotension (<5%)	Idiopathic/drug related/neurodegenerative disease
Syncope (1%)	Arrhythmias, aortic stenosis; vasovagal and carotid sinus disease
Other (~5%)	Hysterical; malingering; vision

Key points in history

Single or recurrent	Each fall increases risk of future falls by fourfold
Explained or unexplained	Unexplained – more likely to be neurocardiac
Blackout or no blackout	Blackout likely to be neuro-cardiovascular disease
Indoors or outdoors	Indoors more likely to involve environmental factors
Gait difficulties	More likely to be locomotor or neurologic cause

It is important to distinguish between syncope and non-syncope. The latter is suggestive of primary brain disorder such as epilepsy.

Introduction

Thirty percent of people over 65 years and living in the community fall each year. Of those in long-term care, 70% fall each year. Falls are complex. Typically, the cause involves a number of elements that coalesce. Most have more than one cause. In addition, risk factors may play a vital role in their genesis. A systematic approach is required (Fig. 18.1).

Risk factors for falls

- Visual impairment
- Arthritis
- Depression and dementia
- Age over 80 years.

Determine the cause(s) of the fall

History

Where?	Indoors or outdoors – indicates degree of mobility
	May need occupational or physiotherapy
What?	Symptoms preceding fall:

	Dizziness or blackouts	Possible neuro; cardiovascular or epilepsy
	Palpitations	Cardiac? Conduction disease

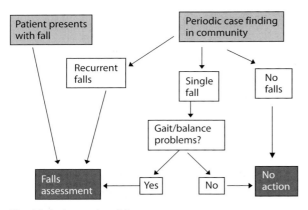

Fig. 18.1. Approach to falls.

Symptoms after fall:

	Urine loss	Epilepsy
	Arm/leg weakness	Stroke
	Amnesia for fall	Carotid sinus syndrome
How?	Leg/foot gave way	Musculoskeletal – OA
	Missed step	Vision difficulty – cataracts
	Related to posture	Cardiovascular – drug induced
		Multiple medications
	Hit by bus	Deaf – check hearing

Examination

Check postural blood pressure (especially if on multiple BP lowering drugs)

Feel pulse (cardiac arrhythmia cause)

Auscultate aortic and carotid areas (may have aortic stenosis)

Examine range of movement of lower back and lower limbs for deformity, swelling, tenderness, and movement (arthritis)

Review neurology (power of hip and foot flexors along with sensation)

Vision – check with Snellen chart (binocular glasses are discouraged)

Watch gait – see pattern with and without aid (clue to cause of fall)

Look at footwear (flat shoes are better)

Reduce future falls

Having made an accurate diagnosis of the cause, intervention is based on addressing matters such as improving muscle gait and balance with specific exercise programs. Recognition and removal of hazards in the home can be achieved with occupational therapy help. Modification of offending drugs and treatment of neurologic and cardiovascular causes are vital.

Reduce consequences of falls

Fractures are common and responsible for 3%–8% of all emergency department admissions. A fall leading to a fracture is the commonest trigger for long-term care and is the leading cause of death in older people. Treatment of bone health is important and the National Institute of Clinical Excellence (NICE) has issued clear guidance on use of vitamin D, calcium supplementation, and bisphosphonates post-fracture.

Fear of future falls is common and leads to reduced confidence and impaired quality of life. There are no trials to guide treatment, but group exercises in community or home increase confidence and independence.

Specific conditions: Neural mediated syncope – also known as vaso-vagal syncope (also Chapter 9)

The triggers leading to a drop in pressure by vagal stimulation are wide and varied and may not be easily identifiable. Possible triggers include fear, severe pain, emotional distress, or prolonged standing. Syncope usually occurs when upright and is preceded by a typical prodrome of weakness, sweating, nausea, and a feeling of blood draining away before the syncope. There is pallor and a weak pulse. The patient soon recovers after seconds to minutes in the recumbent position. Vaso-vagal syncope is more common in advancing age. It is a clinical diagnosis. The investigation of choice is tilt testing. Diagnosis is confirmed when symptoms are reproduced and there are no other obvious explanations. Management is empiric and includes avoidance of precipitating events and blood pressure lowering agents where possible, and of too rapid changes in posture. Increasing fluid intake and caffeine will increase vascular tone, and support stockings also help. There is no effective cure.

Orthostatic hypotension

This has also been known as postural hypotension. Clinical features include a feeling of weakness on standing upright, which may lead to syncope. It is

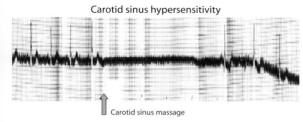

Carotid sinus hypersensitivity

Carotid sinus massage

Fig. 18.2. An ECG tracing demonstrating a prolonged pause of 10 seconds in response to right CSM.

more common with advancing age. For many years no specific pathologic mechanism was identifiable but newer research has described neurodegeneration in the dopamine pathways of the brain with, in some cases, genetic defects of dopamine metabolism. The diagnosis is made on testing the blood pressure (BP) on lying for 5 mins and then on standing. The BP on standing should be measured for as long as it takes to determine the nadir of the fall, which may occur 3–10 minutes later. A symptomatic fall of 20 mmHg or more in systolic or 10 mmg or more in diastolic confirms the diagnosis. Management is both pharmacologic (reduce/avoid offending drugs; consider Midodrine, an alpha agonist) and non-pharmacologic (support stockings, avoid triggers, slow rising from horizontal position).

Carotid sinus syndrome (CSS)

This syndrome accounts for many causes of recurrent unexplained falls (Kenny *et. al.* 2004). It presents with unexplained falls in which there is no recollection "of hitting the ground." Studies have suggested it can account for up to 40% in some series. Investigation is by carotid sinus massage (CSM) using a standard protocol. If there is a carotid bruit, carotid Doppler must be performed prior to testing. CSM testing is positive if the typical symptoms are reproduced. CSM requires vertical massage of the right carotid sinus for 5 seconds by applying firm backward pressure on the sinus against vertebrae. After a pause, this is repeated on the left. A positive CSM is regarded as a pause of 3 or more seconds (cardio-inhibitory) and/or a drop in systolic blood pressure of >50 mmHg (vasodepressor). The cardio-inhibitory type is treated with a dual chamber pacemaker (Fig. 18.2).

There is no effective cure for the vasodepressor type, although selective serotonin reuptake inhibitors have been tried with some benefit (Fig. 18.2).

Situational syncope

Situations include micturition, defecation, coughing, and occasionally laughing and swallowing. The history is usually clear, but one must ask the correct questions to elucidate the story. It is rare in the general population. The mechanism is assumed to be excess vagal stimulation. On straining at stool, there is raised intra-abdominal pressure producing vagus nerve activation and subsequent drop in pulse and cardiac output leading to syncope. Cough syncope mimics a Valsalva maneuver. No investigations are necessary. The outcome is excellent with avoidance of triggering stimulation by cough suppression or sitting down to urinate.

Drop attacks

This describes an uncommon situation when the patient falls without warning and with no loss of consciousness. Patients describe their knees buckling for no reason and falling forward without protection. The falling down suggests a loss of muscle tone. They are able to get up immediately. The mechanism is unknown and the diagnosis is clinical. There is no effective treatment, but the outcome is typically benign save for bruises and cuts.

Miscellaneous causes of collapse presenting as a fall

Other conditions leading to fall or collapse include epilepsy, cerebrovascular events, and arrhythmias. In epilepsy, the characteristic features include tongue biting, incontinence, and tonic clonic movements. In cerebrovascular events, there are additional focal signs in the neurology examination. Transient arrhythmias such as ventricular tachycardia may cause falls. It is unusual for supraventricular rhythm disturbance to cause a fall. The history may provide pointers such as sudden onset of impending collapse with pallor indicating a drop in cardiac output due to the rhythm disturbance. In all these causes the treatment of the specific medical condition will reduce future collapses.

Key learning points in falls assesment

1. Determine the cause (s) of the fall – possible in 98% of cases
2. Reduce future falls where possible – by treating cause(s), especially gait and balance retraining
3. Reduce the consequences of future falls – this principally means fear of falls and bone health

Incontinence
Urine Incontinence
Urinary Incontinence clinical analysis

Loss of urine		Acute /temporary or new onset *or* Chronic/for some time	Reversible **(Dippers)** Longer persisting **Stress/Urge/ Overflow/ Functional**
Nature of loss	**Questions**	**Answers**	**Due to**
	How much	Small or large amounts	**Stress or urge**
	How is it lost	On coughing	**Stress**
		On rushing to toilet / frequent toileting	**Urge**
		With large abdomen with painless loss	**Overflow**
		Inappropriate loss	**Dementia**

Acute reversible causes of urinary incontinence

D   Delirium (acute confusional state)
I   Infection or fecal impaction
P   Pharmacological (diuretics)
P   Psychological (depression)
E   Estrogen deficiency (atrophic vaginitis)
R   Restricted (mobility/access)
S   Sugar in urine (diabetes mellitus and other causes of polyuria)

Reversible causes should always be sought and excluded before labeling a person with chronic urinary incontinence.

Chronic causes of urinary incontinence
Types of UI

Stress: minor increases in abdominal pressure cause drops of urine to leak.

Urge: sudden precipitous urgency to pass water due to involuntary detrusor contractions.

Overflow: there is neurological damage to the nerve supply to the uro-genital tract leading to inability of the bladder to empty.

Functional: the cause for the UI is not related to any local pathology.

Causes of UI

Urge: Over-active bladder due to detrusor instability/prostatism.

Stress: Obstetric/gynecological surgery/post-menopausal perineal floor disuse.

Overflow: Spinal cord nervous disease.

Functional: Dementia (central nervous diseases).

Introduction

Incontinence is defined as the involuntary loss of urine. It is common and 12% of the community dwelling population suffer the problem. The incidence increases to 70% in long-term care institutions. The medical, psychological, social, and economic costs are considerable. These include recurrent urinary tract infections, depression, social isolation, and the cost of pads. Patients may not present with symptoms of urine control because they expect it as part of old age. Understanding of the patho-physiology of conditions that cause incontinence has improved leading to improved management.

It is crucial to determine transient reversible causes of UI from chronic long-term causes.

History

How long: acute or chronic

How UI occurs: dribbles (stress) or having to rush (urgency)

Associated symptoms: vaginal itch (vaginal atrophy); vaginal discharge (cancer); "lump coming down" (prolapse)

Past history: obstetric history and gynecology surgery; medications;

Functional history: mobility and ability to self-care; memory assessment

Examination

- Cardiac examination
- Abdominal examination – bladder enlargement (overflow)
- Vaginal bi-manual examination – condition of vaginal tissues and prolapse (atrophy)
- Get patient to cough on standing if possible and observe the urethral meatus (for drips = stress UI)

- Anal tone during rectal examination and perineal sensation (spinal cord disease)
- Review range of movement of lower back and limbs (arthritis)

Investigation	Why
Urinalysis/MSU	UTI/diabetes
Urine cytology	Bladder tumor
U&E, creat, PSA	Renal failure/benign prostatic hypertrophy
Blood glucose	Diabetes
Post-void Residual	Obstruction/over-active bladder (OAB)
Ultrasound	Tumor/stone/obstruction
Cystoscopy	Anatomical pathology of tract/tumor/stricture/stone
PAD testing & charts	Amount of loss/when
MRI spine	Spinal cord pathology

Other more specialized tests such as urodynamics have no place in routine UI assesment.

Genuine stress incontinence

This is common in women over 60 years. There is leakage of small amounts of urine on coughing or laughing, or when constipated because of forward pressure of the full rectum on the bladder. It occurs when intravesical pressure is greater than urethral pressure. The urethral sphincter is commonly damaged in vaginal childbirth, weakens post-menopause, and is disrupted in prolapse of uterus or urethra.

- Management includes removing or reducing anything that increase abdominal pressure such as constipation.
- Specifically, pelvic floor exercises with or without biofeedback have been shown to be effective. Success depends on persisting with the program of exercises.
- Surgical techniques have also improved and have focused more on the management of intrinsic urethral sphincter incompetence. This involves injecting inert substances to increase the bulk of the sphincter, improving its ability to hold urine in the bladder. Collagen is used, but it degrades and repeat injections are needed. Colposuspension is also effective in some cases.

Over-active bladder (OAB)

This is the second commonest cause of chronic UI. There is a need to rush to the toilet as soon as the urge to pass urine is felt and those affected may not make it in time. The amount of urine lost is much greater than with stress. Frequency is a common complaint as is disturbed sleep because of night-time passing of urine. Frequently, both stress and urge incontinence co-exist. This makes separation difficult on history alone. For reasons which are not clear, the detrusor muscle resets its intrinsic pressure so that the muscle contracts at much lower volumes. As it contracts involuntarily there is a sense of impending urine loss hence the urge feeling.

Management includes non-pharmacologic behavioral feedback techniques aimed at retraining the bladder capacity to hold urine using a regular bladder drill programme. This includes fluid restriction and modification including avoiding alcohol or caffeine after supper. Pharmacologic treatment is helpful and frequently first line.

Drugs used in OAB
- Flavoxate
- Imipramine
- Oxybutynin
- Propantheline
- Propiverine
- Tolteradine
- Desmopressin

All of the above, apart from desmopressin, are anticholinergic agents. Some are more selective at inhibiting the muscarinic subtype receptors involved in micturition (m3) than others. All produce side effects expected when acetylcholine is blocked – dry eyes, dry mouth, constipation.

Desmopressin, an antidiuretic hormone analog, leads to reduction in urine formation. It is used to reduce night-time disturbance from OAB. Dilutional hyponatremia frequently occurs from water retention and needs to be managed accordingly with dose titration.

Surgery has a small role. Myomectomy (removal of part of the detrusor bladder muscle) can reduce the frequency of contractions. The operation is called a clam cystoplasty. It is reserved for severe, intractable cases.

Medications
Many medications cause or worsen UI.

Where possible, modification of medications can be important in reducing or eliminating UI. The list below (Table 18.1) is not exhaustive, but should encourage the student or doctor to question every

Table 18.1. Drugs that can cause or exacerbate UI

Drugs	Mechanism
Diuretics	Excess urine production (except low dose thiazides used for BP control)
NSAIDs	Fluid retention
Calcium blockers	Fluid retention and leg edema
Lactulose	Increase glucose level
Alcohol and caffeine	Induce diuresis
Alpha-blockers	Relax urinary sphincter (used in treatment)
Anti-psychotics, and major tranquilizers and hypnotics (e.g. benzodiazepines)	Increase confusion/delirium and cause bradykinesia
Over-the-counter (OTC) drugs which might include caffeine/liquorice	Induce diuresis

medication including over-the-counter drugs and complementary medicines. The association may not be immediately obvious. For example, many slimming aids contain diuretics.

Vaginal atrophy

Vaginal atrophy occurs to a lesser or greater degree in all post-menopausal women not taking estrogen replacement therapy. Loss of estrogen leads to loss of normal columnar tissue. Secretions are reduced and the friability of the tissue is increased. Consequently, the skin can become dry and itchy and is more prone to local infection. It is important to use water-based gel during vaginal exam. Management is simple and effective – locally applied vaginal estrogen cream relieves the itch and will frequently improve UI.

Vaginal and urethral prolapse

This occurs more as a contributory element to chronic UI. The complaint is more of "something coming down" than of UI. However, there will usually be some urinary symptoms. Diagnosis is by examination of the posterior and anterior vaginal wall. Loss of support from pelvic floor ligaments occurs after childbirth and is exacerbated after menopause. A ring pessary is very helpful in those with prolapse as part of their UI and especially helpful in those not suitable for surgery.

Spinal cord disease

Sacral nerves S2–S4 supply the bladder and any pathology of these nerves within or outside the cord can lead to UI.

Causes of sacral nerve involvement
- Osteoarthritis
- Cord demyelination (due to multiple sclerosis – UI is a common occurrence in MS patients)
- Cord tumors (rare)
- Plexopathy due to cancer (very rare)
- Peripheral neuropathy (most commonly due to diabetes)
- Idiopathic

Fecal incontinence (FI)

FI is less common than UI. It is said to occur in 2% of the population, but in up to 10% of care home residents. The causes are similar to UI.

Acute
Constipation leading to overflow.

Chronic
- Stroke
- Rectal cancer/colitis
- Local neurologic disease

Constipation
This is very common. In severe cases incontinence occurs as more liquid higher up runs over harder motion and presents as liquid motion. On rectal examination, hard stool is detected and cure is resolution of the constipation.

Spinal disease
This includes a variety of conditions that affect the terminal spinal cord such as tumor, hemorrhage or very rarely, syringomyelia. Peripheral lesions are more common and include local carcinoma invasion of the sacral plexus of nerves and peripheral neuropathies due to diabetes. Treatment will include specific treatments for the condition. General treatments will include constipation medications linked to manual bowel evacuation.

Key Points
Incontinence is more common than appreciated

Incontinence causes much indignity and reduced quality of life

Ask all patients about UI and FI

All patients can benefit from proper assesment and treatment

There are increasingly effective treatments

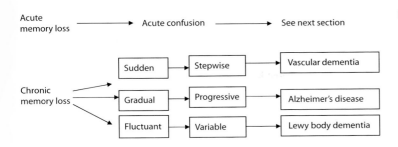

Fig. 18.3. Memory loss.

Memory loss (Fig. 18.3)

Introduction

Impairment of memory is common with advancing age. In many cases this does not imply dementia. The syndrome of age-related cognitive decline affects all persons. This must be distinguished from dementia.

Dementia

As we live longer, surviving cancer and cardiovascular disease, the prevalence of dementia increases from 1% in 60–64-year-olds to 35% in over-90-year-olds. It is defined as global impairment of intellect, memory, and reasoning without any alteration in level of consciousness. There are a number of definitions of dementia. Many of these have been developed mainly for research.

The causes of dementia are listed with prevalence data for UK in Table 18.2. It is increasingly important to distinguish between the various types of dementia because of emerging therapeutic options. Alzheimer's disease (AD) is the most common form and is a cortical dementia. By contrast, Lewy body dementia is increasingly recognized and is a sub-cortical dementia.

Criteria for diagnosis of dementia

- Evidence of decline in memory (impaired learning of new material and/or evidence of impaired recall of previously learned information)
- No impairment of consciousness
- Decline in emotional control or motivation or change in social behavior
- Present for at least 6 months
- No evidence of another reversible cause

Newer tests (Table 18.2 and Fig. 18.4) such as those below may improve our diagnostic accuracy.

Alzheimer's disease

AD is the commonest form of dementia (see Table 18.1). The principal histologic findings are intracellular neurofibrillary tangles (NFT) and extracellular deposition of beta amyloid between neurons. These changes lead to increased inflammation, fibrosis, and cell death with consequent synaptic loss. Familial cases of Alzheimer's disease present at a young age, typically less than 65 years. Gene mutations called presenilin 1 and 2 have been detected in such families.

The predominant areas of the brain affected are the parieto-temporal regions including the hippocampus. The clinical consequence of this damage is increased loss of recent memory along with an increasing inability to retain new information (parietal lobe). Visuo-spatial problems also occur because of loss of connections within the posterior cerebral cortex. Language is preserved but word finding difficulties emerge. The biochemical theory of Alzheimer's disease is that of an acetylcholine (Ach) deficiency syndrome due to progressive selective neuronal loss, following the observation that inhibition of Ach, using scopolamine, a postsynaptic Ach blocker, causes memory loss. Ach is synthesized by the enzyme choline acetyltransferase. Ach is then released by the presynaptic neurons into the cleft. It stimulates both pre- and postsynaptic muscarinic and nicotinic receptors.

The effect of Ach is terminated by synaptic uptake or breakdown by acetylcholinesterase. Consequently, drug therapy has targeted (i) increased presynaptic Ach (ii) enhanced Ach duration in cleft, or (iii) post-synaptic receptor stimulation (Fig. 18.5).

Non-pharmacologic treatment

It is important to pay attention to:

- Improving orientation by use of clocks and other time questions
- Providing a supportive and understanding environment

Table 18.2. Types and incidence of irreversible dementias

TYPE	% of cases	Genetics	Drug therapy
Alzheimer's disease	50–60	Yes	Donepezil Rivastigamine Galantamine Antipsychotics for behavioral symptoms
Vascular dementia	25–30	No	No specific treatment Risk reduction of BP and strokes
Lewy body dementia	10–15	No	No specific treatment Avoid neuroleptic drugs Behavior treated with donepezil/hypnotics
Pick's disease	<11	No	No
Dementia with Parkinson's disease	<5	No	No
Alcoholic dementia with Korsakof's psychosis	<5	No	No
HIV dementia	<1	No	Treat HIV disease and other cerebrotrophic diseases
Prion diseases, e.g. Creutzfeld–Jacob disease	<1	? Yes	No

Table 18.3. Tests of higher brain function

Commonly used clinical scales – take 5–10 min to perform	
Mini mental state examination or abbreviated mental score	Cognition and memory
Neuro-psychiatric inventory	Behavioral symptoms
Geriatric depression score or Hamilton depression score	Mood
Bristol activity of daily living scale or Barthel Index	Functional capacity
Research scales – take up to 1 h to perform	
Alzheimer's disease assesment score for cognition	
Alzheimer's disease assesment score for behavior	
Hachincki score for vascular disease	Etiology score

- Maintaining adequate nutritional intake
- Providing stimulating and organized activities daily

The above treatments are supportive. They do nothing for the deficits in dementia. However, there are newer drugs available to treat AD.

Pharmacologic treatment

There are four drugs: Memantine is a glutamate antagonist, which protects and preserves neurons from excito-toxicity and cell death. It is not used much but it may have a role as additive therapy to the other drugs. Its main side effect is agitation.

Donepezil, rivastigmine, and galantamine act by reversible inhibition of acetyl cholinesterase (AchEI). This leads to increased concentration of synaptic Ach. Side effects are typical of excess Ach – nausea, diarrhea, occasional vomiting.

Donepezil, rivastigmine, galantamine, and memantine have shown statistically significant increases in memory using the Alzheimer's disease assessment scale – cognitive section (ADAS-cog). Randomized trials have showed improvement in behavior using various rating scales. None has improved the quality of life.

In the trials, all drugs were given double blind for up to 26 weeks only. Open label follow up exists over several years but there is concern about using such drugs for a long time.

Because of these concerns, active monitoring is recommended. The National Institute of Clinical Excellence in the UK (NICE) has issued guidance about initiation and follow-up:

- Assessment by specialist with experience in such patients
- Use of scales (MMSE, behavioral scale, and a carer stress scale)
- Follow-up for efficacy and tolerability
- Shared care with primary care is encouraged (Fig. 18.6)

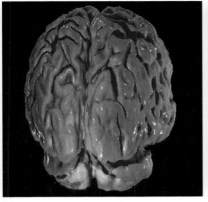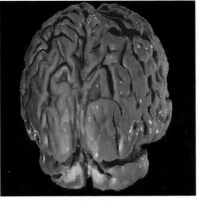

Fig. 18.4. Functional magnetic resonance images of dementia subject (left) and normal subject (right). The image distinguishes differences in brain activity on stimulation. (Image: Professor SHD Jackson, King's College, London.)

Non-responders   Responders

Table 18.4. Investigations of chronic memory loss

Blood count	Anemia
Renal function	Chronic renal disease
Liver function	Acute or chronic liver disease
Thyroid function	Hypothyroidism
Serum calcium level	Hypercalcemia
Syphilis test; HIV test	Syphilis or HIV disease
ESR/CRP	Arteritides
Vitamin B12/serum folate	Nutritional deficits
CT/MRI brain	Brain tumors/hydrocephalus
MSU	Urine infection

Note:
Other tests are indicated based on clinical history and may include EEG or lumbar puncture for spinal fluid analysis.

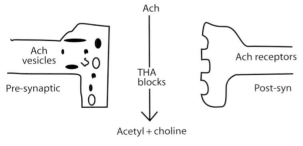

Fig. 18.5. Scheme of mechanism of action of all acetylcholinesterase inhibitors (THA = tacrine).

Patients who do not respond to a lower dose are increased to maximal tolerated doses. Thereafter, a failure of response leads to discontinuation of the drug. Such a decision should be made in consultation with patients and their principal carers. Patients and carers should be warned of an anticipated decline regardless of treatment, as there is no cure for progressive neuronal loss.

Vitamin E

Vitamin E has been studied in many conditions including dementia. It acts as an antioxidant. Randomized controlled trials of vitamin E have hinted at some neuroprotective effect, but it cannot be recommended for use in AD because of limited evidence.

AD and psychotic symptoms

There is little evidence to guide the use of drugs for managing psychotic symptoms that cannot be controlled by behavioral modifications. This partly reflects the lack of adequate trials. Haloperidol is a widely used and safe traditional alternative. There is evidence for the use of the newer antipsychotics such as respiridone.

Key points in AD
- The choice of drugs for the management of AD is limited
- The amount of improvement is variable
- Response to drug treatment:
  - 30% deteriorate in spite of drug treatment
  - 40% respond with real clinical improvement
  - 20%–30% respond with an increase in scores from baseline but with uncertainty about true benefit
- Responders cannot be predicted in advance
- A therapeutic trial in patients in whom compliance is assured seems appropriate

Vascular dementia (VD)

Vascular dementia is also known as multi-infarct dementia. VD occurs due to progressive damage by

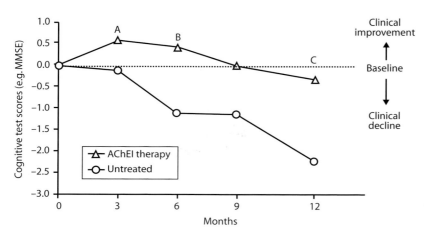

Fig. 18.6. Schema of effect of acetyl cholinesterase inhibitors (ACEIs) on cognition. All similar Alzheimer disease drugs have produced a similar composite graph of the effect on cognition.

atherosclerotic disease in the brain. This occurs in hypertensives, those with high cholesterol, diabetes, and those who smoke. Either large or more typically small strokes lead to sudden stepwise loss of brain function – some of which may return. Over time, many such patients deteriorate and present with dementia symptoms. Brain scans demonstrate multiple lesions in a random and widespread fashion.

Cardiovascular risk factors should be treated aggressively, targeting:

- Elevated cholesterol
- Atrial fibrillation
- Raised blood pressure
- Diabetes mellitus control
- Smoking cessation

There is no evidence to indicate that specific drugs can be used to treat VD. However, recent trials of a combination of perindopril and indapamide reduced the occurrence of stroke in patients with previous stroke disease. Cholesterol-lowering drugs have also been shown to reduce stroke event rate. It is presumed that reduction of repeated strokes will reduce development of VD.

Memantine is licensed for the treatment of VD and AD in the UK. It acts by inhibition of GABA excitotoxic neurotransmitter.

Key points in VD

- Reduce vascular risk factors
- Trials are ongoing into specific drugs for VD

Lewy body dementia (LBD)

This is an increasingly recognized form of dementia. It is typified by symptoms similar to AD but fluctuating

cognition, symptoms similar to Parkinson's disease, prominent early visual hallucinations, and higher rate of falls then AD to VD. Typically, the patients react very badly to use of traditional antipsychotics such as haloperidol. This reaction has assumed a pathognomonic aspect of LBD. Lewy bodies are normally occurring proteins. Pathologically, there is significant excess deposition of Lewy bodies in cells to a far greater amount than in AD. The exact nature of the Lewy bodies and why there is a predilection for the basal ganglia system is not clear. Rivastigmine has been shown in one trial to be helpful in LBD. Atypical antipsychotic drugs such as quetiapine or olazapine should be used for behavioral management. Like other forms of dementia, LBD is progressive and incurable. Increasing care needs frequently necessitate moving the patient to a care home.

Fronto-temporal dementias (FTD)

All are characterized by symptoms similar to AD, but with an early prominent element of emotional inappropriateness out of keeping with the rest of the disease. Genes associated with familial FTD have been isolated (function unknown). These are rare forms of dementia and include Pick's disease. Management is mainly non-pharmacologic as there are no drugs licensed for use in FTDs to date. Methods include reality orientation, structured living pattern, Social Services input (respite, additional allowances, care packages for personal and domestic support), and most importantly linking in with local carer groups such as the Alzheimer's Society.

Miscellaneous causes

Normal pressure hydrocephalus or non-communicating hydrocephalus is a rare condition described in the 1960s. It presents as progressive dementia with

Table 18.5. Causes of acute confusion

Infection	Associated with temperature	
Metabolic	Associated with renal failure with dehydration, renal disease, and obstruction	
	Associated with hypercalcemia	
Drug or alcohol related		
	Withdrawal of alcohol	Usual clear history or obvious intoxication
	Medication	Take history from GP, family
	Over the counter or recreational drugs	Always consider
Endocrine		
	Hypothyroidism	
	Hyperthyroidism	
	Hypoglycemia	
	Adrenal insufficiency	
Nutritional		
	Vitamin B12 deficiency	Common in old age
	Thiamine deficiency	Common in alcoholics
Acute brain injury	Associated with stroke, head injury, epilepsy, and infection	
Miscellaneous	Constipation	
	Anemia	
	Extracranial neoplasm with paracrine effects	

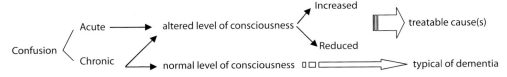

Fig. 18.7. Confusion.

prominent early ataxia and urinary incontinence out of proportion to the degree of dementia. It occurs when there is an acquired imbalance between CSF formation and CSF removal leading to accumulation of CSF in the brain and compression of brain tissue. Diagnosis is by brain scanning. Management is by insertion of a ventricular–peritoneal shunt to decompress the brain. Many patients respond well to this.

Pugilistic dementia is associated with excessive head injury such as boxing. Whether head trauma actually causes it is not clear.

Down syndrome dementia occurs when the affected person lives long enough. This is because the trisomy 21 over-expresses the pre-amyloid precursor gene and its protein, which leads to excess amyloid deposition in the brains of such children.

Alcohol dementia occurs when alcohol is taken in excess over many years. The damage is due to alcohol neurotoxicity along with nutritional depletion of vitamin B1 (thiamine) crucial to methyl transport. It is irreversible.

HIV dementia occurs as the virus is neurotrophic and can lead to neuronal cell death. It is rare now due to effective drug therapy.

Confusion (Fig. 18.7)

Confusion may be acute or chronic. Acute confusion is also known as delirium or toxic confusion or acute confusional state (Table 18.5). When it is chronic, it is best viewed as an element of a dementing illness (see above).

The confused patient is very common in hospital. Up to 30% of all acute hospital admissions have acute confusion at some time during their admission, frequently on presentation to the hospital. Its prevalence

Table 18.6. Investigations of the confused patient

In all patients	Where indicated by assesment
FBC and blood film and	
U&E	
LFTs	ANA, ANCA, Immune complexes
TFTs	Random cortisol
Calcium	MRI
ESR	EEG
MSU and sputum culture, Gram stain	Auramine stain for *Mycobacterium*
Chest X-ray	Drug toxicology urine screen
ECG	Stool culture
CT brain	

increases in those age over 65 yrs. With aging, the brain becomes less able to withstand any form of insult. Infection is the most common cause but typically, in the acutely confused patient, a number of insults will be relevant to the presentation.

On meeting the confused person for the first time it is vital to collect as much information as possible (Table 18.6).

- Is it acute/new or a worsening of chronic confusion?
- Is it of sudden onset?
- What is the history of the acute event?
- Are there any obvious precipitants, e.g. prescription drugs/over the counter medications?
- Has there been any foreign travel?

It is vital to:

- Determine the cause of the acute confusion (possible in all cases)
- Reverse the cause where possible (possible in many cases)

Drugs

Many drugs can cause acute confusion and this text cannot hope to cover all. Any newly commenced medication can either contribute to confusion or cause confusion.

Undertake a critical review of all medications with the aim of stopping all unnecessary medications.

Common groups of drugs	Examples
All opiate or codeine-based analgesics	Codeine
All central acting drugs	Diazepam
All cardiac drugs	Furosemide
All acetylcholine inhibitors	Tolteradine

Subdural hematoma

The patient presents with a gradual change in behavior, altered level of consciousness with typically agitation at night and drowsiness by day. There may be psychomotor retardation. The story of a fall (s) is not immediately obvious, as the fall may have occurred some time ago. It is common amongst older people – as are falls. There is blood in the subdural space compressing the brain, and if severe, leading to midline shift on brain scanning (CT or MRI), which is the investigation of choice to make the diagnosis. Management depends on severity and presence of co-morbid disease. Where it is deemed appropriate, decompression by burr hole surgery is very effective.

Anemia

Anemia commonly worsens confusion. The effect is related to the rate of change in hemoglobin and the vulnerability of the brain to hypoperfusion due to reduced oxygen-carrying capacity. Correction of anemia to a level of >10 g/dl will reduce confusion and improve delirium, although it is never the primary cause.

Further Reading

Falls

NICE falls and osteoporosis guideline (www.nice.org.uk/falls and osteoporosis)

J Am Geriatr Soc 2001; 49: 664. Falls guideline

SLIPS Project (www.slips-online.co.uk)

Incontinence

International Continence Society (www.icsoffice.org/)

Memory loss

Drugs for dementia 2006 (www.NICE.org.uk)

Cochrane Library (www.cochrane.org/)

McKeith *et al. Neurology* 1996; 47: 113

Confusion (delirium)

Inouye *et al. N Engl J Med* 2006; **354**, 1157–1165

British Geriatric Society delirium guideline, 2006 (www.bgs.org.uk)

The critically ill patient

Richard Leach

Contents

The acutely unwell patient

Assessment and resuscitation to correct deranged physiology must precede diagnosis in the acutely unwell patient. Initial diagnostic uncertainty and the need for immediate therapeutic action define critical care medicine. Many of the relevant conditions are discussed in other chapters.

Recognition

Early recognition of deterioration is paramount and should prompt immediate action to correct abnormal physiology and prevent damage to vital organs including the brain, kidneys and gastro-intestinal systems. Recognition is not difficult when the critical illness is already far advanced as in patients with (a) sudden, catastrophic deterioration; (b) those presenting with established illness in the emergency room and (c) with advanced, previously unrecognized, progressive deterioration on the ward. In these, organ damage may be already apparent and is difficult to reverse, but immediate action may prevent worsening. It is failure to recognize progressive deterioration (i.e (c) above), whilst under medical supervision, and to undertake appropriate early preventative action that are common causes of morbidity and mortality.

Prevention of organ damage is better than cure. Identifying "at-risk" patients (including medical and surgical emergencies, the elderly, post-surgical subjects, trauma victims, and those requiring massive blood transfusions) allows complications to be anticipated and prevented. These "at-risk" patients must be monitored, deterioration recognized, and appropriate action initiated early. Early warning scoring systems promote detection and trigger intervention. The modified early warning score "MEWS" is in common use: temperature, blood pressure, heart rate, respiratory rate, urine output, and consciousness level are scored 0–3 depending on the derangement. The scores are summed, and if >4 require staff to summon medical assistance from outreach teams (e.g. Patient At Risk Teams (PART) or Medical Emergency Teams (MET)) composed of senior nurses and doctors familiar with management of acutely unwell patients.

Initial assessment and management: the A, B, C, D system

Figure 19.1 illustrates the immediate assessment and management of acutely ill patients and is based upon the recommendations of a number of life support programmes including the ALS, ALERT, ATLS and the "Care of the Critically Ill Surgical Patient" course. It is designed to ensure patient safety and survival rather than a diagnosis.

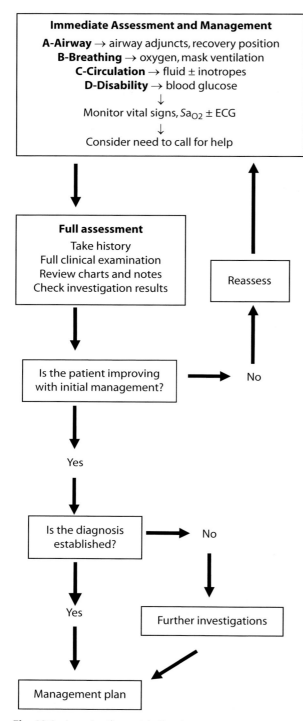

Immediate Assessment and Management
A-Airway → airway adjuncts, recovery position
B-Breathing → oxygen, mask ventilation
C-Circulation → fluid ± inotropes
D-Disability → blood glucose
↓
Monitor vital signs, Sa_{O_2} ± ECG
↓
Consider need to call for help

Full assessment
Take history
Full clinical examination
Review charts and notes
Check investigation results

Reassess

Is the patient improving with initial management?   No

Yes

Is the diagnosis established?   No

Yes

Further investigations

Management plan

Fig. 19.1. Assessing the acutely ill patient.

Asking the patient "How are you?" or "Are you alright?" provides important information. A normal response indicates that the airway is patent and that the patient is breathing, conscious, and orientated. A patient having difficulty speaking, or speaking in short sentences suggests serious breathlessness. No response indicates serious illness or unconsciousness. Assessment starts with the detection and simultaneous treatment of life-threatening emergencies. It uses the familiar ABC system: A-Airway, B-Breathing, C-Circulation, in this order, as airways obstruction causes death faster than disordered breathing which in turn causes death faster than circulatory collapse. Wherever possible, simple monitors including pulse oximeters, cardiac monitors, and non-invasive blood monitoring should be used to assist assessment as soon as is safely possible.

Airway

Obstruction of the upper airway is a medical emergency. It may be partial or complete and can occur at any level. Upper airways obstruction may be due to aspiration of solid particulate matter (e.g. partially masticated food, coins, teeth, vomit, blood, or gastric fluid). Laryngeal edema may be due to allergy, burns, or inflammation and laryngeal spasm due to stimulation by foreign bodies, blood, or secretions. Tracheobronchial obstruction includes aspiration of particulate matter, bronchospasm, or pulmonary edema. In the drowsy or sedated patient the tongue may obstruct the pharynx as it falls backward when the normal muscle tone is reduced (Fig. 19.2). Persistent airways obstruction causes a rapid fall in arterial oxygen tension (PaO_2), progressive hypoxic brain injury, coma, and death.

Recognition of airways obstruction is based on the "look, listen and feel" approach:

- *Look*: If there is respiratory effort. Complete airways obstruction causes paradoxical chest and abdominal movement, increased use of the accessory (e.g. neck, shoulder) muscles of respiration, and tracheal tug. Central cyanosis is a late sign. The mouth should be examined for the cause of the obstruction including foreign bodies and secretions.
- *Listen*: In complete obstruction there are no breath sounds. In partial obstruction air entry is reduced and noisy (e.g. snoring when the tongue is obstructing the pharynx, stridor with obstruction at the level of the larynx).

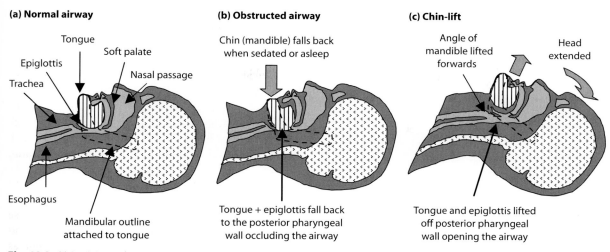

(a) Normal airway

Tongue
Soft palate
Epiglottis
Nasal passage
Trachea

Esophagus

Mandibular outline
attached to tongue

(b) Obstructed airway

Chin (mandible) falls back
when sedated or asleep

Tongue + epiglottis fall back
to the posterior pharyngeal
wall occluding the airway

(c) Chin-lift

Angle of
mandible lifted
forwards

Head
extended

Tongue and epiglottis lifted
off posterior pharyngeal
wall opening the airway

Fig. 19.2. Maintaining a clear airway.

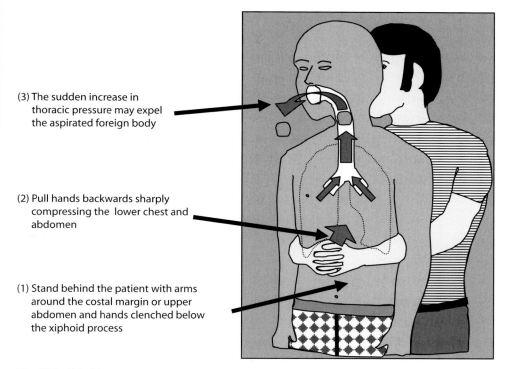

(3) The sudden increase in
thoracic pressure may expel
the aspirated foreign body

(2) Pull hands backwards sharply
compressing the lower chest and
abdomen

(1) Stand behind the patient with arms
around the costal margin or upper
abdomen and hands clenched below
the xiphoid process

Fig. 19.3. Heimlich maneuver.

- *Feel*: Movement of air is detected by placing cheek or hand in front of the patient's mouth.

Aspiration of partially masticated food is the most common cause of acute airways obstruction, giving rise to the "café coronary." Following complete occlusion, the subject is unable to speak or breathe and rapidly becomes cyanosed. If a sharp blow to the back of the chest fails to dislodge the particle, the Heimlich maneuver should be attempted (Fig. 19.3). The attendant stands behind the patient with arms around the upper abdomen, adjacent to the costal margin, hands clenched below the xiphoid process. The hands

575

(a) Oropharyngeal airway in place

Rigid (Guedel) airway holds
tongue forward

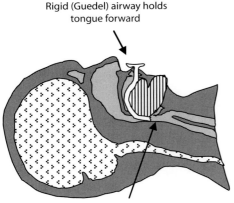

Tongue and epiglottis held forward
providing a channel for air passage

(b) Nasopharyngeal airway in place

Soft tube passes beyond
base of tongue

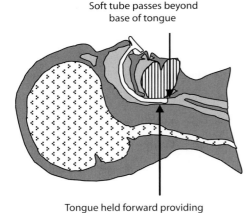

Tongue held forward providing
a channel for air passage

Fig. 19.4. Pharyngeal airways.

are pulled sharply backwards, compressing the upper abdomen and lower costal margin. The sudden increase in thoracic pressure may dislodge the obstructing particle, which is exhaled.

In many cases, use of simple measures to open the airway is all that is required. These include the chin lift manoever (Fig. 19.2) or insertion of an oropharyngeal (Guedel) airway (Fig. 19.4). If the oropharyngeal airway insertion is not possible (i.e. clenched teeth), the use of a soft nasopharyngeal airway may help. Tracheal intubation may be required if these fail. This may be performed without medication if the patient is *in extremis* or is having a cardiorespiratory arrest. If the patient is responsive and anesthetic drugs

Thumb and forefinger hold mask
tightly over nose and mouth

Head
extended

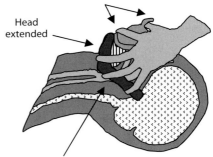

Three remaining fingers pull mandible
forward opening the airway

Fig. 19.5. Mask ventilation.

are required, an anesthetist or a physician with airways skills must be sought. Meanwhile, simple positioning of the head and orophargyngeal mask ventilation with 100% oxygen using a bag–valve–mask system (Fig. 19.5) should be used. As a last resort, an emergency cricothyroidectomy should be attempted. A large bore needle is inserted through the cricothyroid membrane, which is palpable just below the thyroid cartilage. This will only be successful if the obstruction is at the level of the larynx. Oxygen should be fed down the needle or tube. Urgent rigid bronchoscopy and/or thoracic surgery is required to remove the obstruction.

Breathing

Respiratory distress and inadequate ventilation are also detected by a "look, listen and feel" approach:

- *Look:* Respiratory rate is the most useful sign that breathing is compromised and rates higher than 12–20 are a useful warning sign that the patient may suddenly deteriorate. Inadequate breathing may be detected by looking for central cyanosis, distressed breathing, increased work of breathing, and abnormal chest wall movement (i.e. depth of breathing and equality of movement on each side of the chest). Chest wall deformity, jugular venous pressure (JVP), inspired oxygen concentration (Fi_{O_2}), saturation (Sa_{O_2}), and abdominal distension (that may impede respiratory movement) should be noted. The pulse oximeter cannot detect raised Pa_{CO_2} and the Pa_{O_2} may be normal in a patient receiving oxygen in the presence of a high Pa_{CO_2}.

Table 19.1. Typical physical signs in respiratory disorders

	Consolidation	Pneumothorax	Pleural fluid	Collapse
Movement	↓ on affected side	↓ on affected side	↓ on affected side	↓ on affected side
Trachea	Central	Central or shifted to unaffected side	Central or shifted to unaffected side	Shifted towards affected side
Percussion	Dull	Hyper-resonant	Stony dull	Dull
Breath sounds	Bronchial	Reduced/absent	Reduced/absent	Bronchial/reduced

- *Listen*: for airways noise (e.g. rattling secretions), stridor, and wheeze both with and without a stethoscope. Assess presence and quality of breath sounds to determine underlying lung disease.
- *Feel*: for the position of the trachea to detect mediastinal shift, depth and equality of movement, and percuss for hyper-resonance (e.g. pneumothorax) and dullness (e.g. pleural fluid, consolidation). Table 19.1 illustrates typical physical signs in respiratory disorders.

The management of individual respiratory disorders is discussed elsewhere. Every critically ill patient should receive oxygen to prevent end-organ damage. The aim is to achieve a Pa_{O_2} of 13 kPa (Sa_{O_2} 96%–98%) and at least 8 kPa ($Sa_{O_2} >$92%). To accomplish this, most acutely unwell patients should be given high flow oxygen ($>$10 l/min; $Fi_{O_2} >$60%) administered through a reservoir, non-rebreathing mask.

In patients with COPD or type-2 respiratory failure, high oxygen concentrations may precipitate carbon dioxide retention. Nevertheless, hypoxia must still be prevented to avoid end-organ damage. Initial O_2 therapy (i.e. before blood gas measurements are available) is started at an $Fi_{O_2} \sim$40% and to maintain the Sa_{O_2} at $\sim$88%–92%. After blood gas measurement, controlled oxygen therapy using a fixed performance (24%–35%) Venturi mask is preferable using the lowest oxygen concentration to achieve an Sa_{O_2} of 88%–92% ($Pa_{O_2} >$8 kPa). A higher Sa_{O_2} has no advantages but may cause or worsen hypercapnia and respiratory acidosis. Arterial blood gases must be monitored regularly. If Pa_{CO_2} rises ($>$10.5 kPa), pH falls ($<$7.25), or drowsiness or fatigue occurs, non-invasive ventilation (NIV) should be considered.

Circulation

Hypovolemia is the primary cause of shock until proven otherwise. In surgical patients, hemorrhage, which is not always easily identified, must be considered. Unless there are signs of cardiogenic shock, any patient with cool peripheries and tachycardia should be given intravenous fluid.

As previously; assess the circulation with the "look, listen and feel" approach:

- *Look* for cool, pale limbs and digits, peripheral cyanosis, under-filled veins, and signs of hemorrhage. The capillary refill time is the time for color to return to a finger tip held at heart level after pressing for 5 seconds (normally $<$2 s). Confusion and reduced urine output are additional features of poor cardiac output.
- *Listen* for heart valve leaks and blood pressure (BP). It is essential to remember that the BP may be normal initially as compensatory mechanisms (i.e. increased peripheral resistance) maintain the BP despite a low cardiac output. Cardiac output has to fall by more than 20% (i.e. equivalent to the acute loss of a liter of blood) before the blood pressure begins to fall. However, the pulse pressure (the difference between systolic and diastolic pressure; normally $\sim$40 mmHg) may narrow during arterial vasoconstriction (e.g. during hypovolemia or cardiogenic shock), whereas diastolic BP may be low during arterial vasodilation (e.g. sepsis).
- *Feel* the peripheral and central pulses for rate, rhythm, and equality. Thready, fast pulses indicate a poor cardiac output, whereas a bounding pulse suggests sepsis.

Initial stabilization of circulation depends on the cause of failure. Immediately life-threatening conditions including hemorrhage, cardiac tamponade, and massive pulmonary embolism must be treated. The aim is to replace fluid, control bleeding, and restore cardiac output, BP, and tissue perfusion. Good venous access must be established using wide-bore peripheral and central venous cannulas. In the absence of cardiac

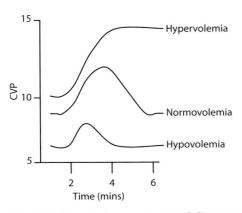

Fig. 19.6. The central venous pressure (CVP) response to a 500 ml fluid challenge.

Table 19.2. Common causes of unconsciousness

Profound hypoxemia
Hypoglycemia
Hypercapnia
Sedatives or analgesics
Cerebral hypoperfusion
Anesthetic agents

failure (i.e. failure to detect a raised jugular venous pressure (JVP) or coarse bilateral basal crepitations on lung auscultation), a crystalloid fluid challenge of 0.5–1 l should be given and the response assessed in terms of pulse rate, BP, and chest auscultation for crepitations. The response of the central venous pressure to a fluid challenge is a useful measure of the patient's fluid status (i.e hypovolemic, normovolemic, or hypervolemic) as illustrated in Fig. 19.6. Aim to restore blood pressure to the patient's normal or achieve a systolic BP >100 mmHg.

If no improvement with initial fluid challenge, repeat and reassess. If continuing fluid resuscitation fails to stabilize the vital signs or the patient develops cardiac failure, alternative means of improving cardiac output and tissue perfusion must be considered (i.e. inotropes and vasopressors). If vital signs return to normal but large volumes of fluid are necessary, reassessment for fluid loss is essential. If hemorrhage is suspected, send blood for cross-matching. At this stage blood should also be sent for routine investigations including FBC, biochemistry, and clotting profiles.

D-Disability

Rapid assessment of neurologic status is performed by examining the pupils and by whether the patient is alert, responds to voice or pain or is unresponsive (Glasgow Coma Scale (GCS)). Hypoglycemia must be excluded with dextrostix or glucometer. If below 3 mmol/l, give 50 ml 20% glucose intravenously. Severe or refractory hypoglycemia (e.g. sulphonylurea overdose) requires glucagon or hydrocortisone. These patients must be admitted for blood sugar monitoring

(± glucose infusions). Table 19.2 illustrates other common causes of unconsciousness. Examine for injury, ischemia, or trauma (e.g. unrecognized fractured hip). Patients with reduced conscious levels (GCS < 8) should be managed on a high dependency unit (HDU) or intensive care unit (ICU).

Unconscious patients with spontaneous ventilation and circulation are best nursed in the lateral recovery position (Fig. 19.7). They are at risk of airways obstruction in the supine position due to the tongue obstructing the pharynx. Airway protective reflexes may be insufficient to prevent inhalation of secretions or vomit. If there is risk of cervical injury, the patient should be left supine with constant attention to ensure airway patency. If the patient must be turned, they should be log rolled into the lateral recovery position.

Full patient assessment

Following initial assessment, the patient should be improving and cardio-respiratory function should have stabilized. Help should have been summoned. At this stage, full assessment is required. If the diagnosis has not been established further investigation may be required. If the diagnosis is clear, the management plan must be communicated to the medical team and documented in the notes.

The hypotensive patient

Hypotension (i.e. low blood pressure) is a common occurrence both within and outside the hospital. It is often preceded by warning signs of tachycardia or bradycardia, nausea, and a cold "clammy" sweating. Most have experienced these symptoms, i.e. vaso-vagal hypotension. Hypotension is a late sign of compromised circulation as increased peripheral resistance maintains the blood pressure despite low cardiac output. Hypotension results in poor perfusion and damage to major organs, including the brain and kidneys. It should be regarded as an emergency requiring immediate intervention and a search for the cause.

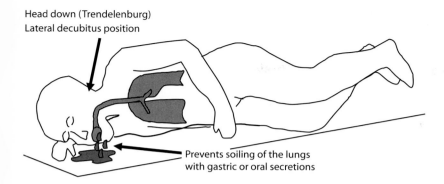

Head down (Trendelenburg)
Lateral decubitus position

Prevents soiling of the lungs
with gastric or oral secretions

Fig. 19.7. The recovery position: head down (Trendelenburg) lateral decubitus position.

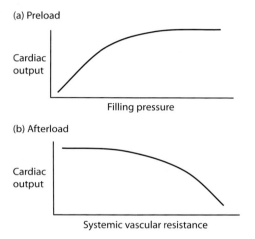

(a) Preload

Cardiac output

Filling pressure

(b) Afterload

Cardiac output

Systemic vascular resistance

Fig. 19.8. Cardiac output response of the normal heart to preload and afterload.

Blood pressure is determined by cardiac output and vascular resistance. Hypotension results if cardiac output or vascular resistance fall, or both. Three factors determine cardiac output:

- **Preload**: is the "filling pressure" of the heart and reflects the amount of blood returning to the right side of the heart from the tissues. The relationship between preload and cardiac output is shown in Fig. 19.8(a). If filling of the heart falls, so will cardiac output. Hypovolemia due to fluid loss is the commonest cause of a fall in preload. Reduction of vascular resistance (vasodilation) and altered distribution of circulating blood volume cause relative hypovolemia and a fall in cardiac output. This may be due to sepsis, allergic reactions, drugs, or epidural analgesia.
- **Contractility**: is a measure of the strength of cardiac contraction. If the heart is unable to pump and contractility is reduced, cardiac output will

fall. Reduced cardiac contractility may be due to arrhythmias, myocardial infarction, severe sepsis, valve dysfunction, pulmonary embolism, or cardiac tamponade.

- **Afterload**: the resistance to ejection of blood from the heart. It approximates to "vascular resistance." If vascular resistance rises, cardiac output falls (Fig. 19.8(b)). In practise, hypotension is rarely due to an increase in vascular resistance. In contrast, a fall in vascular resistance causes hypotension, often associated with increase in cardiac output. The commonest cause of a fall in vascular resistance is sepsis. It causes hypotension with a high cardiac output. A reduction in sympathetic nervous stimulation also reduces vascular resistance following high spinal cord damage or some drugs.

Organ oxygenation is dependent on the flow of blood to tissues, which relies on a mean arterial blood pressure greater than 55–65 mmHg in most organs, where the mean BP = diastolic BP + (systolic BP − diastolic BP/3). Hypotension will cause the following effects:

- **Renal**: if mean renal BP falls below ~60 mmHg, glomerular filtration decreases and urine production falls. Thus urine output is a good indicator of renal perfusion. If urine output falls below 1 ml/kg per h, it indicates poor renal perfusion. Oliguria (<0.5 ml/kg per h) for more than 2 hours indicates the need for immediate intervention to prevent acute tubular necrosis.
- **Cerebral**: falling conscious level (GCS decreases by >2 points) suggests reduced cerebral perfusion pressure and the need to increase the BP.
- **Heart**: the coronary blood flow depends on diastolic BP. A fall in BP may reduce coronary

579

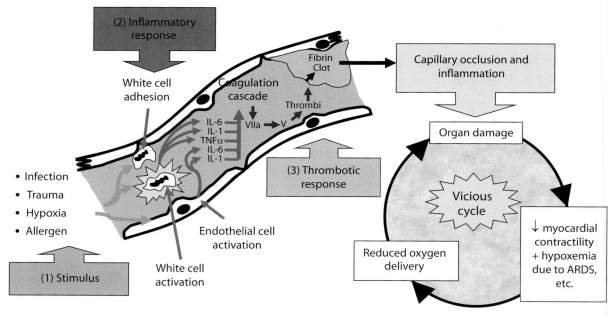

Fig. 19.9. The pathophysiology of shock.

artery filling causing myocardial ischemia or infarction and reduced cardiac contractility.

- *Skin*: a fall in blood pressure reduces skin perfusion and may cause ischemia.
- *Gastro-intestinal tract*: reduced gut perfusion may lead to bowel ischemia and bacterial translocation with subsequent sepsis.

Shock
Definition
Shock is a loose term used to describe the clinical syndrome of hypotension and circulatory failure with inadequate or inappropriately distributed tissue perfusion. The resulting failure to meet tissue metabolic demands causes generalized cellular hypoxia with or without lactic acidosis and tissue damage (Fig. 19.9).

The causes of shock and hypotension can be classified into six categories:

- **Hypovolemic:** major reductions in circulating blood volume caused by hemorrhage, plasma loss, e.g. burns, pancreatitis, or extracellular fluid loss, e.g. diabetic ketoacidosis, trauma.
- **Cardiogenic:** severe heart failure, e.g. myocardial infarction, acute mitral regurgitation.
- **Obstructive:** caused by circulatory obstruction e.g. pulmonary embolism, cardiac tamponade.

- **Septic:** septicemia, e.g. *E. coli, Candida*. Vasodilation, arteriovenous shunting, and capillary damage cause subsequent hypotension and maldistribution of flow.
- **Anaphylactic:** allergen-induced vasodilation, e.g. bee sting, peanut and other food allergies.
- **Neurogenic (spinal):** follows high traumatic spinal cord lesions above T6. Interruption of sympathetic outflow causes vasodilation, hypothermia, and bradycardia, which may be severe if vagal stimulation due to pain or hypoxia is unopposed.

Clinical features
Clinical features include hypotension (systolic BP <90 mmHg), tachycardia (>100 beats/min), oliguria (urine output <0.5 ml/kg per h), rapid respiration (>30/min), and drowsiness, confusion, or agitation. The features depend on the underlying cause and the severity. It tends to be either:

- *"Cold, clammy" shock*: due to hypovolemic, cardiogenic, obstructive, or late septis are associated with cold peripheries due to skin vasoconstriction, weak pulses and low cardiac output, oliguria, peripheral cyanosis, and confusion.
- *"Warm, dilated" shock*: occurs in early septis or anaphylactis and is associated with warm

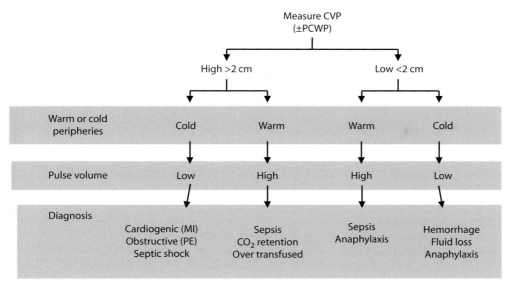

Fig. 19.10. Clinical assessment algorithm.

peripheries and flushing due to vasodilation, bounding pulses, and high cardiac output due to reduced vascular resistance.

Investigations

These include routine hematology, biochemistry, blood gases, cardiac enzymes, lactic acid, and cross-matching if hemorrhage suspected. Circulatory assessment may require intra-arterial blood pressure, CVP, and ECG monitoring. Additional measurements may include cardiac output, systemic vascular resistance, pulmonary capillary wedge pressure, and central venous oxygen saturation (Sv_{O_2}). Chest or abdominal radiographs may be required. Microscopy and culture of blood, sputum, and urine may be indicated.

Clinical assessment

The clinical features, CVP, and systemic vascular resistance (SVR) define the cause of shock (Fig. 19.10). The CVP, pulmonary capillary wedge pressure (PCWP), and SVR are useful when clinical signs are difficult to interpret. For example:

- CVP: *(a) reduced* in hypovolemic and anaphylactic shock
  (b) elevated in cardiogenic and obstructive shock
  (c) low, normal or high in septic shock
- SVR: *(a) high* in cardiogenic shock with sympathetic mediated vasoconstriction
  (→ "cold, clammy" patient)

(b) low in septic vasodilation due to release of inflammatory mediators
(→ "warm, dilated" patient).

Simple hemodynamic patterns may aid diagnosis in the acutely unwell hypotensive patient:

➢	Hypovolemic shock	→	low CVP/ PCWP	+	low CO	+	high SVR
➢	Cardiogenic shock	→	high CVP/ PCWP	+	low CO	+	high SVR
➢	Septic shock	→	low CVP/ PCWP	+	high CO	+	low SVR

Complications

Shock with circulatory failure and tissue hypoxia results in multi-organ failure including acute respiratory distress syndrome (ARDS), systemic inflammatory response syndrome (SIRS), acute renal failure, disseminated intravascular coagulation (DIC), hepatic failure, and mucosal ulceration. A cycle of increasing "oxygen debt" and "shock-induced" tissue damage develops as decreased myocardial contractility and hypoxemia, e.g. due to ARDS, further impairs oxygen delivery and tissue oxygenation (Fig. 19.9). Ischemic damage to the intestinal mucosa causes bacterial and toxin translocation into the splanchnic circulation causing further organ impairment and sepsis. Eventually, "refractory" shock develops with irreversible tissue damage and death.

General management of shock

Aim to correct the underlying cause, reverse "the tissue oxygen debt", and prevent the cycle of progressive organ damage. Management of shock, whatever the cause, has common features:

(1) *Identify the cause*

(2) *Early treatment is vital*: mortality increases if shock lasts more than an hour, giving rise to the concept of "the golden hour." Hypoxemia must be corrected with supplemental oxygen. In the absence of lung disease, severe shock will cause hypoxia due to reduced pulmonary blood flow, ventilation–perfusion (V/Q) mismatch, and a low Sv_{O_2}.

(3) *Resuscitation*: requires appropriate fluid management and is dependent on the cause of shock. For example, hypovolemia with low CVP requires fluid replacement whereas cardiogenic shock due to a myocardial infarction and raised CVP needs fluid restriction, although fluid administration may be required in right ventricular infarction. The time course of the disease is also important. For example, at the onset of septic shock, fluid replacement is essential but, if ARDS develops, fluid restriction is necessary to prevent pulmonary edema.

(4) *Inotropic support*: required when hypotension (mean arterial pressure <60 mmHg) or tissue hypoxemia, e.g. oliguria persists despite adequate fluid replacement, or when fluid resuscitation is contraindicated in cardiogenic shock. The type of inotropic support depends on the cause:

- *In septic shock*, the cardiac output is high but vasodilation with a low systemic vascular resistance may cause hypotension, inadequate tissue perfusion, and organ hypoxia with oliguria and confusion. In this situation, norepinephrine, a peripheral vasoconstrictor (alpha-receptor agonist), increases the vascular resistance, restoring blood pressure and tissue perfusion.
- *In cardiogenic shock*, the cardiac output is low and systemic vascular resistance high. Dobutamine increases myocardial contractility

and causes vasodilation resulting in rising blood pressure and cardiac output.

(5) *Remove circulatory obstructions*: for example (a) thrombolysis in pulmonary embolism; (b) drainage of pericardial effusion causing tamponade; (c) relief of tension pneumothorax compressing the right ventricle of the heart and preventing filling; (d) correction of disseminated intravascular coagulation (DIC) to prevent micro-circulatory obstruction.

(6) *Correction of severe acidosis*: which may impair cardiac contractility, with a sodium bicarbonate infusion. This is controversial but may be considered when pH <7.1 with a normal Pa_{CO_2}, i.e. base excess >−8.

(7) *Intubation and ventilation*: indications for intubation include progressive hypoxemia with Pa_{O_2} <8 kPa on >40% O_2, hypercapnia with Pa_{CO_2} >7.5 kPa, or respiratory rate >35/min. In obtunded patients, the high risk of aspiration necessitates a low threshold for intubation. Ventilatory support reduces work of breathing, improves cardiac function, and increases tissue oxygen delivery. Non-invasive ventilation, e.g. CPAP, may avoid need for intubation. Septic shock management is considered in detail.

Sepsis and the systemic inflammatory response syndrome

Definition

The inflammatory response that characterises "sepsis" is not always due to infection. A potential infective cause is detected in ~60%–70% with severe sepsis and blood cultures are positive in fewer than 25%. Table 19.3 presents definitions used to describe infection, systemic inflammatory response syndrome (SIRS), sepsis, and septic shock.

Epidemiology

Infection and sepsis cause significant morbidity and mortality. In the USA, about 500 000 patients, with an average age of 55 years, develop sepsis each year. It is the leading cause of multiple organ failure, ARDS, acute renal failure, and late death following trauma. In critical care units, 50% require antibiotics and in 50% infection was acquired after admission.

Pathology

The host's immune response is stimulated by invasive microorganisms and/or bacterial endotoxins. Initial cytokine release, e.g TNFα and interleukins, activates

Table 19.3. Terminology for the inflammatory state and sepsis

Infection	Invasion of sterile host tissue by microorganisms
Bacteremia	Viable bacteria in the blood
Systemic Inflammatory Response Syndrome (SIRS)	An inflammatory response to infective and non-infective conditions (e.g. pancreatitis, trauma, burns) defined as ≥ 2 of 4 criteria: 1. Temperature >38 or <36°C 2. Heart rate >90/min 3. Respiratory rate >20/min, $PaCO_2$ <32mmHg 4. White cell count >12 000 or <4000 cells/mm^3 or >10% immature (band) forms
Sepsis	SIRS due to infection
Septic Shock	Sepsis with features of shock (e.g. hypotension, inadequate organ perfusion)
Multiple Organ Dysfunction	Development of impaired organ function in SIRS. Multiple organ failure may follow

polymorphs, platelets, endothelium, complement, and coagulation pathways. White cells adhere to and damage vascular endothelium, allowing fluid and cells to leak into the interstitial space. Release of inflammatory mediators (e.g. nitric oxide (NO), prostacyclin) from the vascular endothelium and activated white cells causes profound circulatory vasodilation and susbsequent hypotension and shock. Damaged endothelium initiates secondary thrombotic activity with micro-circulatory occlusion and further impairment of tissue oxygen delivery. Systolic and diastolic myocardial dysfunction is due to reduced coronary perfusion associated with hypotension and the negative inotropic effects of NO and inflammatory mediators. Impaired tissue oxygen utilization is caused by sepsis-mediated cellular enzyme inhibition. Combined failure of oxygen delivery and inadequate tissue oxygen utilization causes multiorgan dysfunction.

Clinical presentation
Clinical features and potential sources of infection are illustrated in Fig. 19.11. The hemodynamic changes are variable and unrelated to the organism. Hypotension in a vasoconstricted "cold, clammy" patient, can mimic pulmonary embolism or myocardial infarction. Examination may reveal a focus of infection and characteristic clinical signs identify specific infections. For example, nail-bed splinter hemorrhages suggest endocarditis and the purpuric rash of meningococcal septicemia is characteristic (Fig. 19.12). Chest infection is the commonest source of sepsis.

Investigations
Initially, routine blood tests, C-reactive protein, plasma lactate; coagulation profile, and arterial blood gases for acid–base profile. Cultures of blood, sputum, urine, and wound pus *should* be taken before antibiotics, but should not delay therapy, one example being suspected meningococcal septicemia. Investigations include urinalysis, chest radiography, and ECG. Specific investigations (Fig. 19.11) depend on the suspected underlying cause, e.g. ultrasonography in intra-abdominal sepsis.

Management
General measures Supplemental oxygen therapy, respiratory support, e.g. non-invasive ventilation, nutrition, and prophylaxis against stress ulceration and thromboembolism. If the source of infection is identified, it must be treated. For example, unless an empyema or abscess is drained, the sepsis will persist and recur. Temperature, BP, urine output, and saturation must be monitored. When severe, CVP and/or cardiac output, central venous saturation (SvO_2), and lactate must be measured. Biochemistry, white cell count, and C-reactive protein provide information about the course of infection.

Fluid, vasopressor, and inotropic support In early septic shock, widespread vasodilation reduces systemic vascular resistance (SVR) causing hypotension and relative hypovolemia. The associated reduction of left ventricular afterload (see above) increases cardiac output (CO) but inappropriate distribution can cause regional, e.g. splanchnic and renal, ischemia. Initial fluid administration aims to correct hypovolemia, increasing BP and restoring organ perfusion pressures. As sepsis progresses, toxic myocarditis may impair myocardial function resulting in a flat left ventricular stroke function curve (poor contractility) and a fall in CO. Further fluid administration in an attempt to increase cardiac filling pressures only produces small increases of CO and may cause pulmonary edema due to the vascular permeability associated with sepsis. In this situation, vasopressor support with norepinephrine, an alpha-vasoconstrictor agonist, increases SVR, BP, and thus organ perfusion pressure and tissue oxygenation without further fluid administration. The CO may fall as SVR increases

583

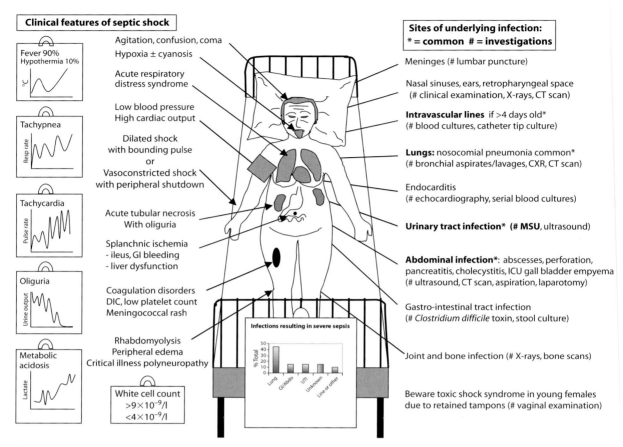

Clinical features of septic shock

Fever 90%
Hypothermia 10%

Agitation, confusion, coma

Hypoxia ± cyanosis

Acute respiratory distress syndrome

Tachypnea

Low blood pressure
High cardiac output

Dilated shock
with bounding pulse
or
Vasoconstricted shock
with peripheral shutdown

Tachycardia

Acute tubular necrosis
With oliguria

Splanchnic ischemia
- ileus, GI bleeding
- liver dysfunction

Oliguria

Coagulation disorders
DIC, low platelet count
Meningococcal rash

Metabolic acidosis

Rhabdomyolysis
Peripheral edema
Critical illness polyneuropathy

White cell count
>9×10⁻⁹/l
<4×10⁻⁹/l

Sites of underlying infection:
* = common   # = investigations

Meninges (# lumbar puncture)

Nasal sinuses, ears, retropharyngeal space
(# clinical examination, X-rays, CT scan)

Intravascular lines if >4 days old*
(# blood cultures, catheter tip culture)

Lungs: nosocomial pneumonia common*
(# bronchial aspirates/lavages, CXR, CT scan)

Endocarditis
(# echocardiography, serial blood cultures)

Urinary tract infection* (# MSU, ultrasound)

Abdominal infection*: abscesses, perforation,
pancreatitis, cholecystitis, ICU gall bladder empyema
(# ultrasound, CT scan, aspiration, laparotomy)

Gastro-intestinal tract infection
(# *Clostridium difficile* toxin, stool culture)

Joint and bone infection (# X-rays, bone scans)

Beware toxic shock syndrome in young females
due to retained tampons (# vaginal examination)

Infections resulting in severe sepsis

Fig. 19.11. The clinical features and potential sources of infection in sepsis.

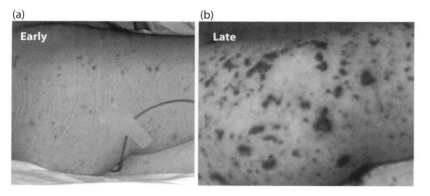

(a) Early (b) Late

Fig. 19.12. Early and late rashes of meningococcal meningitis.

if myocardial performance is impaired. The best approach then, is with inotropic agents: epinephrine, dopamine, or dobutamine, which increase cardiac contractility and maintain CO.

Antibiotic therapy   Initially *empiric* whilst awaiting microbiologic results and sensitivities. The regimen is selected by determining the most likely organisms: where the organism was contracted, in the community or hospital, the probable site of primary infection, and local antibiotic resistance patterns. Hospital-acquired infections usually involve staphylococci and Gram-negative organisms with greater antibiotic resistance than community-acquired organisms. Risk factors for hospital-acquired infections include age, male sex, prolonged admission (>3 days), mechanical ventilation, trauma, catheters, drugs (e.g. steroids), and immunodeficiency.

New therapies Activated protein C (APC) modifies the micro-circulatory thrombotic cascade and prevents ischemia. Relative adrenocortical insufficency is common in severe sepsis and "low-dose" steroid therapy is beneficial when profound hypotension is refractory to vasopressor support. Anti-inflammatory therapies including anti-TNF are unhelpful.

Line-related infection

About 10%–20% of central venous catheters (CVC) become infected and cause sepsis. Non-sterile insertion technique or inadequate line care are the commonest causes, although infection from distant sites (e.g. endocarditis) or contamination from infusions can occur. *S. aureus*, *S. epidermidis* and Gram-negative bacilli, e.g. *E. coli*, are the usual organisms. If line-related infection is suspected with sepsis and positive blood cultures, the cannula is removed and the tip cultured. A new line is inserted at a different site. Empiric antibiotic therapy is started, although fever may resolve spontaneously after removal of a line. Prevention of line infection requires strict aseptic insertion and closed infusion systems. Lines should be removed as soon as possible, preferably within 3 days.

Sepsis prevention and prognosis

Infection control, hand washing, microbiologic monitoring, prophylactic antibiotics for some invasive procedures, and prompt management of suspected infection, e.g. early line changes, are essential. The prognosis in severe sepsis worsens with age, lactic acidosis, low white cell count, cytokine elevation, reduced SVR, and the number of organs failing. Mortality is 40%–60%.

The "blue (cyanosed) and breathless" patient

Hypoxia due to inadequate tissue oxygen for normal metabolism occurs within 4 minutes of failure to deliver oxygenated blood to the organs and tissues. Local oxygen reserves in tissues are small. The causes are as follows:

Respiratory Failure

- *Type I* describes failure of oxygenation and occurs when blood bypasses or is not fully oxygenated in the lungs causing hypoxemia (Pa_{O_2} <8.0 kPa or Sa_{O_2} <90%). The Pa_{CO_2} is normal (~5.3 kPa) or low because ventilation is unchanged or increased due to breathlessness. The causes include ventilation–perfusion (V/Q) mismatch, right to left shunts, diffusion defects, and low inspired oxygen levels (Fi_{O_2}) as at high altitudes. In these circumstances oxygenation can be improved by re-expanding collapsed alveoli, oxygen therapy, and reducing V/Q mismatch.

- *Type 2* describes failure of ventilation with alveolar hypoventilation due to either reduction in respiratory rate or a fall in tidal volume. This increases Pa_{CO_2}, as in Fig. 19.13. The relationship between Pa_{CO_2} and alveolar P_{O_2} ($P_{A_{O_2}}$) is described by the alveolar gas equation (Fig. 19.14). Hypoventilation is the commonest cause of type 2 respiratory failure with failure of alveolar carbon dioxide clearance and arterial hypercapnia (Pa_{CO_2} >6–6.5 kPa) with or without hypoxemia. Hypoventilation results in an alveolar–arterial oxygen difference of <1 kPa. This distinguishes it from other causes of hypoxemia.

Failure of oxygen transport

Due to reduced blood flow, anemia, or hemoglobinopathy. In low output cardiac states high concentration oxygen therapy (Fi_{O_2} >60%) hardly improves oxygenation because hemoglobin is fully saturated and oxygen solubility is low. Such patients require restoration of tissue blood flow by blood transfusion or increase in cardiac output. In carbon monoxide poisoning high-dose oxygen therapy is required despite a normal Pa_{O_2} to reduce carboxyhemoglobin half-life.

Failure of tissue oxygen utilization

This occurs during sepsis or poisoning, as from cyanide, and is due to failure of cellular (mitochondrial) utilization despite good oxygen delivery.

Clinical features

Successful therapy requires recognition of tissue hypoxia. The clinical features are non-specific: altered mental state, dyspnea, hyperventilation, cyanosis, arrhythmias, and hypotension. They are often missed or attributed to other causes.

Cyanosis describes the "blue" discoloration of skin, lips, or tongue which occurs when the blood passing through these tissues contains more than 1.5 g/dl of reduced, deoxygenated hemoglobin which

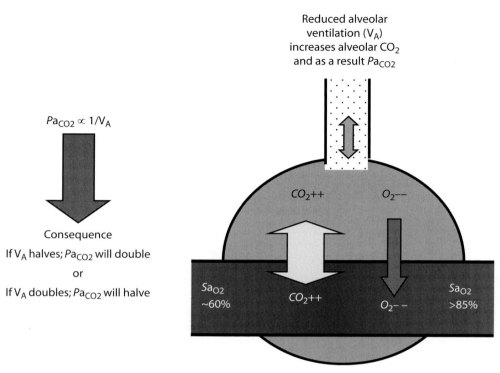

$Pa_{CO2} \propto 1/V_A$

Consequence

If V_A halves; Pa_{CO2} will double

or

If V_A doubles; Pa_{CO2} will halve

Reduced alveolar ventilation (V_A) increases alveolar CO_2 and as a result Pa_{CO2}

CO_2++ O_2--

Sa_{O2} ~60% CO_2++ O_2-- Sa_{O2} >85%

Fig. 19.13. The relationship between alveolar ventilation (V_A) and Pa_{CO_2}.

causes the blood to change from red to deep blue. Cyanosis can be peripheral or central.

- Peripheral cyanosis describes "blue discoloration" of the hands and feet, while the tongue and lips remain "pink." It occurs when the blood flow in the peripheral circulation is slow or reduced due to heart failure, hypovolemia, or cold. This allows time for tissues to extract oxygen from the blood, increasing the concentration of deoxygenated blood and causing tissues to appear blue.

- Central cyanosis causes "blue discoloration" of the tongue and lips as well as the peripheral tissues. It is usually due to a reduction in Pa_{O_2} (or Sa_{O_2}). Common sudden causes include pneumonia, pulmonary edema, acute embolism, severe asthma, pneumothorax. Chronic causes are right to left shunts, polycythemia, COPD, and fibrotic lung disease. Polycythemia results in a large quantity of hemoglobin which includes more than 1.5 g/dl of deoxygenated hemoglobin and so patients look cyanosed but are not hypoxic. In contrast, anemic patients often cannot generate 1.5 g/dl of deoxygenated hemoglobin and do not

appear cyanosed even when hypoxic. Thus, cyanosis does not always indicate hypoxia.

The causes of fall in Pa_{O_2} with associated central cyanosis are:

(1) hypoventilation

(2) ventilation–perfusion (V/Q) mismatch in the lungs

(3) impaired gas transfer in the lungs

(4) right to left intracardiac shunts

Conditions causing hypoxemia include pulmonary edema, pulmonary embolism, and pneumonia. ARDS occurs mainly in the critically ill and is discussed below.

Hypoventilation

Hypoventilation is caused by respiratory muscle weakness, e.g. myasthenia gravis, chest wall deformity, e.g. kyphoscoliosis, impaired respiratory drive, e.g. opioid overdose, CNS disease, and excessive work of breathing, e.g. exhaustion due to airways obstruction. Hypoventilation is characterized by increased alveolar and arterial blood carbon dioxide concentration ($P_{A_{CO_2}}$ and Pa_{CO_2}, respectively). As Pa_{CO_2} rises,

Alveolar Oxygen Tension: as derived from the Simplified Alveolar Gas Equation

$$P_{AO_2} = PI_{O_2} - (1.25 \times Pa_{CO_2})$$

Where

$PI_{O_2} = Fi_{O_2} \times (\text{barometric} - \text{water vapor pressure})$
Breathing air; $PI_{O_2} = 0.21 \times (101 - 6.2) = 19.9 \text{ kPa}$

$$P_{AO_2} \text{ (breathing air)} = 19.9 - (1.25 \times 5.3)$$
$$= {\sim}13.5 \text{ kPa}$$

Alveolar–Arterial Oxygen Tension Difference

$$P(A\text{-}a)_{O_2} = P_{AO_2} - Pa_{O_2}$$
$$= {\sim}13.5 - {\sim}13 = {<}1.0 \text{ kPa (breathing air)}$$

P_{AO_2} = alveolar oxygen tension, PI_{O_2} = Inspired oxygen tension,
Fi_{O_2} = fractional concentration of oxygen in inspired air,
$P(A\text{-}a)_{O_2}$ = alveolar–arterial oxygen tension difference,
Pa_{O_2} = arterial oxygen tension, Pa_{CO_2} = arterial CO_2 tension

---

Fig. 19.14. Alveolar oxygen tension and alveolar–arterial oxygen tension difference.

P_{AO_2} and Pa_{O_2} fall (Fig. 19.14). This hypoxemia can be corrected with higher inspired oxygen concentrations (Fi_{O_2}). To reduce increased Pa_{CO_2}, alveolar ventilation is improved by:

(1) ventilatory support - non-invasive or mechanical, or reversing drug-induced CNS depression e.g. with naloxone for opiate overdosage

(2) reducing airways resistance by bronchodilation and secretion clearance

(3) decreasing work of breathing, e.g. re-inflating collapsed alveoli

(4) improving lung compliance – reducing lung stiffness, e.g. treating pulmonary edema

(5) ensuring good chest wall positioning to improve the mechanical advantage of respiratory muscles

Ventilation–perfusion (V/Q) mismatch

Normally, ventilation (V) and blood flow (Q) are matched ensuring saturation of hemoglobin with oxygen. In pneumonia, areas of consolidated lung are poorly ventilated, whereas blood flow is maintained, resulting in failure of blood to be oxygenated in these areas. In pulmonary embolism blood flow is reduced in relation to ventilation. Blood that fails to be oxygenated passing from the right to the leftside of the heart is termed "shunt" and is normally $<2\%$–3% of total blood flow. The effect of V/Q mismatch is to

Table 19.4. Causes of V/Q mismatch

- Pneumonia
- Pulmonary embolism
- Pulmonary edema
- Acute asthma
- COPD
- Pneumothorax
- ARDS

"shunt" more blood through the lungs (or heart wall defects), resulting in reduced oxygenation and arterial hypoxemia. V/Q mismatch is the commonest cause of arterial hypoxemia and occurs in most acute respiratory diseases (Table 19.4).

Treatment depends on cause. Initially, supplemental oxygen is given to achieve an $Sa_{O_2} > 90\%$ ($Pa_{O_2} > 8 \text{ kPa}$). As the shunt increases (termed shunt fraction), raising the concentration of inspired oxygen (Fi_{O_2}) becomes less effective. Shunts greater than 30% are always associated with hypoxemia (Fig. 19.15(a)). The type of shunt affects the response to supplemental oxygen and Fig. 19.15(b) illustrates the effect of a few areas of marked V/Q mismatch and very reduced ventilation with almost complete shunt compared to many areas of relative V/Q mismatch and relatively poor ventilation but some oxygenation. With V/Q mismatch, the alveolar–arterial oxygen difference ($P_{AO_2} - P_{aO_2}$) tends to be greater than 1 kPa. This assists differentiation from hypoventilation (see Fig. 19.14).

When the shunt fraction is high, treatment is designed to reduce it. In obstructive airways diseases bronchodilators relieve bronchospasm and improve V/Q matching. Similarly, draining a pneumothorax restores ventilation and rapidly corrects V/Q matching. In pneumonia antibiotics aid resolution of consolidation and over longer periods will restore V/Q matching, as will anticoagulation in pulmonary embolism.

Non-invasive ventilation such as continuous positive airways pressure (CPAP) or mechanical ventilation may be required to re-expand collapsed alveoli and restore V/Q matching in some conditions. One of these is ARDS. Changes in posture can improve oxygenation because V/Q matching is not uniform throughout the chest. Lower V/Q ratios occur in dependent regions due to gravity.

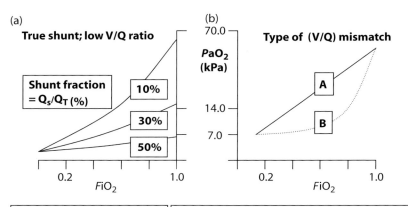

(a)

True shunt; low V/Q ratio

Shunt fraction
= Q_s/Q_T (%)

10%

30%

50%

0.2   1.0

FiO_2

(b)

70.0 —

PaO_2
(kPa)

Type of (V/Q) mismatch

A

14.0 —

B

7.0 —

0.2   1.0

FiO_2

Fig. 19.15. Effect of true shunt (Q_s/Q_t) and V/Q mismatch on the arterial oxygen tension (Pa_{O_2}) and inspired oxygen fraction (Fi_{O_2}) relationship.

Hypoxemia caused by true right to left shunt is refractory to supplemental O_2 when "shunt fraction" exceeds 30%

Reductions in Pa_{O2} caused by V/Q mismatch respond to O_2 but the response depends on whether there are many units with mild V/Q mismatch (A) or a few units with very low V/Q ratios (B)

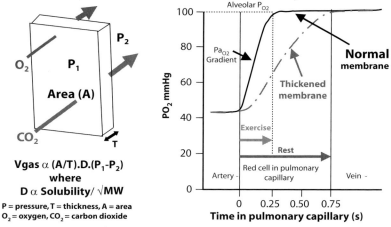

(a) Diffusion through a tissue sheet

P_2

O_2 P_1

Area (A)

CO_2 T

Vgas α (A/T).D.(P_1-P_2)
where
D α Solubility/ $\sqrt{MW}$

P = pressure, T = thickness, A = area
O_2 = oxygen, CO_2 = carbon dioxide

(b) Time course of oxygenation of hemoglobin in the pulmonary circulation

Alveolar P_{O2}

100 —

80 —

Pa_{O2} Gradient

Normal membrane

PO_2 mmHg

60 —

Thickened membrane

40 —

Exercise

20 —

Rest

Artery -

Red cell in pulmonary capillary

Vein -

0 —

0   0.25   0.50   0.75

Time in pulmonary capillary (s)

Fig. 19.16. Diffusion across the alveolar capillary membrane.

Impaired gas transfer

The amount of oxygen diffusing across the alveolar–capillary membrane is inversely proportional to its thickness and proportional to the pressure across the membrane (Fig. 19.16). In pulmonary edema and pulmonary fibrosis the transfer of oxygen from alveolar air to the capillary hemoglobin may be slowed by interstitial or alveolar fluid and fibrous tissue. This is only rarely a significant cause of hypoxemia unless the transit time through the alveolar capillary is substantially shortened (Fig. 19.16). As with V/Q mismatching the alveolar–arterial oxygen difference would be expected to be >1 kPa with impaired diffusion (Fig. 19.14). Supplemental oxygen will partly reverse the hypoxemia due to poor diffusion by increasing the concentration gradient across the membrane. Where a reversible cause can be corrected, like pulmonary edema, it should also be treated.

Right to left cardiac shunts

These occur with congenital cardiac defects, or acquired defects, e.g. post-myocardial infarction. In this situation a proportion of the blood bypasses the lungs completely carrying unoxygenated blood from the right to the left of the heart. It is an extreme form of V/Q mismatching (i.e. true shunt) and oxygen therapy in these patients is ineffective Fig. 19.15(a).

Acute respiratory distress syndrome (ARDS)

ARDS is best defined as "leaky lung syndrome" or "low pressure (i.e. non-cardiogenic) pulmonary edema". It describes acute inflammatory lung injury, often in previously healthy lungs, mediated by a uniform pulmonary pathologic process in response to a variety of direct (i.e. inhaled) or indirect (i.e. blood-borne) insults (Table 19.5).

Table 19.5. Common causes of ARDS

Direct pulmonary insults	Indirect insults
Infection	Sepsis
- pneumonia, tuberculosis	Non-chest trauma,
Pulmonary trauma	Massive transfusion
Toxic gas inhalation	Burns
- smoke, NO_2, Cl_2, phosgene	Pancreatitis
Near drowning	Eclampsia
Gastric aspiration (pH <2)	Drugs (e.g. salicylates)
Oxygen toxicity ($Fi_{O_2} > 0.8$)	Post arrest

During the acute inflammatory phase of ARDS, cytokine-activated neutrophils and monocytes adhere to alveolar epithelium or pulmonary endothelium, releasing inflammatory mediators and proteolytic enzymes (Fig. 19.17). These damage the integrity of the alveolar–capillary membrane, increase permeability and cause alveolar edema. Reduced surfactant production causes alveolar collapse and hyaline membrane formation. Progressive hypoxemia and respiratory failure result from loss of functioning alveoli and ventilation–perfusion (V/Q) mismatch. The later healing, fibroproliferative phase causes progressive pulmonary fibrosis and associated pulmonary hypertension.

Diagnostic criteria

The internationally agreed criteria for the diagnosis of ARDS include the three following criteria:

(1) **Severe hypoxemia**: Pa_{O_2}/Fi_{O_2} <200 (regardless of PEEP) i.e. if Pa_{O_2} is 80 mmHg on 80% inspired oxygen, $Pa_{O_2}/Fi_{O_2} = 80/0.8 = 100$

(2) **Bilateral pulmonary infiltrates on CXR** (Fig. 19.18)

(3) **Normal left atrial pressure**: pulmonary artery occlusion pressure <18 mmHg (i.e. not heart failure)

Acute lung injury (ALI) is the precursor to ARDS. Apart from a lesser degree of hypoxemia, (Pa_{O_2}/Fi_{O_2} <300), the criteria for diagnosis are the same.

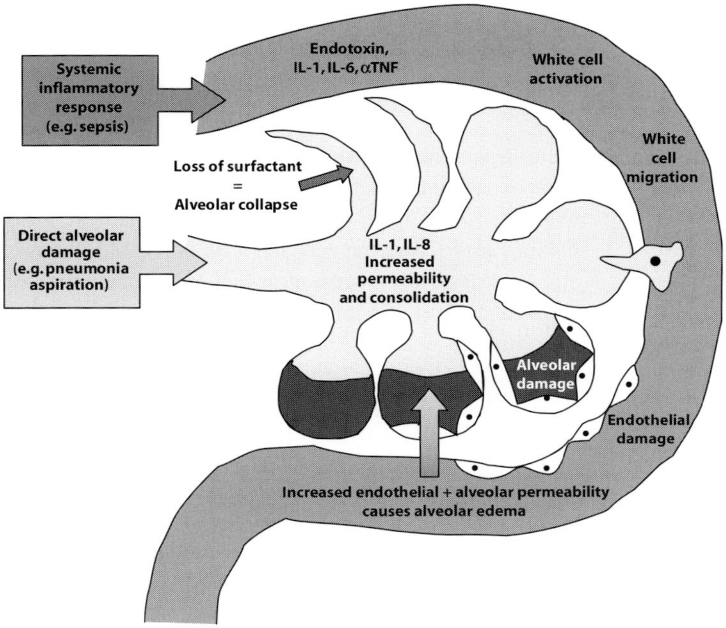

Fig. 19.17. Pathophysiology of ARDS.

Systemic inflammatory response (e.g. sepsis)

Endotoxin, IL-1, IL-6, αTNF

White cell activation

White cell migration

Loss of surfactant = Alveolar collapse

Direct alveolar damage (e.g. pneumonia aspiration)

IL-1, IL-8 Increased permeability and consolidation

Alveolar damage

Endothelial damage

Increased endothelial + alveolar permeability causes alveolar edema

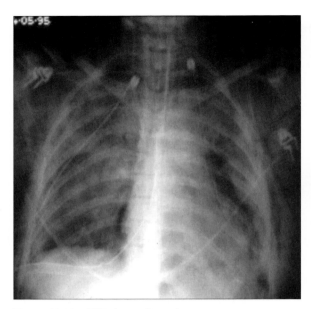

Figure 19.18. ARDS chest radiograph.

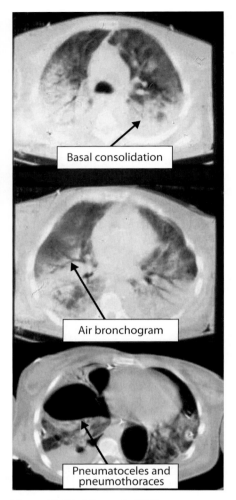

Basal consolidation

Air bronchogram

Pneumatoceles and pneumothoraces

Figure 19.19. CT scans in ARDS.

Epidemiology and prognosis

The incidence of ARDS is about 2–8 cases per 100 000 of the population per year but its precursor ALI is much commoner but frequently unrecognized. Overall, the mortality for ARDS is high at about 30%–40%, but is largely determined by the precipitating condition. ARDS following trauma has a lower mortality rate (~30%) than that associated with aspiration pneumonia (~80%). Both increased age (>60 years) and associated sepsis increase mortality. The cause of death in ARDS is usually multiorgan failure (MOF). Fewer than 20% die from hypoxemia alone.

Clinical features

The clinical course of ARDS has two phases. The *acute inflammatory phase* lasts 3–10 days and results in hypoxemia and multiorgan failure. It presents with progressive breathlessness, cyanosis, tachypnea, hypoxic confusion, and lung crackles. These features are not diagnostic and are frequently incorrectly interpreted as heart failure. During the second *healing, fibroproliferative phase*, lung scarring and pneumothoraces are common. Secondary chest and systemic infections are common in both clinical phases.

Investigation and monitoring

Monitor temperature, respiratory rate, oxygen saturation, and urine output. Hemodynamic monitoring, including central venous pressure, cardiac output, and occasionally left atrial pressure measurement using a pulmonary artery catheter ensures fluid balance and tissue oxygen delivery. Serial blood gases and occasionally capnography (measurement of expired carbon dioxide concentrations) are used to monitor gas exchange. Regular sputum or bronchial lavage can detect secondary infection early. Serial CXRs detect progression of bilateral pulmonary infiltrates (Fig. 19.18). Computed tomography (CT) scans often demonstrate dependent consolidation (Fig. 19.19). Later scans reveal pneumothoraces, pneumatoceles, and fibrosis.

Management

Identify and treat the precipitating cause. In mild disease (e.g. ALI) oxygen therapy, diuretics, and physiotherapy may maintain adequate gas exchange. If respiratory failure progresses, non-invasive ventilation with continuous positive airways pressure (CPAP) recruits collapsed alveoli and improves oxygenation. It may avoid the need for mechanical ventilation. In severe disease, mechanical ventilation with high inspired oxygen concentrations are necessary. Due to the reduced lung compliance caused by interstitial edema and fibrosis, ventilation requires high peak inspiratory pressures (PIP) to achieve normal tidal volumes. High pressures during ventilation can cause lung damage, termed "barotrauma", including pneumothorax, and pneumatoceles (Fig. 19.19). "Volutrauma" describes damage due to overdistention and damage of healthy lung/alveoli associated with the high pressures required to ventilate damaged lung.

General measures Include good nursing, physiotherapy, nutrition, sedation, and infection control. No drug therapy, including early steroids, anti-inflammatory agents, anti-cytokines, or surfactant, is beneficial. After 7–10 days, high dose steroids may reduce development of fibrosis.

Avoid excessive fluid loading This causes alveolar flooding due to characteristic increased alveolar permeability. Maintain perfusion of other organs using the lowest possible cardiac filling pressure, i.e. CVP. In the acute phase, diuretics reduce extravascular lung water and may improve oxygenation. Cardiac output, perfusion pressures, and regional oxygen delivery may have to be maintained at low CVP using inotropic and vasoactive drugs rather than fluid filling.

Mechanical ventilation avoids oxygen toxicity (i.e. Fi_{O_2} <80%) and ventilator-induced lung injury. Both contribute to mortality. The principles are (a) optimize oxygenation; (b) avoid reduced cardiac output due to high intrathoracic pressures; (c) limit pressure induced lung damage. Re-expansion (recruitment) of collapsed alveoli (Fig. 19.17) is achieved with high positive end expiratory pressures (PEEP >10 cm H_2O) and long inspiratory to expiratory (I : E) times (i.e. 2 : 1 instead of the normal 1 : 2). Ventilator-induced lung damage is reduced and survival improved with "protective" ventilation strategies which use low tidal volumes (6 ml/kg) and low PIP (<30 cmH₂O). The carbon dioxide retention, termed "permissive hypercapnia," resulting from this low tidal volume strategy is usually tolerated with adequate sedation. No specific ventilatory mode is superior but pressure-controlled ventilation is favored.

Additional measures Improve V/Q matching and reduce shunt fraction. Prone positioning can improve oxygenation. This is because blood flow is greatest in the dependent areas and in ARDS consolidation is also dependent. V/Q matching can thus be improved by prone nursing so that non-consolidated, ventilated lung (i.e. which was previously dorsal) is now dependent and perfused. Bronchoscopy improves ventilation and V/Q matching by removing sputum plugs and secretions. Inhaled nitric oxide increases perfusion of ventilated alveoli by vasodilating vessels in these alveoli producing short-lived improvement of oxygenation with no survival benefit. Extracorporeal membrane oxygenation (ECMO) techniques that oxygenate blood or remove carbon dioxide are effective in children but not adults. Chest drainage of air leaks, including pneumothorax and pneumatoceles, which are common during the late fibroproliferative phase of ARDS, is essential to optimize oxygenation. These air leaks are often difficult to detect on CXR and the importance of CT scanning to localize and drain these has only recently been appreciated (Fig. 19.19).

The oliguric/anuric patient

Poor or deteriorating urine output (i.e. <0.5 ml/kg per h) is an early sign of deterioration and the cause must be corrected quickly. Urine output is normally ~1 ml/kg per h if:

- Renal blood flow and mean arterial pressure are adequate.
- The kidneys are healthy and functionally normal.
- There is no obstruction to urine flow.

Oliguria describes the production of <400 ml of urine a day, and anuria no urine production. The initial management of the oliguric patient is summarized in Fig. 19.20. The causes of poor urine output include

(1) **"Pre-renal" renal disease:** due to reduced renal blood flow or hypotension
(2) **"Renal" renal disease:** due to intrinsic renal disease including nephrotoxic damage due to drugs (e.g. non-steroidal anti-inflammatory agents) or glomerulonephritis
(3) **"Post-renal" renal disease:** due to urinary tract obstruction

Pre-renal disease

Mean arterial blood pressures (MAP) of 60 to 160 mmHg ensure a constant renal blood flow of

Step 1

Palpate the abdomen
for a distended bladder

Step 2

Insert a urinary catheter
or flush catheter if already *in situ*

Step 3

Send urine sample for osmolality
and sodium analysis

Step 4

If no urinary obstruction
give fluid challenge

Step 5

If fluid challenges fail to
maintain systolic BP >100 mmHg
consider CVP line and inotropes

Step 6

If oliguria persists consider
cautious use of diuretics (e.g. fursemide)
BUT remember that
diuretics can cause
further renal impairment

Step 7

Check drug chart for nephrotoxins
and stop them

Step 8

If hypotension or oliguria persist
call for senior assistance

Figure 19.20. Management of oliguria.

Table 19.6. Urinalysis in patients with oliguria

	Osmolality (mOsm/l)	Urinary sodium (mmol/l)
Inadequate perfusion	>450	<20
Renal damage (e.g. ATN)	~280	>20

(ADH), and aldosterone, to restore blood pressure. Antidiuretic hormone (ADH) and aldosterone increase renal salt and water retention increasing circulating blood volume and renal blood flow. This results in a reduced volume of highly concentrated urine with increased osmolality and a low sodium. (Table 19.6).

If oliguria is pre-renal, due to hypotension or reduced cardiac output, it may be reversible with fluid resuscitation and restoration of mean arterial pressure >65 mmHg, cardiac output, and renal blood flow. This is achieved by increasing cardiac filling pressures. Administer a bolus of 0.5–1 l of crystalloid fluid, e.g. 0.9% normal saline, and reassess blood pressure, filling pressures, and urine output. Aim for a urine output >0.5 ml/kg per h. Peripheral vasoconstriction, empty peripheral veins, and a low central venous pressure indicate dehydration and the need for further fluid. Even patients with heart failure should receive a small bolus of fluid (~250 ml) with careful monitoring to assess whether hypovolemia is the cause of poor urine output. If blood pressure remains inadequate because of cardiac failure or sepsis, inotropes, e.g. dobutamine, and vasopressors, e.g. norepinephrine are required.

Renal disease

Poor urine output or a rising urea and creatinine may be due to intrinsic renal disease. The commonest cause of sudden oliguria is acute tubular necrosis (ATN), which is usually due to delayed or inadequate treatment of renal hypoperfusion and hypotension. Nephrotoxins may also be responsible. Charts should be reviewed for any drugs that may damage the kidneys, e.g non-steroidal anti-inflammatory agents, contrast media, gentamicin, penicillins, cephalosporins, and furosemide (especially with gentamicin).

In renal disease and acute tubular necrosis osmolality of urine is similar to plasma (~280 mOsm/l) and urinary sodium is high due to loss of kidney concentrating ability (Table 19.6). In acute glomerulonephritis the renal tubules continue to function

about 1–1.5 l per minute. If MAP falls below the lower limit of autoregulation or cardiac output decreases, renal blood flow and perfusion decrease rapidly and autonomic and endocrine responses are activated, including release of epinephrine, antidiuretic hormone

well and produce urine with high osmolality and low sodium (<20 mmol/l). Oliguria due to renal impairment requires diagnosis and treatment of the underlying disorder, e.g. glomerulonephritis, whilst ensuring renal perfusion by maintaining blood pressure and cardiac output. Maintaining urine output with furosemide can be counterproductive. It may delay diagnosis of the cause of the oliguria and sometimes can be nephrotoxic, causing interstitial nephritis.

Post-renal urinary tract obstruction

Urinary tract obstruction may cause acute anuria or oliguria. Palpate for distended bladder suggesting urethral obstruction. In men, the commonest cause is prostatic hypertrophy. A urinary catheter should be inserted and urine sent for analysis. If already in place, exclude catheter obstruction by flushing. If no urinary flow, renal ultrasound will exclude obstruction of ureters and assess the size/texture of the kidneys.

Hyperkalemia, metabolic acidosis, and fluid overload will develop if oliguria persists and renal disease progresses. Hyperkalemia ($K^+ > 6.5$ mmol/l) is corrected with insulin–dextrose infusions and calcium resonium enemas to prevent cardiac arrhythmias. Metabolic acidosis may be controlled with sodium bicarbonate. Fluid overload and edema require fluid restriction. If renal impairment progresses accumulation of creatinine, hyperkalemia, and fluid overload will necessitate invasive renal replacement therapy with dialysis or hemofiltration.

The "obtunded" patient with acutely disordered conscious level

Many acutely unwell patients become confused, disorientated, and "obtunded" with a reduced level of consciousness. A reduction in consciousness level is associated with potential airways obstruction, loss of the gag and cough reflexes, and increased risk of aspiration of upper airways secretions and gastric contents. There are many potential causes for reduced consciousness (Table 19.7).

The Glasgow Coma scale (Table 19.8) assesses conscious level. The normal points score is 15. It is best measured following treatment of hypotension and hypoxemia. Patients with a score less than 8–9 may require intubation because risk of aspiration is high. Formal anesthetic induction is required.

Blood glucose levels should be assessed immediately and treated with 50 ml 20% glucose solution intravenously if below 3 mmol/l. Hypoxia, hypercapnia,

Table 19.7. Causes of reduced conscious level

Hypoxemia
Hypotension
Hypoglycemia
Drugs (e.g. opiates)
Epilepsy
Hypothermia
Hypothyroidism
Cerebral infection
Hypercapnia
Stroke (e.g. CVA)
Hypercapnia
Liver failure
Cerebral neoplasm

Table 19.8. The Glasgow Coma Scale

Eyes	Open	Spontaneously	4
		To verbal command	3
		To pain	2
		No response	1
Best motor response	Verbal command	Obeys	6
	Painful stimuli	Localizes pain	5
		Flexion-withdrawal	4
		Flexion-decorticate	3
		Extension-decerebrate	2
		No response	1
Best verbal response		Oriented, converses	5
		Disoriented, converses	4
		Inappropriate words	3
		Incomprehensible sounds	2
		No response	1
Total			3–15

and hypotension all decrease conscious level and may worsen cerebral injury and edema. Airway, breathing, and circulation must be secured and high-dose supplemental oxygen (Fi_{O_2} 60%–100%) given with intravenous fluid to correct hypotension. If no cervical cord injury is suspected, the patient should be positioned in the left lateral decubitus position to protect the airway. In suspected raised intracranial pressure, nursing is 30° head up, but in the acute situation the horizontal recovery position avoiding head down is preferred to reduce risk of aspiration. Drug-induced CNS depression should be reversed, e.g. naloxone for opiate overdosage.

The pupils may provide clues. Bilateral dilation occurs with sympathetic drugs, e.g. tricyclic antidepressants, and sympathetic overactivity, e.g. anxiety. Pupillary constriction occurs with opiates and brainstem (usually pontine) infarcts. Unilateral, unreactive, dilation indicates a space-occupying lesion such as hematoma, abscess, or tumor and is a neurosurgical emergency.

Blood tests should include toxicology, thyroid function tests, liver function, and blood cultures, CSF, and head, chest, or other imaging. Suspected intracerebral bleed, space-occupying lesion, or raised intracranial pressure requires a CT brain scan. Patients with an unprotected airway should be intubated and monitored for the scan.

Ongoing management

Management of the critically ill patient requires a multidisciplinary team, good communication, careful documentation, leadership, decision-making, and clear objective plans. Help should always be sought in good time and communication with relatives should be considerate, honest, and consistent.

The ethics of "do not resuscitate" (DNR) decisions, withholding and withdrawal of treatment are major issues in the management of critically ill patients.

Further reading

Dellinger RP, Carlet JM, Masur H *et al.* Surviving Sepsis Campaign guidelines for management of severe sepsis and septic shock. *Crit Care Med* 2004; **32**(3), 858–873.

Leach RM *Critical Care Medicine at a Glance* Oxford, UK: Blackwell Publishing, 2004.

National Heart, Lung and Blood Institute Acute Respiratory Distress Syndrome Clinical Trials Network. Pulmonary artery versus central venous catheter to guide treatment of acute lung injury. *N Engl J Med* 2006; **354**, 2213–2224.

Severe respiratory failure: advanced treatment options. *Crit Care Med* 2006; **34**, S278–S2790.

The acute respiratory distress syndrome network. Ventilation with lower tidal volumes as compared with traditional tidal volumes for acute lung injury and the acute respiratory distress syndrome. *N Engl J Med* 2000; **342**, 1301–1308.

Vincent JL, Gerlach H. Fluid resuscitation in severe sepsis and septic shock; an evidence-based review. *Crit Care Med* 2004; **32**, S451–S454.

Teresa Beynon

Contents

Introduction

In England and Wales approximately 500 000 deaths are recorded each year (Fig. 20.1).

Although diseases of the circulatory system are the most frequently recorded cause of death overall, under 75 years of age cancer is the most commonly recorded cause of death (Fig. 20.2).

Most deaths take place in hospital with a much smaller percentage at home (Fig. 20.3). This means that care of the dying patient is part of the daily work of most health professionals, whether working in a hospital or primary care.

Defining "dying"

Dying: No cure known. Usually describes the last few days of life.

Terminally ill: The disease is incurable and will result in death.

Palliative: Treating the symptoms of the disease rather than the disease itself.

Many diseases eventually result in death, either from the disease itself or from its consequences. Cancer can be cured, particularly if diagnosed early enough. For example:

Lymphoma – often very sensitive to chemotherapy

Breast cancer – if diagnosed and treated early

The time scales for the disease or its consequences causing death vary enormously (Fig. 20.4).

Where cure is not possible, the aim of management is usually to reduce the intensity of symptoms related to the disease. This can prolong life as well as improve the quality of life.

Diagnosing dying

The diagnosis of "dying" is usually made when, following a full assessment of the illness, there are no known medical treatments that will reverse the progression of the disease or reverse the damage caused by the illness. At this stage the patient may be described as entering the "terminal stage" of their disease. Treatment is then described as palliative (or sometimes supportive) care. "Dying" can be a difficult diagnosis and is one doctors do not always feel confident to make. The reasons for this are complex (Box 20.1).

Palliative care

Aims to improve quality of life for patients and their family when they face life-threatening illness (Fig. 20.5).

"You mean Macmillan nurses?"

"That's just pain control"

In the Western world many treatment options are available for people with cancer and other life-threatening diseases. Palliative care is needed because

595

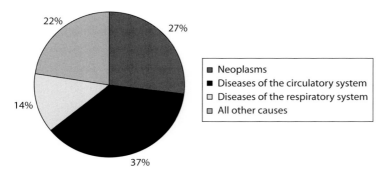

Fig. 20.1. Common causes of death in England and Wales (2004). *Source: Office of National Statistics (ONS) DH2 no.31.*

Legend:
- ■ Neoplasms
- ■ Diseases of the circulatory system
- □ Diseases of the respiratory system
- ▨ All other causes

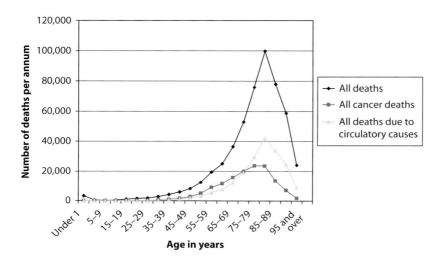

Fig. 20.2. All deaths compared to the commonest causes of death by age. *Source: Office of National statistics Series DH2 no. 31.*

Legend:
- All deaths
- All cancer deaths
- All deaths due to circulatory causes

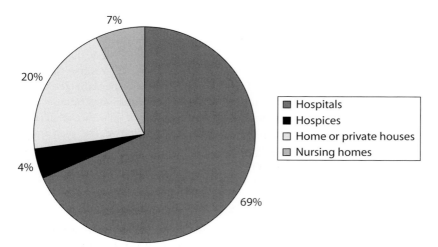

Fig. 20.3. Place of death in England and Wales (2003). *Source: Office of National Statistics DH2 Series 30 (2003).*

Legend:
- ▨ Hospitals
- ■ Hospices
- □ Home or private houses
- ▨ Nursing homes

many people with a cancer diagnosis will be incurable from the time of diagnosis or will develop recurrence of their cancer following an apparently curative surgical resection or initial response to treatment.

In much of the rest of the world, people are frequently in the advanced stages of cancer when first seen by a medical professional (WHO). Where medical treatment is expensive or not available, the only

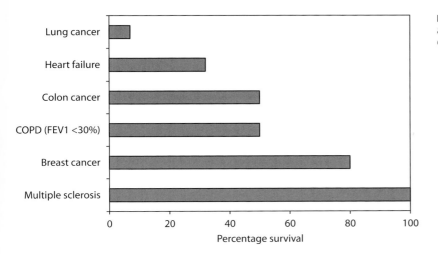

Fig. 20.4. Percentage survival 5 years after diagnosis for 'incurable' medical conditions.

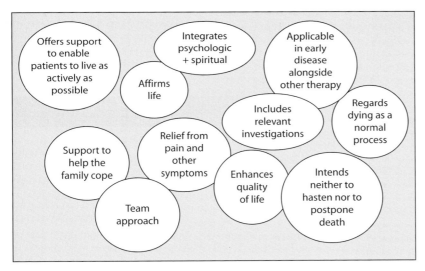

Fig. 20.5. World Health Organization definition of palliative care.

Box 20.1. Why it might be difficult to diagnose dying

Doctors are trained to cure.
Death feels like failure.
Uncertainty about whether all treatment options have been considered.

realistic treatment option may be pain relief and palliative care.

Cancer
Determining the "stage" of cancer
Identifying the nature and extent of the disease is important. Confirming a diagnosis of cancer with histology is advised (Fig. 20.6).

Staging determines how advanced the cancer is and whether it might be cured. It is recommended before treatment is commenced except in immediately life-threatening situations. Whenever someone with cancer presents to a doctor, the extent of the cancer and any previous treatments should be reviewed (Table 20.1). This ensures people are neither under- nor over-treated.

Site
Some cancers are incurable from the time the diagnosis is made, usually because the site of the tumor determines symptoms (Box 20.2).

Cancers detected early through screening programs or which present early because of their position are more likely to be cured. Surgery is a definitive treatment for early stage cancers and may result in

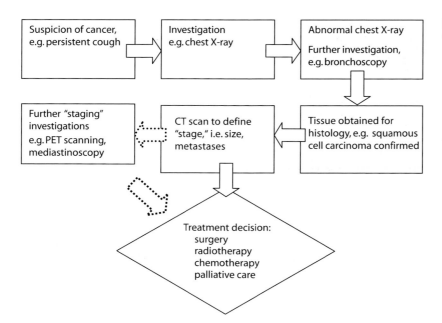

Fig. 20.6. The process of investigating cancer.

Table 20.1. Determining the stage of the cancer

Questions to yourself when assessing a person with cancer	Description
Site of cancer	Origin or site of the cancer will often determine how treatable it is
Staging cancer	TNM classification (size and spread)
Pathology of the tumor	Cell type, degree of differentiation
Previous oncologic treatments	Includes surgery, radiotherapy, chemotherapy, and hormone therapies
Current "fitness" of the patient	Standard scales exist, e.g. Karnofsky, ECOG, or WHO scale
Co-morbid conditions	Other diseases which may affect the oncologic treatment that can be given

Box 20.2. Effect of site of cancer on stage and outcome of cancer treatment

Early presentation	Late presentation
Screening *e.g. breast*, may be palpable Curative surgery possible	Asymptomatic until advanced, *e.g. lung*, may be asymptomatic sometimes weight loss
	Surgery rarely possible Relatively chemoinsensitive
Chemosensitive *e.g. teratoma*, may be palpable – very chemosensitive	*e.g. pancreas*, weight loss, and jaundice
Cure likely	Cure unlikely

cure. Unfortunately, some cancers present too late to be completely removed surgically and consequently tend to have a poorer prognosis.

Chemotherapy is an excellent treatment for certain cancers.

Pathology of the tumor

The degree of differentiation of the tumor cells will tend to predict the prognosis; poorly differentiated tumors usually indicate a poorer outcome. The type of tumor cell will also determine the likely response to radiotherapy and chemotherapy. Certain types of cancer frequently respond well to chemotherapy whereas others generally respond poorly. In adenocarcinoma degree of differentiation is based on number of glands seen. Well differentiated carcinoma has more distinct glands, poorly differentiated less distinct (Fig. 20.7).

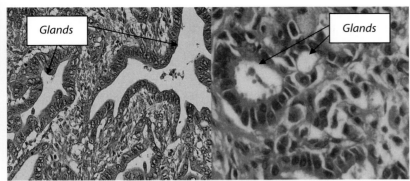

Glands

Glands

Well differentiated   *Poorly differentiated*

Fig. 20.7. Adenocarcinoma of the esophagus.

Example: chemosensitivity by site

Adenocarcinoma of ovary – responds well to chemotherapy

Sarcoma (any site) – responds poorly to chemotherapy

Staging cancer

A standard classification system is used to stage cancer, the commonest of which is the TNM system (Table 20.2) (Murtagh *et al.*, 2004). Larger tumors, nodal spread, and metastases all suggest a poorer prognosis.

Table 20.2. TNM classification

TNM classification	Describes	Staging
T	Size of primary tumor. Higher numbers indicate larger tumors	0–4
N	Extent of lymph node spread Higher numbers indicate more distant node involvement	0–3
M	Metastases: absent (0) or present (1)	0–1

Previous oncologic treatments

A complete history of the treatments so far will help in assessing what further treatment options might be available.

Oncologic treatments are described as either radical or palliative (Table 20.3).

Radical treatment

Aimed at cure

Usually given over a longer period (weeks)

More side effects (toxicity) accepted

Example: radical radiotherapy

For early stage lung cancer

Given over 6 weeks to maximum tolerated dose

May develop esophagitis or skin burns

Palliative treatment

Aims to provide relief of symptoms

May prolong the length of life through reducing tumor burden and complications of the disease

Table 20.3. Oncologic interventions

Type of treatment	Radical	Palliative
Surgery	Complete resection of the tumor with margins clear of cancer cells	Bypass procedures to alleviate a symptom, e.g. stenting a bile duct to relieve jaundice
Radiotherapy	Aimed at cure. Usually for several (4–6) weeks	Aimed at relieving a symptom, e.g. bone pain from metastases. Usually 1–10 treatments
Chemotherapy	Curative, e.g. lymphoma Neoadjuvant: prior to surgery Adjuvant: following surgery	Aims to reduce symptoms. May prolong life. Less toxicity from treatment acceptable
Hormone blockade	Breast and prostate cancer which are hormone sensitive may be dramatically improved, e.g. Tamoxifen, Zoladex	Hormone therapy may dramatically reduce symptoms, e.g. bone pain in metastatic disease
Bisphosphonates	Prophylaxis to reduce the number of fractures particularly in breast cancer and multiple myeloma	Treat hypercalcemia and bone pain
Radioactive sources	e.g. Iodine used to treat thyroid cancer due to preferential uptake in the thyroid gland	e.g. Strontium used to treat bone pain from bone metastases particularly in prostate cancer

Usually given over a shorter period of time (days)

Lower level of side effects considered acceptable

Palliative radiotherapy

For bone pain caused by lung cancer which has metastasized

One to two treatments common

Performance status

Oncologists use a scale to determine a patient's fitness for chemotherapy. This is usually described as "performance status" as it describes average daily activity. The most commonly used scale in the United Kingdom is the World Health Organization (WHO) performance scale (also known as the Eastern Cooperative Oncology Group (ECOG) scale) (Box 20.3). A patient with a performance status of 3 or 4 would not usually be considered able to tolerate a course of chemotherapy.

Co-morbid conditions

Concurrent conditions and increasing age do not exclude people from oncologic therapy but may mean the treatment has to be modified.

Box 20.3. World Health Organization performance status scale

0 Normal activity
1 Restricted but ambulatory; able to carry out light work
2 Self-caring, ambulatory; up and about >50% of the day
3 Limited self-care; confined to bed or chair >50% of the day
4 Completely disabled, no self-care; completely confined to bed or chair

---

Impact of concurrent conditions on treatment options

Example: Severe chronic obstructive airways disease

+

Technically surgically respectable lung tumor

↓

Unfit for surgery

Example: Chronic renal failure or heart failure

↓

Limits choice of chemotherapy agents

When to involve oncology

Following an histopathologic diagnosis of cancer, all patients should be discussed in a multidisciplinary meeting (Fig. 20.8). Radiology, e.g. X-rays and CT scans, and isotope scans, e.g. bone scans, PET scans, should also be reviewed. A treatment plan will be agreed and recorded before being discussed with the patient. This discussion reassures the clinician, patient, and carers that all possible treatments have been considered.

Deciding that the prognosis is poor

Studies identifying poor prognostic factors suggest that, although clinician estimates are the most accurate guide, they tend to overestimate prognosis. The best estimate is probably based on a combination of experience and assessment of physical symptoms (Box 20.4). Research is continuing into how to predict prognosis more accurately, since this may influence the choice of treatment.

Not cancer

Determining the prognosis in patients who do not have a diagnosis of cancer can be much more difficult.

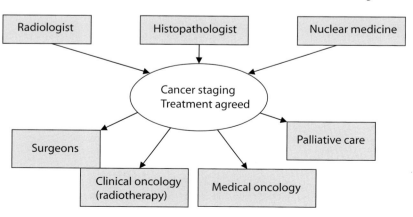

Fig. 20.8. The multidisciplinary team.

The course of a chronic illness is often much less predictable and may follow a pattern of increasing debility (Fig. 20.9).

For instance, in Fig. 20.9 below the "dips" will often coincide with hospital admissions. With cancer the course of the disease tends to be more predictable (or perhaps more familiar) with a tendency for the person's physical health to mirror disease progression.

Managing "dying"

Assessment of the dying patient should include a review of physical, psychologic, social, spiritual, and financial needs. It should also include considering the needs of the family and friends of the dying person.

General principles of symptom management

Assessment of a palliative care patient should begin with open questions regarding the patient's problems or concerns (Table 20.5). These may be physical but may also include other areas such as the need for more information, financial worries, or concerns about their family.

Common symptoms

Studies report similar frequencies of symptoms in cancer patients and non-malignant disease. All symptoms in a cancer patient may be caused by the cancer itself, cancer treatment, the consequences of the cancer, or by another condition (Fig. 20.10).

Pain

Pain is the commonest and often the most feared symptom in people with cancer. A good history, thorough examination, and appropriate investigation of the pain (or pains) is needed in all palliative patients.

Clinical features
"It hurts"

Pain An unpleasant sensory and emotional experience associated with actual or potential tissue damage.

Pain is usually described by its site, intensity, and the organ or tissue from which the pain originates, if this can be determined (Table 20.5).

Some pains can be described as "mixed" pains, with more than one of these components. It may be difficult to distinguish between the different types and more than one type of analgesic or co-analgesic (p. 606) may be required. Take a full history of the pain including the features outlined in Box 20.5.

Epidemiology
Most patients with cancer report pain at some time during their disease. At presentation this may be as

> **Box 20.4.** Physical symptoms that suggest a poor prognosis in cancer patients
>
> Dyspnea
> Anorexia
> Poor performance status (3–4)
> Inability to take food or fluid
> Deteriorating consciousness level
> Dry mouth

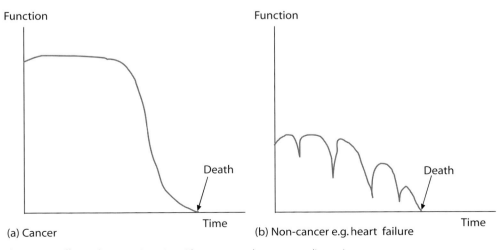

(a) Cancer

(b) Non-cancer e.g. heart failure

Fig. 20.9. Differing disease trajectories with a cancer and non-cancer diagnosis.

Table 20.4. Principles of symptom management

Assess	Explore	Manage
Physical	What is the presenting symptom? Ask about other common symptoms Examine/investigate if this helps to clarify the cause	*General* Listen Give information Explain
Psychologic	Do they know the diagnosis? What coping strategies are they using? Are these working?	
Social	Who is available at home? e.g. family, friends Existing support services? e.g. district nurse What is their housing like?	*Specific* Treat reversible underlying cause where possible
Financial	Are they working or retired? What impact has their illness had on finances?	
Spiritual	What gives their life meaning? Do they have a religious faith?	
Impact on family/carers	How are they coping? Do they need additional support?	*Symptomatic* Non-pharmacologic Pharmacologic
Information	Is there a need for more information/explanation?	

Table 20.5. Describing different types of pain in cancer

Type of pain	Patient says	Special features	Example
Visceral	"Dull ache" 'Throbbing'	Occurs around damaged organ	*Carcinoma of the colon*
Bone	"Dull ache"	In or around a bone. Pain may radiate and often increases on movement	*Metastasis in femur will cause local pain but also cause pain radiating towards the knee when weight-bearing*
Nerve	"Stabbing" or "shooting"	May have a change in sensation (numbness or "pins and needles") or function (weakness)	*Pain radiating down the arm due to brachial plexus involvement*
Soft tissue	"Soreness"	Often helped by topical treatments	*Mucositis from chemotherapy*

Mechanism

Understanding the reason for the pain is helpful for the clinician in determining which treatments can be used to palliate the underlying disease and which medication will most quickly relieve the current pain (or pains). Not all pain is caused by the cancer itself (Fig. 20.11).

Investigations

Taking a good history is part of the investigation. Ask about any associated features. Examine the site of the pain to define its anatomic location. Existing radiologic investigations may help to confirm the origin of the pain. If no existing investigation explains the reason for the pain, further investigation such as an X-ray of the painful area or a CT scan may be warranted to determine the cause, particularly if the pain is of recent onset (Fig. 20.12).

Management

Explaining the cause of the pain to the patient is part of managing the pain. Explanation:

- Reduces unnecessary anxiety about possible reasons for the pain
- Enables the patient to understand and come to terms with the diagnosis. It may be possible to reassure if the pain is not related to cancer.
- To discuss treatment that might be of help.

low as 25%. Two-thirds of people with pain will have more than one pain. Similar figures are reported for hospitalized non-cancer patients.

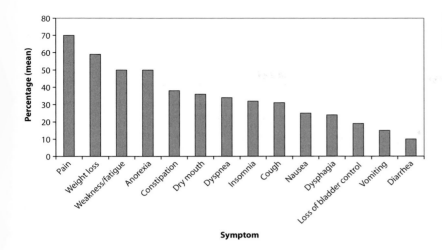

Fig. 20.10. Reported frequencies of physical symptoms experienced by cancer patients in the literature.

Box 20.5. PQRST characteristics of pain		
P	Palliative (relieving) factors	What makes it better?
	Provocative (aggravating) factors	What makes it worse?
Q	Quality	What does it feel like?
R	Radiation	Does it spread anywhere else?
S	Severity	How bad is it? Score out of 10.
		Does it stop you doing anything? (e.g. disturbs sleep)
T	Timing	Is it there all the time?
		Is it worse at any particular time of day or night?

Note:
Source: modified from Twycross (1999).

Example: Radiotherapy can relieve bone pain caused by cancer, but will not usually help pain caused by osteoarthritis.

In many situations management for the pain will also include treating the underlying disease.

Example: *Carcinoma of the prostate with bone metastases*

(1) Treat the underlying disease – antiandrogen hormone therapy

(2) Advanced or hormone resistant disease – radiotherapy or bisphosponates for bone pain

The bone scan shown in Fig. 20.13 is typical of carcinoma of the prostate which has metastasized to bone. Sites of increased cancer activity are shown by the darker areas, which are called "hot." Long bones and ribs are rarely "hot" on a bone scan. The only other explanation for this would be a healing fracture. Not all sites showing increased activity will cause pain; however should any of them coincide with a painful site, radiotherapy is indicated.

Management
The cornerstone of pain management is the World Health Organization (WHO) analgesic ladder (Fig. 20.14).

All pain killers (analgesics) should be given:

- by mouth (orally) wherever possible and
- at regular intervals (regularly) according to the duration of the drug (rather than on an "as needed" basis).

Example: oral and regular medication
Acetaminophen 1 g qds (4 times a day) p.o.

Morphine is the "gold standard" strong opiate and should be the first strong opiate used in most circumstances.

At each step of the analgesic ladder, a co-analgesic may also be needed.

Co-analgesic A drug whose principal action is not as an analgesic but which has pain relieving properties.

Example: co-analgesic Amitryptyline (tricyclic antidepressant) used to relieve nerve pain, e.g. post-herpetic neuralgia.

603

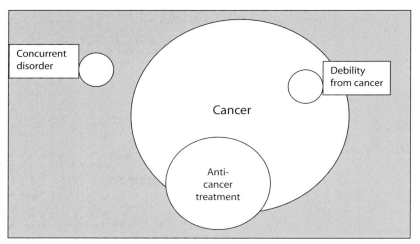

Fig. 20.11. Relative proportions of causes of pain in advanced cancer. (Data source: Grond *et al.*, 1996)

Data source: Grond[8]

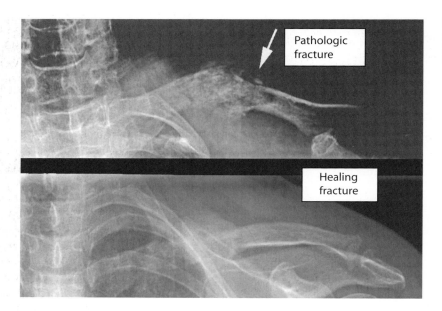

Fig. 20.12. Example of a useful radiologic investigation showing pathologic fracture of the clavicle before and 6 weeks after radiotherapy.

"Difficult" pain

Certain types of pain can be particularly difficult to control. Help from a pain or palliative care service may be needed for these types of pain.

- Pain on movement ("incident" pain) e.g. pathologic fracture of vertebra
- Nerve (or neuropathic) pain e.g. infiltration of brachial plexus

Infiltration of nerves with a local anesthetic can provide useful pain relief. An epidural is the most commonly used local anesthetic technique.

Outcome

Between 25% and 100% of people with cancer have pain (Fig. 20.15). Using appropriate methods for pain relief, significant reductions in pain can be made (Fig. 20.15).

Fatigue

"A subjective state of overwhelming, sustained exhaustion and decreased capacity for physical and mental work, that is not relieved by rest."

"Feeling tired," "No energy."

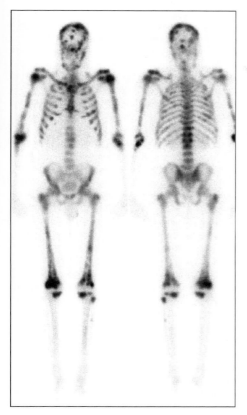

Fig. 20.13. Bone scan showing diffuse bone metastases particularly in skull, ribs and long bones.

Fatigue is common in cancer patients. Often, no specific underlying cause is found.

Clinical features

Cachexia, anorexia, and fatigue tend to occur together.

Cachexia

Anorexia

Muscle wasting

Weight loss

Fatigue

Epidemiology

About 55% of cancer patients (10%–35% of a general practice patient population) describe themselves as fatigued or lacking in energy. Fatigue increases with progression of cancer. Its presence often heralds a poorer prognosis, although some people experience fatigue throughout the course of their illness.

Mechanism

There are a large number of possible causes of fatigue. Explore reversible causes in the history, examination, and investigations. In the history ask about recent anti-cancer treatment, particularly about chemotherapy. Consider low mood; 25%–50% of people with cancer are depressed and this will exacerbate fatigue (Box 20.6).

Investigation

Investigation should normally include a full blood count and corrected calcium levels. Renal failure and diabetes are common, often induced by the cancer or

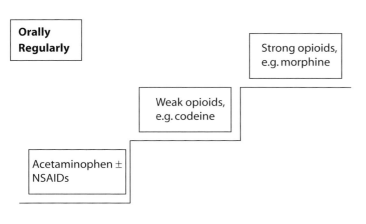

Fig. 20.14. The World Health Organization analgesic ladder.

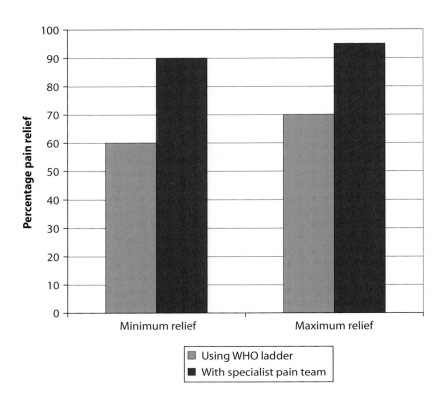

Fig. 20.15. Percentage pain relief obtained applying the analgesic ladder and specialist pain services.

its treatment. Hypothyroidism is a possible cause, particularly in the elderly.

Management

Treat any reversible abnormalities found on hematologic or biochemical testing. Antidepressant or anxiolytic therapy, and psychologic or pscyhiatric support may be required. If no reversible cause is found, a 1-week trial of corticosteroid therapy can be considered. There has been recent interest in modified exercise programes.

Example: corticosteroids e.g. Dexamethasone may improve fatigue.

Outcome

The benefits of the appropriate management of fatigue have not been carefully evaluated.

Loss of appetite

Anorexia

Formal definition: "An involuntary decline in food intake."

"I just don't feel like eating."

Clinical features

Anorexia (or loss of appetite) is loss of the desire to eat or just not feeling hungry. Often people lose the pleasure of eating too. A careful history will sometimes reveal underlying nausea, or nausea induced by the smell of food. Carers can become extremely worried when someone is eating less, fearing that they will starve.

Epidemiology

Over half of patients with cancer will have anorexia.

Mechanism

Anorexia most frequently occurs without an identifiable underlying cause. However, explore the following possibilities when someone complains of reduced appetite or loss of pleasure in eating (Table 20.6).

Squashed stomach syndrome Mechanical compression of the stomach due to an increase in the volume of intra-abdominal contents.

Example: ascites

Investigations

Explore what someone means when they describe loss of appetite. Examination of the gastro-intestinal tract

Box 20.6. Causes and management of fatigue in cancer

Cause		Management
Chemotherapy	Anemia	Transfuse
Marrow suppression		Stop offending medication
		Radiotherapy – if tumor is bleeding
Bleeding		Consider fibrinolytic agents
Chronic disease		Reduce dose of chemotherapy next cycle
Bone metastases	Metabolic	Treat hypercalcemia
or	Hypercalcemia	Intravenous fluid + bisphosphonate
PTH secreting tumor		
Corticosteroids	Hyperglycemia	Review steroids
		Insulin may be needed
		Discontinue or reduce dose if possible
Adapting to diagnosis	Mood changes	Psychologic assessment
	Depression	Antidepressants or anxiolytics
	Anxiety	
Debility	Deconditioning	Modified exercise program
Cytokines	Cachexia	Modified exercise program, corticosteroids
Pain	Insomnia	Review analgesics
Anxiety		Explore concerns
		Short-acting anxiolytics

Table 20.6. Reversible causes of anorexia

Causes of anorexia	Caused by	Secondary to
Painful mouth	Infection Mucositis	*Candida* ("thrush") Chemotherapy
Nausea	May be mild but sufficient to prevent hunger	See reasons for nausea (Box 20.8)
Early satiety	Gastric stasis	Opiates "Squashed stomach syndrome"

including the mouth is necessary. Investigations are rarely helpful in managing this symptom.

Management

Steroids can help to stimulate appetite if no alternative explanation for loss of appetite is found. Corticosteroids or progesterones may be used. All steroids can be harmful, particularly if prescribed over long periods of time. The expected benefits of prescribing steroids must be balanced against potential side effects. Side effects and effectiveness of both types of steroid are dose related.

Corticosteroid, e.g. dexamethasone
Avoid in diabetes mellitus and previous history of peptic ulcer
Usually effective in 3–5 days

Progesterone, e.g. Megestrol acetate
Avoid if history of thromboembolism
Effective in 1–2 weeks
Produces weight gain

Small, easily digestible but frequent meals are advised. Dietary supplements are often suggested but are of unproven benefit. Food supplements are often suggested although there is little evidence to support their use. Fish oils may be helpful.

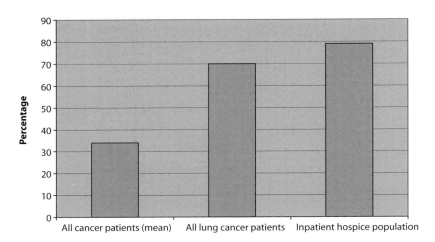

Fig. 20.16. Percentage of people describing themselves as breathless.

Outcome

Fifty percent of people will have some improvement in their appetite in response to steroid therapy.

Breathlessness

"An unpleasant awareness of difficulty in breathing."
  "Just can't get my breath,"
  "suffocating," or "choking."
  Breathlessness can be an extremely distressing symptom. Patients will sometimes describe a fear of not being able to take another breath.

Clinical features

Breathlessness is a subjective sensation; therefore people who feel breathless do not necessarily appear so. Conversely, people who have signs of breathlessness (increased respiratory rate, cyanosis, use of accessory muscles), if chronically dyspneic, may not *feel* short of breath, as they have accommodated to the sensation.

Epidemiology (see Fig. 20.16)

Mechanism

There are many causes of breathlessness in advanced cancer. They usually relate to the underlying disease but may also be caused by co-existing non-cancer diagnoses.

Investigations

Knowledge of the diagnosis and current stage of disease is helpful. Review the current medication. Ensure co-existing respiratory problems are optimally controlled. Take a full history of the breathlessness from the patient (Box 20.7).

Box 20.7. Assessing breathlessness	
Activity	How much is possible? e.g. talking, stairs
Breathing	When did it start to get worse?
Cough	Productive or dry?
Drugs	Does any medication make it better? e.g. salbutamol
Exercise	Does it make it worse?

Previous medical history e.g. chronic obstructive pulmonary disease, heart failure.
  Physical examination may point to an underlying cause. A full blood count may be helpful if there is a possibility of anemia either from the disease or treatment. A raised white cell count may point to infection. A chest X-ray will often be helpful in confirming a pleural effusion or infection. It may be necessary to request an ultrasound or CT scan to define the change that has caused the increase in breathlessness.

Management

Always explain the reason for breathlessness. Offer reassurance that choking or suffocating is unlikely.

Treat reversible causes aspiration of a malignant pleural effusion can provide rapid relief.
  In most situations infection should be treated and use of bronchodilators optimized. If the cause of the shortness of breath cannot be reversed, morphine in low doses can be helpful. There is good evidence that both oral and parenteral morphine produce a small but significant reduction in the sensation of breathlessness. This has been tested in people with cancer

and in chronic obstructive pulmonary disease and does not appear to increase carbon dioxide retention. Anxiolytics such as benzodiazepines are sometimes used to treat dyspnea, although little evidence is available to support this practice.

No reversible causes for breathlessness identified Low dose morphine 2.5–5 mg 4-hourly orally.

The use of a fan or oxygen may be helpful. Relaxation and breathing techniques have been shown to be of benefit.

Outcome
Breathlessness is generally a poor prognostic sign; however, treatment of the underlying cause, if this is possible, can control this symptom for many months.

Nausea and vomiting
Nausea
"An unpleasant feeling of the need to vomit."
"I feel sick."

Vomiting
"The forceful expulsion of gastric contents through the mouth."

Clinical features
Nausea and vomiting may be accompanied by autonomic symptoms such as sweating, salivation, or pallor. Both symptoms can occur without the other being present.

Epidemiology
Nausea is more common than vomiting. Nausea is recorded in 25% of cancer patients, vomiting in 15%.

Mechanism
As with the other symptoms, it is important to determine the likely cause, because this will most likely result in successful treatment (Box 20.8).

Investigations
Investigations should be directed toward determining the cause if this is not already known. Check for the three "Ms": recent changes in medication, common metabolic disturbances, and disease progression which may be causing new symptoms (Box 20.8). Remember the cause may be unrelated to the cancer.

Biochemical tests such as urea and electrolytes may be important to establish whether fluid replacement is needed. Calcium should be checked. Other investigations will depend on the putative underlying cause. CT scan of the brain may reveal metastases as a cause of nausea.

Box 20.8. Possible causes of nausea/vomiting

Medication	Chemotherapy
	Analgesics
Metabolic	Hypercalcemia
	Renal failure
More disease	Bowel obstruction
	Increased intracranial pressure

Management
Treat the underlying cause if possible, as well as offering an appropriate antiemetic. Consider the patient's overall condition and the potential long-term benefits before embarking on surgery or radiotherapy. Symptom relief can usually be achieved using medication: hypercalcemia with intravenous fluids and bisphosphonates; surgical bypass for malignant obstruction.

Choice of antiemetic is dependent on the presumed underlying cause and its mode of action (Table 20.7). On occasions, a combination of antiemetics is required to achieve good symptom control.

If someone is vomiting persistently or unable to take oral medication, antiemetics should be administered subcutaneously to ensure absorption. In the palliative care setting a syringe driver, a battery-operated device that delivers the medication at a controlled rate over a 24-hour period, will often be suggested for ease of administration.

Outcome
In hospice inpatients 70%–80% of nausea and vomiting is controlled within 24 hours.

The last 48 hours
Are they dying?
Making a decision that someone is likely to die within the next few days includes a review of their condition in the context of their disease as a whole. This is important whether the diagnosis is cancer or another disease (Box 20.9).

These criteria should be used as a *guide* only and should be used to encourage a multidisciplinary discussion about the role of future active treatment. Discussion should also take place with the family or carers and, if possible, with the patient. If a decision is made to provide palliative treatments only, it is usually appropriate to complete a "not for cardiopulmonary resuscitation" order.

Table 20.7. Management of nausea and vomiting

Suspected cause	Proposed action of antiemetic	Antiemetic of choice
Drug induced, e.g. opioids Metabolic, e.g. renal failure Malignant bowel obstruction	Activity at chemoreceptor trigger zone Noxious stimuli transmit signal to higher centers	Haloperidol
Gastric outflow obstruction/stasis Constipation Gastric irritation	Stimulates stomach and upper bowel activity	Metoclopramide Omeprazole
Raised intracranial pressure Vestibular disorders	Steroids reduce cerebral edema and are antiemetic through an unknown mechanism Cyclizine has antihistamine activity at higher emetic centers	Dexamethasone Cyclizine
Highly emetogenic chemotherapy Anticipatory nausea/anxiety	5HT3 activity stimulated by chemotherapy Reduces nausea caused by anxiety by activity at higher centers	Ondansetron Lorazepam
Intractable vomiting	Mixed activity	Levomepromazine

Box 20.9. Signs that suggest death is likely within the next few days

Patient bedbound
Semiconscious
Difficulty swallowing medication
Only able to take sips of fluid

Symptom management

At this stage, management should be directed towards ensuring maximum comfort. The goals of care for the last days of life are described in the Liverpool Care Pathway (LCP 2004) for the dying (Fig. 20.17), an integrated care pathway which is used in the majority of hospitals in England.

There are 18 goals of care encompassed by the LCP. These are divided into categories that cover the period before death and the period immediately afterwards. The aims are to ensure that all aspects of care are routinely explored.

Goals of care encompassed by the LCP

Physical
  Review of current drugs.
  Subcutaneous as needed medication prescribed, e.g. for pain.
  Stop unnecessary interventions, e.g. 4-hourly temperature.

Psychological/religious/spiritual
  Assess ability to speak English.
  Assess insight of patient and carer.
  Assess religious spiritual needs of patient and carer.

Communication
  How next of kin wish to be informed of death.
  Relevant written information.
  GP informed of condition.
  Plan of care explained to and understood by patient and family.

Care after death
  GP informed.
  Procedure followed for laying out.
  Process after death explained to family.

  The pathway encourages review of current treatment and relevant prescribing. It also encourages communication with the patient, family, and their general practitioner regarding impending death. Discussion should take place with family members regarding their wishes surrounding the patient's death, including specific religious rituals.

Religious rituals surrounding death
  Roman Catholic: Last rites prior to death.
  Islam: Non-Muslims should wear gloves handling body.
  Judaism: Body to be buried within 24 hours of death.

Deciding the appropriate place of care

The majority of people with cancer will spend most of their last year of life at home. The majority will also choose to die at home if at all possible, although most still die in hospital (Fig. 20.18).

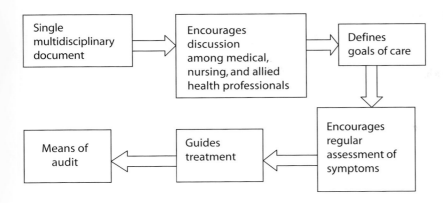

Fig. 20.17. The Liverpool care pathway (LCP).

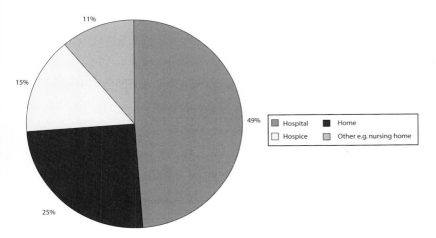

Fig. 20.18. Place of death for people with cancer.

Hospital death

Many patients are admitted to hospital due to deterioration in their condition or because of an increase in a symptom, for example breathlessness. It may become clear either on or during the admission that the person is dying. They may at this stage be too ill to be transferred home or to a hospice and death consequently takes place in the hospital.

Example: change in symptom requiring hospital admission

Advanced carcinoma of lung

Increasing breathlessness

Cause unclear ?pleural effusion ?chest infection

Hospital admission for investigation and management

Chest X-ray – infection

Antibiotics started

Deterioration after 48 hours

Diagnosis of dying made

Patient too unwell to discharge home

It is important that, as soon as it is recognized that someone is dying, appropriate discussions take place with the patient and family, so that, if someone wishes to go home to die they may do so.

Home death

It is important that a discussion regarding the preferred place of care and of death takes place. This both establishes the patient's wishes and ensures that they are aware of their prognosis. At times, this is a difficult discussion but is necessary (Table 20.8).

The place someone wants to be cared for may change as the disease progresses and as circumstances change. What may have felt possible can become increasingly difficult as the reality of caring for someone over a long period of time sinks in. Relatives and friends can become physically and emotionally exhausted at the increasing

Table 20.8. Advantages and disadvantages of alternative places of care

	Hospital	Home	Hospice
Advantages	Medical and nursing expertise readily available. Burden of care removed from family. Patients and families may feel safer.	Often patient's choice. Familiar surroundings. Non-medical environment. Family life maintained. Patient/family control. Familiarity with professional staff, e.g. GP, DN.	Immediate access to specialist, multiprofessional team. Higher staff/patient ratio. More peaceful environment. Greater awareness of patient/family needs – more supportive environment. Bereavement support readily available.
Disadvantages	Often more cure than care oriented. Failure to anticipate death. Patient/family isolation on a busy unit. Nursing care may be limited by resources. Symptoms can be poorly controlled. Unfamiliarity with and rapidly changing staff. Family may not be encouraged to participate in care of the patient. Visiting hours may be restricted. Difficulties of travel to hospital for families.	Good symptom control may be harder to achieve. Professional help not always as accessible as patient/carer would like. Family anxiety. Financial consequences for carer, e.g. may need to give up work. Disruption of family life for other family members.	Hospices sometimes perceived as "a place to die" so some are reluctant to be admitted. Unfamiliar surroundings. Some hospices perceived as catering for a specific group, e.g. white, middle class, Christian. May not meet the needs of ethnic minority groups. Majority of patients admitted to hospices still have a cancer diagnosis.

Box 20.10. Factors associated with home death

Stated patient and carer preference
Presence of more than one carer
Higher socioeconomic status
Longer disease trajectory
Proximity to a hospital or hospice
Supportive family physician
Availability of specialist equipment
Adequate community support
Good symptom control
Involvement of a palliative care service
Male gender
Being married
Younger age

---

demands of looking after a dying person, despite the desire to do so. In these circumstances admission to hospice or hospital may be needed (Box 20.10).

Facilitating a discharge home from hospital for a home death
To ensure a successful discharge from hospital to die at home, it is important to consider symptom control, and social and emotional support. These assessments can be done concurrently, in order to avoid unnecessary delays. It is essential to contact the general practitioner before discharging a seriously ill person home.

Assessing the palliative care patient for discharge
Symptom control
- Are symptoms adequately controlled?
- If yes – who will review and when?
- If no – should discharge be delayed to improve symptoms?
- Has all required medication been prescribed including as needed drugs?
- By what route is medication being given? If subcutaneously (syringe driver), a district nurse needs to be contacted.

Emotional needs
- Have you adequately explored the patient's concerns about a home death?
- Have you adequately explored the carer's concerns about a home death (often these are greater than the patient's)?
- What other family/social support is available at home?
- Is any additional psychologic support needed?

Social needs
- Involve nursing team in discussions regarding nursing care needs
- What accommodation does the patient have, e.g. stairs?

Physiotherapist
Occupational therapist
Social worker
District nurse
Palliative care team
GP
Marie Curie Night Nursing service
Others, e.g. Crossroads, Befriending service

- Is there a need and space for specialist equipment?
- What can the patient do, e.g. self caring, help needed with personal care?
- Often assessment of social care needs are made by other health professionals but it is important to remember to ask them! (Box 20.11)

What to do when someone dies at home

Relatives and carers need to know what to do in these circumstances. Explain that they need to:

- Call the GP to certify death and complete a death certificate.
- Discuss laying out the body – families may wish to be involved in this, although more commonly this would be done by the funeral director.
- Call a funeral director, who will remove the body from the house.
- Register the death at the local registry office within 5 days of the death.

Hospice death

Only a small number of cancer deaths take place in a hospice and an even smaller number of non-cancer deaths occur in this environment (Fig. 20.18). Hospice care at the end of life is associated with improved pain and symptom control, increased availability of psychologic care, and higher carer satisfaction.

Organ donation

At times people request that their body be used to benefit medical science or they may wish to donate their organs for use by others. There are contra–indications to certain types of donation, of which it may be helpful to be aware.

Diseases which preclude organ donation:

Neurologic, e.g. Alzheimer's, dementia, motor neurone disease, Creutzfeldt–Jakob disease

Diseases of unknown etiology
Hepatitis B and C
Leukemia
HIV

Patients with cancer may donate

- heart valves
- corneas
- tendons
- bone
- skin

Procedure for donation

Death should have been certified by a doctor and recorded in the medical notes.

Some patients will want to discuss organ donation prior to death. If this has not happened, written or verbal consent should be obtained from the next of kin. If the next of kin is unable to attend the hospital, the person taking verbal consent should record this in the notes. Relatives need to be made aware of the need for HIV and hepatitis testing. If the patient's case is referred to the coroner, permission should be sought for organ donation via the coroner's officer.

Bereavement and grief

Bereavement (loss)

"Losing something or someone to which or to whom one has an attachment."

In the context of incurable advanced disease there is loss associated with deteriorating health as well as death and dying. Receiving news of a life-threatening illness has been described as being like an "emotional hydrogen bomb," often shattering plans for the future and introducing new fears. Serious illness challenges the often-held belief that we are immortal, that death is defeat, rather than seeing it as a fundamental part of life. It may also force a change in role, degree of independence and may have financial consequences.

Grief

"The psychological and emotional reaction which accompanies bereavement."

There is no specified "normal" length of time that a grief reaction should last. The grief process usually begins at the time when a serious illness is diagnosed. A period of adjustment will follow, often followed by further grief reactions as the illness progresses. A person's response to the current loss will be strongly influenced by the strategies used to deal with previous losses.

Anticipatory grief

"Doing the work of grieving in anticipation of the impending loss."

The more proactive we are in dealing with "abnormal" anticipatory grief reactions, the more likely it is that a normal grief reaction will follow.

There is often a mixture of feelings surrounding the knowledge that someone close to you is dying. There are many challenges facing the "being bereaved."

Challenges facing those "being bereaved"

Change in role, e.g. widowhood.

Contact with numerous health professionals.

Potential difficulties communicating with dying person, e.g. protecting one another is common.

Incidence

Bereavement and grief accompany all serious illness. The patient, the family, and friends all have to cope with loss, although the type of loss is different for each person involved due to numerous factors, so responses may differ.

Clinical features

All health professionals should be able to identify someone who is struggling to come to terms with loss so that appropriate specialist support can be offered if necessary. Relatives and friends may be very distressed at this time and it can be difficult to distinguish between the normal emotions surrounding grief and those which are less "usual." Some risk factors for an "abnormal" or maladaptive grief process are listed in Table 20.9.

Reactions to loss may include all or some of the emotions described in Fig. 20.19.

People may feel more than one apparently contradictory emotion at the same time.

Anger: that the person has died and left them.

Relief: that the person has died and is free of pain.

Management

(1) Listen: make an assessment regarding how the person is coping with loss. Most people adjust normally following bereavement.

(2) Feelings: acknowledge whatever feelings are expressed. Explain that some distress associated with illness is normal. Acknowledge problems and affirm and encourage positive ways of coping.

Table 20.9. Factors that may suggest the risk of an "abnormal" bereavement

Relationship to person	Physical relationship (e.g. spouse, parent)
	Quality of relationship (positive or negative?)
Support structures	What other family is there? (A genogram can be helpful.)
	Are there are conflicts /unresolved issues?
Other sources of stress	Financial worries? Single parent?
Circumstances of death	Sudden or unexpected death increases risk
History of grieving	How have they coped with previous losses? e.g. divorce, loss of a job
Personality	"Controlled" people
	Thinkers who have difficulty expressing emotion
Psychiatric history	Previous history increases risk, e.g depression
Social factors, e.g. alcohol or drug use, gender	What other stressors are there in their lives?
Belief systems	Making sense of what is happening to them.
	May be in the context of religion.

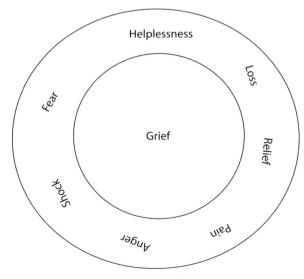

Fig. 20.19. Potential emotions in grief.

(3) Affirm and encourage positive coping strategies Example: "I'm sure that it helped him to know that you were there with him when he died."

(4) Families: different family members may cope very differently. Encourage awareness of each others' needs within the family.

(5) Avoid glib or patronizing statements. You probably don't know how someone feels, even if you have had the same experience!

(6) If you are concerned that someone is having difficulty coping with grief, support services are usually available through the palliative care team or psychologic support services.

Acknowledgments

Some of the material in this chapter is taken from material compiled for undergraduate teaching at Guy's, Kings and St. Thomas' Medical School, King's College, London by Dr. Polly Edmonds and Dr. Rachel Burman.

The X-rays, scans, and pathology slides are courtesy of Consultant colleagues at Guy's and St. Thomas' NHS Foundation Trust: Dr. Shareen Ahmed, Dr. Hattie Deere, and Dr. Sally Barrington.

Further reading

Butters E, Pearce S, Ramirez A, Richards M. Assessing symptoms and concerns in patients with advanced cancer: the development of a check list for use in clinical practice. Unpublished work 2005.

Grond S, Zech D, Difenbach C, Radbruch L, Lehmann KA. Assessment of cancer pain: a prospective evaluation in 2266 cancer patients referred to a pain service. *Pain* 1996; **64**:107–114.

Hoskin P, Makin W. *Oncology for Palliative Medicine.* Oxford University Press, 1998.

Liverpool care pathway for the dying 2004. www.lcp-mariecurie.org.uk.

Murtagh FE, Preston M, Higginson I. Patterns of dying: palliative care for non-malignant disease. *Clin. Med.* 2004;4:39–44.

Office of National Statistics. www.statistics.gov.uk.

Twycross R. *Introducing Palliative Care.* Radcliffe Press Ltd, 1999.

World Health Organization. www.who.int/cancer/palliative.

Index